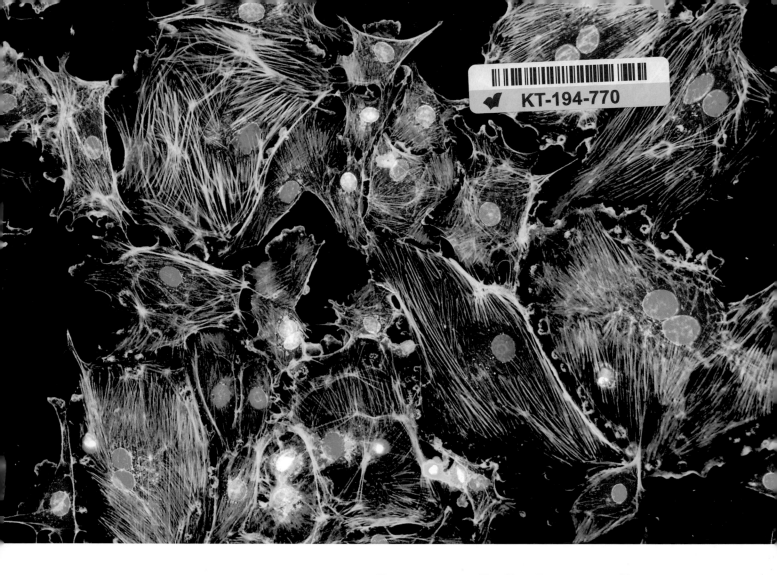

Functional histology
2e

Jeffrey B Kerr PhD

Associate Professor
Department of Anatomy and Developmental Biology
Monash University, Melbourne, Australia

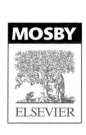

MOSBY

ELSEVIER

Sydney   Edinburgh   London   New York   Philadelphia   St Louis   Toronto

To my wife, Marlene, and my son, Jamie

ELSEVIER

Mosby is an imprint of Elsevier

Elsevier Australia. ACN 001 002 357
(a division of Reed International Books Australia Pty Ltd)
Tower 1, 475 Victoria Avenue, Chatswood, NSW 2067

National Library of Australia Cataloguing-in-Publication Data

Kerr, Jeffrey B.

Functional histology / Jeffrey B. Kerr.
2nd ed.

ISBN: 978 0 7295 3837 4 (pbk.)

Includes index.
Bibliography.

Histology—Atlases.

611.0180222

Publisher: Sophie Kaliniecki
Developmental editor: Sunalie Silva
Publishing Services Manager: Helena Klijn
Edited by Deborah McRitchie and Carol Natsis
Proofread by Teresa McIntyre and Kerry Brown
Illustrations by Joseph Lucia
Cover, internal design and typesetting by Modern Art Production Group
Index by Merrall-Ross International
Printed by 1010 Printing International Ltd.

Contents

Preface vii
Acknowledgments viii

1 The cell 1
2 Origin of tissue types 61
3 Blood 77
4 Epithelium 95
5 Connective tissue 117
6 Muscle 137
7 Nervous system 161
8 Circulatory system 189
9 Skin 207
10 Skeletal tissues 223
11 Immune system 257
12 Respiratory system 287
13 Orodental and salivary tissues 305
14 Gastrointestinal tract 323
15 Liver, gall bladder, and pancreas 355
16 Urinary system 373
17 Endocrine system 393
18 Female reproductive system 413
19 Male reproductive system 441
20 Special senses 469

Appendix: stains 491
Index 492

Preface

This second edition has been revised and updated to add, where necessary, new discoveries in tissue and cell biology based upon recent advances published in the biomedical science literature. Although histology remains a key element in medical and allied health training, increasingly it is integrated into the curriculum rather than taught as a stand-alone subject. However, presentation of concepts and details of histological importance cannot readily be fragmented and reassembled piecemeal to match, for example, a specific case-study or problem-based scenario. Hence, each chapter conforms to the traditional approach used in the basic medical sciences of reviewing the histology from a functional perspective, and relating this to a particular set of tissue types or organ system.

Although histological knowledge provides the basis for the study of pathology for medical/dental/veterinary programs, histology has become increasingly important for students, postgraduates, and postdoctoral fellows pursuing basic biomedical research. Identification of cell and tissue phenotypes in normal and experimentally altered situations is vital for interpretation of function, and is equally important in studies of pre- and postnatal development. Chapter 2 aims to meet this requirement.

Overall, this new edition was prepared for those with an interest in biological science as applied to the health professions, and for the research community who together make the discoveries that contribute to advances in our knowledge of how cells and tissues function. Where relevant, the biology of organs or organ systems is reviewed in relation to their physiology and biochemistry, followed by information about the contributions of individual cells and the tissues that they form.

Reading a book like this is only part of the secret to success in learning histology. Examining sections with a microscope or studying digital images and identifying what is observed and how it functions is the real test of your knowledge. If this book helps in achieving these outcomes it will have fulfilled its aim of contributing to biomedical education.

JB Kerr 2009

Acknowledgments

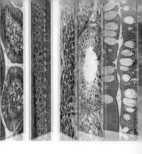

A large measure of the motivation to revise and update this work has come from interactions with the teaching of medical and science students, in addition to working with research assistants, postgraduate students, and postdoctoral scientists. Hardly a week goes by without somebody posing a question that requires more than the commonly accepted answer. In this regard, their enquiring minds act as the stimulus to find answers that are not simply looked up in a standard textbook but sought in the contemporary literature. Often the answers are found in original research articles or recent reviews. There is no doubt that attempting to answer questions such as "What is it that we are looking at?" or "What is its function?" demands informed responses. In this context, I thank all of those above.

Numerous figures have been provided by fellow academics and scientists, and I thank them all for their generosity together with acknowledgment of the original sources of the illustrations. The cover image was supplied courtesy of Rishi Raj, Olympus Australia.

I thank the publisher, Elsevier Australia, for the opportunity to prepare a second edition. Helena Klijn, assisted by Carol Natsis, managed to coordinate and direct the assembly of text and illustrations into the page design with tireless efficiency that made my job that much easier, and I thank them for their efforts.

Finally, this work would have had no prospect of completion without the support of my family, Marlene and Jamie. To them I record my gratitude for their patience and understanding.

JB Kerr 2009

REVIEWERS

Christine Lunam, BSc (Hons), PhD
Senior Lecturer, Anatomy & Histology
Flinders Medical Science & Technology,
School of Medicine, Flinders University,
Adelaide, Australia

Julie Haynes, BSc, PhD
Senior Lecturer, Anatomical Sciences
School of Medical Sciences, University of Adelaide,
Adelaide, Australia

R Claire Aland, BSc (Hons I), PhD, GCE (Tert)
Lecturer, Division of Basic Medical Sciences (Anatomy),
St George's, University of London, England

Christopher R Murphy, BSc, PhD, DSc
Bosch Professor of Histology & Embryology Professor
of Female Reproductive Biology
Sydney Medical School, The University of Sydney,
Sydney, Australia

Anthony Woods, BA, BSc (Hons), PhD, MAIMS
Associate Professor
School of Pharmacy & Medical Sciences,
University of South Australia, Adelaide, Australia

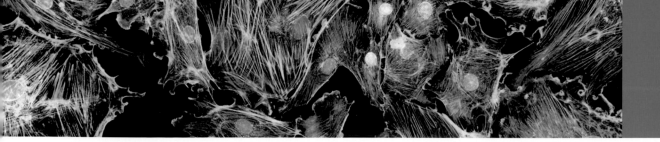

The cell

The study of cells has had a long history since their first description in 1665 by Robert Hooke, who examined thin slices of dried cork. In 1831 the cell nucleus was recognized as distinct from the cytoplasm. By 1839 animal and plant tissues were known to be composed of cells, giving rise to the cell theory: all organisms consist of cells, and the cell is the structural unit of life. In 1855 Virchow concluded that "every cell arises from a pre-existing cell." This idea was revolutionary for pathology and for the origin of all cells, which we now know arise ultimately from the ovum and sperm.

This chapter presents an overview of the structure and workings of the cell. Research in cell biology largely follows a reductionist approach—discovering all the parts as a means of understanding how they work. Presenting a comprehensive review of the "parts list" for cells is overwhelming and beyond the scope of this book. For more information on the molecular biology of the cell and the enormous "facts base" associated with new discoveries of cell function, the reader should consult the numerous texts on cell biology and relevant journals.

Cells may be classified into two basic groups:
- *Prokaryotes*—bacteria, subdivided into eubacteria and archaea
- *Eukaryotes*—all other living cells, i.e. protozoa, fungi, plants, and animals.

Traditionally these divisions among cells have been considered separate, but there is growing evidence, discussed later, that suggests that this distinction is not quite as clear-cut as previously thought.

Prokaryotes have a plasma membrane but their DNA (deoxyribonucleic acid) is not contained in a nucleus, and their cytoplasm generally, but not always, lacks internal organization.

The most important structural feature of eukaryotic cells is the collection of intracellular membranes segregating the cell into a range of identifiable components. The two major components are the nucleus and the cytoplasm. The tissues of mammals have hundreds of different cell types (many of which are developmental or regional variants of particular types of cells) and a wide variety of extracellular materials, recognizable using a light microscope (LM).

The old cliché that size is important is certainly true in histology. It is often forgotten or not known that an appreciation of relative size is important for the interpretation of tissue sections. This sense of scale fosters an understanding of which structures can reasonably be expected to coexist, or to be found within or outside of another structure, or which structures have limits to their smallest or largest dimensions. Commonly used dimensions are given in Figure 1.1, and examples of the considerable size variations of cells and tissues are given in Figure 1.2.

Unit	Subunits	Example
1 cm	10 mm	Organs or parts thereof
1 mm	1000 μm	Small organisms
0.1 mm	100 μm	Tissue components
1000 nm	1 μm	Cell organelles, bacteria
1 nm	10 Å	Molecules
0.1 nm	1 Å	Atoms

▲ **Fig 1.1** Units of dimension in histology and cell biology.

Cells and tissues	Dimension	Cells and tissues	Dimension	Cells and tissues	Dimension
Long axon	1 m	Fertilized ovum	200 μm	Hepatocyte	25 μm
Longest muscle cell	30 cm	Arteriole	30–200 μm	Neutrophil	12 μm
Graafian follicle	2 cm	Seminiferous tubule	180 μm	Capillary	4–10 μm
Liver lobule	0.7–2 mm	Human oocyte	100–150 μm	Erythrocyte	7 μm
Thick skin epidermis	1.5 mm	Thin skin epidermis	100 μm	Platelet	2–3 μm
Villus	1 mm	Megakaryocyte	50–70 μm	Mitochondrial width	0.5 μm
Bronchiole	0.5–1mm	Luteal cell	30–50 μm	Resolution light microscope	0.2 μm
Osteon	200 μm	Pancreatic acinus	40 μm	Plasma membrane	10 nm

▲ **Fig 1.2** Typical dimensions in histology.

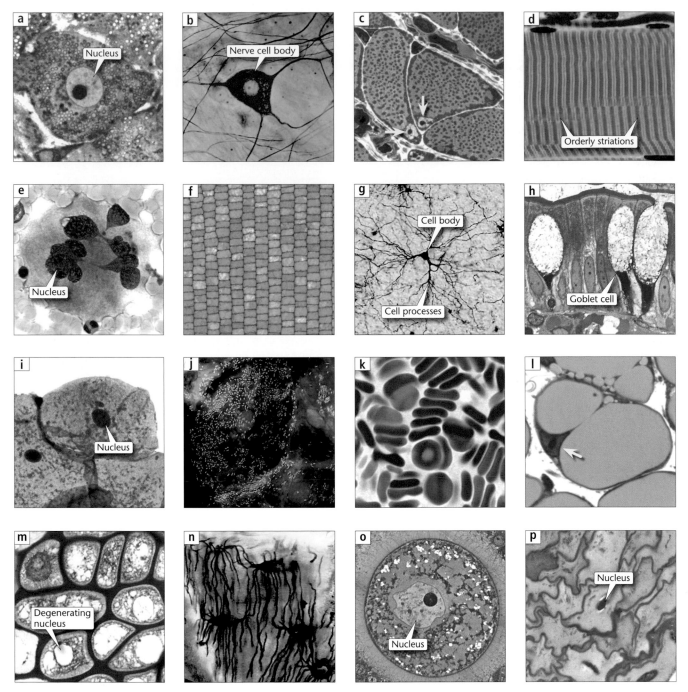

▲ **Fig 1.3a** Typical cell with large nucleus, central nucleolus, and extensive cytoplasm. **b** Nerve cell body with thin dendritic processes. **c** Skeletal muscle cells with peripheral nuclei (**arrows**). **d** Skeletal muscle cell with cytoplasm filled with orderly contractile proteins. **e** Megakaryocyte with lobulated nucleus. **f** Lens fibers seen end-on, lacking nuclei. **g** Glial cell in the brain. **h** Tall goblet-shaped cells of the gut. **i** Flat epithelial cells of the buccal mucosa. **j** Oral bacteria (orange) and buccal cells (green). **k** Red blood cells. **l** Fat cells with peripheral nucleus (**arrow**). **m** Cartilage cells with extracted degenerating nuclei. **n** Osteocytes of bone with many cytoplasmic extensions. **o** Oocyte with central nucleus and abundant cytoplasm. **p** Skin cells with shrunken degenerating nuclei.

Most cell types have a nucleus and cytoplasm (Fig 1.3a–p), but there are exceptions: red blood "cells," many fibers of the lens, and the cornified layer of skin have no nuclei. Blood platelets are cytoplasmic fragments and also lack a nucleus.

Fundamental functional properties of cells include:
- A genetic program
- Motility and dynamic change
- Growth and reproduction
- Communication
- Energy to drive metabolism
- Self-regulation.

The animal cell consists of the nucleus and the cytoplasm, each of which shows a recognizable range of morphological features, which in general make them relatively easy to identify, even in very different cell types. The environment in which many cells reside is by definition extracellular, and it too exhibits a variety of components that are somewhat difficult to identify owing to a rather amorphous appearance or apparent lack of structure. In learning how to discriminate between the structures within, on the surface of, and external to the cell, consider the following categories:

- **Nucleus:** This membrane-bound sac contains the genetic information in the chromosomes. Often round or oval-shaped, the nucleus can have many different forms depending upon the cell type in which it is found (e.g. highly lobulated in an eosinophil, flat and pyramidal for a sperm cell, thin and elongated in gut absorptive cells) (Fig 1.4a–c).
- **Cytoplasm:** A so-called ground substance, or cytosol, occupies the cytoplasm that surrounds the nucleus. It consists of a sol-gel fluid mixture of water and proteins (together about 85% of total cell weight), nucleic acids, complex sugars, lipids, inorganic ions, and many small metabolites. Suspended in the cytosol are the organelles, a group of tiny, mainly membrane-bound components, capable of carrying out specific metabolic functions. Inclusions, also in the cytosol, are metabolically inert, representing stored or accumulated products that may be temporary features of the cytoplasm. The cytoskeleton provides an internal supporting and structural framework for the cell, enabling cell mobility and plasticity (Fig 1.5).

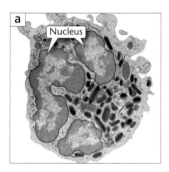

▲ **Fig 1.4a Lobulated nucleus.** White blood cell (eosinophil), showing a lobulated nucleus of three parts. In humans the nucleus is bilobed, and in thin sections such as this for electron microscopy the lobes appear separated. × 5,500.

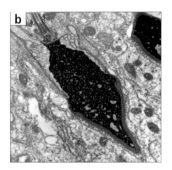

▲ **Fig 1.4b Pyriform nucleus.** Human spermatid, showing a pyriform nucleus with highly condensed chromatin. × 9,000.

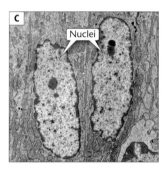

▲ **Fig 1.4c Elliptical nuclei.** Elongated elliptical nuclei typical of absorptive cells of the intestinal epithelium. × 2,500.

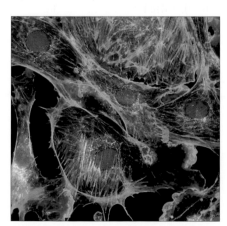

◀ **Fig 1.5 Cytoskeleton** of endothelial cells stained with fluorescent dyes, showing microfilaments (fluorescein green), microtubules (rhodamine red) and nucleus (DAPI blue). × 1,050.

- **Cell surface:** The outer border of the cell is the cell membrane or plasma membrane. It is responsible for regulating the entry and exit of substances, together with providing specializations whereby cells gain attachment to one another. Surface specializations are common features of cells (e.g. finger-like projections or motile apparatus) (Fig 1.6).
- **Extracellular material:** This may be fluid-like (e.g. blood plasma) or consist of lymph or tissue fluid. Other extracellular material consists of fibers such as the connective tissues made of collagen or elastin that reside within a gel-type matrix rich in macromolecules such as proteoglycans and glycoproteins (Fig 1.7a & b).

CELLS ARE AMAZINGLY COMPLEX

Most images of cell ultrastructure are two-dimensional representations recorded with the transmission electron microscope (EM) (Fig 1.8). The often remarkably beautiful electron micrographs of the three-dimensional morphology of cells, recording surface features and sometimes internal components, are the creation of the scanning EM. The availability of confocal fluorescence microscopy and digital deconvolution microscopy has greatly improved our appreciation of the structural makeup and function of cells. Advances in technology that permit examination of living cells with four-dimensional microscopy (three dimensions of space plus time) will further enhance our understanding of the biology of cells.

How then can we relate two-dimensional micrographs of cells to the actual living state? There are two considerations here:
1. Is what we see a true picture of how the cell is constructed?
2. What is it actually like inside a cell if we magnify it enormously?

The answer to the first question is yes. The proof comes from two pieces of evidence. Firstly, in living isolated cells analyzed by high-resolution light microscopy such as phase contrast or interference contrast, the shapes, sizes, and locations of numerous components are very similar to the same parameters seen in fixed, dead cells prepared for electron microscopy.

Secondly, and more convincing, is that when living tissues are very rapidly frozen by contact with liquid nitrogen/propane/ethane/helium, a depth of tissue up to 50 μm can be instantaneously preserved with no ice crystal contamination. When the frozen stabilized cells are carefully thawed and examined by cryoelectron tomography, their ultrastructure is very similar and often identical to cells prepared by conventional chemical fixation methods (Fig 1.9, see page 6).

The answer to the second question is very surprising—the complexity is astounding. Perhaps this should be anticipated because, as a living entity, a cell is a dynamic structure constantly maintaining internal order. If a cell were not highly ordered, it would resemble a disorganized blob of matter consisting of mostly water and a huge conglomeration

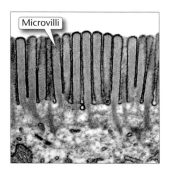

▲ **Fig 1.6 Microvilli** are examples of specialized cytoplasmic extensions that serve to increase the surface area of the plasma membrane, in this case for absorption of materials. Intestinal epithelial cells each have several thousand microvilli. × 15,000.

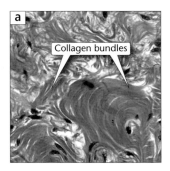

▲ **Fig 1.7a Extracellular materials.** Extracellular materials consisting of bundles of collagen fibers, which are synthesized by the fibroblasts embedded within. Hematoxylin and eosin (H&E), paraffin, × 300.

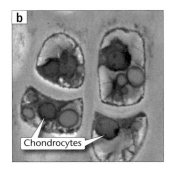

▲ **Fig 1.7b Extracellular materials.** Extracellular matrix surrounding several chondrocytes (cartilage cells). The matrix is homogeneous and consists of collagen and proteoglycans. Toluidine blue, araldite, × 700.

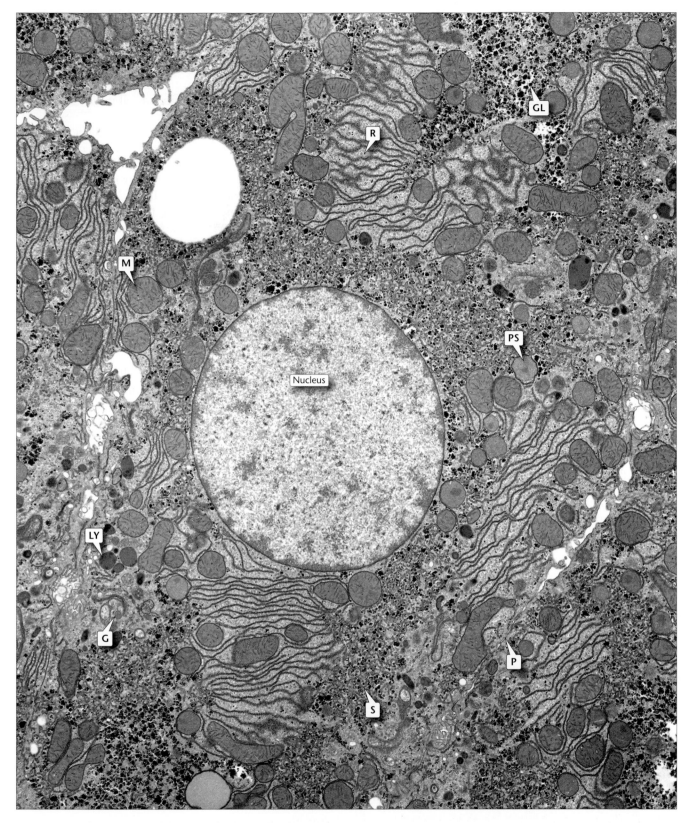

▲ **Fig 1.8 Ultrastructure of a very thin (60 nm) section of a liver cell.** It exemplifies many of the subcellular components found in mammalian cells. As a typical liver cell is about 25 μm in diameter, more than 400 serial sections would need to be assembled to view the whole cell. Surrounding the central nucleus, the cytoplasm is crowded with many membrane-bound organelles and inclusion bodies: mitochondria (**M**), rough endoplasmic reticulum (ER) (**R**), smooth ER (**S**), lysosomes (**LY**), glycogen (**GL**), Golgi (**G**), plasma membrane (**P**), peroxisomes (**PS**). × 9,700.

of macromolecules. Cells therefore generate order out of chaos much as a factory is highly structured to carry out hundreds or millions of separate tasks that together are designed to produce an end product. We refer to chaos as *entropy*, a concept described by the second law of thermodynamics: everything tends towards disorder.

Order versus chaos

Just how do cells deal with entropy? By way of analogy, the home handyperson has a workshop in which the tools are (ideally) carefully located where they can be readily accessed. The tools do not arrange themselves neatly on their pegboards and shelves; rather the handyperson is responsible for their orderly positions and this requires expenditure of energy—energy creates order out of chaos. The home handyperson may have 50 or even 100 tools, but a cell has about 10 billion protein molecules to look after. The entropic possibilities that challenge a cell every minute/hour/day of its life are colossal.

Cells maintain order out of molecular chaos through complex bioengineered components and, by acquiring and expending energy, ensure that the right molecules get to the right places at the right times. They do this by creating compartments within the cell. Many cells have similar subdivisions that remain separate yet function in cooperation. This ensures normal pathways of processing essential raw materials, synthesis of these into macromolecules, transport, response to stimuli, defense against attack or pathogens, replacement of worn-out parts, changes in shape—and the list goes on.

Compartments and packaging

Returning now to the original question of what does all this organization look like inside the cell, a good idea of what goes on has been gained, in large part, from the discoveries made with the EM. This can be illustrated by taking two examples of cells that are reasonably familiar to most students of biology: the liver cell (Fig 1.10a) and the exocrine (secretes via a surface) pancreatic cell (Fig 1.10b). Both cell types contain abundant supplies of organelles (mini-organs) made of membranes as well as variable amounts of non-membranous components.

With a few relatively straightforward mathematical formulas, the area and volumetric proportions or percentages taken up by the membranous components can be estimated from analysis of the two-dimensional images made with the EM. Other formulas can estimate the relative surface densities (i.e. how much

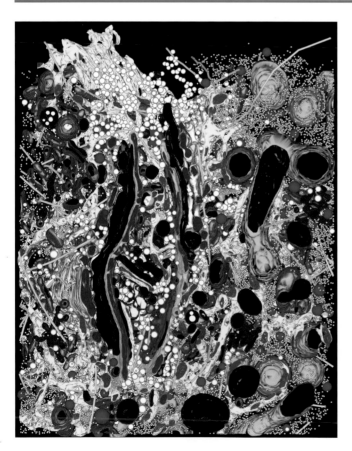

◄ **Fig 1.9 A three-dimensional model of a Golgi region (vertical membrane stacks) in an insulin-secreting cell.** This is based upon three serial 400 nm sections cut from a high-pressure frozen, freeze-substituted, and plastic-embedded cell. This image represents 12 μm³ reconstructed by dual-axis electron tomography. Color codes: Golgi—green, maroon, light and dark blue; endoplasmic reticulum—yellow; mitochondria—green; free ribosomes—orange; microtubules—bright green; dense core vesicles—bright blue; clathrin-negative vesicles—white; clathrin-positive vesicles/membranes—bright red; clathrin-negative membranes/vesicles—purple. x 13,000. (Courtesy B Marsh, Institute for Molecular Bioscience, University of Queensland; from data published in: Marsh BJ, et al. Organellar relationships in the Golgi region of the pancreatic beta cell line, HIT-T15, visualized by high resolution electron tomography. PNAS 2001; 98:2399–406.)

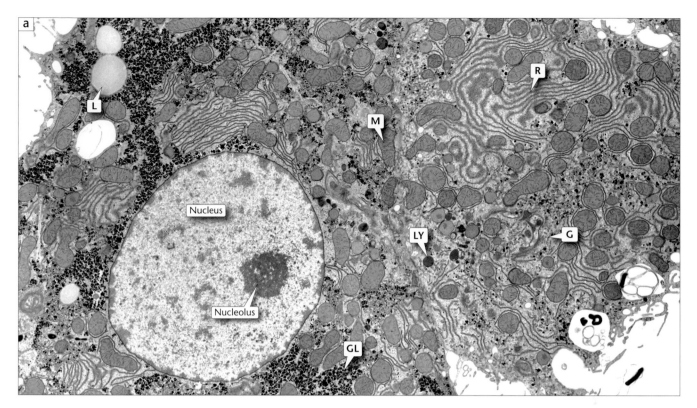

▲ **Fig 1.10a Ultrastructure of a hepatocyte**, showing cellular machinery associated with the many metabolic functions of the liver: rough ER (**R**); mitochondria (**M**); glycogen (**GL**); lysosomes (**LY**); Golgi (**G**); lipid (**L**). × 5,500.

▼ **Fig 1.10b Ultrastructure of a exocrine pancreatic cell**, showing membrane compartments associated with secretion of enzymes: rough ER (**R**); Golgi (**G**); condensing vacuoles (**C**); zymogen granules (**Z**). × 11,000.

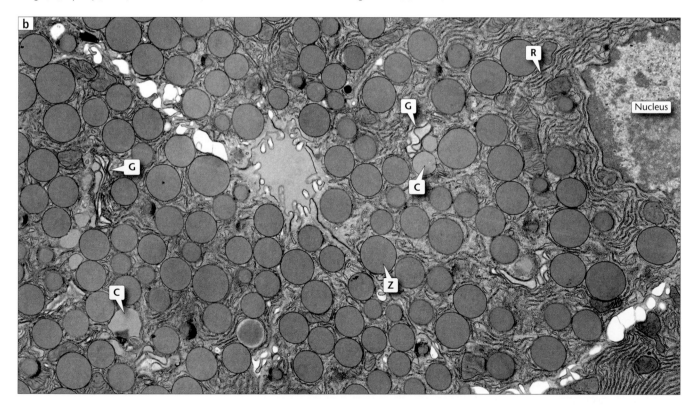

surface area of a particular organelle type occupies a given volume of the cell).

The calculations yield numbers, of course, and while these facts may be found in most books of cell biology, the quantity of membrane and the extent of the compartmentalization is not commonly appreciated. Membrane area within cells is usually reported as area density, with the unit of $\mu m^2/\mu m^3$ or more simply μm^{-1} (Fig 1.11).

Many cell types have membrane densities of 20–40 μm^{-1}, but the implications of measurements using this unit are not clear to most readers. If we note that 1 μm^{-1} is equivalent to 1,000 square meters

per liter, however, it is clear that eukaryotic cells have enormous amounts of membrane.

But just how big is "enormous"? Certainly the detailed diagrams of cell ultrastructure do not convey a sense of just how much is inside a cell, and even electron micrographs cannot do this satisfactorily because they are images of extremely thin slices through the cell. In fact the EM picture of a whole cell that is 20 μm in diameter represents only one four-hundredth or 0.0025% of the total width of the cell.

Figure 1.12 compares the basic quantitative data for a liver cell, pancreatic cell, and testicular Leydig cell.

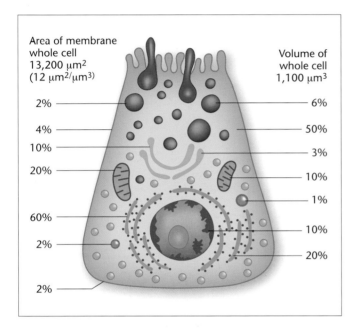

◀ **Fig 1.11 Diagram of a typical exocrine cell such as a protein-secreting pancreatic acinar cell.** Average cell volume is 1,100 μm^3 (percentage volumes of organelles shown on the left). Total surface area of cell membranes is 13,200 μm^2 (percentage surface membrane areas shown on the right). These morphometric estimations illustrate how much membrane can be packaged into a relatively small volume.

Area of membrane whole cell 13,200 μm^2 (12 $\mu m^2/\mu m^3$)

Volume of whole cell 1,100 μm^3

Left	Right
2%	6%
4%	50%
10%	3%
20%	10%
	1%
60%	10%
2%	20%
2%	

	Surface area of membranes in μm^2		
Membrane type	**Liver cell (volume 5,000 μm^3)**	**Pancreatic exocrine cell (volume 1,000 μm^3)**	**Testicular Leydig cell (volume 4,000 μm^3)**
Plasma membrane	2,200	650	2,400
Rough endoplasmic reticulum	38,000	7,800	770
Smooth endoplasmic reticulum	18,000	100	32,000
Golgi	8,000	1,300	900
Mitochondria outer	8,000	500	2,600
inner	35,000	2,200	5,600
Nucleus	220	90	220
Secretory vesicles	not determined	380	not determined
Lysosomes	450	not determined	500
Peroxisomes	450	not determined	600
Endosomes	450	not determined	200
Total	110,000	13,000	46,000
If cell enlarged to a golf ball, total membrane surface area in square meters	737 m^2 27 × 27 m	436 m^2 21 × 21 m	385 m^2 19.5 × 19.5 m

▲ **Fig 1.12** Quantitative comparison of amounts of membrane types in three different cells (data based upon morphometric analysis of electron micrographs).

The cells have different volumes and even more variation in the total surface area of membranes, ranging from 13,000 to more than 100,000 μm². Big numbers indeed, but unfamiliar units of measurement can betray the true scale, so what do these data mean? Imagine each cell enlarged to the size of a golf ball. The liver, pancreatic, and Leydig cells would have respective total membrane surface areas equivalent to 737, 436, and 385 square meters, respectively. For comparison, the area of a singles tennis court is 196 square meters.

The ultrastructure of cells therefore reveals an amazing degree of internal complexity, but membrane occupancy is only part of the story.

The crowded cytoplasm

With an understanding of the concept of membrane area within the cell, the next step is to consider how these membranes are distributed and how they localize in particular domains. Biology textbooks often refer to the cell cytoplasm as the cytosol, or "ground substance," said to consist mostly of water, with inorganic ions and organic macromolecules.

The cytosol is a sol–gel mixture resembling a watery gel. Conventional electron micrographs show that the space in between the visible cytoplasmic components looks rather empty, consistent with its high water content. The reality, however, is rather different (Fig 1.13). By analogy, take the example of an aliquot of blood, which is centrifuged to spin down and separate the formed elements (erythrocytes) from the leukocytes and blood plasma. The plasma so formed is a clear, pale-yellow fluid that nevertheless contains proteins (albumin, globulins, fibrinogen) and other solutes, gases, nutrients, and hormones, dissolved or suspended in water. Cytoplasm is no different in this respect. About 90% of blood plasma is water; 70% of total cell mass is water and 26% is comprised of macromolecules.

The aqueous phase of cells contains most of the molecules that participate in intracellular reactions and it is but one of the properties of water—its cohesive nature—that makes it the prime molecule of life. The cytosol is a very crowded environment. Proteins and ribonucleic acids (RNAs) are found at a concentration of about 300 mg/mL; in terms of mass this is equivalent to dissolving one aspirin tablet in just 1 mL of water, quite a strong brew.

Understanding how all the billions of macromolecules interact at the right time and the right place is beyond the scope of this discussion, but it can be said that the cytosol plus the membrane compartments within it is much more than a fluid-filled bag.

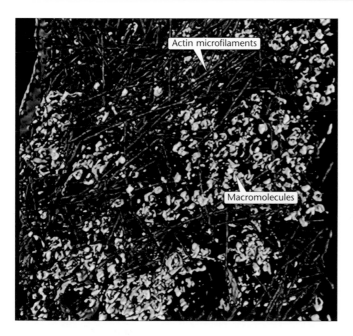

Actin microfilaments

Macromolecules

◀ **Fig 1.13 Three-dimensional reconstruction of part of the cytoplasm of a slime mold cell visualized by cryoelectron tomography.** Multiple images are recorded over a range of tilt angles and assembled by computer. Linear red structures are the cytoskeleton (actin), ribosomes/macromolecules are green, and membranes are blue. × 100,000. (Courtesy O Medalia, Max Planck Institute of Biochemistry, Germany.)

ORGANIZATION OF THE CELL

Plasma membranes

The plasma membrane is a dynamic, fluid boundary comprising a lipid bilayer 8–10 nm thick, with proteins extending through both layers or attached to external or internal surfaces. In electron micrographs it appears trilaminar, displaying two dense lines (lipid bilayer) separated by a lighter central zone (Fig 1.14a & b). The lipid defines membrane form, being capable of deformation and resealing, and prevents the escape of water-soluble components from the cell. Membrane proteins provide mechanisms for transport of molecules across the lipid bilayer (Fig 1.14c), serving as receptors and structural supports for the internal cytoskeleton, and participate in membrane-associated enzyme reactions. Macromolecules and larger entities (vesicles, microorganisms, or cell debris) are ingested or secreted across the plasma membrane via endocytosis or exocytosis. In the former process, membrane segments pinch off forming internalized vesicles; in the latter, substances for secretion are packaged into vesicles, which fuse with the plasma membrane and subsequently release their contents outside the cell.

> **Tip:** Although the plasma membrane is only 10 nm wide, borders may be seen between adjacent cells in paraffin sections using the LM. This is because the image consists of two plasma membranes and stained extracellular materials between the cells.

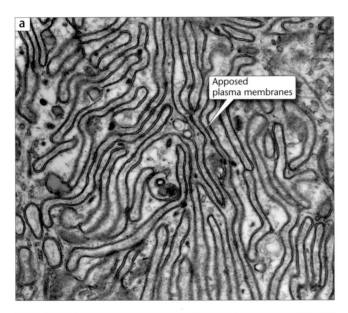

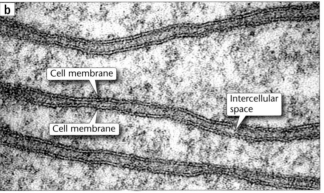

◄ **Fig 1.14a Ultrastructure of the complex interdigitations of plasma membranes of several epithelial cells of the small intestine.** The highly folded and parallel plasma membranes create a considerable lateral surface area for the cells. Sodium and chloride ions move from the cytoplasm into the narrow intercellular spaces and facilitate copious reabsorption of fluids from the gut lumen into the vascular system. × 20,000.

◄ **Fig 1.14b Ultrastructure of plasma membranes,** showing a trilaminar appearance of two dense lines (about 3 nm) separated by an electron-lucent zone (4 nm). These structures represent deposition of osmium, one of the fixatives used in tissue preparation, in the outer ends of phospholipids, and the central pale zone is their unstained hydrocarbon chains. The gray region between membranes is the intercellular space. × 160,000.

Internal structures

The many internal components of the cell can be categorized in various ways, but essentially they are subdivided into elements that perform metabolic, synthetic, energy-dependent, and energy-generating functions, as well as those that are not involved with active metabolism. The first category consists of the organelles, all of which are visible by light microscopy of tissue sections or cell cultures, specially stained or after labeling with fluorescent dyes. Organelles are unique to eukaryotic cells. An "organelle," actually vesicles enclosed by membrane, has been found in a bacterium. These organelles contain specific enzymes, and very similar structures exist in one eukaryotic parasite. The divergence between prokaryote and eukaryote cells may be less clear-cut than previously thought; recent evidence indicates that some cytoskeletal filaments believed to be unique to eukaryotic cells also exist in prokaryotes.

Nucleus

As the storehouse for genes, the nucleus is the organelle responsible for maintaining the blueprint for the construction and function of the cell. Many different molecules are exchanged between the nucleus and the cytoplasm, and, similar to most other components in the cytoplasm, the nucleus is highly dynamic, disintegrating during cell division but reforming when new cells are created and at the end of mitosis.

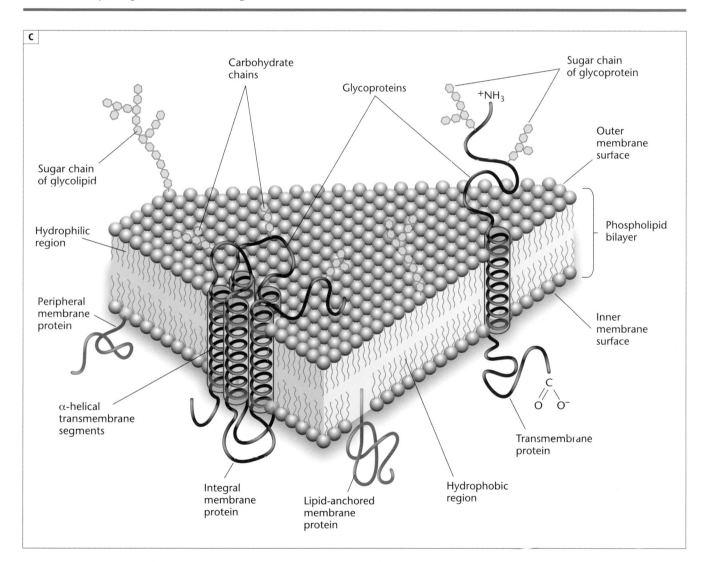

▲ **Fig 1.14c Diagram of the plasma membrane**, consisting of a lipid bilayer of phospholipids with hydrophilic and hydrophobic ends respectively facing externally and internally. Embedded proteins are oriented similarly, and most of these are glycoproteins exhibiting carbohydrate side chains. Functions of proteins include those acting as enzymes, attachment sites for the cytoskeleton, or receptors or transport activity, the latter two types spanning the whole membrane.

Usually 5–10 μm in diameter, the nucleus is bounded by a nuclear envelope consisting of inner and outer nuclear membranes separated by a perinuclear space of about 30 nm (Fig 1.15a). The outer membrane may be studded with ribosomes and can be continuous with the membranes of the rough endoplasmic reticulum (rough ER); thus protein synthesis may occur very close to the nucleus. In plasma cells (synthesizing immunoglobulins), the perinuclear space is often distended with protein secretion (Fig 1.15b).

On the nuclear side is a thin zone of filamentous protein meshwork, termed the *nuclear lamina*, that supports nuclear shape. The lamina may be connected with the nuclear matrix, which is a network of filaments thought to maintain shape and act as an internal skeleton, and is possibly involved with chromosome mobility.

Nuclear pores

These are special openings or channels that span the nuclear envelope and provide entry and exit routes linking the nuclear environment with the cytoplasm. Nuclear pores allow the entry of enzymes/proteins from cytoplasm for chromosome replication and transcription, and the export of RNA and partly made ribosomes needed by the cytoplasm. The distribution of nuclear pores is akin to the arrangement of holes in a kitchen colander, in which a half-sphere is perforated with many small holes that act as sieves (Fig 1.16).

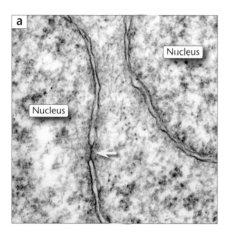

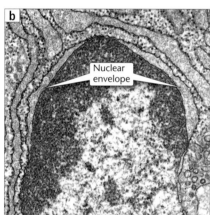

◄ **Fig 1.15a Ultrastructure of the nuclear envelope**, consisting of inner and outer membranes separated by a 10–30 nm space. The membranes are interrupted by a nuclear pore (**arrow**) appearing as a single, dense diaphragm. In three dimensions, the pores are tiny barrel-shaped structures that allow exchange of materials between the nucleus and cytoplasm. × 54,000.

▲ **Fig 1.15b Ultrastructure of the nuclear envelope**, with the outer nuclear membrane showing ribosomes and the perinuclear space distended with particulate material. This arrangement illustrates the continuity of the nuclear envelope with the rough endoplasmic reticulum. × 22,000.

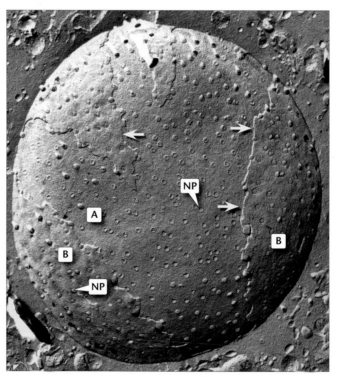

▲ **Fig 1.16 Ultrastructure of a freeze-fracture preparation** of the inner (**A**) and outer (**B**) nuclear membrane showing many nuclear pores (**NP**) that number several thousand per nucleus. At these sites, A and B membranes are fused. Pores are cylinders that assemble from both sides of the nuclear membrane and provide a route for entry and exit of many macromolecules. **Arrows** indicate the interface between the two membranes. × 13,500. (Courtesy L Orci, University of Geneva; from Orci L, Perrelet A. Freeze-Etch Histology. Heidelberg: Springer-Verlag, 1975.)

There may be several thousand pores per cell nucleus.

A nuclear pore resembles an alloy car wheel—a ring with spokes. Like a camera iris diaphragm, the central hole can open or close to regulate the passage of variably sized molecules.

The nuclear envelope can be ripped up—it is literally torn in many cells. Why? When cells divide, the envelope must be dismantled to allow freedom for replicated chromosomes to attach to microtubules that pull the chromosomes to opposite poles of the cell. This separates the chromosomes into the two daughter cells. A likely model is discussed later in the section on cell division.

Nucleolus

This is the ribosome factory of the cell, and there may be more than one nucleolus per cell. It is an example of three-dimensional compartmentalization within the nucleus, where ribosomal RNA (rRNA) gene clusters of several chromosomes together create a domain dedicated to rRNA synthesis and early ribosome production. Nucleolar size is correlated with its level of activity. Cells with high rates of protein synthesis have large nucleoli that may occupy 20% or more of nuclear volume (Fig 1.17).

About 2 μm in diameter, the nucleolus consists of fibrillar, spherical elements linked with a granular network sometimes called the nucleonema (Fig 1.18a & b). The former contains DNA coding for rRNA, and the latter are granules of rRNA molecules that are packaged with proteins (imported from the cytoplasm, but see below) to form ribosome subunits. These are transported through the nuclear pores to the cytoplasm. Mutant embryos that lack nucleoli cannot synthesize rRNA and die in early development.

Recent studies have identified hundreds of proteins in the nucleolus, many of which have known functions in ribosome assembly; others may be involved with hitherto unsuspected roles. Evidence is emerging that translation can occur in the nucleus, a notion that is quite unorthodox. The cytoplasm is supposed to be protected from the synthesis of faulty proteins, which could occur if incompletely processed messenger RNAs (mRNAs) were translated inside the nucleus. If nuclear translation is a common phenomenon, it suggests that the nucleus/nucleolus offers an additional opportunity for the cell to check the integrity of mRNAs before they are "let loose" in the cytoplasm.

The nucleus also contains numerous other small structures variously called speckles, gems, cleavage bodies, and Cajal bodies. The latter have been linked with assembly and modification of RNA-processing molecules, but definitive evidence is lacking.

Chromatin and chromosomes

In appropriately stained sections viewed with the LM, the chromatin within the nucleus of non-dividing (interphase) cells consists of faint particulate

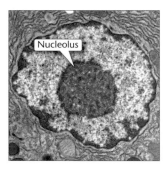

▲ **Fig 1.17 The nucleolus** is the site for synthesis of rRNA and ribosome subunits; it contains genes from multiple chromosomes that encode the rRNAs. Genes for transport RNA (tRNA) are also found in the nucleolus. When ribosome biogenesis is a major requirement for the cell, the nucleolus is large, as in this case. The nucleolus is not detectable in the absence of ribosome production and disappears during mitosis. × 6,000.

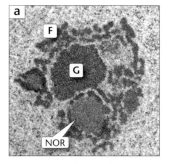

▲ **Fig 1.18a Nucleolus of segregated morphology**, showing nucleolar-organizing regions (**NOR**) of rRNA genes, and granular (**G**) and fibrillar (**F**) components for assembly of the RNA and ribosomal proteins that together are exported from the nucleus to the cell cytoplasm. × 8,000.

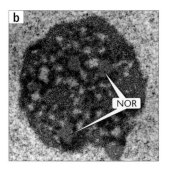

▲ **Fig 1.18b Detail of compact nucleolar structure** showing several nucleolar-organizing regions (**NOR**), and the nucleonema network of fibrillar and granular components. × 11,000.

matter together with conspicuous clumps of dense material. The former is called *euchromatin* (genes actively transcribed) and the latter is referred to as *heterochromatin* (transcriptionally inactive). Both types constitute the interphase chromosomes, each of which is segregated into particular domains or territories within the nucleus. Interchromosomal domains contain RNAs destined for export from the nucleus. Chromosomes are not intertwined and thus avoid the problem of disentanglement (and possible breakage) prior to their segregation during mitosis. The relative abundance and distribution patterns of chromatin is often characteristic of particular cell types and facilitates their identification (Fig 1.19a & b). Just prior to cell division the chromatin becomes highly compacted into recognizable chromosomes (Fig 1.20a & b). Chromatin consists of DNA intimately associated with histones (basic proteins of five major

types), together with many other non-histone protein complexes. There is about twice as much protein as DNA in chromatin, and about 10% of the mass of a chromosome consists of RNA chains formed by transcription of its DNA.

The smallest unit of chromatin organization is the nucleosome, about 10 nm in diameter, in which about 146 base pairs of double-stranded DNA are wrapped around a core of four pairs of histone proteins. A shorter segment of linker DNA, about 10–80 base pairs in length, connects neighboring nucleosomes. The packaging and arrangement of nucleosomes and chromatin is illustrated in Figure 1.21. Each chromosome is therefore a single large nucleosomal fiber. Few ultrastructural details are apparent when chromatin in non-dividing cells is examined in conventional tissue sections with electron microscopy. This is because the molecular structure of chromatin

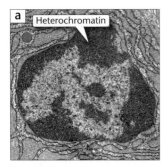
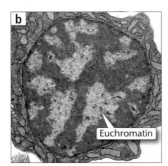

◀ **Fig 1.19a & b Variations in heterochromatin content and distribution**, showing association with the nuclear membrane and condensation throughout the nucleus, which suggests compaction of chromatin during prophase of mitosis. The less dense regions of nuclear material represent euchromatin, where chromatin is decondensed and available for transcription. × 8,000.

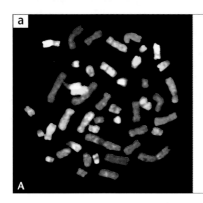
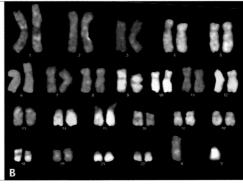
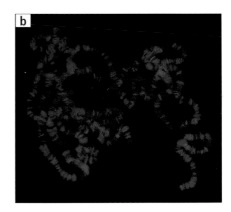

▲ **Fig 1.20a Chromosomes** visualized with fluorescence in situ hybridization (FISH) method where chromosome-specific fluorescent complementary DNA probes label each of the 24 chromosomes a different color. **A** normal male metaphase; **B** karotype arranged according to size and centromere position. (Courtesy R Anderson, MRC Radiation and Genome Stability Unit, Harwell, UK.)

▲ **Fig 1.20b Large polytene chromosome** from *Drosophila* consisting of striking band patterns, here double labeled with a Hoechst fluorescent dye (blue) representing most of the DNA. Interband regions (red) stained with Chromator antibody represent protein maintaining chromosome structure. × 700. (Courtesy KM Johansen, Iowa State University; J Cell Science 2006; 119:2332–41.)

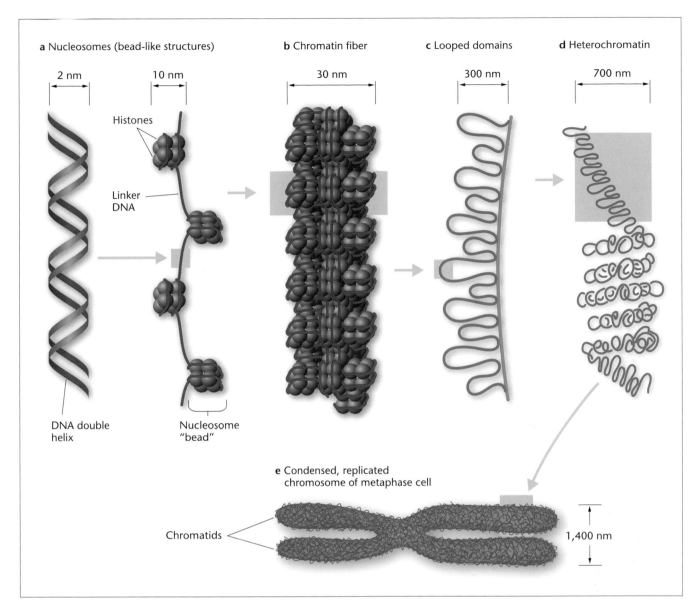

a Nucleosomes (bead-like structures) **b** Chromatin fiber **c** Looped domains **d** Heterochromatin

2 nm 10 nm 30 nm 300 nm 700 nm

Histones

Linker DNA

DNA double helix

Nucleosome "bead"

e Condensed, replicated chromosome of metaphase cell

Chromatids

1,400 nm

▲ **Fig 1.21 Diagram of the hierarchical organization of the chromosome. a** DNA in duplex strands is wound around histone proteins similar to beads on a string; **b** supercoiled assembly into a chromatin fiber; **c** fibers looped and anchored to a protein scaffold; **d** highly folded into dense heterochromatin; **e** compacted into a recognizable arm of the chromosome.

is so tightly compacted that individual components are rarely seen. In specially prepared specimens of isolated chromosomes from which histone proteins have been removed, the uncoiled DNA is visible at the ultrastructural level (Fig 1.22). The three-dimensional structure of nucleosomes can be extended to the atomic level using X-ray crystallography/diffraction methods (Fig 1.23). EM images reveal the extraordinarily tight packaging of DNA in chromatin, which compacts about 1.8 meters of DNA inside a nucleus that is only 5–6 μm in diameter. A single chromosome 4–5 μm in length may contain 10 cm of DNA, representing a compaction factor of 20,000.

In relation to the whole human genome, less than 2% represents genes that code for RNA and proteins, called exons, which are separated by non-coding intervening sequences, called introns. About half the genome consists of repeat DNA sequences that may exist in millions of copies. The functions of repeated DNA and most of the non-coding gene sequences in the other half of the genome are unknown.

Genes are believed to be clustered not on the basis of their function, but rather in relation to when they are expressed (e.g. during cell differentiation). Genes are thus not arranged randomly along a linear genome.

Numerous efforts have been made to sequence and characterize the human genome, and several chromosomes such as 5, 16, and 19 have been targeted (see http://www.jgi.doe.gov/). Chromosome 5 is a large chromosome with 923 protein-coding genes and vast regions of non-coding DNA (called gene deserts) that are conserved across many vertebrates. Gene deserts are believed to regulate functional genes that are physically separated. Chromosome 16 has 880 genes and has many regions copied to other parts of itself or to other chromosomes. It has genes associated with breast cancer and Crohn's disease. Chromosome 19 has about 1,460 genes, including those coding for heart disease and diabetes. It has about twice the average gene density of the genome.

Chromatin has special domains. Only the heterochromatin is easily seen by microscopy because its high density (and thus affinity for stains) represents a condensed state in which the DNA is not or never transcribed. It is often partly tethered to the nuclear envelope. Heterochromatin represents only 10% of the entire genome and contains few functional genes, but many sequences of repetitive DNA. Most of the heterochromatin is of the constitutive type, permanently compacted and containing so-called junk DNA, which is transcriptionally silent. The centromeres and telomeres (Fig 1.24) are surrounded by constitutive heterochromatin and depend upon repeated DNA sequences for chromosome cohesion, segregation, and stability. Telomeres seal and stabilize the ends of chromosomes but, in somatic cells, telomeric DNA cannot be fully copied prior to cell division. After a finite number of cell divisions, the length of the telomere is reduced to the point where it no longer protects the end of a chromosome. This causes abnormal chromosome stickiness/fusions and cell death. Heterochromatin designated as the facultative type contains chromatin that is transiently compacted and specifically inactivated, depending on the cell type and its function. An example is the inactivation of one of the X chromosomes in cells of females. In contrast, euchromatin is not seen in the LM, and only as faint particulate matter in the EM; it represents accessible DNA that is available for transcription.

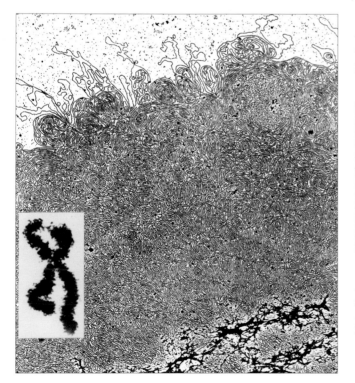

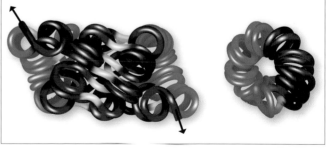

◀ **Fig 1.22 Ultrastructure of part of a chromosome** after the histones were extracted, allowing the DNA to uncoil into 4 nm filaments. x 10,000. (Courtesy U Laemmli, University of Lausanne, Switzerland.)

▲ **Fig 1.23 Models of DNA in the nucleosome**, about 30 nm in width, showing a solenoid-type arrangement in a supercoiled organization. DNA of the core is colored magenta red and blue, and linker DNA is yellow. (Modified from Dorigo B, et al. Science 2004; 306:1571–3.)

DNA sequencing in humans, other animals, and plants has been proclaimed as a breakthrough in molecular biology coupled with computer technology, but just how important is it to know the sequences of the three billion base pairs of adenine, guanine, cytosine, and thymine? Consider the enormous complexity of the human brain and nervous system. The brain is the most complex 1.5 kg mass known in the universe, but does the DNA in its cells alone direct its construction and function? IIow do 25,000 human genes determine 100 billion neurons, 10 times this number of glial cells, and 10^{15} connections in the nervous system? The regulatory mechanisms certainly cannot be the same as the nematode worm's 18,000 genes that control its 959 somatic cells. Obviously, complex regulatory mechanisms are crucial in determining how, when, and to what extent genes are expressed throughout the life of an organism. The sequencing of the genome, a massive research effort to date, is the prelude to discovering what role the genes really have in controlling the cell itself and its interactions with other cells and the extracellular environment

(proteomics, metabolomics, physionomics). These studies will take much longer than genome sequencing—decades at the very least.

Rough (or granular) endoplasmic reticulum

The rough ER consists of narrow tubular membranes or flattened membrane sacs called cisternae. Its designation as "rough" is from the attachment of ribosomes on the outer membrane, which gives it a studded appearance (Fig 1.25a & b). It is the affinity of the ribosomes for basic dyes such as hematoxylin, methylene blue, and toluidine blue that enables the location of rough ER to be marked within the cell cytoplasm. The cisternae and/or membranes form a continuous network in one or more regions of cytoplasm, the quantity of which is indicative of the level of synthesis and secretion of protein by the cell. Parts of the rough ER are continuous with the outer nuclear envelope, and tubular ER membranes are the source of a new nuclear membrane during telophase/cytokinesis in cell division.

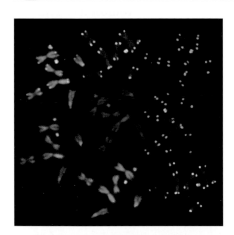

◀ **Fig 1.24 Fluorescent-labeled chromosomes and telomeres sealing their ends.** Telomeres have tandemly repeated, simple-sequence DNA loops that prevent unwanted chromosome fusions. Dividing somatic cells progressively lose their telomeres and die, but most cancer cells have a type of polymerase enzyme called telomerase that replicates the telomere DNA. This ensures prolonged proliferation of the cancer cell. Some embryonic cells and male germ stem cells possess telomerase, ensuring their long-term ability to divide. × 1,300. (Courtesy M Gatti, University of Rome "La Sapienza," Italy.)

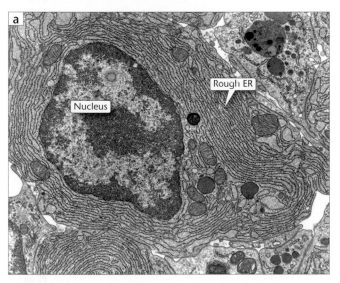

▲ **Fig 1.25a Ultrastructure of a plasma cell**, showing exceptionally abundant cisternae of rough ER surrounding the nucleus. This organelle is required for the synthesis of immunoglobulin proteins that are secreted as antibodies. × 8,000.

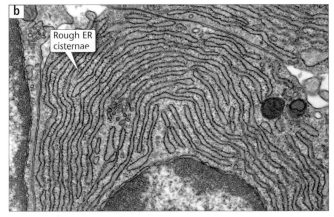

▲ **Fig 1.25b Ultrastructure at higher magnification of rough ER membranes**, showing attached ribosomes and narrow and dilated segments of the parallel membranes. In conjunction with mRNA, the ribosomes assemble amino acids into growing polypeptide chains, which are extruded into the lumen of the rough ER and folded to form the particular conformation of the protein. These proteins may be retained by the reticulum or exported for further modifications. × 16,000.

Purpose of the rough ER

The attachment of ribosomes to the membrane allows the newly synthesized polypeptides to:

- be incorporated and anchored into membrane that is required as new membrane is formed (e.g. other membrane-bound compartments)
- accumulate within the lumen of the rough ER to be secreted as soluble proteins (e.g. antibodies) (Fig 1.26) or packaged into secretory vesicles containing proteins/enzymes (e.g. in cells of pancreas or salivary glands).

Free ribosomes in the cytoplasm are called polyribosomes, and are unattached ribosomes in clusters linked by mRNA resembling beads on a string. Proteins made on free ribosomes are generally destined to stay in the cytoplasm or be routed to mitochondria, peroxisomes, and the interior of the nucleus.

Protein synthesis

The mechanisms by which ribosomes act as protein synthetic "machines" are discussed in detail in cell biology texts. A summary of protein synthesis and sorting is presented in Figure 1.27. Originating from the nucleolus, the rRNA molecules are assembled with proteins (from the cytoplasm) to form small (40S) and large (60S) ribosomal subunits that are exported to the cytoplasm. These subunits unite to form complete ribosomes when they become bound to mRNA whose nucleotide sequence is derived from the transcription of genes encoded within DNA. Translation of the code specified in mRNA requires access to and correct assembly of amino acids, one by one, into a growing polypeptide chain. Transfer RNA (tRNA) molecules bring specific amino acids to the site where a ribosome is bound to a start codon of the mRNA. The latter is specifically recognized by the anticodon region of the tRNA. In this way, amino acids linked to tRNAs are matched up to mRNA codons, enabling the translation of the nucleotide sequence into a polypeptide sequence. The ribosomes act as molecular machines moving along the mRNA directing the synthesis of a polypeptide. Many small polypeptides are synthesized in minutes, larger types within several hours. As the amino acids are assembled together by peptide bonds, the elongating chain is extruded from a tunnel in the core of the ribosome. Bulk synthesis of identical polypeptides is achieved by many ribosomes moving along the same mRNA, "reading" the codon sequences and producing the same polypeptide.

For peptides required by most membrane compartments of the cell, the ribosomes and their early-forming polypeptides become associated with the ER, forming rough ER. The function of rough ER is to process the growing peptides into proteins that are required for the synthesis of new membranes or for further modifications and transport within membrane-bound vesicles to organelles such as the Golgi complex or the lysosomal system.

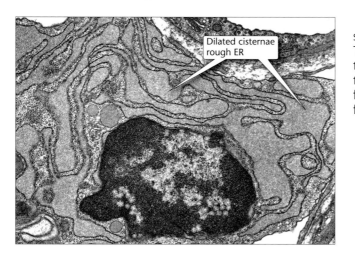

Dilated cisternae rough ER

◀ **Fig 1.26 Ultrastructure of rough ER in a plasma cell,** showing dilated membranous sacs containing fine granular material. This morphology reflects the intense protein synthesis necessary for the production of antibodies (immunoglobulins). In these proteins, the heavy and light chains are linked together within the rough ER, followed by glycosylation and then export to the Golgi apparatus for further modification before secretion. × 10,000.

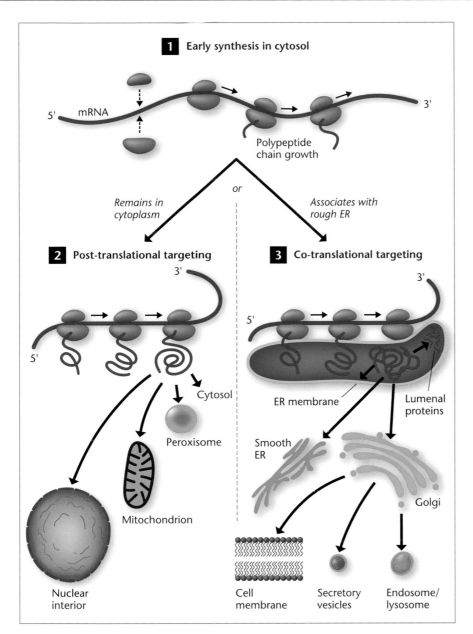

1 **Early synthesis in cytosol**

5' mRNA 3'

Polypeptide
chain growth

*Remains in
cytoplasm*

or

*Associates with
rough ER*

2 **Post-translational targeting**

3'

5'

Cytosol

Peroxisome

Mitochondrion

Nuclear
interior

3 **Co-translational targeting**

3'

5'

ER membrane

Lumenal
proteins

Smooth
ER

Golgi

Cell
membrane

Secretory
vesicles

Endosome/
lysosome

▲ **Fig 1.27 How proteins are sorted in the cytoplasm. 1** Newly forming peptides grow in length into polypeptides. **2** Proteins destined for the cytoplasm or nucleus continue synthesis on free ribosomes in the cytoplasm. When translation is complete, the proteins remain in the cytoplasm or are transported to designated organelles, depending on their types. **3** If proteins are required for the endomembrane system or secretion from the cell, the ribosomes associate with the ER, and protein synthesis continues within the lumen. The fully formed polypeptide is used for the ER or transported to designated membrane compartments.

In both cytosolic and ER-associated protein synthesis, the nascent polypeptides must undergo folding and modification of their molecular composition to achieve a final three-dimensional configuration that is essential for their particular function. If synthesized in the cytosol, proteins are fully translated and folding and/or modification occurs in the cytosol after release from the ribosome.

Proteins destined for the nucleus, mitochondria, or peroxisomes are said to exhibit post-translational import to these organelles. They are sorted to these destinations by specific signal sequences forming part of the protein itself.

For proteins synthesized on the rough ER, the transfer of the growing polypeptide is called cotranslational import, because entry of the polypeptide

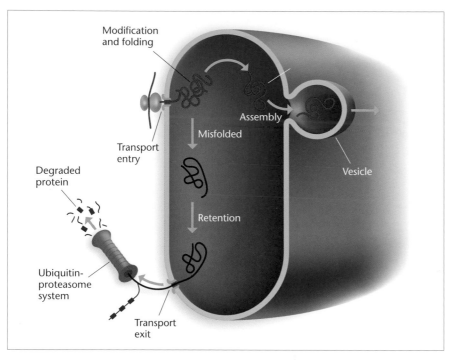

◀ Fig 1.28 Diagram of peptide synthesis and folding. Peptide chains in the lumen of the rough endoplasmic reticulum are assembled, processed and folded, then packaged in vesicles destined for the Golgi complex. Proteins not correctly folded are detected and then diverted by the rough ER into the proteasome, the cellular protein executioner.

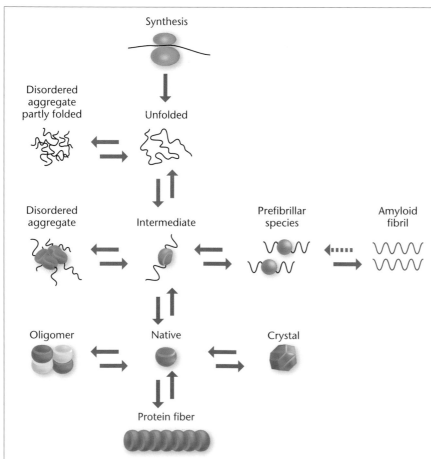

◀ Fig 1.29 Variations of the fate of proteins. Newly synthesized peptides are processed into a native state that is thermodynamically stable, forming crystals, oligomers, or fibers. Alternate pathways result in abnormal folding, denaturation, or disorderly assemblies of globular proteins. Any of these aberrations may give rise to malfunction and disease.

into the ER lumen occurs at the same time as it is being synthesized. In addition, the rough ER is responsible for cotranslational folding of the growing polypeptide. This crucial process is carried out by a wide range of molecular chaperones and folding catalysts; correctly folded proteins are directed to the secretory pathway (to the Golgi complex), but incorrectly folded proteins are diverted to cytoplasmic proteasomes for degradation (Fig 1.28). The rough ER thus performs a "quality check" of translated proteins. Misfolded proteins can escape degradation if the ER and/or cytosolic processing is dysfunctional, and these disordered proteins may give rise to diseases as diverse as cystic fibrosis, some cancers, and neurodegenerative disorders including Alzheimer's and Parkinson's diseases and type II diabetes (Fig 1.29). In some cell types, the proteins assembled within the rough ER are not continuously secreted but show transient storage or aggregation without being degraded. An example is the plasma cell, where immunoglobulin protein accumulates in distended rough ER prior to release (Fig 1.26).

Smooth endoplasmic reticulum

This consists of interconnected tubular membranes or flattened concentric membrane cisternae that vary greatly in quantity and distribution (Fig 1.30a & b). Functions include synthesis of lipids and steroids (steroidogenic cells of the adrenal glands, ovary, testis), detoxification of harmful substances that include a variety of drugs such as barbiturates and alcohol (in the liver), carbohydrate metabolism (also in the liver), and storage and release of calcium (in cardiac and skeletal muscle). The smooth ER is a rich source of proteins/enzymes involved with these activities.

Steroidogenesis and drug detoxification require the hydroxylation reaction, the addition of hydroxyl groups to organic substrates. The steroid hormones made in the smooth ER remain hydrophobic (i.e. they are lipid soluble but not water soluble). In contrast, the hydroxylation of drugs increases their solubility in water and assists uptake by the blood and elimination from the body.

Carbohydrate metabolism in the liver by smooth ER enzymes causes breakdown (catabolism) of stored glycogen in hepatocytes to yield glucose, which helps maintain blood glucose levels within a narrow range. Glycogen in the liver is stored as granules associated with the smooth ER and is easily seen in the EM.

Uptake and storage of calcium in heart and skeletal muscle cells is essential for contraction of muscle fibers. In muscle, the smooth ER is extensive and organized into the sarcoplasmic reticulum, a network of smooth membranes that occupy spaces between individual myofibrils. When calcium floods into the cytoplasm around the myofibrils, it triggers the interactions between actin and myosin, and initiates their motor function.

> **Tip:** The endoplasmic reticulum is a dynamic organelle. It is essential for protein synthesis (rough ER), steroid synthesis and drug detoxification (smooth ER), calcium storage and release (sarcoplasmic reticulum), and reconstitution of the nuclear membrane late in mitosis.

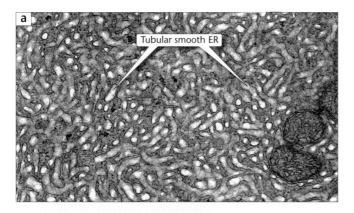

◀ **Fig 1.30a Ultrastructure of smooth ER in a cell synthesizing steroid hormones.** Typically, if the tissue is fixed by perfusion, the smooth ER presents as a tightly packed mass of tubular-type membranes. If the tissue is immersion-fixed, the tubules of smooth ER breakdown to form thousands of vesicles representing a morphological artifact. × 25,000.

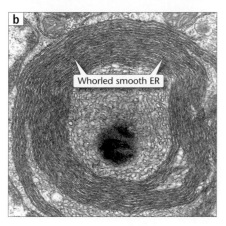

◀ **Fig 1.30b Ultrastructure of smooth ER, showing a whorled appearance of concentrically stacked membranes.** This type of organization is common in active steroidogenic cells, such as luteal and Leydig cells. Recent data suggest that interactions between proteins on the cytoplasmic surface of the membranes maintain the whorled morphology. × 20,000.

Golgi apparatus

Arguably the most complex and interesting of the organelles, the Golgi is the major sorting apparatus in the cytoplasm. It consists of stacks of membranes that form curved cisternae which are often localized to one pole of the cell. In EM sections several Golgi stacks may be visible, indicative of the Golgi's existence as multiple units concentrated to particular domains in the cytoplasm (Fig 1.31).

The Golgi apparatus is a highly dynamic organelle. It is critical for the processing of macromolecules that it receives from the cytosol or other membrane compartments, as well as for sorting proteins and lipids for delivery to specific destinations. Both of these functions are coordinated within the Golgi cisternae and in the numerous membrane vesicles with which it is associated. Enzymes located at specific sites within the Golgi serve to glycosylate proteins that it receives and to sulfate sugar molecules and selected proteins. This processing is accompanied by sorting and then exporting these macromolecules within vesicles that have one of two fates: transport to other organelles within the cell, or delivery to the plasma membrane where, for example, the vesicle cargo is discharged as a secretory product.

New membrane vesicles from other regions of the cell may fuse with the Golgi, and at the same time membrane vesicles bud off from the Golgi for transport elsewhere. Thus, the Golgi is surrounded by numerous transport vesicles.

The convex face of the Golgi, usually close to the rough ER, is called the *cis* or forming face, whereas the concave face is referred to as the *trans* or maturing face (Fig 1.32). The cis face, middle cisternae, and trans face membranes are biochemically and functionally distinct, and carry out the activities listed above, including cleaving protein precursors into active peptides and lipid synthesis.

A central sorting station

Movement of materials from the ER to the Golgi complex and then to the plasma membrane is called *anterograde transport* (e.g. the assembly, packaging, and transport of secretory granules in typical exocrine glands). As granules fuse with the plasma membrane, a piece of membrane that originated from the ER becomes part of the surface membrane. To maintain roughly the same total membrane surface area, the cell recycles membrane back into the cytoplasm. This is termed *retrograde transport*, where vesicles flow back to the Golgi and then to the ER.

Thus the Golgi becomes the central sorting station, shuttling membranes between the ER, vesicles, and the plasma membrane (Fig 1.33). The position of the Golgi is maintained within the cell at the same time as it is deformed and pulled apart by the constant yet orderly addition and loss of its membranes, in much the same way as a tubular "liquid plasma" light continuously recycles blobs of colloid suspended in fluid. The location of the Golgi in the cell is controlled by the cytoskeleton, specifically microtubules and actin together with their specific motor proteins. These elements not only serve to maintain a dynamic equilibrium between stability and plasticity of the Golgi, but they are also essential for the shuttling/transport of imported and exported vesicles.

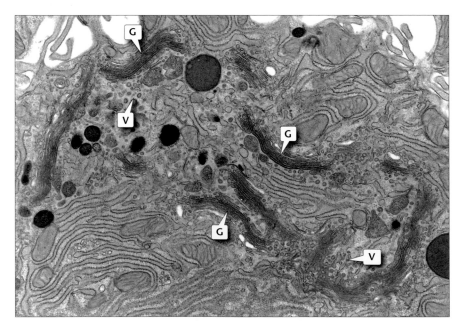

◀ **Fig 1.31 Ultrastructure of several profiles of the Golgi complex.**
Membranes of the Golgi apparatus (**G**) consist of parallel stacks of smooth membranes or cisternae, associated with many vesicles (**V**). The Golgi performs many functions, including uptake, modification, transport, and release (as secretory vesicles) of nascent proteins received from the rough ER; production of lysosomes; and serving as a sorting point in the endocytotic pathways and the regulated and constitutive secretory pathways. × 17,000.

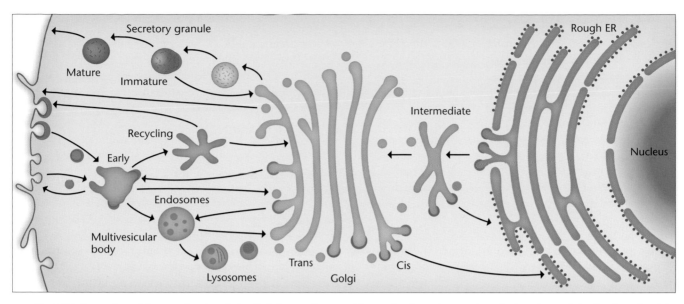

▲ Fig 1.32 Central position and role of the Golgi complex. Membranes shown as vesicles are transported and recycled between the ER, the Golgi, and the secretory and lysosomal compartments. The forming, or cis, face of the Golgi interfaces with the ER, and the maturing, or trans, face is highly interactive with vesicle transport for secretory pathways and ingestion of extracellular or intracellular materials via the endosome–lysosome compartments.

The mechanisms that regulate the location and destination of vesicles and their proteins include specific markers or tags on the proteins or on the membranes and the length of membrane domains. Using these characteristics, the Golgi becomes the principal organelle in sorting and packaging the traffic through the various membrane compartments.

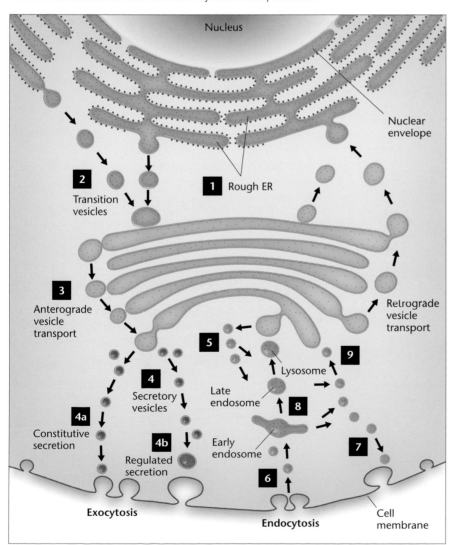

◀ Fig 1.33 Details of the transport of vesicles within the cytoplasm.
1 Rough ER for synthesis of peptides for metabolism and lipids for membranes.
2 Transport of vesicles to the Golgi.
3 Movement of vesicles through or in association with Golgi cisternae.
4 Despatch of mature protein-containing vesicles to the secretory pathways for release by exocytosis. **5** Transport of hydrolytic enzymes to the endosome–lysosome compartments. **6** Uptake of extracellular materials via endocytosis and routing to endosomes. **7** Recycling of ingested and excess membranes to the plasma membrane. **8** Endosomes mature into primary and secondary lysosomes. **9** Recycling membranes back to the Golgi complex and then the ER.

Transport mechanisms

Movement of vesicles through the Golgi is thought to occur by a combination of two mechanisms, the vesicular transport and the cisternal maturation models (Fig 1.34). In vesicular transport, the membrane stacks are stable, with shuttle vesicles budding from one cisterna and fusing with another in the cis–trans (forward) direction. The cisternal maturation model, for which there is compelling evidence, proposes that the cisternae themselves mature and migrate from the cis to the trans face. In both models resident proteins and lipids are recycled backwards via a separate series of vesicles.

The key role of the Golgi in the sorting and transport of protein-containing vesicles in the whole cell is seen in Figure 1.35a. These vesicles have the following major destinations:

1. Apical or basolateral plasma membranes
2. The endosome–lysosome system
3. Secretory granules
4. Retrieval from the cell surface with recycling back to endosomes or Golgi, or transport across the cell to the opposite surface, a process called transcytosis.

Vesicles involved with these pathways acquire special protein coats recruited from the cytosol. There are three main types of coated vesicles: COPI-coated (COP = cytosolic coat protein), COPII-coated, and clathrin-coated (lattice type). They serve to convert flat membranes into round buds and help select particular cargoes within the formed vesicles. Coated vesicles participate in export and import pathways in the cell. COPI is involved in intra-Golgi transport and retrograde transport from the Golgi to the rough ER. COPII vesicles move anterogradely from

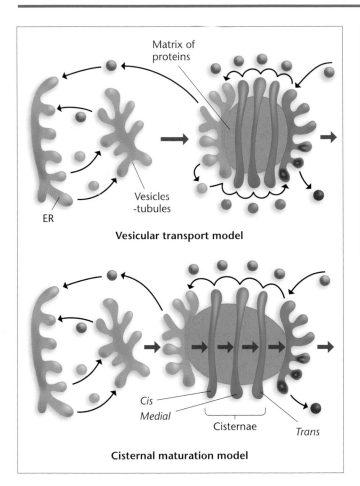

▲ **Fig 1.34 Two models of protein trafficking through the Golgi apparatus.** In the **vesicular transport model**, the Golgi membranous cisternae remain in place with no displacement. Forward-moving vesicles bud and fuse with cisternae in the cis-to-trans direction and retrograde-moving vesicles in the opposite direction. In the **cisternal maturation model**, vesicles from the endoplasmic reticulum fuse with the Golgi cisternum, which itself matures through the cisternal stacks, reaching the trans face, where it fragments. Coated-protein vesicles recycle resident Golgi membranes in a retrograde direction.

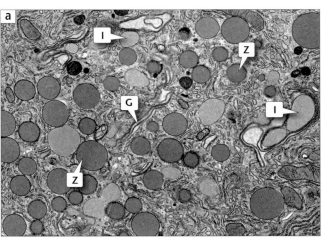

▲ **Fig 1.35a Cytoplasm of a pancreatic exocrine cell.** Note several profiles of Golgi apparatus (**G**) and their association with newly forming secretory vesicles, termed immature zymogen granules (**I**). These contain dozens of proteins being processed into digestive enzymes that, with time, are concentrated into numerous mature zymogen granules (**Z**). Zymogen granules are stored in the cell until discharged by exocytosis in response to appropriate stimuli. × 9,500.

the rough ER to the Golgi, and clathrin-coated vesicles are restricted to post-Golgi pathways. Soon after its formation, the vesicle loses its coat and the disassembled proteins are available for new vesicle budding.

Uncoated vesicles reach their correct targets by means of a specific tag or receptor on the vesicle that is recognized by a complementary receptor on the target membrane of another organelle or the plasma membrane. Vesicles are tethered to their target, then dock with it, followed by fusion of membranes between the vesicle and the target.

The Golgi in secretion and absorption

The Golgi plays a central role in secretory cells by determining when and how a protein secretory product is released from the cell. The release can be continuous or controlled (Fig 1.35b).

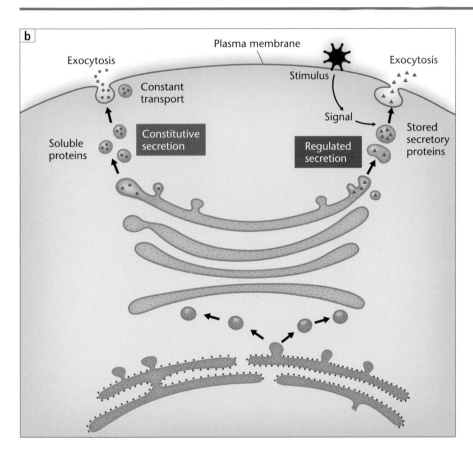

▲ **Fig 1.35b Constitutive versus regulated secretion.** Constitutively secreted proteins within Golgi-derived vesicles are continuously transported to the cell surface, fuse with the plasma membrane, and are released from the cell. In regulated secretory processes, vesicle formation and release of their contents is controlled by specific stimuli acting upon the cell. The secretory vesicles mature in the cytoplasm, accumulating concentrated stores of proteins that are exocytosed from the cell in response to specific signals.

Constitutive secretion means the steady streaming and continuous discharge of secretory vesicles or granules at the plasma membrane surface. All cells require this pathway. *Regulated secretion* is shown by cells that secrete products on demand, usually in response to a specific stimulus (e.g. insulin secretion by beta cells in the pancreatic islets of Langerhans, histamine release by mast cells, and digestive enzyme secretion by pancreatic acinar cells) (Fig 1.36a & b). As the proteins are assembled, packaged, and discharged from the Golgi, they are put into condensing vesicles, where the proteins are concentrated and undergo proteolytic processing. The vesicles become mature secretory vesicles, or zymogen granules, which are temporarily stored in the cytoplasm awaiting the discharge signal. Fusion of the limiting membrane of the zymogen granules with the plasma membrane is called *exocytosis* (Fig 1.37).

By tracing the uptake and fate of radiolabeled amino acids into protein-secreting cells, EM analysis using the technique of autoradiography has determined that it takes about 1.5 hours for an exogenous amino acid to appear within zymogen granules.

Fusion of zymogen granules with the cell surface increases the surface area of the plasma membrane. In actively secreting pancreatic cells, about 900 µm² of additional membrane are added to the apical membrane, which has a surface area of only 30 µm². Clearly this is a potential problem, but it is solved by the ability of the cell to internalize excess membrane as quickly as it is added—a process of recycling that is a type of *endocytosis*. A pancreatic cell may recycle all its surface membrane in 90 minutes, a macrophage in 30 minutes.

Cells that have absorptive functions engage in endocytosis, and again this involves the Golgi, which balances the anterograde and retrograde flow of membranes between itself and the plasma membrane. Absorptive cells include those, for example, in the gut and kidneys, and phagocytic cells like macrophages.

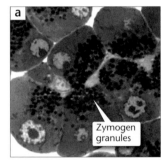

▲ **Fig 1.36a Light micrograph of a pancreatic acinus**, containing exocrine secretory cells with dense apical granules, called zymogen granules. These granules are derived from the Golgi complex, and are packages containing several dozen digestive enzymes. Toluidine blue, araldite, × 1,100.

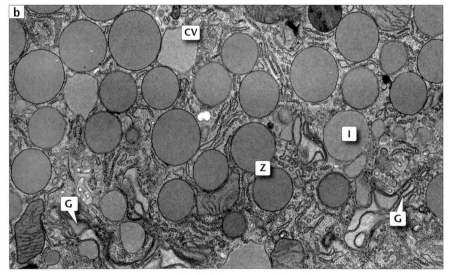

▲ **Fig 1.36b Ultrastructure of the formation of zymogen granules.** Emerging from the Golgi apparatus (**G**) are irregularly shaped condensing vacuoles (**CV**) that contain processed enzymes. CV round up, forming immature (**I**) and mature zymogen granules (**Z**), recognized by their increasing density and compaction of their proteins. × 16,000.

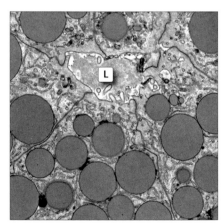

▲ **Fig 1.37 Ultrastructure of zymogen granules** subjacent to the acinar lumen (**L**) and poised for release by exocytosis. When granule membranes fuse with the apical cell membrane, the granule contents are discharged, evidence of which is the particulate material within the lumen. × 8,500.

Endocytosis is a way in which a small segment of plasma membrane folds inwards then pinches off to contain substances that were in the extracellular space (Fig 1.38). The vesicles so formed have many different fates, depending on the cell type. One example is their union with endosomes (immature lysosomes) made by the Golgi and then, if the material is foreign, it is degraded.

The Golgi's identity crisis

Of all the current research on the Golgi apparatus, one function that remains controversial is the question of its autonomy/life history. When a cell divides, the Golgi seems to disappear. There are two schools of thought about this: either the Golgi disperses into protein segments that mostly go to the ER but some make their way into the daughter cells, where they might be a template for rebuilding the Golgi; or the Golgi proteins disassemble into the ER but, after cell division is complete, the ER produces the Golgi proteins that reassemble into the characteristic Golgi apparatus.

Mitochondria

Mitochondria, the cellular centers of energy production and other essential metabolic reactions, are commonly considered to be the classic kidney-bean-shaped organelle. Yet these structures are very polymorphic, are often long, snake-like tubules, sometimes branched, and at times extend networks reaching into the extremities of the cell. We tend to think that mitochondria are particularly abundant inside the average cell because many of them can be seen in the thin sections examined in the EM. Liver cells, for example, are thought to contain 500–1000, but this estimation may not be correct. In a few

studies with EM that have reconstructed the topology of the mitochondria, and in phase-contrast LM views of living cells, the mitochondria often show large, branching networks in a state of dynamic flux, pinching off and fusing.

Generally about 0.5–1 μm in width, the EM reveals the often complex internal morphology of mitochondria, recognized as four compartments (Fig 1.39). The *outer membrane* is permeable to many molecules that pass into and exit from the organelle. The *inner membrane* is extensive and folded back on itself, creating tubes or plate-like structures called cristae, which contain respiratory chain enzymes that produce adenosine triphosphate (ATP). These proteins are visible in the EM as many particles attached to the large surface area afforded by the cristae. ATP provides chemical energy to drive biochemical reactions, the details of which are concerned with the chemistry of aerobic respiration. An *intermembrane space* occurs between the outer and inner membranes. The mitochondrial *matrix* is inside the inner membrane in the core of the mitochondrion. It contains enzymes and DNA (less than 1% of total cellular DNA with just 37 genes) that codes for RNAs and protein subunits of just 13 membrane proteins. Most of the 900 or so gene products in the mitochondrion are coded for by nuclear DNA.

Mitochondria arise only by growth and division of preexisting mitochondria. Almost all mitochondria in the zygote arise from the ovum and very rarely from the sperm. A maternal mutation in mitochondrial DNA will be passed on to all children, but only daughters will transmit it to their progeny. Malfunctions of mitochondrial pathways can cause diseases, many of them involving the brain and skeletal muscle, with a prevalence of up to 15 cases per 100,000 people.

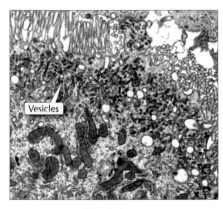

▲ **Fig 1.38 Ultrastructure of apical cytoplasm**, showing a variety of vesicles, many of which are clathrin-coated vesicles generated in situations of receptor-mediated endocytosis. × 4,000.

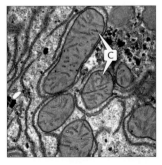

▲ **Fig 1.39 Ultrastructure of typical orthodox mitochondria**, showing lamellar cristae (**C**) and small granules in the matrix. Reactions of the tricarboxylic acid cycle and fatty acid oxidation in the matrix supply electrons to the cristae (an ion gradient), which reduces O_2 and generates ATP (chemical potential energy for the cell). Granules contain stored cations such as calcium. × 16,000.

Main structural variations of mitochondria are recognized by their cristae. In the orthodox type, cristae are lamellar and widely separated, while the cardiac muscle type have abundant and tightly packed cristae (Fig 1.40). In contrast, steroid-type cristae are mainly tubular, with a large surface area to accommodate enzymes associated with steroidogenesis (Fig 1.41). The inner membrane of steroid-type cristae converts cholesterol to pregnenolone, the precursor of further steroid synthesis. Steroidogenesis can be stimulated 10 to 100-fold within minutes by steroidogenic acute regulatory protein (StAR) and may be rapidly terminated by control of the availability of cholesterol. This permits the rapid regulation of circulating steroid hormone levels and explains in part why steroidogenic cells store minimal amounts of hormone.

Cellular respiration is aerobic. Oxidation drives the electron flow associated with the cristae membranes to an electron acceptor, accompanied by generation of ATP. Electrons come from the metabolism of carbohydrates, and oxygen is the electron acceptor, which is reduced to water. The energy of the electrons drives proton pumps within the cristae, which in turn drive the production of ATP.

In muscle, the complete oxidation of one molecule of glucose generates 36 molecules of ATP.

Digestive processes
Endosomes and lysosomes

Endosomes and lysosomes exist as several classes of organelles involved with internalization of extracellular material, recycling of membranes, and breakdown of macromolecules. Endosomes belong to the endocytic membrane system that arises from assembly of Golgi-derived vesicles and internalized plasma membrane, the latter often in the form of endocytic vesicles (Fig 1.42). The functions of endosomes include the recycling of membranes between the Golgi and the plasma membrane and their maturation into

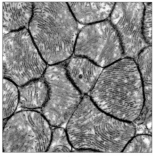
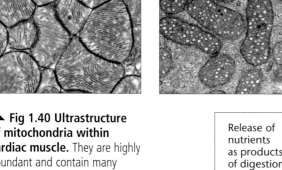

◀ **Fig 1.41 Ultrastructure of mitochondria in a steroidogenic cell.** The mitochondrial cristae are typically tubular, presenting a large surface area for certain enzymes associated with steroid synthesis. The inner mitochondrial membrane converts cholesterol to pregnenolone, the enzyme activity being hormone-dependent and, thus, the mitochondrial reaction is a rate-limiting step in the further synthesis of other steroids. × 15,000.

▲ **Fig 1.40 Ultrastructure of mitochondria within cardiac muscle.** They are highly abundant and contain many tightly packed cristae, which are required to generate ATP in sufficient quantity to sustain the energy consumed during continuous and cyclical cell contraction. Each mitochondrion may produce 250,000 electrons per second using pyruvate formed during glycolysis. × 13,000.

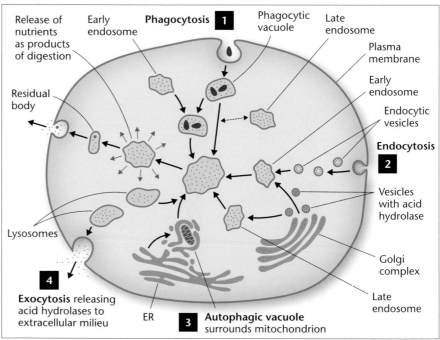

▲ **Fig 1.42 Summary of the various pathways of digestion involving the endosome–lysosome system. 1** Phagocytosis of cell debris or microorganisms, showing vacuole formation and conjunction with hydrolytic enzyme-rich endosomes. **2** Endocytosis of small vesicles and routing to, and amalgamation with, the endosomal system. **3** Autolysis of redundant or dysfunctional intracellular materials and sequestration to endosomes. **4** Release of hydrolytic enzymes from the endosome–lysosome system for extracellular digestive functions.

lysosomes. These activities provide a balance between the turnover of membranes required for secretion (constitutive or regulated) and those necessary for carrying macromolecules into the cell by passive or induced mechanisms (endocytosis). Endosomes are therefore supplementary sorting stations related to the Golgi complex. Resident or acquired components that are damaged or no longer needed are sequestered to lysosomes for destruction.

Lysosomes contain several dozen types of digestive enzymes, called acid hydrolases, and are formed as a final maturation step originating from the Golgi complex and from endosomes (Fig 1.43).

The mechanisms by which extracellular materials or portions of the plasma membrane are internalized by endocytosis can be divided into two main categories: *phagocytosis* is the uptake of large particles (includes microorganisms and cells or parts thereof) and

pinocytosis is the uptake of fluid and solutes (Fig 1.44).

Phagocytosis occurs mainly in cells specialized to scavenge debris, pathogens, or dying cells. Examples are neutrophils of the blood and, in extracellular tissues, macrophages/monocytes, and other cells including many epithelial cells. The clearance of debris and apoptotic cells (cells programmed to die) by phagocytosis is important for the tissue restructuring that accompanies development, inflammatory responses, normal cell turnover, and various immune responses.

Pinocytosis operates in all cells and occurs by several basic mechanisms. Macropinocytosis occurs by "membrane ruffling," when an extension of the plasma membrane samples comparatively large volumes of the extracellular environment and internalizes this into a large endocytic vesicle. Caveolae are small, flask-shaped invaginations of

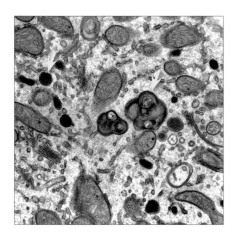

◀ **Fig 1.43 Lysosomes (arrows)**, showing a range of densities and partly digested membranous materials. They contain hydrolases and lipases and arise as the endpoint of the endocytic pathway for degradation of intra- and extracellular components. × 12,000.

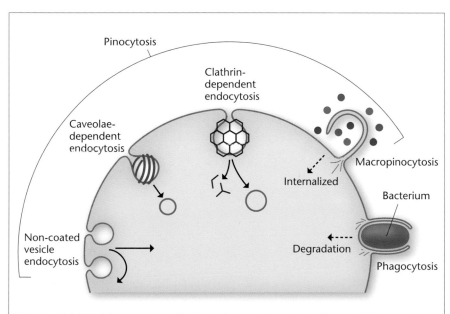

◀ **Fig 1.44 Portals of entry into the cell through the plasma membrane.** Endocytosis via non-coated vesicles serves to retrieve membranes or uptake of fluid. Caveolae are invaginations of membrane coated with caveolin protein, and occasionally may form vesicles. Clathrin-coated vesicles form uncoated vesicles after shedding their clathrin protein coat, and then join with the endosome system. Ruffled membranes may form large endocytic compartments (macropinosomes) as the tip of the ruffle fuses with the plasma membrane. Larger particles (bacteria, cell fragments) internalize using actin-dependent processes and are common in phagocytic cells such as macrophages/monocytes and neutrophils.

plasma membrane that participate in endocytosis by, as yet, poorly understood mechanisms (Fig 1.45). Caveolae occur in many cells and are abundant in endothelial cells. Their function and relationship to "caveosomes" is controversial, since knockout-deficient mice have no special phenotype other than a respiratory disorder caused by lung fibrosis.

Clathrin-mediated endocytosis is well characterized and occurs in all cells, where it serves to internalize macromolecules by means of specific receptors on the plasma membrane. It is best known for uptake of essential nutrients such as low-density lipoprotein and transferrin. It is often referred to as "receptor-mediated" endocytosis, but this is not strictly accurate because most pinocytosis involves receptor–ligand interactions. The budding pits acquire a protein coat of clathrin, a three-pronged structure called a triskelion that assembles into clathrin cages (Fig 1.46). Coated vesicles lose their clathrin and are directed to endosomes for processing of the receptor–ligand complexes. Finally, cells constantly take up extracellular fluid by non-selective mechanisms, a process termed *fluid phase endocytosis*. The vesicles so formed may occupy a few percent of surface membrane area, but they exist for only several minutes. Taken together, all these endocytic mechanisms may be responsible for complete recycling of the plasma membrane in just 2 hours.

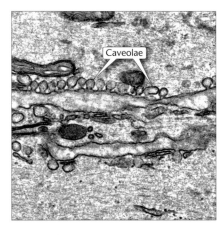

◀ **Fig 1.45 Ultrastructure of caveolae**, recognized as tiny flask-shaped vesicles associated with the plasma membrane. Caveolae are endocytic vesicles coated with caveolin protein and are present on many cells. Their exact function remains poorly understood except in endothelial cells, where they are thought to contribute to bulk fluid-phase uptake. × 32,000.

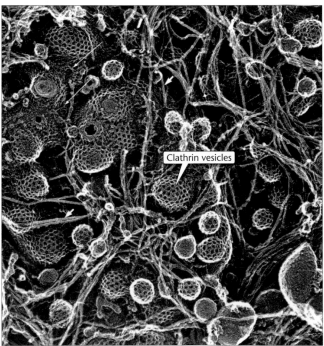

◀ **Fig 1.46 Ultrastructure of a quick-freeze, deep-etch preparation of the cytoplasmic surface of a liver cell**, showing many clathrin-coated vesicles forming by endocytosis from the plasma membrane. Clathrin lattices resemble a cage and their self-assembly around coated pits (which contain extracellular materials) facilitates endocytosis of the pits into vesicles. Removal of clathrin coats from vesicles allows vesicles to reach their target, often the endosomes. A clathrin protein is a three-pronged structure, called a triskelion, and may be recycled back to the plasma membrane. × 60,000. (Courtesy J Heuser, Washington University School of Medicine, USA; Cell 1982; 30:395–406.)

Fate of digested materials

Materials that are subject to digestion by lysosomes can be degraded and reused by the cell, and are occasionally exported into the extracellular fluid or remain within the cell as identifiable undigested matter (Fig 1.47).

Two types of mature lysosomes can be distinguished, depending on their origins. *Heterophagic lysosomes* contain substances of extracellular origin delivered via the various pathways of pinocytosis or phagocytosis. When large particles such as bacteria or dead cells are ingested, the surrounding endocytic vesicle so formed is called a phagosome that fuses with lysosomes for degradation. The soluble products of digestion that are formed after lysosomal hydrolysis may be reused as a source of nutrients for the cell.

Undigested materials that cannot be further broken down remain as residual bodies (Fig 1.48) and are recognizable with electron microscopy as dense membrane-bound elements that contribute to pigment accumulation in cells and perhaps cellular aging.

Autophagy, or self-digestion, is a type of internal degradation/recycling in which intact organelles, membranes, or large parts of the cytoplasm are broken down by lysosomes (Fig 1.49). *Autophagic lysosomes* are the second type of mature lysosome and

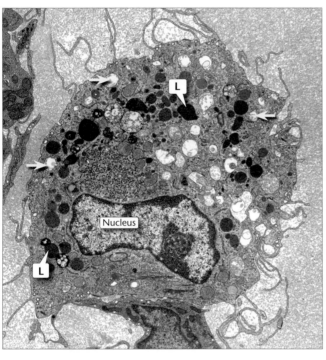

▲ **Fig 1.47 Ultrastructure of a macrophage**, showing many dense lysosomes (**L**), and endosomes (**arrows**) that contain ingested materials from vesicles arriving through endocytic pathways. Macrophages may be very highly phagocytic and thus are richly equipped with endosome–lysosome compartments. × 5,300.

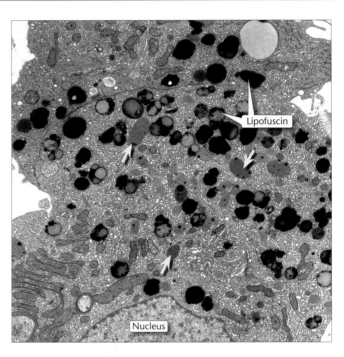

▲ **Fig 1.48 Ultrastructure of lipofuscin pigment inclusions** (may also be called residual bodies), seen as composites of lipids and dense undigested materials that remain after processing through the lysosomal system. Less-dense organelles representing mature lysosomes are shown (**arrows**). × 6,300.

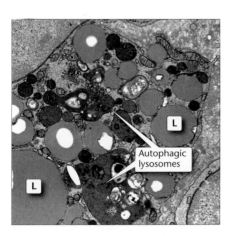

◀ **Fig 1.49 Ultrastructure of autophagic lysosomes.** This organelle, a derivative of endosomes, contains many hydrolytic enzymes residing within an acidic environment (about pH 5) that also contains intracellular materials sequestered for digestion. Lysosomal enzymes are made in the Golgi complex and are delivered to early endosomes within vesicles. The endosomes gradually mature into lysosomes. Lipid droplets (**L**) also shown. × 6,700.

contain materials of intracellular origin. This occurs as cells are developing and remodeling their machinery or when tissues undergo extensive remodeling.

All eukaryotic cells carry out autophagy. Essentially it is a process of cell survival that maintains normal cellular homeostasis. It is especially important for intracellular quality control in the liver, nerve cells, and cardiac muscle. The relationship between autophagy and apoptosis (self-killing) is complex, because the two pathways are regulated by common factors and each can modify the activity of the other. Apoptosis is discussed later in this chapter.

Peroxisomes

Resembling lysosomes in appearance, peroxisomes are membrane-bound organelles about 0.5 µm in size (Fig 1.50). They are responsible for detoxification, degradation of alcohol, fatty acid oxidation and metabolism of nitrogen-containing compounds. Peroxisomes contain oxidases (often visible in the organelle as a crystal) that generate potentially harmful hydrogen peroxide (H_2O_2). They also contain catalase, which immediately degrades hydrogen peroxide to oxygen and water. Thus, hydrogen peroxide never leaves the peroxisome and its toxic properties are prevented from entering the cytoplasm. It has been

suggested that peroxisomes multiply by biogenesis— they are derived from preexisting peroxisomes, or assemble by a series of vesicle fusions. Recent evidence suggests that peroxisome membrane components may be derived from the endoplasmic reticulum. Disorders of peroxisome function or their biogenesis, some of which are fatal genetic disorders, are associated with neurological disorders.

Cytoplasmic inclusions

In contrast to organelles, which are mini-organs within the cell that participate in essential metabolic reactions, inclusions are generally inert elements in the sense that they are not critically important for the viability of the cell.

Glycogen

Stored as macromolecular assemblies of polymers of glucose, this inclusion is electron-dense and appears as small granular rosette structures about 0.1 µm in diameter (Fig 1.51). Glycogen is abundant in liver, cardiac, and skeletal muscle. In hepatocytes, glycogen is found close to smooth ER, which has enzymes that produce free glucose for transport out of the cell into blood vessels for blood glucose regulation.

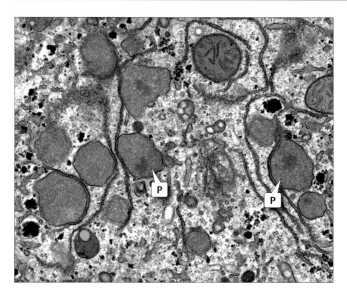

▲ **Fig 1.50 Ultrastructure of peroxisomes.** Formerly called microbodies, the peroxisomes (**P**) are membrane-limited organelles (about 0.5 µm in diameter) containing enzymes that use oxygen to oxidize substrates and produce hydrogen peroxide (H_2O_2), which is decomposed by catalase. They are essential in lipid metabolism, synthesizing myelin sheath components, and they degrade very-long-chain fatty acids. Peroxisomes, abundant in liver cells, are thought to derive from both the rough ER and cytoplasmic proteins, and increase in number by fission. × 21,000.

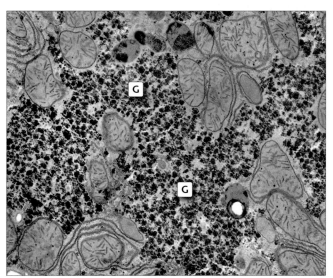

▲ **Fig 1.51 Glycogen**. Glucose is stored in the cytoplasm as polymers of glycogen (**G**), forming granule clusters, or rosettes. Glycogen is broken down to glucose, which can be released into blood or, by glycolysis, supply substrates for the citric acid cycle in mitochondria. × 14,000.

Lipid

Lipid may be stored in many different cells and especially in adipocytes, where this inclusion dominates the whole cytoplasm and may attain a diameter of 100 μm. Lipids include fatty acids, cholesterol, phospholipids and glycolipids, and other classes. Many are stored forms of energy; some are for building membranes, others for steroid hormone synthesis. In non-adipocytes (Fig 1.52), lipid mostly appears as spherical droplets of variable diameter (0.5–5 μm) with a homogenous moderate electron density not surrounded by membrane (Fig 1.53a & b). Their abundance is commonly inversely proportional to the metabolic activity of the cell (i.e. more lipid = a quiescent phase).

In adipose cells where lipid occupies 90% or more of the cell, the cytoplasm becomes a thin, outer rim with the nucleus compressed to one edge. This morphology applies to white fat, the most common type. The other type is brown fat, and the cell has many small lipid inclusions. Brown fat is a source of heat production.

Pigments

If substances remain indigestible following their association with the lysosomal system, the "leftovers" are referred to as residual bodies (see above) that may or may not be membrane bound.

They contain dense molecules that appear brown by light microscopy and are called lipochrome or

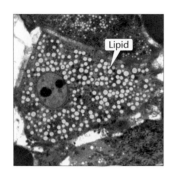

▲ **Fig 1.52 Cell of the corpus luteum** with an abundant supply of lipid inclusions scattered through the cytoplasm. Lipid droplets such as these represent stores of cholesterol for steroid hormone synthesis. Toluidine blue, araldite, × 700.

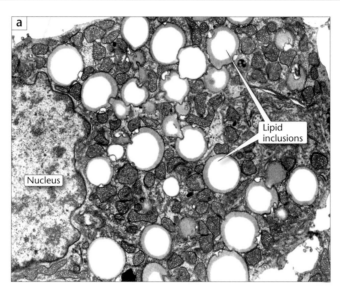

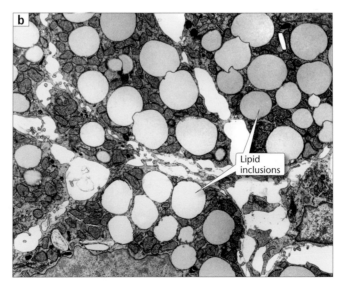

◀ **Fig 1.53 Ultrastructure of lipid inclusions.**
a Partly extracted during tissue processing, × 6,000. **b** With a homogeneous appearance, × 5,500. Lipids/fats may be stored as triglycerides, cholesterol, or its esters in lipid inclusions, are variable in diameter, and are not membrane bound. Lipids are used to fuel oxidative metabolism in mitochondria (to produce ATP). Lipid inclusions are common in liver cells and alveolar glands of breast, and are stored in quantity in adipose cells; they also occur in steroidogenic cells (such as adrenocortical, luteal and Leydig cells), supplying cholesterol for steroid synthesis. Phagocytosis of degenerating cells may result in the accumulation of lipid inclusions as a by-product of digestion.

lipofuscin pigment. Ultrastructurally, aggregations of dark blobs are seen, representing pieces of membranes, often in compressed or contorted shapes. Lipofuscin is the end product of lipid peroxidation and it may be abundant in aged cells. Melanin is another type of pigment responsible for skin, hair, and iris color (Fig 1.54) and is found in the retina and substantia nigra of the brainstem.

Crystals

Crystals are quite an uncommon inclusion, yet some cells always contain them. Eosinophils have cytoplasmic granules with small crystalloids of protein that are toxic for parasites (Fig 1.55). Bone consists of hydroxyapatite crystals embedded in collagen within the extracellular matrix.

Spermatogonia and Sertoli cells in the testis contain needle-like crystals about 2–3 μm in length. Large crystals, up to 20 μm in size, are found in the cytoplasm of the human Leydig cell (Fig 1.56). The function of these protein-rich inclusions is obscure.

> **Tip:** A generic model of a cell shows internal compartments—the nucleus, the organelles, the inclusions, and the aqueous environment in which they are suspended, the cytosol. Compartments carry out specific functions, are usually interactive and interdependent, and play critical roles in import, export, synthesis, and digestion.

Cytoskeleton: cell support, shape, and motility

The term *cytoskeleton* infers a structure of some rigidity, but this is only partly correct. Recall that the ultrastructure of cells as revealed by the EM is a representation of a living, dynamic object that has been killed. Its structure has been preserved, but what we see is a "freeze-frame" image of a formerly moving object. Cells are continuously mobile structures that adjust their shapes, surface membranes, and internal architecture using the properties of the cytoskeleton (Figs 1.57, 1.58).

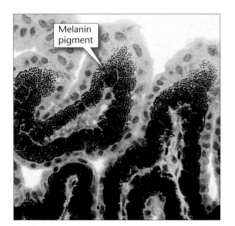

◀ **Fig 1.54 Pigmented cells in the ciliary body of the eye.** The pigment consists of melanin granules in a layer that is continuous with the pigment layer of the iris and retina. Pigment absorbs stray light passing through the eye. H&E, acrylic resin, × 350.

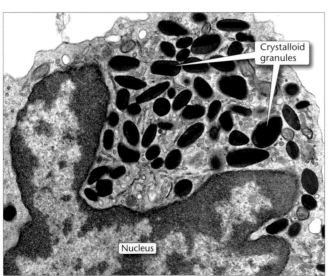

▲ **Fig 1.55 Ultrastructure of crystalloid bodies in granules of an eosinophilic leukocyte.** These crystals contain protein involved with the destruction of parasites by the eosinophil. × 13,000.

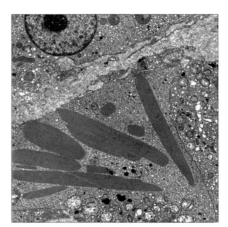

▲ **Fig 1.56 Large crystalloid inclusions in the cytoplasm of a Leydig cell in the human testis.** These protein-rich crystals have a regular lattice substructure, although their function remains obscure. × 2,700.

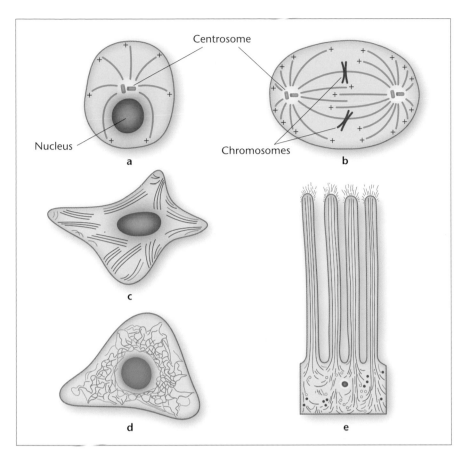

◀ **Fig 1.57 Overview of the cytoskeletal system. a** Microtubules arising from a centrosome. **b** Microtubules making up the spindle in a dividing cell. **c** Microfilaments of actin. **d** Intermediate filaments encircling the nucleus. **e** Actin filaments in the core of microvilli.

▼ **Fig 1.58 The microfilament cytoskeleton of bovine arterial endothelial cells** labeled with fluorescent dyes. Microtubular networks are labeled red, actin microfilaments are green and nuclei are labeled blue. × 800. (Courtesy Rishi Raj, Olympus Australia.)

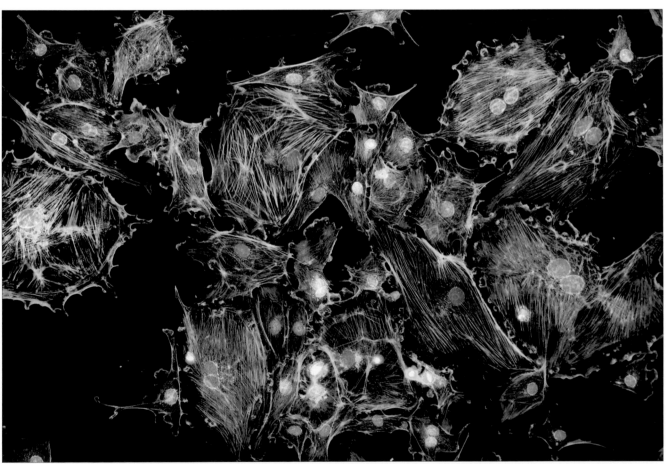

On a nanometer scale, the cytoskeleton confers stability when required, but it also allows plasticity throughout the cytosol (e.g. when a cell divides), and it achieves this by generating as well as resisting mechanical loads. The shape of a cell thus depends upon a balance between internal tension and compression and, in part, this is achieved by the constant assembly and disassembly of all elements of the cytoskeleton. Special motor proteins that use parts of the cytoskeleton as guidance tracks carry out movement of organelles and macromolecules through the cytoplasm.

The three main subdivisions of the cytoskeleton (Fig 1.59) are:
- *Microtubules*—hollow protein cylinders 25 nm in diameter; involved in motility and maintaining cell shape; resist compression
- *Microfilaments*—polymers of actin 7 nm in diameter; play a major role in motility and forming meshwork/bundles; resist tension
- *Intermediate filaments*—coiled proteins 10 nm in diameter; provide a dynamic scaffold and mechanical strength; resist tension.

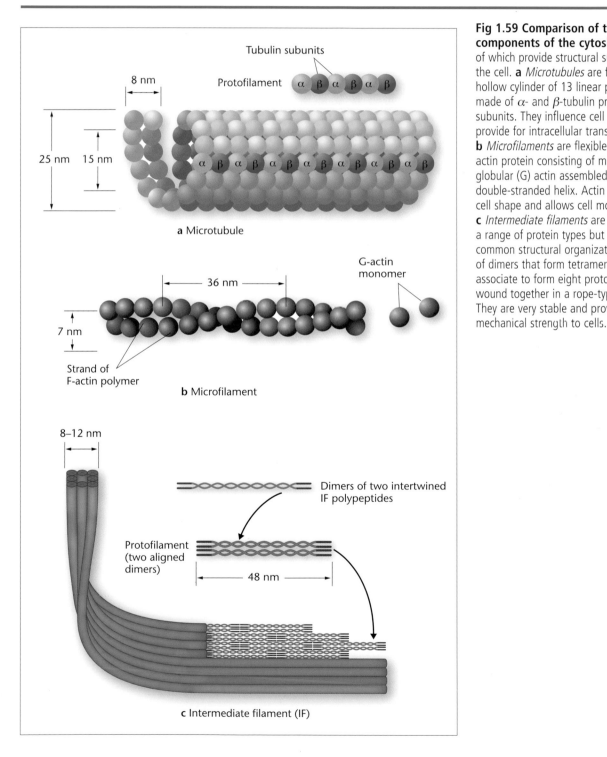

Fig 1.59 Comparison of the three components of the cytoskeleton, all of which provide structural support to the cell. **a** *Microtubules* are formed by a hollow cylinder of 13 linear protofilaments made of α- and β-tubulin protein subunits. They influence cell shape and provide for intracellular transport.
b *Microfilaments* are flexible polymers of actin protein consisting of monomers of globular (G) actin assembled to form a double-stranded helix. Actin determines cell shape and allows cell movement.
c *Intermediate filaments* are made from a range of protein types but share a common structural organization consisting of dimers that form tetramers. These associate to form eight protofilaments wound together in a rope-type structure. They are very stable and provide mechanical strength to cells.

All of these cytoskeletal elements pervade the cytoplasm, forming a complex three-dimensional meshwork that supports macromolecules and the membrane compartments. The abundance of the cytoskeleton is quite impressive, even though for most cells it remains undetected in electron micrographs. The meshwork is so fine that the pore size is only about 50 nm and particles larger than this must be transported actively rather than by simple diffusion. A ribosome at 30 nm would pass through the cytoplasm, but all membrane-bound structures would be restricted or otherwise controlled in movement.

Microtubules

These dynamic hollow cylinders of tubulin protein are continually forming and disassembling, with a half-life of only several minutes providing so-called dynamic instability. Microtubules (MTs) assemble by polymerization of tubulin dimers that confer polarity—tubulins assemble quickly at the plus (+) end whereas the minus (–) end is slow growing. Minus ends are usually anchored at centrosomes and the MT grows out into the cytoplasm led by the plus end. In living cells, the plus ends switch between intervals of growth and rapid shrinkage, hence the term *dynamic instability* (Fig 1.60a). Microtubules occupy large regions of cytoplasm and may appear straight or curved, probably due to compressive forces that tend to cause bending (Fig 1.60b).

MTs are essential in mitosis where they separate the duplicated chromosomes and remodel the cell as it splits in two.

Drugs that disrupt MT assembly are useful in the treatment of certain cancers. Colchicine, a plant alkaloid, works in this way, as does nocodazole, a synthetic drug that is used in research since its action is reversible when removed. Vinblastine and vincristine (from the periwinkle plant) cause abnormal MT aggregation and are used as chemotherapeutic agents because they destroy mitotic spindles and can stop cell division. These compounds are called antimitotic drugs. Taxol, from the yew tree, stabilizes the MT for prolonged periods, thereby interfering with cell division, which makes it a useful

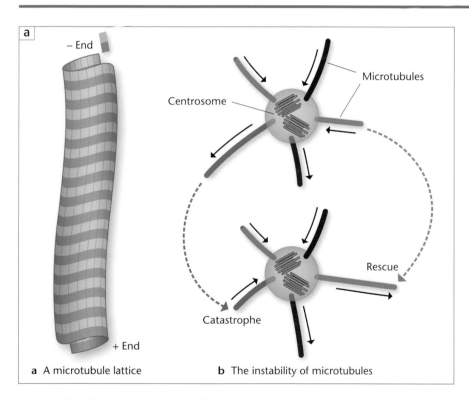

a A microtubule lattice   b The instability of microtubules

◀ **Fig 1.60a Microtubule dynamics.**
a Microtubules self-assemble from tubulin protein subunits at each end: the plus end with a cap of β-tubulin, the minus end with a cap of α-tubulin. Microtubules thus have structurally different ends and are polarized, giving them directionality. **b** Minus ends anchor to a centrosome but plus ends switch between slow growth and rapid shrinkage. Shrinkage is called catastrophe, and growth is called rescue. The blue microtubule is initially growing (upper diagram) but at a later time (lower diagram) undergoes catastrophe. The olive green microtubule is initially shrinking (upper diagram), but later shows rescue (lower diagram).

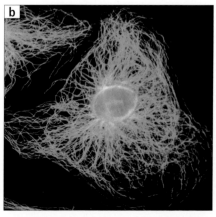

◀ **Fig 1.60b Microtubular networks** labeled with a green fluorescent dye. Minus ends of microtubules are located near the cell center, with plus ends at the cell plasma membrane. Together with molecular motors, microtubules act as tracks for the conveyance of cargoes through the cytoplasm. Nuclei are labeled blue. × 1,800. (Courtesy J Zbaeren, Inselspital, Bern, Switzerland.)

37

chemotherapeutic agent (the taxane antimetabolites) and experimental tool.

In most cells MTs are linked with MT-associated proteins (MAPs), which increase the stability of MTs in, for example, nerve axons, maintenance of cell polarity, and remodeling of the elongating cytoplasm in the developing sperm tail.

MTs are the tracks along which organelles, vesicles, and proteins are mobilized within the cell. Transport within nerve axons may involve a distance of a meter (for the sciatic nerve), although, for most cells, moving an object from A to B spans only a few micrometers.

MAPs are motor proteins, energized with ATP, that move along the MTs with their attached cell components. The dynein class of MAPs tend to carry their cargo toward the center of the cell, whereas kinesin-type motor proteins transport in the opposite direction. Both also control the locations of ER, Golgi, mitochondria, and lysosomes (Fig 1.61). These molecular motors have a heads-on-stalk morphology, where the head binds to the track and the stalk binds to cargo or other motors (Fig 1.62). Motors move in small steps where the head subunits appear to proceed "hand over hand." Some motors, such as

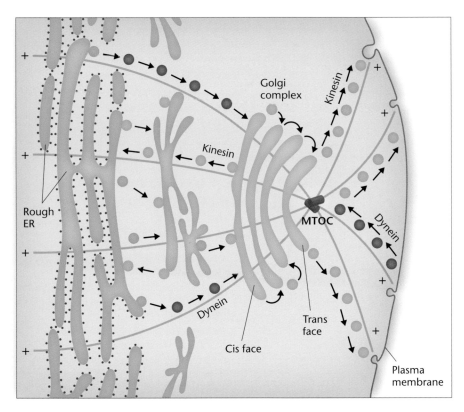

◀ **Fig 1.61 Diagram summarizing the location and role of microtubules**. Originating from a microtubule organizing center (**MTOC**: a pair of centrioles), the microtubules (MTs) act like tracks for the transport of vesicles (colored circles) using MT-associated motor proteins (MAPs) such as dynein and kinesin. MAPs "walk" along the MTs carrying their cargo, using ATP for energy supply. Other types of MAPs serve to stabilize or disassemble the MTs. Together MAPs not only act as carriers but also determine the positions of membrane compartments within the cell.

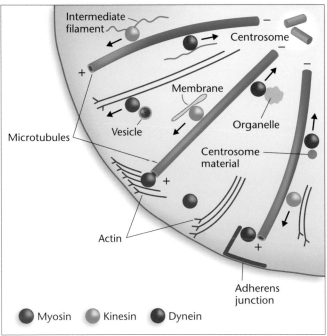

◀ **Fig 1.62 Transport mechanisms using the cytoskeleton.** Kinesin and dynein are microtubule motor proteins that attach filaments, membranes, or macromolecules and transport them along the tracks provided by the polarized microtubules. Kinesin moves in the anterograde direction along the microtubules, dynein in the opposite direction. Myosins move on actin filaments in muscle cells but they also transport organelles. All three motor classes use ATP hydrolysis as an energy source for movement.

dynein, are geared for a range of stepping distances (8–32 nm), with smaller steps able to generate more powerful strokes.

In mitosis, the MTs grow from centrosomes (see below) to form the familiar spindle that anchors plus ends to the kinetochore region of chromosomes and guides them to the daughter cells. This is achieved by growth and shrinkage of attached MTs (Fig 1.63). Some spindle MTs do not attach to chromosomes but overlap: motor proteins act to slide overlapping antiparallel MTs past each other, pushing the spindle poles apart. Others arising from the separated centrosomes radiate outwards to the fixed cell cortex, where resident motors like dynein pull the poles apart as cytokinesis proceeds.

Centrosome

MTs originate from a centrosome, which is the microtubule-organizing center (MTOC) of the cell. In interphase cells, a centrosome is seen close to the nucleus. It consists of two centrioles with surrounding pericentriolar material that acts as a focus and an anchor for the construction of new MTs that radiate out from the centrosome (Fig 1.64). Centrioles are made of a hollow cylinder of nine pairs of triplet microtubules about 0.25 μm long and oriented 90° to each other. Centrosomes become most apparent during the formation of the mitotic spindle, having duplicated between interphase and prophase of the cell cycle. Cells are capable of assembling centrioles *de novo*, arising from a cloud of pericentriolar material.

Centrioles are not always required for the formation of the centrosome: they do not occur in plant cells or in some animal oocytes that divide after destroying their centrioles earlier in meiosis. Early embryos divide by mitosis in the absence of the centrosome.

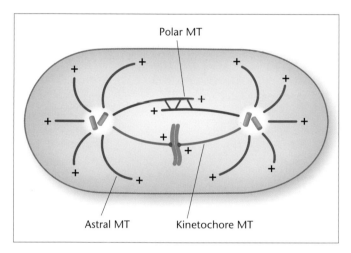

▲ **Fig 1.63 Diagram of the arrangement of microtubules in mitosis.** Centrosomes are located at opposite poles of the cell, where they form anchoring points for the negative ends of radiating arrays of astral microtubules (MTs) collectively called asters. MTs that grow toward the chromosomes form a spindle and are of two types; kinetochore MTs attach to chromosomes and will in time pull the two sister chromatids toward opposite spindle poles; polar MTs are unattached but overlap and slide past each other to further separate the centrosomes.

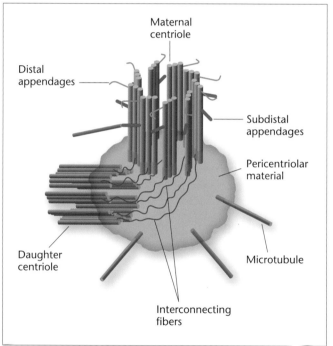

Fig 1.64 Diagram of the centrosome showing the alignment of a pair of centrioles connected by pericentriolar material (PCM). Centrosomes are microtubule organizing centers about 0.5 μm in overall size. Microtubules are anchored to and originate from the PCM and the maternal centriole. Non-dividing cells have a single centrosome, which is duplicated when DNA is copied prior to mitosis.

Microfilaments

Microfilaments are the major cytoskeletal proteins of most cells and consist of thin, linear, flexible fibers of actin assembled into a tight helix up to several microns in length. Their linearity is maintained by tension similar to a suspensory cable.

They form three-dimensional networks, cross-linked with binding proteins that form triangulated complexes (Fig 1.65). Actin shows reversible polymerization and is especially abundant beneath the plasma membrane, where it provides support, regulates cell shape, and modulates the mobility of the cell surface, for example, when cells are required to crawl. The assembly of actin occurs in two steps. Firstly monomers assemble into trimers (nucleation) that act as a seed, and secondly more monomers are added to the seed (polymerization) and thus elongation is initiated. Actin filaments have a growing "barbed" plus end and a "pointed" non-growing minus end, these structures being revealed by their arrowhead morphology when stained with myosin protein. For slow growth, actin subunits are added to the growing end while subunits are removed from the minus end in a process referred to as treadmilling. For protrusion of spike-type filopodia, bundles of actin assemble from dendritic actin networks subjacent to the plasma membrane to form extruded cones that project the cytoplasm outwards (Fig 1.66). In the case of the broad, flat lamellipodia, actin forms highly branched brush-type structures where new filament growth occurs as a branch on the side of an existing filament. Assembly of growing ends of actin filaments is assisted by several proteins and ATP embedded within the subunits. Filament growth is terminated before filaments become too long to push.

The scaffold thus formed pushes along a broad length of plasma membrane, and the force applied may be assisted by unbending of curved actin filaments.

In vivo, actin filaments are anchored to adherens junctions between cells that resemble a belt of adhesion around the apposed sites of contact. When cells such as fibroblasts are cultured in vitro they stick to the plastic substrate at certain points on their surface. The attachment sites are associated with concentrations of actin filaments, which form bundles, called stress fibers, that anchor the cell and exert tension against the substratum. Points of adhesion consist of integrin receptors and act as traction sites for cell migration (Fig 1.67). Some cells like fibroblasts move slowly, whereas others such as neutrophils are fast-moving; the mechanisms controlling these different velocities are not well understood.

The drug cytochalasin (a fungal metabolite) inhibits actin formation. Phalloidin and phallacidin (from the most poisonous of the mushrooms) blocks actin disassembly, thus stabilising the actin network, which makes this drug a useful marker for actin if labeled with a fluorescent dye.

Microfilaments are well known for their role in actin–myosin muscle contraction; for amoeboid movement or mobility of cultured cells over a surface; for cytoplasmic streaming—a flow of cytoplasm in some plant and animal cells; and for creating the cleavage furrow that divides the cytoplasm during cytokinesis. In the latter case a ring of actin filaments is constructed just beneath the plasma membrane, assisted by organizing proteins called formins. The ring constricts like a tightening belt when the filaments slide over each other, similar to muscle contraction. This activity is assisted by myosin proteins.

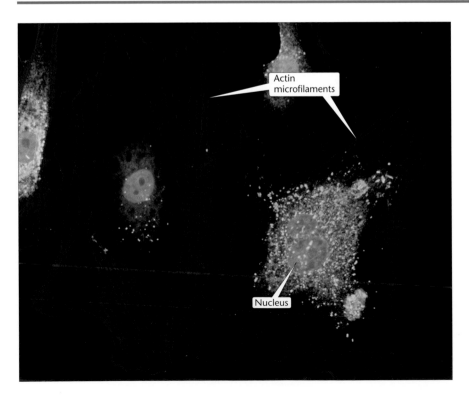

Actin microfilaments

Nucleus

◀ **Fig 1.65 Microfilaments of actin labeled with a red fluorescent dye.** Actin proteins are assembled as polymers, which form thin, flexible fibers, seen here as ordered networks and bundles. Actin bundles are often near the plasma membrane, where they act to determine cell shape. By assembly and disassembly, actin polymers regulate cell mobility such as in crawling cells, where they support cytoplasmic extensions such as filopodia and lamellipodia. × 1,600. (Courtesy J Zbaeren, Inselspital, Bern, Switzerland.)

Intermediate filaments

These are the most stable and least soluble of the cytoskeletal proteins, encoded by more than 65 genes. The proteins self-assemble and polymerize into 10 nm filaments. Their structure takes the form of eight protofilaments intertwined like a rope. These dynamic rather than static structures form elaborate and complex reticulated networks, usually in the perinuclear region, and radiate throughout the cytoplasm (Fig 1.68). Intermediate filaments (IFs)

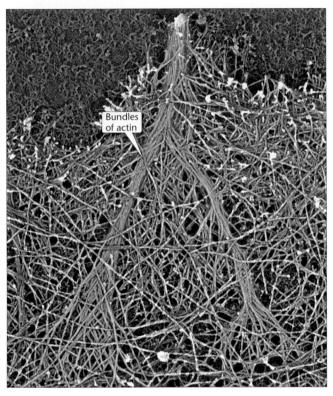

▲ **Fig 1.66 Platinum replica electron micrograph of a cytoplasmic filopodium,** showing a core of actin filaments consisting of two sub-bundles, colored blue for clarity. The actin roots are splayed, blending with the deeper network. Actin filaments assemble into Y-shaped junctions, which contribute to protrusion of the filopodium. × 45,000. (Courtesy T Svitkina, University of Pennsylvania; J Cell Biology 1999; 145:1009–26.)

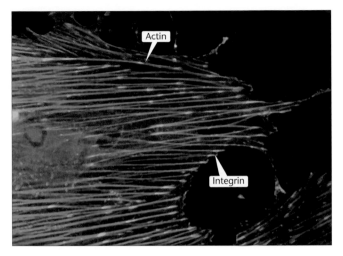

▲ **Fig 1.67 Actin filaments and attachment sites.** Fluorescence micrograph of actin filaments (green) and their association with substrate attachment sites of integrin (orange). Movement of the cytoplasm to the right is achieved by leftward displacement of actin driven by myosin, and, using the attachment sites, actin elongates to the right, thus extending the cytoplasm. × 2,000. (Courtesy K Burridge, University of North Carolina, USA.)

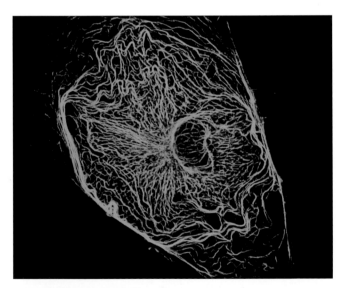

▲ **Fig 1.68 Intermediate filaments.** Confocal image of intermediate filaments of a human lung epithelial cell tumor line (type II pneumocyte) stained with anti-Keratin18. Intermediate filaments are stable structures extending from a ring around the nucleus and associate with plasma membrane desmosomes. They provide mechanical strength to cells. × 1,400. (Courtesy E Flitney, Northwestern University, Feinberg School of Medicine, USA.)

support the microfilament cores anchoring the microvilli of intestinal absorptive cells (Fig 1.69). There are five main categories of IF: four are found in the cytoplasm (cytoskeletal types) and one in the nucleus, the nuclear lamins. Most cytoskeletal IFs are keratin proteins, also called tonofilaments, which are abundant in epithelial cells. Hard keratins form hair, nails, and horns. The others are vimentin (connective tissues/fibroblasts), desmin (muscle cells), glial fibrillary acidic protein (in the cells that support neurons), peripherin (in some neurons), neurofilament proteins (in nerve cells particularly in long axons), and nestin (in embryonic nerve cells). IFs provide mechanical strength to cells. In neurons, the synthesis of new IF proteins occurs in the cell body, but the protein subunits may be required at the distal regions of dendrites and axons. This axonal transport is mediated by MT motor proteins.

Detection of these different IF subtypes is a useful way of characterising cancer since tumor cells retain their IF proteins from their tissue of origin.

Keratin IFs connect with desmosomes, the special intercellular contacts/junctions that make cells stick together. These IFs provide a mechanical link between adjacent cells such as in epithelial tissues, with skin being a particularly good example of cells that are tightly bound together to provide a barrier function. Recent studies have shown that some bacteria have a protein called crescentin that is similar to eukaryotic IFs. This protein confers a curved morphology to these bacteria.

Cell surface: interactions with external environment

Many cells show elaborate modifications to their plasma membrane necessary for changing shape, for mobility, and for exchange of materials with the external environment. Particular specializations of the plasma membrane take the form of minor or major extensions that are visible by light microscopy. Three classes of surface specializations are reviewed: microvilli, cilia and flagella, and stereocilia.

Microvilli

Microvilli are minute (1 μm long) surface projections of the apical plasma membrane that greatly increase surface area for absorption. They are found in numerous cell types and are particularly abundant lining the luminal surface of the intestine. They are visible in the LM as a thin, striated, or "brush" border (Fig 1.70). In electron micrographs they consist of innumerable finger-type projections (Fig 1.71) with a combined intestinal surface area of about 200 m². The core consists of vertical actin microfilaments attached to the tip and anchored to the subjacent cytoplasm by a network of horizontal contractile microfilaments called the terminal web (Fig 1.72). Contraction of this web causes the microvilli to spread apart, thus increasing the space between them to facilitate absorption of luminal contents. Contraction and lengthening of microvilli also assists with mixing of nutrients.

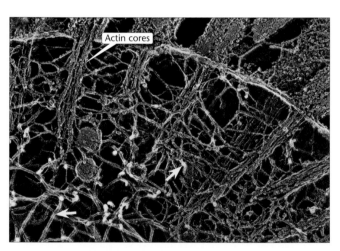

▲ **Fig 1.69 Terminal web region supporting microvilli of intestinal epithelial cell**, examined by the quick-freeze, deep-etch, rotary-replication method. The actin filament cores of microvilli are connected and anchored to a rich network of intermediate filaments (**arrows**). × 67,000. (Courtesy J Heuser, Washington University, School of Medicine, USA; J Cell Biology 1981; 91:399–409.)

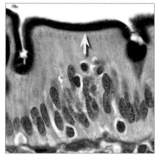

▲ **Fig 1.70 "Brush border."** Light micrograph of the "brush" border of the apical surface of the intestinal epithelium, consisting of innumerable microvilli (**arrow**). Magenta stain represents mucus-type materials. PAS, paraffin, × 450.

Cilia and flagella

Cilia and flagella are the motile surface projections of cells (Fig 1.73). Cilia are found lining the trachea and bronchi or the uterine tube, and flagella form the long tail of the spermatozoa. They share a common structure and differ only in size (cilium = 2–10 μm; flagellum = 50 μm), number per cell, and mode of beating. Many cells have primary cilia that consist of one or two cilia, which are thought to be temporary structures that act as a type of cellular antenna to detect external signals and pass them to the cell nucleus (Fig 1.74). Cilia on epithelial cells bend

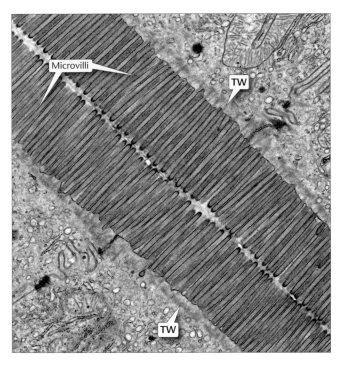

▲ **Fig 1.71 Ultrastructure of microvilli on the apical surface of intestinal epithelial cells.** Each microvillus shows a core of actin filaments that extend into the cytoplasmic region called the terminal web (**TW**). This region has a range of cytoskeletal filaments that serve to anchor the microvilli. × 12,000.

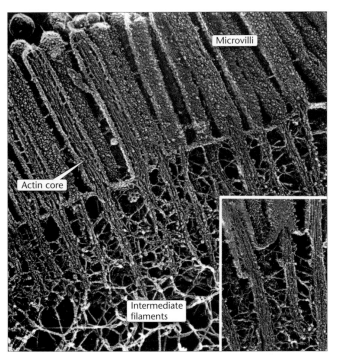

▲ **Fig 1.72 Microvilli of intestinal epithelial cell**, visualized by fixation and quick-freeze, deep-etch, rotary-replication method. The core of actin filaments in the microvilli extends as bundled rootlets into the cell cytoplasm, which shows fine fibrils between bundles and a deeper network of thicker intermediate filaments. × 47,000. (Courtesy J Heuser, Washington University, School of Medicine, USA; J Cell Biology 1982; 94:425–43.)

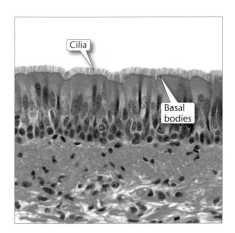

▲ **Fig 1.73 Cilia extending from the apical surface of epithelial cells**, resembling the hairs of a brush. The dense line deep to the cilia is formed by rows of basal bodies that anchor the cilia. H&E, acrylic resin, × 300.

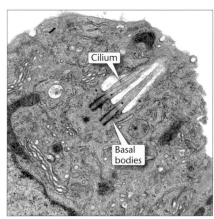

▲ **Fig 1.74 A pair of primary cilia emerging from underlying basal bodies, which are modified centrioles.** During interphase, the centriole approaches the plasma membrane and is the source of the axonemal core of the cilium. Isolated cilia act as cellular antennae, which sense the extracellular environment and transduce signals to the cell. × 9,000.

43

to-and-fro in a synchronous wave that effectively moves surface particles, cells, debris, or mucus in one direction. The flagellum moves by waves of bending, much like a whip.

The core of cilia and flagella consists of the axoneme, a cylinder of microtubules formed into nine doublet MTs surrounding a central pair of single MTs, the so-called 9 + 2 arrangement. The outer MTs are connected to the central pair by nine radial spokes, and projecting outwards from the outer MTs are side arms of dynein (Fig 1.75a & b). With the energy generated by local ATP hydrolysis, the dynein arms momentarily attach and detach from the adjacent doublet MT, similar to a ratchet mechanism. The MTs do not change in length; thus one doublet slides past another. When MTs slide past each other on one side of the axoneme, this activity causes a forward power stroke, followed by doublet activity on the opposite side that causes the return stroke.

The clinical significance of cilial/flagellar dysfunction is seen in Kartagener's syndrome (a rare autosomal recessive genetic disorder), in which dynein arms are absent. This results in bronchiectasis (pulmonary problems with congestion of mucus), infertility (immotile sperm or failure of implantation of a conceptus owing to abnormal oviduct function), and sometimes situs inversus (congenital lateral inversion of organs such as right-sided heart, left-sided liver, right-sided spleen).

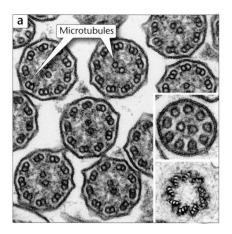

◀ **Fig 1.75a Ultrastructure of cilia in cross-section**, showing the 9 + 2 arrangement of microtubules making up the axoneme core, × 33,000. The upper inset shows 9 single outer microtubules and a central pair at the tip of the cilium, × 38,000. The lower inset shows the anchoring basal body of 9 triplet microtubules, × 55,000. (Courtesy Pavelka M, Roth J. Functional ultrastructure. Wien: Springer-Verlag, 2005).

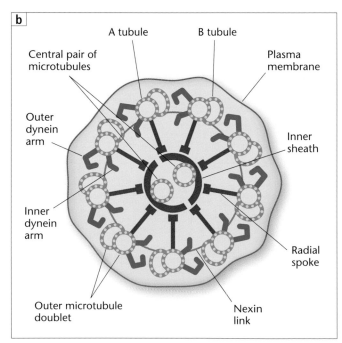

◀ **Fig 1.75b Diagram of the axoneme of a cilium with central pair and outer doublet microtubules.** ATPase activity in dynein arms initiates sliding of outer doublets relative to each other, resulting in bending of the cilium. Cilia beat in the same direction slightly out of phase, resulting in movement of materials (mucus, particles, cells/cell debris) upon their surface.

Stereocilia

Stereocilia are long tufts of immotile microvilli and are found lining the epididymis, where they assist with fluid absorption originating from the testis as it produces the fluid in which the sperm are suspended (Fig 1.76). These stereocilia may be 25 µm long.

Stereocilia are also found in the inner ear, where they have sensory roles in hearing and maintenance of equilibrium. They project into a gelatinous layer, which, when displaced by linear acceleration, bends and triggers a nerve impulse to the brain, which responds by correction of body position. We know when an elevator is moving (in a straight line), even though we detect no visual signals. Angular accelerations in the semicircular canals operate similarly, which is why astronauts may experience motion sickness in zero gravity.

Hair cells in the cochlea also consist of stereocilia that initiate the sensation of hearing as they respond to vibrations in the lymph, into which they project.

Cell junctions: attachment and communication

Most cells are packed together intimately within tissues and require some mechanism to remain closely associated and to communicate. Free, non-attached cells such as those found in blood, cells of the tissue spaces that originate from blood, and cells that are separated by extracellular matrix all retain the property of adhesion and interaction with other cells.

Cells establish contact and exchange signals via specialized cell junctions that have distinctive morphologies, regardless of the type of cell. Intercellular junctions are found in the plasma membrane. Four main types are described (Fig 1.77). Some cells exhibit all classes of junctions, some express one or two types, and some cells show regional or polarized locations of junctions, depending on their particular location and function.

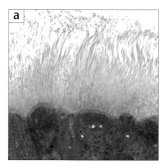
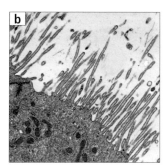

◀ **Fig 1.76 Stereocilia.** Light micrograph (**a**) and electron micrograph (**b**) of stereocilia on the apical surface of epididymal epithelial cells. Stereocilia resemble microvilli with a core of actin filaments, but lack an axoneme and are non-motile. Stereocilia of auditory hair cells are responsible for the sense of hearing. **a** Toluidine blue, araldite, × 800; **b** × 7,000.

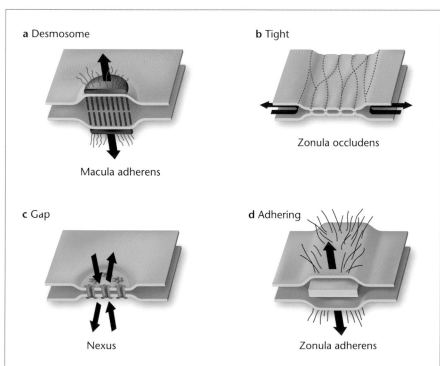

◀ **Fig 1.77 Diagrams of the four types of intercellular junctions.** These are found between many cell types and particularly between epithelial cells respectively for: **a** localized attachment by desmosomes, **b** barrier function by tight junctions, **c** exchange of molecules by gap junctions, **d** broad bands of adhesion by adhering junctions.

45

Zonula occludens

More commonly known as a tight junction, the zonula occludens (ZO) is a region of adjacent cells where their apposed plasma membranes are joined together or fused in sharply defined ridges (Fig 1.78a–c). Ridges are interconnected or interwoven, creating a belt-type zone of fusion lines around the circumference of the cells. Imagine two sheets of corrugated iron aligned so that the ridges touch and are fused. Lengths of fusion represent occlusion barriers, which prevent the passage of substances.

The tight junctions formed by ZOs are especially prominent between the cells of the intestine, occurring in the lateral cell membranes just deep to the apical surface. By effectively obliterating the intercellular space, they block the passage of fluids, molecules, and ions between adjacent cells, which would otherwise render the cell layer leaky for substances in the gut lumen. ZOs thus block paracellular transport.

The position of ZOs forms a barrier, so luminal contents must be absorbed by the intestinal cells to enter the gut epithelial layer (i.e. transcellular transport). More ridges = better seal = tighter junction.

The ZO within the lateral plasma membrane acts like a fence segregating stretches of membrane that have different functions (e.g. the apical cell membrane facing the lumen has a different molecular composition to the membrane on the lateral and basal aspects of the cell). This assists with maintenance of cell polarity, both functionally and structurally.

ZOs occur in many epithelia (e.g. bladder, seminiferous epithelium of testis), in cells of ducts, and between cells of the liver and pancreas.

Zonula adherens

Adhesive junctions link cells together and anchor the actin network of microfilaments of one cell to another. The zonula adherens (ZA) serves to maintain cell and tissue integrity against mechanical stress. ZAs may occur in series with ZOs, or individually in cells such as cardiocytes or skin cells (Fig 1.79). A space of 20 nm separates the two halves of the ZA, spanned

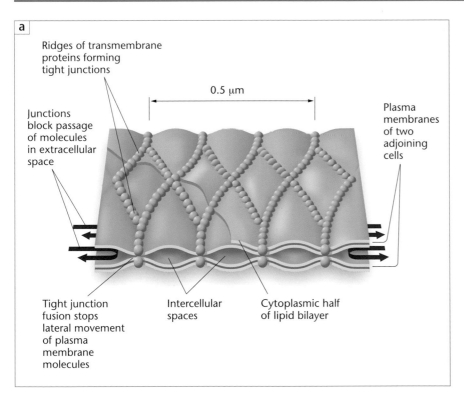

a

Ridges of transmembrane proteins forming tight junctions

0.5 µm

Junctions block passage of molecules in extracellular space

Plasma membranes of two adjoining cells

Tight junction fusion stops lateral movement of plasma membrane molecules

Intercellular spaces

Cytoplasmic half of lipid bilayer

▲ **Fig 1.78a Diagram of a tight junction (zonula occludens),** consisting of multiple fusion sites between apposing cell plasma membranes. Such sites contain transmembrane proteins, which form interconnected ridges applied to the contour of the plasma membrane.

b

Zonula occludens

Zonula adherens

▲ **Fig 1.78b Detail of zonula occludens,** showing fusion points between adjoining plasma membranes and zonula adherens (ZA). The gap between the membranes is occupied by cadherin receptor proteins, which bind the membranes closely. The ZA is associated with bundles of actin filaments, which link the cadherins. × 60,000. (Courtesy P Cross, Stanford University, USA.)

▶ **Fig 1.78c Freeze-fracture electron-microscopic view of the tight junctions (zonula occludens) in the intestinal epithelium.** Junctions appear as anastomosed strands interconnected to form an irregular network of grooves in the outer half-membrane of the cell. The grooves represent sites of membrane fusions. Freeze fracture, × 39,000.

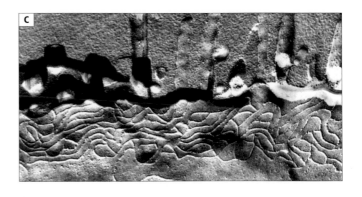

c

by a single type of adhesion molecule of cadherin. In many epithelia, the ZA is like a belt running around the circumference of the cell near the apical surface. It forms a strong adhesion between adjacent cells. On the cytoplasmic side is a parallel region of anchoring proteins that connect to the actin filament network, which transmits force across the lateral plane of the epithelium.

Desmosome

A desmosome is a type of adhesive junction that resembles a button, hence its other name macula adherens, or spot desmosome. Desmosomes are found on lateral cell membranes, appearing like a series of spot welds, with adjacent membranes separated by 25 nm but filled with a dense core of adhesion proteins (Fig 1.80a & b). Desmosomes contain two classes of cadherin adhesion molecules that reinforce and sustain intercellular adhesion. On the cytoplasmic side is the attachment plaque, into which the intermediate filaments are anchored. This links the cytoskeleton of one cell to its neighbor and thus enhances torsional strength. Desmosomes are very abundant between certain epithelial cells of the skin, where they bind cells together and provide the strength required to maintain the skin as a thick, impervious layer that resists wear and tear. They are prevalent also between cardiac muscle cells, resisting shear stress in this tissue.

Hemidesmosomes are found at the base of epithelial cells where they associate with the basal lamina via focal adhesion through integrins that connect to intermediate filaments within the cell cytoplasm.

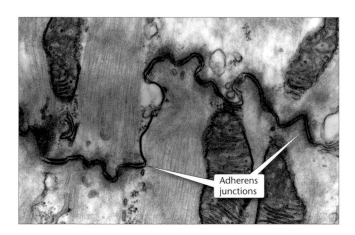

▲ **Fig 1.79 Ultrastructure of adherens-type junctions (arrows) between apposing cardiac muscle cells.** The intercellular space contains the adhesion molecule cadherin, and the junctions are sites of attachment for cytoplasmic actin filaments. The junctions provide for adhesion between the cells. × 26,000.

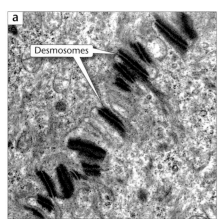

▲ **Fig 1.80a Ultrastructure of desmosomes between two keratinocytes.** These are localized points of attachment for cells with adhesion-type proteins in the intercellular space flanked by dense plaques that attach to cytoplasmic intermediate filaments. × 13,000.

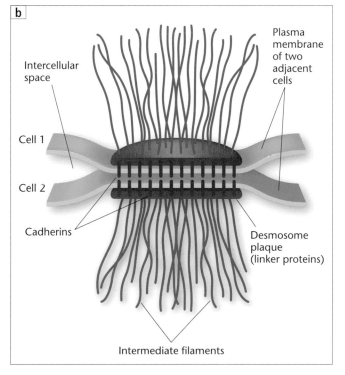

▲ **Fig 1.80b Diagram of desmosome structure**, showing the attachments of intermediate-type filaments (keratin, desmin, or vimentin) into the desmosome plaque. The desmosome thus links adjacent cells through their association with the cytoskeleton of each cell. Desmosomes are very abundant between the spinous/prickle cells of the epidermis.

Nexus

The nexus, or gap/communicating junction, is where the intercellular space is narrowed to about 3 nm and provides for a point of cytoplasmic contact between two adjacent cells. The contact or communication is formed by tiny, hollow cylinders called connexons, which consist of connexin proteins (Fig 1.81a & b). They provide a selective signaling route that depends upon the molecular identity of the connexins. These junctions allow the exchange of ions and small molecules such as cyclic nucleotides and are critically important for physiological coupling of cells, as shown by connexon knock-out and knock-in models. Gap junctions occur as circular zones between cells and are about 1 μm in diameter. They may reduce resistance to current flow, which is very important in cardiac muscle, for example, where rapid excitation passes from cell to cell to provide coordinated and simultaneous contraction through atrial and ventricular muscle cells.

Tip: Unlike unicellular organisms with no permanent associations, multicellular organisms have cells that join together to form tissues, and thus organs. Cells join via a variety of junctions that provide for membrane adhesion, fusion, and intercellular communication. Most junctions link to the cytoskeleton, which in turn creates a continuous cell-to-cell cytoskeletal network.

CELL PROLIFERATION AND THE CELL CYCLE

Tissues produce new cells in several circumstances:
- *Organ development and growth* associated with increases in cell number
- *Renewal and replacement* of cells that are continually lost
- *Regeneration* after natural or induced tissue loss.

Cell proliferation is normally controlled such that the number of new cells made matches the number

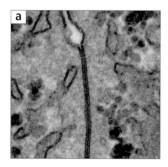

◀ **Fig 1.81a Ultrastructure of a gap junction (nexus),** where the apposed plasma membranes are separated only by a gap of 2–3 nm. This close association is bridged by minute channels that permit exchange of ions and small molecules (about 1 kDa or 2 nm in size), making cells permeable. Gap junctions may be up to several micrometers in diameter on the cell surface. × 65,000.

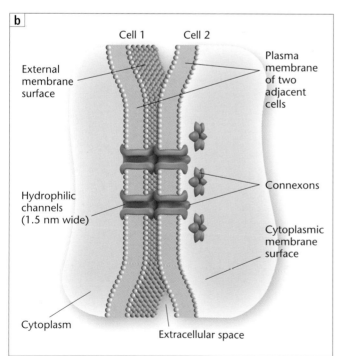

◀ **Fig 1.81b Diagram of gap junction structure,** showing communicating channels of connexons that vary in number up to thousands per junction. Connexons open and close and thereby control cell permeability.

needed for growth and the replacement of worn-out cells. Some cells never proliferate, whereas others may only survive for a few days and must be replaced continuously. Tissues can be categorized into three groups according to their proliferative capacity:

- *Permanent tissues*, in which there is no cell division, or regeneration—for example, the human brain shows no capacity for spontaneous neuronal turnover. If cells in permanent tissues are destroyed they may be replaced by less-specialized cells (e.g. dead cardiac muscle cells are replaced by fibroblasts). Other examples of non-renewable tissues are cells in the core of the adult lens of the eye and the postnatal population of female germ cells in humans and most mammals, which are gradually depleted from the ovaries with age.
- *Stable tissues* containing cells that do not normally divide, but may regenerate if damaged—for example, the liver, in which cell proliferation occurs after partial destruction or partial surgical removal.
- *Labile tissues*, in which there is a steady replacement of cells lost—for example, surface epithelia, sebaceous gland, bone marrow, and male germ cells.

The cell cycle

The cell cycle is divided into two main phases that can be recognized by cytological features: the *M phase* is when a cell divides into two daughter cells and is referred to as mitosis; *interphase* occurs when the cell is non-dividing and occasionally is called the "resting phase."

Many cells divide by mitosis to produce two new daughter cells that are identical to the older parent cell, whereas others, such as stem cells, produce another stem cell and a cell that is committed to further differentiation.

In mitosis, two components of cell division are involved, karyokinesis (nuclear division) and cytokinesis (cytoplasmic division), together occupying a brief period of time, usually one hour, of proliferative activity making up M phase. In interphase, the time that a cell may be at rest varies in duration from a day or so (in rapidly proliferating cells) to decades or a lifetime for cells in a permanent tissue.

Interphase

Interphase has three intervals (Fig 1.82): G_1 *(or first gap) phase*; *S phase* for synthesis of DNA, during which the DNA content of the nucleus is doubled and chromosomes are replicated; and G_2 *(second gap) phase*, or interval before the M phase. Often the cell cycle occurs in 24 hours, but not all cells proceed through the cycle at this rate. Some cells may remain in G_1 for weeks, years, or permanently, and in this arrested state they are considered to be in a special G_0 phase. Chromosome replication in S phase results in the formation of two identical "sister chromatids" for each chromosome: for human cells, 46 double chromosomes composed of 92 chromatids are formed.

M phase

Passing through the G_2 phase, the cell enters the M phase, during which four stages or phases are

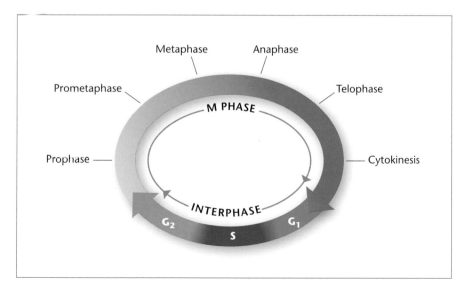

▲ **Fig 1.82 The cell cycle and mitosis.** A cell enters mitosis (M phase) at prophase (condensing chromosomes) and proceeds to pro/metaphase (equatorial alignment), anaphase (separation), telophase (reformation of nuclei), and cytokinesis (division of cytoplasm). In G_1 (gap phase) the cell pauses prior to entering S phase (DNA is copied) and then G_2 (another gap), where DNA synthesis is checked for accuracy. Then the cell enters M phase again.

recognizable (Fig 1.83a–f, Fig 1.84a–h). The purpose of mitosis is to use a bipolar network of MTs, resembling a spindle in shape, to attach and separate the pairs of sister chromatids to opposite poles of the spindle, whereby they decondense to form two new nuclei of the daughter cells. During *prophase*, chromosomes condense and pairs of chromatids join at the centromere, beside which lies a MT-binding site (kinetochore), one for each chromatid. A pair of centrioles moves toward opposite poles of the cell and, with the breakdown and disappearance of the nuclear membrane, about 20 of the many spindle MTs from the centrioles capture and attach to each of the kinetochores. This distinguishes *prometaphase*, and the chromosomes are moved to the center of the cell via the MTs. In *metaphase*, pairs of sister chromatids (chromosomes) align along the cell equator, forming a "metaphase plate" suspended by the MT spindle. In *anaphase*, chromatid pair adhesion is lost and chromatid pairs separate, moving toward opposite cell poles created by shortening of the spindle MTs. It is also at anaphase that the chromosome–spindle complex

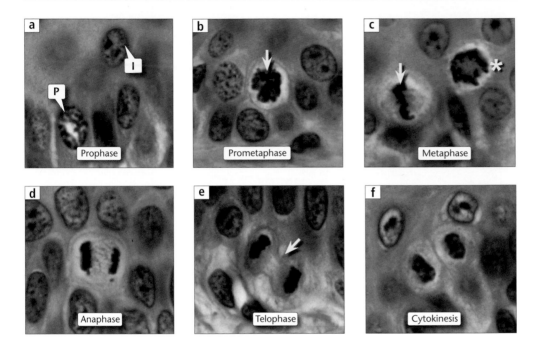

▲ **Fig 1.83 Stages of mitotic division. a** *Interphase and prophase:* Interphase cells (**I**) show a nucleus, nucleolus, and diffuse chromatin. In prophase (**P**), chromosomes condense and each has duplicated in the preceding S phase into two chromatids. **b** *Prometaphase:* Disappearance of the nuclear membrane, with chromosomes (**arrow**) becoming centralized in the cell owing to attachment with spindle microtubules. **c** *Metaphase:* Chromosomes aligned equatorially viewed side-on (**arrow**) and at a 90° angle (**✱**) through the polar axis of the cell. **d** *Anaphase:* Separation of chromosomes into two sets of chromatids (now called chromosomes), pulled apart by spindle microtubules. **e** *Telophase:* Two sets of chromosomes forming presumptive nuclei; cytoplasm showing a cleavage furrow (**arrow**). **f** *Cytokinesis:* Two new nuclei are formed with decondensing chromosomes; the cleavage furrow now splits to give separate daughter cells. H&E, paraffin, all × 1,000.

sends a signal to the cell cortex, which establishes a contractile ring of actin filaments. The ring later becomes the site of the cleavage plane for separation of the daughter cells. Finally, at *telophase*, chromosomes aggregate at the poles, decondense to form heterochromatin–euchromatin, and the nucleolus and nuclear membrane reform. Cleavage of the conjoined daughter cells now follows during cytokinesis, and the two new cells enter G_1 of the cell cycle. In male germ cells, cytokinesis is incomplete, daughter cells remaining connected by cytoplasmic bridges.

As the spindle is assembled during prophase it is thought that MTs and dynein stretch the nuclear membrane, which then tears, causing inflow of cytoplasm. Completion of chromosome condensation and spindle formation between the centrosomes then follows (Fig 1.85). When a new nuclear membrane is reformed during telophase and cytokinesis, membranes of tubular ER bind to chromatin, which cover the chromatin surface with a membrane network. Tubules are stabilized, converted into sheets, and merged, resulting in a closed nuclear envelope.

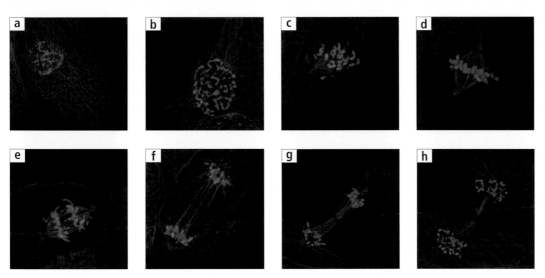

▲ **Fig 1.84 Phases of mitosis.** Fluorescence images of chromosomes stained blue with microtubules red. **a** Interphase. **b** Prophase. **c** Prometaphase. **d** Metaphase. **e** Early anaphase. **f** Late anaphase. **g** Telophase. **h** Cytokinesis. × 900. (Courtesy Pollard T, Earnshaw W. Cell biology. Philadelphia: Elsevier, 2002.)

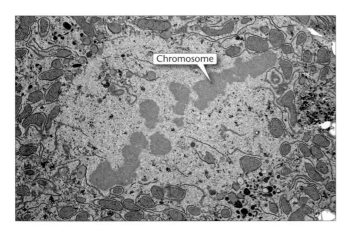

◀ **Fig 1.85 Ultrastructure of a metaphase cell**, showing equatorial alignment of chromosomes and absence of the nuclear membrane, which began its disintegration at prometaphase. The breakdown of the nuclear membrane is thought to occur in response to tension created by attachment to molecular motors of dynein associated with microtubules. Stretching the membrane and its nuclear lamina causes perforation and subsequent flooding of cytoplasmic proteins into the nuclear space. × 4,200.

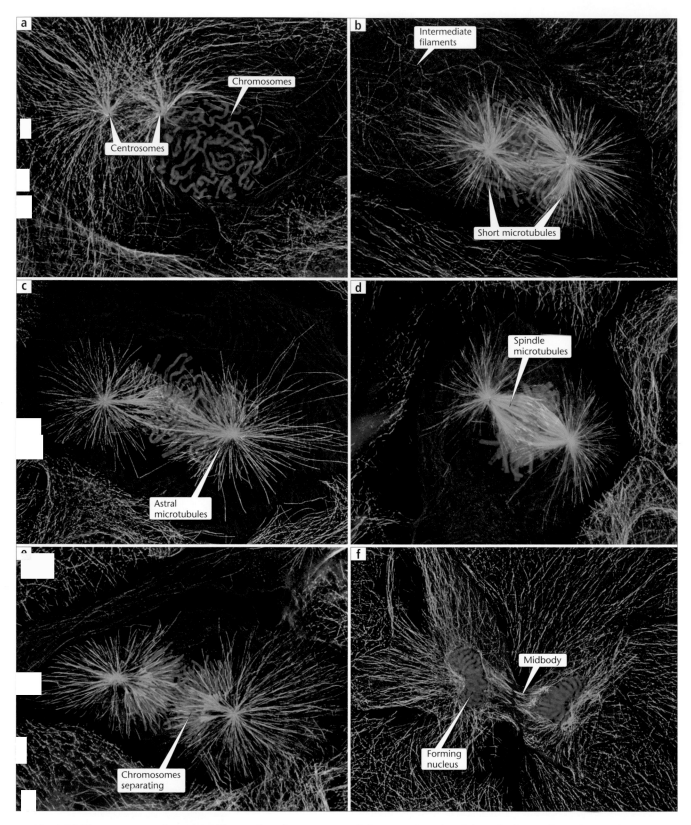

▲ **Fig 1.86 Fluorescence microscopy illustrating the dynamics of the mitotic spindle.** Microtubules are green, chromosomes are blue, intermediate filaments are red. **a** Late prophase with long microtubules radiating from the centrosomes. **b** Early prometaphase with short microtubules. **c** Mid-prometaphase with separation of centrosomes forming asters (starburst-shape) that define opposite poles of the cell. **d** Metaphase showing formation of the mitotic spindle, with microtubules gaining attachment to chromosomes. **e** Anaphase, where microtubule dynamics separate duplicated chromosomes. **f** Telophase–cytokinesis, showing bundles of microtubules (termed the midbody) between the newly forming nuclei. 1,600. (© Rieder C, Wadsworth Center, New York, USA.)

Spindle formation, chromosomes, and cleavage

Formation of bipolar spindles is directed by the centrosomes that serve as nucleation sites for MT growth, many of which grow and shrink until they capture a chromosome (Fig 1.86a–f). The second method of spindle formation is directed by the chromosomes, around which MTs assemble and attach to kinetochores. MT motors also bind chromosome arms, enabling them to be transported along spindle MTs. The spindle consists of four sets of MTs: astral MTs link poles to the cell cortex; chromosomal MTs link the chromosomal arms to poles; kinetochore MTs connect poles to kinetochores; and interpolar MTs link the two poles (Fig 1.87). When aligned at the equator, chromosomes are thought to stabilize MTs that trigger the formation of actin–myosin complexes of the contractile ring, which will become the constriction furrow at the division plane of cytokinesis. Chromosomes segregate to the poles via shortening of their attached MTs (segregation velocity is about 0.1 µm/s) and antiparallel sliding of interpolar MTs, together with shortening of astral MTs, moves the poles further apart during anaphase.

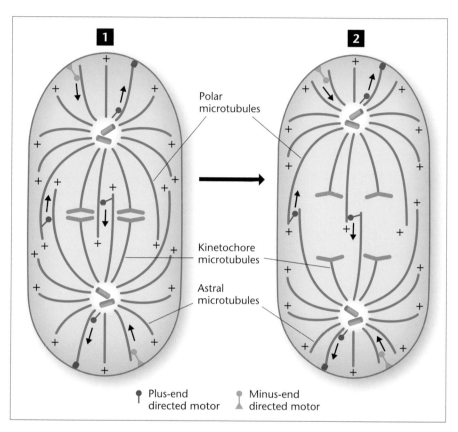

▲ **Fig 1.87 Involvement of microtubules (MTs) and microtubule motors in events at anaphase. 1** Kinetochore MTs attach to chromosome centromeres, forming the kinetochore. Polar MTs overlap and astral MTs are anchored to the plasma membrane. **2** Microtubule motors of polar MTs cause MTs to slide past each other, pushing spindle poles (paired centrioles of the centrosome) apart, and motors of astral MTs pull the spindle poles toward the cell extremities. During this phase of mitosis the microtubules are dynamic; kinetochore MTs shorten, polar MTs elongate, and astral MTs also shorten.

The constriction ring compresses the spindle into a narrow intercellular bridge containing the midbody (Fig 1.88). When the bridge is severed, plasma membrane separates the two daughter cells after their chromosomes have been partitioned into new nuclei during telophase (Fig 1.89).

Cell cycle checkpoints

Specific biochemical steps control the progression of cells through the cell cycle, acting as checkpoints of arrest or advancement. The control system for "stop" or "go" involves cyclic changes in cyclin-dependent protein kinases (Cdks), which phosphorylate proteins regulating key events in all phases of the cell cycle. Cdk activity, as its name implies, depends upon proteins called cyclins. They bind to Cdks and initiate their enzyme activity. Cyclins rise and fall in concentration during the cell cycle.

There are four main checkpoints (Fig 1.90):

- G_1 restriction point monitors cell size and metabolic status
- S phase check for DNA damage (not shown)
- G_2 phase check for DNA integrity and for completion of DNA replication
- Spindle-assembly/metaphase checkpoint during mitosis, which delays the transition to anaphase until all chromosomes are aligned correctly at the metaphase spindle equator.

Meiosis: the key for genetic diversity

Meiosis is a special type of cell proliferation restricted to male and female germ cells, resulting in the formation of haploid cells with half the normal number of chromosomes. For the ovary, the outcome of meiotic maturation of the germ cells is usually a single oocyte that is ovulated on a monthly cycle. In the testis the germ cells proceed through meiosis to produce many millions of haploid spermatozoa each day.

Meiosis involves two successive cell divisions after a single episode of DNA replication, ensuring that four haploid cells are formed from every individual

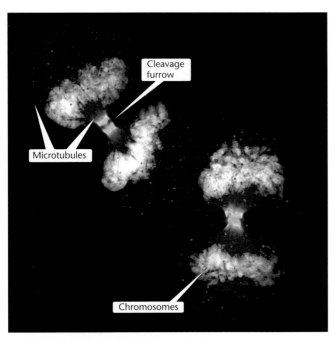

◀ Fig 1.88 Fluorescence deconvolution microscopy of mitotic HeLa cells at late telophase expressing green-fluorescent-protein (GFP)-tagged human Aurora B. Microtubules shown in red, inner-centromere protein in blue, Aurora B-GFP in green, and DNA in white. Aurora B is a protein kinase acting as a chromosome passenger protein for control of microtubule attachment to kinetochores. It organizes the microtubules of the central spindle and the cleavage furrow as shown here. × 2,000. (Courtesy Andrews P, University of Dundee, Scotland; Nature Cell Biology 2003; 5:101.)

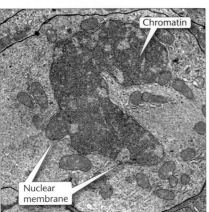

◀ Fig 1.89 Ultrastructure of a cell post cytokinesis, showing how the nuclear membrane is reforming around the condensed chromatin to adopt the characteristic morphology of a nucleus. The outer nuclear membrane has ribosomes on its cytoplasmic surface, which indicates that the rough ER contributes to the reconstitution of the nuclear membrane. × 6,500.

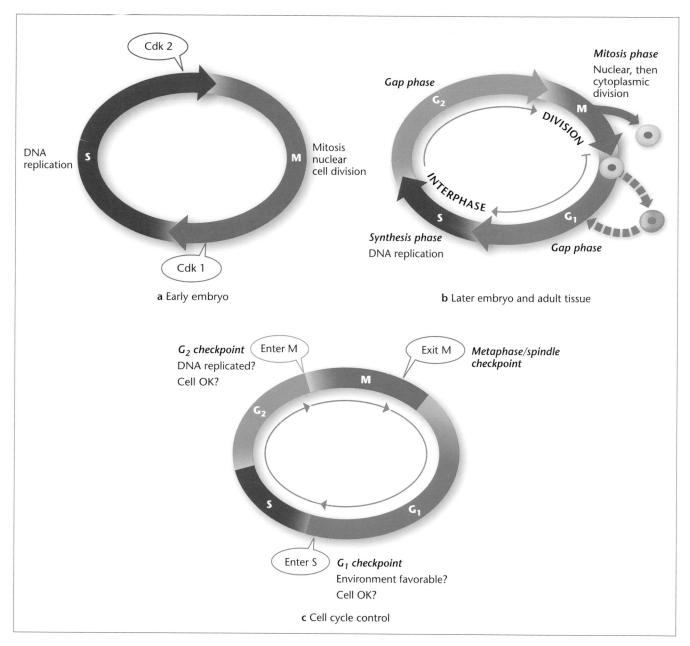

a Early embryo

b Later embryo and adult tissue

c Cell cycle control

▲ **Fig 1.90 Control of the cell cycle. a** In the embryo, cells undergo mitosis and immediately enter S phase for new DNA synthesis. Progression is mediated by cyclin-dependent kinases (Cdks), which are activated when bound to cyclin proteins, so named for their cyclic fluctuating activities in the cell cycle. Cdks phosphorylate target proteins that are essential for membrane, spindle, and chromosome alterations during the cell cycle. **b** Typical cell cycle of four phases, where non-dividing cells are in interphase (i.e. the period between mitoses); in some tissues the cell leaves the cycle at G_1 (or G_2) to become quiescent for long periods or permanently. The decision to continue or exit the cell cycle is regulated by positive or negative signals arising from adjacent cells, circulating factors, or the metabolic status of the cell. **c** Checkpoints during the cell cycle are where the status of the cell is monitored before it proceeds to the next phase. G_1 checkpoint (or restriction point) governs entry into the DNA synthesis phase and is influenced by growth factors, cell size, and nutrient supply. G_2 checkpoint controls entry into mitosis by checking that DNA synthesis is complete. Metaphase/spindle checkpoint monitors that all chromosomes are attached to the spindle prior to chromosome separation during anaphase.

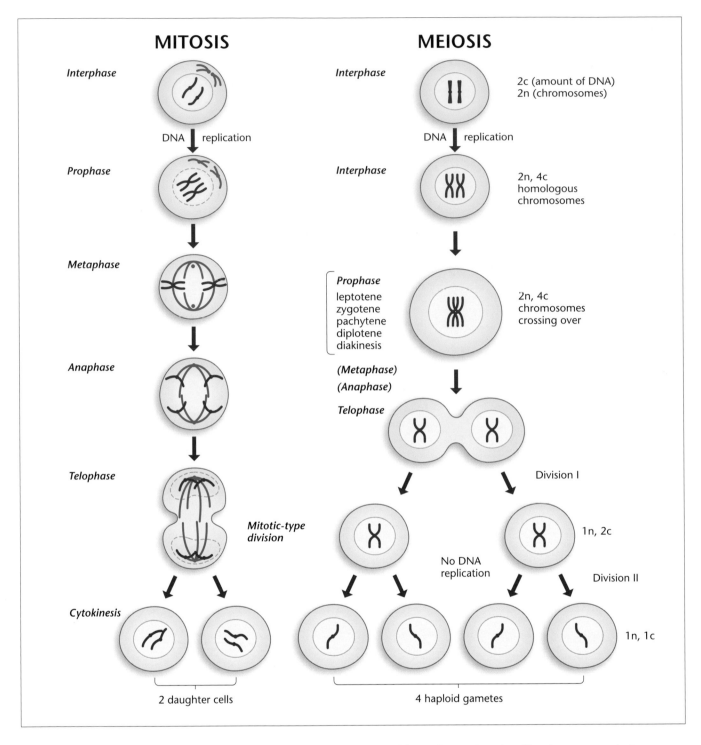

MITOSIS

Interphase

DNA | replication

Prophase

Metaphase

Anaphase

Telophase

*Mitotic-type
division*

Cytokinesis

2 daughter cells

MEIOSIS

Interphase

2c (amount of DNA)
2n (chromosomes)

DNA | replication

Interphase

2n, 4c
homologous
chromosomes

Prophase
leptotene
zygotene
pachytene
diplotene
diakinesis

2n, 4c
chromosomes
crossing over

(Metaphase)
(Anaphase)

Telophase

Division I

1n, 2c

No DNA
replication

Division II

1n, 1c

4 haploid gametes

▲ **Fig 1.91 Comparison of mitosis and meiosis.** For clarity, two chromosomes are shown for mitosis and one pair of homologous chromosomes is shown for meiosis. Each stage is readily visible in histologic sections. The stimulus to enter the cell cycle and undergo mitosis can originate externally, or may arise inside the cell. In the former case, mitogens include growth factors, proteins, and steroid hormones. Within the cell, the genome contains proto-oncogenes (controlling normal proliferation) and tumor-suppressing genes (anti-proliferative). Mutation of proliferation genes results in oncogene expression where cell proliferation is enhanced, causing cancers. During the cell cycle, the amount and activity of cyclin proteins and their dependent kinases regulate progression through interphase and mitosis by dissolving the nuclear membrane, compacting the chromosomes, controlling protein production vital to the cell cycle, and possibly regulating the assembly of the mitotic spindle.

cell that enters meiosis. Meiosis contributes to the genetic variability of progeny by pairing of homologous (male- and female-derived) chromosomes, and mixing and recombining segments of the genetic code that originates in the male-derived and female-derived chromosomes found in a normal diploid cell. Following reciprocal recombination, the chromosomes are segregated into separate cells.

Females have 23 homologous chromosome pairs and males have 22, because the sex chromosomes, X and Y, are morphologically different. One consequence of sharing genetic material is evident in siblings that are not identical twins: phenotypically and genetically they share certain characteristics, which, in turn, are shared with their biological parents and family lineage. In meiosis, this is achieved in two ways. First, the male and female sets of similar chromosomes are distributed randomly to the cells produced by the first meiotic division, which, for humans with 23 genetically different chromosomes, could produce over 8 million genetically different gametes. Second, the ova and spermatozoa represent an even greater range of genetic makeups, because during prophase of the first meiotic division genetic recombination of segments of homologous chromosomes ensures exchange of genes. In this way all gametes derived from an individual are genetically related but contain slightly different gene sequences based on a common genetic program inherited from their ancestors.

Two phases of cell division

Meiosis proceeds through two phases of germ cell maturation and division (Fig 1.91). In division I, prophase is extended in time into five stages defined by the histologic appearance of the chromosomes:

leptotene, zygotene, pachytene, diplotene, and diakinesis. Metaphase, anaphase, and telophase then proceed, followed by division II, which resembles mitotic division, except that chromosomes are not replicated. Four haploid cells (23 chromosomes) are produced. In the ovary, the oocytes are arrested late in prophase I until the oocyte is ovulated, when meiosis resumes. This suspension of meiosis may last for up to four decades, from the time of birth to shortly before menopause (see Ch 18). In the testis, the germ cells enter meiosis continuously at puberty and require about 24 days to complete meiotic maturation (see Ch 19).

Recombination exchanges genes

The exchange of segments between homologous chromosomes results in new versions of chromosomes. For exchange to occur, the homologs must be brought into close association and held there as pieces of chromosomes are swapped. Early pairing and alignment occurs during *leptotene*, followed in *zygotene* by synapsis, where progressive chromosome alignment is engineered by proteins of synaptonemal complexes that extend the whole length of paired chromosomes (Fig 1.92). Crossing over and exchange of chromosome segments in *pachytene* forms linkages or bridges called chiasmata. In *diplotene* chromosomes desynapse, then in *diakinesis* homologs are held together only by chiasmata; the homologs in each pair separate at anaphase and migrate to opposite spindle poles, whereupon meiosis I is completed during telophase and cytokinesis.

Among the chromosomes there are approximately 50 crossing-over sites, which enable mixing of the genetic constitution that is expressed in successive

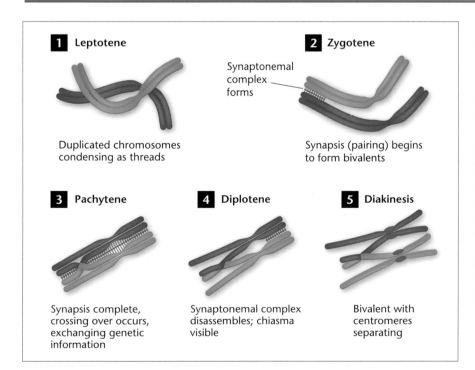

1 Leptotene

Synaptonemal complex forms

Duplicated chromosomes condensing as threads

2 Zygotene

Synapsis (pairing) begins to form bivalents

3 Pachytene

Synapsis complete, crossing over occurs, exchanging genetic information

4 Diplotene

Synaptonemal complex disassembles; chiasma visible

5 Diakinesis

Bivalent with centromeres separating

◀ **Fig 1.92 Behavior of chromosomes during meiotic prophase. 1** At leptotene, double chromosomes, each of sister chromatids, are visible as thin threads. **2** At zygotene, homologous chromosomes (maternal and paternal origin) pair up along a central synaptonemal complex, forming a bivalent of four chromatids. **3** At pachytene, chromosomes are compacted and pairing is complete, allowing for exchange of chromosome segments by crossing over. **4** At diplotene, synaptonemal complexes disappear, and chromosomes separate but are joined at chiasmata where segments have been exchanged. **5** At diakinesis, chromosomes are very short, centromeres separate further, and homologs are only attached by chiasmata. After diakinesis the nuclear envelope disintegrates, a spindle forms, and the cell proceeds into anaphase.

generations by sexual reproduction. The outcome or benefit is similar to reshuffling a pack of playing cards: all cards are retained but their associations have variable significance for how a game is played.

CELL DEATH

Cells degenerate and die either as a natural physiologic process in tissue growth, remodeling, or cyclic replacement, or in response to damage, injury, or some pathologic situations. Dying cells show structural alterations that follow two main pathways: necrosis and genetically programmed cell death, which occurs through a process called apoptosis. The literature describes up to 10 different pathways of cell death that are genetically programmed (Nomenclature Committee on Cell Death).

Necrosis occurs in response to disturbances of the extracellular environment, and usually clumps of many cells all die together, showing swelling, rupture, and leakage of cell contents into the surroundings. Nuclei may remain relatively intact but ultimately lose their ability to be stained by DNA intercalating dyes (karyolysis) due to dissolution of their content (Fig 1.93). Cells that have undergone necrosis and their debris are ultimately removed via phagocytosis by adjacent cells or infiltrating macrophages, but the products of necrosis usually induce an acute inflammatory response.

Apoptosis is commonly, although not universally, a type of physiological cell death that is part of a controlled process. The death of most cells by apoptosis is also known as programmed cell death, although it can be induced by exposure to cytotoxic stimuli, such as treatment with certain chemicals or drugs. Apoptosis is a result of a chain reaction of signaling pathways that can be initiated by extrinsic or intrinsic factors. It occurs in embryogenesis and organogenesis and in tissues of adult animals as a counterbalance to cell proliferation to maintain homeostasis when epithelial cells undergo normal degeneration, and in development and growth of tumors. Thus the birth and death of cells is normally kept in balance. Hypothetically, unopposed cell proliferation until old age would result in 2 tonnes of bone marrow and lymph nodes, and a gut 16 km long.

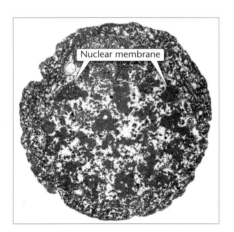

◀ **Fig 1.93 Ultrastructure of a necrotic cell,** showing how the entire cell morphology is undergoing disintegration, with only the remnants of the nuclear membrane and chromatin visible. Cell death by necrosis is a response to non-specific tissue injury such as ischemia. 4,700.

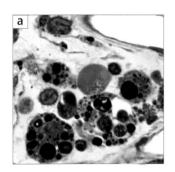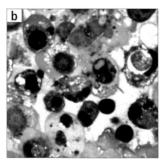

▲ **Fig 1.94 Histology of cells dying by apoptosis. a** Nuclei are intact, but the cytoplasm contains condensations of degenerating organelles. **b** Nuclei show clumping of chromatin, giving rise to densely stained "pyknotic bodies." Cells dying by apoptosis typically are rounded with clumps of nuclear and cytoplasmic materials often fragmented into multiple apoptotic bodies. Apoptosis may be experimentally induced but is a normal physiologic process of cell elimination, particularly in tissues that undergo remodeling, growth, or cyclic development and degeneration. This is also referred to as cell suicide or programmed cell death (i.e. planned cell depletion). Toluidine blue, araldite, × 700.

Apoptotic cells shrink, and organelles compact and may split away, forming individual apoptotic bodies (Fig 1.94a & b). Nuclear chromatin condenses into clumps (the so-called pyknotic nucleus), caused by shredding of DNA into segments of about 150–180 base pairs by endonuclease enzymes. The nucleus may fragment (karyorrhexis) and the apoptotic cell or bodies are rapidly phagocytosed by macrophages or neighboring healthy cells (Fig 1.95a–c), thus precluding induction of an inflammatory response. Apoptosis appears to be a relatively inconspicuous type of cell death because the process takes only 4–6 hours. Rapid disposal of apoptotic cells by phagocytes, epithelial cells, fibroblasts, or endothelial cells may disguise significant rates of cell loss in apparently normal tissues.

Switching on the self-destruct program

Intense interest in the cell and molecular biology of apoptosis has been in part due to its relevance to cancer. Elimination of mutated cells with abnormal growth prevents tumor development. The p53 protein is the product of a tumor-suppressing gene, and inactivating mutations are implicated in about 50% of human cancers. It is a transcription factor that is normally dormant, but when activated it switches on hundreds of proteins that inhibit the cell cycle and/or induce apoptosis. The deadly effects of p53-induced apoptosis are mostly, if not exclusively, mediated by transcriptional induction of two pro-apoptotic members of the Bcl-2 protein family (follicular B cell lymphoma), Puma and Noxa. Regulators of apoptosis include the Bcl-2 family of proteins that either protect against (Bcl-2, Bcl-x_L, Bcl-W, Mcl-1, A1) or promote (Bax, Bak, Bok, Bad, Bik, Hrk, Bid, Bim, Puma, Noxa, Bmf) cell suicide.

The so-called executioners of cells are the caspases, a group of aspartate-specific cysteine proteases responsible for the morphological changes that occur during the later stages of apoptosis. Caspases can be activated directly by the receptor-mediated/extrinsic pathway or by the intrinsic mitochondrial pathway where pro-apoptotic proteins cause release of cytochrome c into the cytoplasm. This induces the caspase destruction reaction.

As apoptotic cells undergo degeneration, they shrink in size as a result of efflux of potassium ions. Condensation and fragmentation of the cell into numerous membrane-bound apoptotic bodies necessitates disposal of the debris. Display of phosphatidylserine on the plasma membrane of apoptotic cells acts as an "eat me" signal for phagocytes, which recognize, engulf, and remove the debris, avoiding an inflammatory response without leakage of apoptotic cell content.

Defects in apoptotic cell death have been implicated in a range of diseases. Abnormal survival of cells that should normally undergo programmed death can cause cancer or autoimmune disease. Moreover, abnormal resistance to apoptotic stimuli is thought to be responsible for resistance of refractory tumors to anti-cancer therapy. Conversely, inappropriate death of cells that should normally be long-lived has been implicated in the etiology of degenerative diseases, such as neurodegeneration, muscular degeneration, or ischemic heart disease.

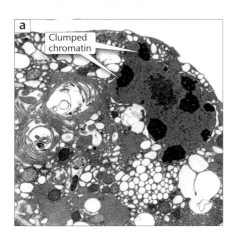
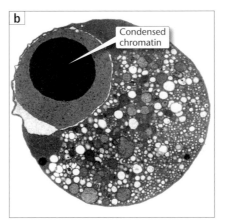
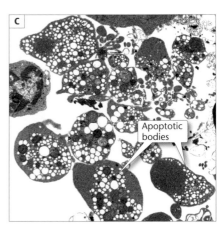

▲ **Fig 1.95a Ultrastructure of early apoptosis.** Chromatin is aggregated into distinct clumps. In the cytoplasm, vesicles are swollen, and organelles show disorganization including bizarre membranous whorls. Clumping of chromatin is a result of DNA being shredded into 150–180 base pair segments by endonucleases, encoded by several genes known to be activated during tissue development. × 5,000.

▲ **Fig 1.95b Ultrastructure of apoptosis.** After DNA cleavage in apoptotic cells, the chromatin usually aggregates into a single entity. Many other enzymes and hydrolases disrupt cytoplasmic organelles, resulting in bizarre morphology. The degraded cell is phagocytosed by macrophages or adjacent normal cells. × 5,000.

▲ **Fig 1.95c Ultrastructure of late apoptosis.** The dying cell has split into numerous parts, which are visible by light microscopy as apoptotic bodies. The fragmented parts are removed by phagocytosis of nearby cells which, depending on the tissue, may be macrophages or epithelial cells, but this clearance of debris is not accompanied by an inflammatory response. × 3,600.

Origin of tissue types

MULTICELLULARITY

A common approach in reviewing histology in the anatomical context is to give an overview of the comparative architecture of the adult organs or organ systems based upon their characteristic tissues and cells. This may provide a useful way of integrating cell biology with physiology and pathology, but it assumes that students have acquired a thorough understanding of the cellular and non-cellular components that make up the tissues found in all organs. Just as a house is made of foundations, walls, windows, a roof, and many internal components, an organ is similarly constructed by assembly of basic parts, the identity of which is founded upon a knowledge of the essential components that, together with "custom-made" variations, are designated as the primary tissue types. But an important question arises: where do these primary tissue types come from? The answer to this question is found in embryology books, rarely in histology texts.

It is important to realize that the tissues, as collections of cells and extracellular materials, are themselves the products of a cell development program that begins in the embryo. These formative cells show specialized rearrangements, which later differentiate and grow into the primary tissues. As embryogenesis proceeds into the fetal period, the developing tissues themselves are subject to regional specializations that ultimately form organs with characteristic morphology and function.

Cells of the early embryo

Among the trillions of cells in the adult body, only two cells (one oocyte and one sperm) are required to unite at the time of conception to form a single cell, called the zygote (the fertilized egg), which marks the beginning of several days of cleavage of the embryo. Through many cell divisions, migrations, growth, and differentiation (cells specialized to perform unique functions) during both intrauterine life and postnatal development, new cells eventually develop into tissues and organs.

The answer to the question above regarding the origin of tissue types is that the embryonic germ layers, of which there are three major types, are the progenitors of the primary tissues. The germ layers develop from the blastocyst, an early embryo first recognized about 5 days postconception (Fig 2.1a–g).

This early conceptus is a hollow ball of cells containing an inner cluster of cells called the inner cell mass (ICM). The ICM contains the embryonic stem (ES) cells, which represent the starting point for all the subsequent cells that will form the germ layers and, in turn, the primary tissue types and organs.

Development of the embryo

Traditionally the first 2 weeks of human development (i.e. starting with a zygote, which divides to form cells called blastomeres) are referred to as the pre-embryonic period. This is because, during week 3, the growing conceptus produces specific cellular components, which individually and reproducibly form designated tissue types and eventually organs. Thus, in the past, the formation of the embryo during the embryonic period (weeks 3–8) has been characterized by the development of most internal and external structures leading to early organ formation, folding, and head, trunk, and early limb development. At around week 9, the embryo enters the fetal period, the term fetus referring to a recognizable human being.

The development of in vitro fertilization (IVF) and the intense interest in stem cells and cloning has led to a revision of the definition of an embryo. Embryos or "early embryos" are now recognized not solely on the basis of their cell numbers or morphology, age, or overall size (Fig 2.2), but whether or not these collections of cells are potentially capable of growing into more specialized organisms that have the characteristics of the traditionally defined "embryo," "fetus," or indeed fully formed newborn individuals.

In the current literature, any of the stages of zygote cleavage (cell multiplication) up to and beyond the first 2 weeks of development (for humans) are referred to as embryos, with the term fetus used after 8 weeks.

Germ layers contribute to primary tissues

As the blastocyst implants into the endometrium of the uterus, the inner cell mass differentiates into two layers: the epiblast, which is the embryonic lineage; and the hypoblast (also known as the primitive endoderm), which will give rise to the extraembryonic tissue of the yolk sac. These two cell layers form a bilaminar embryonic disc (Fig 2.3a–d).

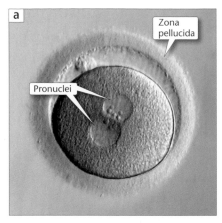

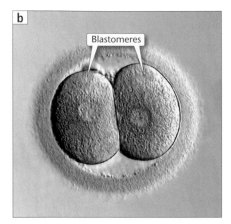

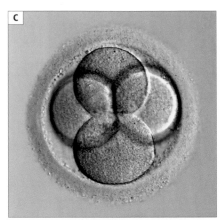

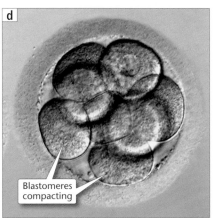

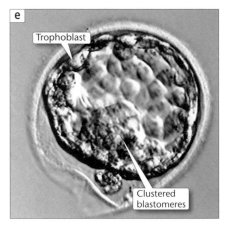

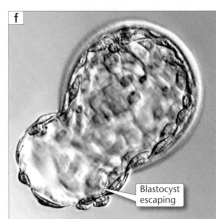

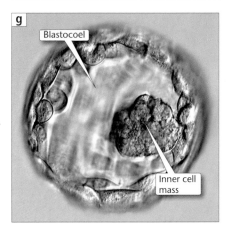

◀ **Fig 2.1 Cleavage stages of the human embryo. a** Newly fertilized human oocyte showing two pronuclei derived from the sperm and oocyte nuclei. Pronuclei make contact and fuse, and their chromosomes intermingle, forming the zygote, which is poised to commence cell division. The zygote is surrounded by a shell rich in glycoproteins (formed initially in early folliculogenesis), deep to which is a polar body. **b** First cleavage, which gives two cells termed blastomeres, day 1 after fertilization. Blastomeres divide every 12–18 hours, with the embryo increasing in size. **c** Day 2, showing four blastomeres. **d** Day 3 or 4 showing eight blastomeres, which are sometimes referred to as the morula (mulberry). Blastomeres increase cell-to-cell contact to become compacted. **e** About day 5, showing cavitation of the embryo, now called a blastocyst, with clustering of blastomeres forming the inner cell mass. Peripheral blastomeres form the trophoblast/trophoectoderm cells (contribute to placenta), external to which is the degenerating zona pellucida. **f** The blastocyst is seen escaping through the zona pellucida, a process occasionally called "hatching." **g** Compaction of the inner cell mass at a polar location within the fluid-filled cavity termed the blastocoel. Cells of the inner cell mass are not identical with regard to their developmental fate. At this stage the blastocyst implants into the endometrium. (Images courtesy L Veeck, Cornell University, New York, USA; from An atlas of human blastocysts. New York: Parthenon, 2003.)

Developmental stage	Days after fertilization	Morphology	Size
Zygote, then 2–4–8 cells	1–2	Solid ball of cells (blastomeres)	Up to 30 μm
Blastocyst 50–60 cells	4–5	Cavity and inner cell mass*; outer trophoblast forms	100 μm
Late blastocyst 100 cells	8–10	Inner cell mass* + hypoblast	200–500 μm
Growing blastocyst now implanted in uterus	12–14	Bilaminar embryonic disc (epiblast* + hypoblast)	1–2 mm
Gastrulation	15–16+	Trilaminar embryonic disc Epiblast → ectoderm** Mesoblast → mesoderm** Hypoblast → endoderm**	2 mm+

* Embryonic stem cells
** Three germ layers

▲ **Fig 2.2** Cell types and characteristics of the early embryo.

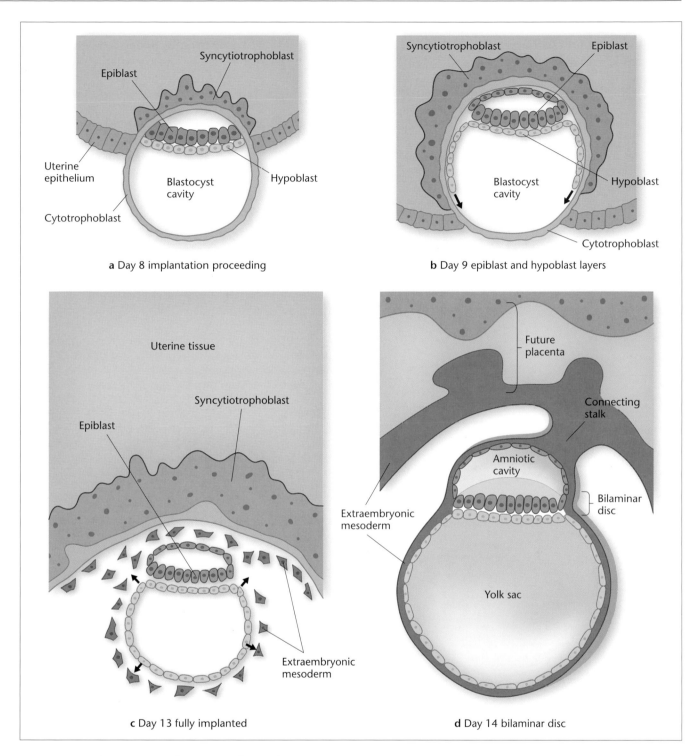

a Day 8 implantation proceeding

b Day 9 epiblast and hypoblast layers

c Day 13 fully implanted

d Day 14 bilaminar disc

▲ **Fig 2.3 Implantation and formation of the bilaminar disc. a** The implanting blastocyst invades the endometrium, with the trophoblast now differentiated into a single cell layer termed the cytotrophoblast. Within the endometrium its outer layer is invasive and its cells form a syncitium (a multinucleated mass of cytoplasm) referred to as the syncytiotrophoblast. The inner cell mass shows two cell types: the upper layer is the epiblast, and the hypoblast layer faces the blastocyst cavity. **b** Formation of a small cavity above the inner cell mass, which is the amniotic cavity that will hold amniotic fluid. The hypoblast produces cells of the extra-embryonic membrane that lines the blastocyst cavity, contributing to the early formation of the yolk sac. The syncytiotrophoblast continues to expand into the endometrium and will contribute to formation of the placenta. **c** Now fully implanted, the epiblast and hypoblast layers are identified and are separated by a basal lamina. The hypoblast-derived cells have formed a new cavity, the early yolk sac, the fluid in which provides nutrition for the embryo prior to a functional placenta. The growing syncytiotrophoblast, with intercalated projections of cytoblast cells forming chorionic villi, is the source of human chorionic gonadotropin (hCG). It maintains the corpus luteum of the ovary supporting the endometrium and its presence in urine is an early indicator of pregnancy. **d** At about day 14 the embryo is recognized as a bilaminar disc of epiblast and hypoblast, with cavities above and below it. The amnion is connected by a stalk to the chorion, consisting of the primary villi, syncytiotrophoblast, and maternal blood vessels. (Modified from Carlson BM. Human embryology and developmental biology, 3rd edn. Philadelphia: Mosby, 2004.)

The epiblast layer contains ES cells, which, via proliferation and differentiation during the period of gestation, give rise to the three germ layers—*ectoderm*, *mesoderm*, and *endoderm*— from which all the tissues of the fetus and adult are formed (Fig 2.4). The germ cells in the ovary (ova) and in the testis (sperm), which via union form the zygote, are themselves derived from primitive sex cells that appear among endodermal cells in the 4-week-old embryo. These are the primordial germ cells (PGCs). It is believed that the progenitors of these cells arise from perhaps a dozen or so cells within the epiblast.

The three embryonic germ layers grow and contribute to the four primary tissue types characteristic of vertebrates, including humans. Cells within a germ layer divide and differentiate to take on the phenotype and functions of *one or more* primary tissue types. Interactions between these cells and those of the other germ layers induce a cascade of cell specializations and tissue differentiations that eventually constitute the various organ systems.

The primary tissue types are epithelium, connective tissue, muscle, and nerve (Fig 2.5).

In addition, an important group of cells termed the *neural crest* appears during week 4 and becomes widely distributed throughout the body (see below).

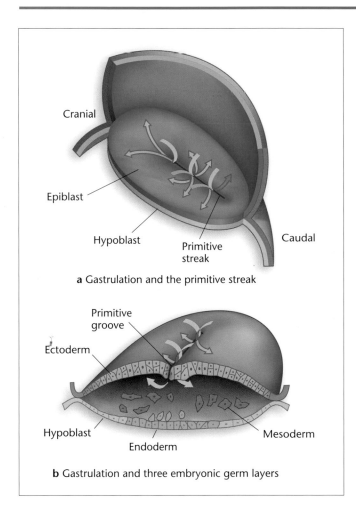

a Gastrulation and the primitive streak

b Gastrulation and three embryonic germ layers

◀ **Fig 2.4 Gastrulation and the three embryonic germ layers. a** Gastrulation is the process by which the bilaminar disc is converted into a trilaminar disc. This occurs from days 15 to 17. A thin band of epiblast termed the primitive streak appears caudally. It is the result of proliferation and migration of epiblast cells toward the midline of the bilaminar disc. The primitive streak defines the cranial to caudal axis of the embryo, left and right sides, and ventral and dorsal surfaces. **b** The streak becomes a narrow depression, called the primitive groove, into which some epiblast cells migrate. These cells detach and differentiate into a layer of cells that replace hypoblast cells to form the endoderm germ layer. Other migrating cells from the primitive groove are located between the former epiblast and hypoblast to form the embryonic germ layer termed mesoderm. Cells remaining in the epiblast will form the ectoderm layer. Ectoderm, mesoderm, and endoderm are the founders of all the tissue and organs of the fetus.

Most organs are formed from several germ layers. The nervous system is neuroectodermal, but the brain also has blood vessels, which are not ectodermal. The intestine is endodermal with respect to its inner lining, but its connective tissue and muscular coats are mesodermal, and the nerves that invade it are ectodermal. The terms ectopia, heterotopia, and aberrance of tissues are used to describe the development of tissues in locations where they are not normally found—for example, ectopia of the testis (maldescent/cryptorchidism), heterotopic foci of gray matter of the central nervous system (arrest of migrating neuroblasts in developing brain), and aberrant location of pancreatic tissue in the stomach wall (Meckel's diverticulum). Metaplasia is the transformation of a differentiated tissue of one type into a differentiated tissue of another kind (e.g. development of bone in skeletal muscle, bronchial respiratory epithelium replaced by squamous epithelium).

Germ layer derivatives

Ectoderm, mesoderm, and endoderm formed in week 3 give rise to the primordia of all tissues and organs during weeks 4–8. The cells of each germ layer grow and form patterns that define the body architecture and the various organ systems (Fig 2.6).

Neural crest

The neural crest is comparable to a fourth germ layer since it gives rise to a remarkable variety of cells and tissues (Fig 2.7). The crest is a transient group of mobile neuroectodermal cells arising between the neural ectoderm (which forms the central nervous system) and the somatic ectoderm (which forms the epidermis). Neural crest cells delaminate from the developing neural tube and migrate along defined pathways to reach their final destinations, chiefly the trunk and the head.

These cells are multipotent cells that differentiate into many cell types: in the head they contribute to skeletal and dental tissues; in the trunk they contribute to the peripheral nervous system, dorsal root ganglia, sympathetic trunk and ganglia, the adrenal medulla, gut autonomic ganglia and amine precursor uptake and decarboxylation (APUD) cells; in the ectoderm they contribute to the melanocytes of skin. Neural crest cells are considered to be a stem-cell-like population.

Primary tissue types				
Embryonic germ layer	Epithelium	Connective	Muscular	Nerve
Ectoderm	✓	In head region	–	✓
Mesoderm	✓	✓	✓	–
Endoderm	✓	–	–	–

▲ **Fig 2.5** Primary tissue types.

Germ layers		
Ectoderm	**Mesoderm**	**Endoderm**
Brain, spinal cord, peripheral nerves	Connective tissue	Epithelial lining of gut, lungs
Skin, hair, nails	Cartilage	Substance of tonsils, thyroid/parathyroid
Breast	Bone	Thymus
Pituitary gland	Muscle	Liver, gall bladder, pancreas
Tooth enamel	Vascular system	Epithelial lining bladder/most urethra
Sensory epithelium of the eyes/ears/nose	Kidneys	Epithelial lining of tympanic cavity and antrum, auditory tube
Neural crest cells that form most ganglia/melanocytes/adrenal medulla	Ovaries, testes, ducts	
Coverings of the peripheral nerves	Lining for heart, chest, abdominal cavities	
Coverings of the brain, spinal cord	Spleen	
	Adrenal cortex	

▲ **Fig 2.6** Organ and tissue derivatives of the three germ layers.

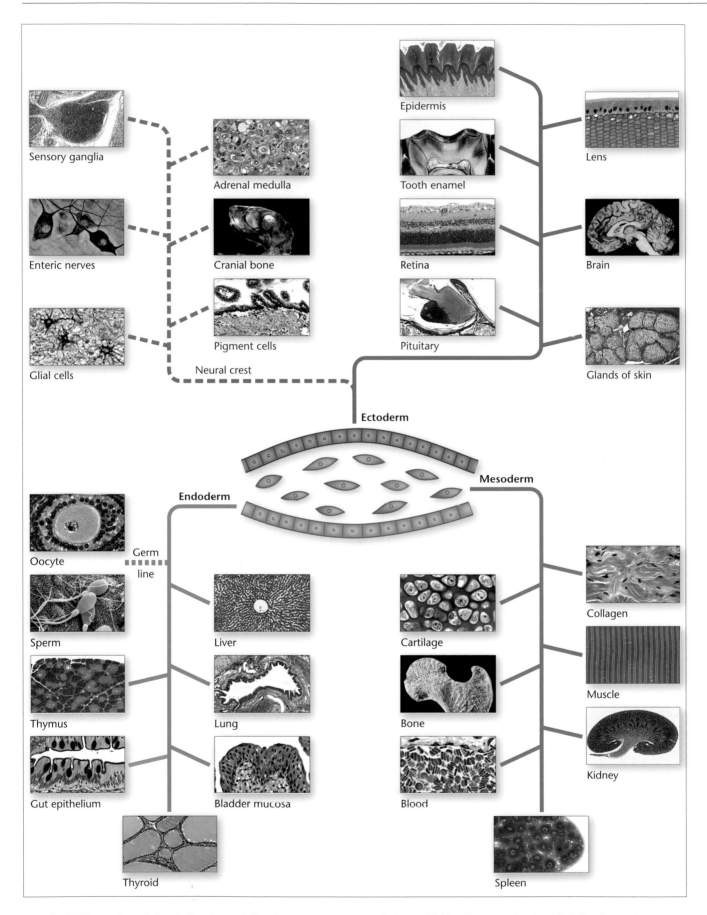

▲ Fig 2.7 Examples of the derivatives of the three embryonic germ layers: ectoderm, mesoderm, and endoderm. The process of gastrulation, whereby the germ layers are formed, results in establishing fate maps for the cells belonging to the germ layers. These pathways are responsible for determining the blueprint that specifies tissue lineages.

Stem cells

It is within a variety of tissues in postnatal life that adult stem (AS) cells are found. These serve the purpose of self-renewal and division into more specialized cell types characteristic of the tissues that replenish the existing types of cells that have a limited lifespan. AS cells occur in organs such as skin, the gut, bone marrow, brain, and spinal cord. The differences between ES cells, AS cells, and embryonic germ cells (EG; cells derived from primordial germ cells) both in vivo and in culture have implications for development of pathologies, and potential for disease treatment. Some terms commonly used to refer to the developmental potential of cells are given in Figure 2.8.

CELLS AND EXTRACELLULAR COMPONENTS

It is essential to understand and be able to recognize what is a cell and what, by logical extension, is not a cell (i.e. extracellular, or non-living, material). All tissues are made of cells plus extracellular material. It doesn't matter if the tissue is rock-hard such as bone, or a liquid such as blood or peritoneal fluid—all tissues contain cells and extracellular components. Bone has osteocytes embedded in hard (extracellular) bone matrix. Blood has red and white cells and platelets suspended in a fluid medium of plasma. Peritoneal fluid contains small numbers of white blood cells in extracellular tissue fluid.

Differentiating between cells and non-cellular components can be troubling initially, because it takes time to become familiar with the differences. A secret to success lies with an appreciation of the generic morphological properties of all cells and the various structural appearances of everything that clearly is not cellular. This task does *not* depend upon memorizing the shapes, sizes, and relative abundance of all the hundreds of different cell types in the human body.

All cells have common structural features that can be observed in histologic sections, including:
- A central nucleus, which is usually darker (purple/blue with hematoxylin and eosin [H&E] staining) than the rest of the cell
- A surrounding cytoplasm, which is usually paler (pink with H&E staining) than the nucleus
- A boundary, which is a contrasting color compared with adjacent structures, either other cells or extracellular material. However, this boundary is not really the cell membrane, which is only 10 nm thick, but may represent the two cell membranes of neighboring cells plus intercellular materials.

In practice, when differentiating between cells and non-cellular elements, it is important to keep three things in mind:
- Variations in cell size
- Variations in how the section passes through the tissue
- Variations in cell shape when looking at a two-dimensional view of three-dimensional objects.

Term	Definition
Blastocyst	Embryo before implantation; contains outer trophoectoderm cells allowing implantation, and the inner cell mass (ICM), within which are embryonic stem cells.
Cell fate	Developmental potential of a cell in the embryo or in an ectopic (extrauterine) site.
Epigenetic	Heritable and reversible changes in gene function but no change in DNA sequence. Involves modifications of DNA or protein binding to DNA sequences.
Lineage	Natural progression from immature cell type to one or more differentiated cell types.
Lineage restriction	Inability of one lineage to give cell types to another.
Multipotent	Able to give rise to more than one differentiated cell type, e.g. bone marrow hemopoietic cells produce erythrocytes and white blood cells.
Plasticity	Ability to cross lineage boundaries.
Pluripotent	Able to give rise to all cell types found in embryo and adult. Examples of pluripotent stem cell lines: embryonic stem cells from inner cell mass; embryonic germ cells from primordial germ cells; embryonal carcinoma (EC) cells obtained from components of adult testis tumors.
Progenitor cells	Can include stem cells or their progeny (can divide but cannot self-renew; can form more differentiated cell types).
Stem cell	A cell capable of self-renewal and differentiation.
Teratocarcinoma	Gonadal tumor with a range of tissues derived from three germ layers, e.g. bone, epithelia, ganglia, muscle, cartilage, glands. Cells of the tumor are formed from pluripotent EC cells, which themselves are derived from primordial germ cells.
Therapeutic cloning	Reprogramming adult cell nucleus by transfer into cytoplasm of the enucleated oocyte.
Totipotent	Able to give rise to all cell types. Only the fertilized egg and early cleavage stage blastomeres are truly totipotent. Cells of the inner cell mass and embryonic stem cells cannot differentiate into cells of the trophoectoderm lineage.
Unipotent	Stem cells that produce only one type of differentiated cell, e.g. spermatogonia of the testis produce sperm.

▲ **Fig 2.8** Useful definitions of terms used in embryology and developmental biology.

Some examples

- **Squamous-type cells** (epidermis, endothelium lining vessels, mesothelium) can be very flat, elongated structures resembling a fried egg or a paving stone or a spindle (in the case of smooth muscle). The nucleus is likewise often very thin and flat, with perhaps hardly any surrounding cytoplasm (Fig 2.9a). *Spherical, cuboidal,* or *columnar cells* are named by their shape and have readily visible nuclei (Fig 2.9b).
- **Irregular, stellate** or very **elongated cells** (there are many examples) may have unusual shapes but they still contain a nucleus. The nucleus may not always be visible because it is not included in the thin slice (5–10 μm only) that makes up the tissue section. This is particularly evident when, for example, the section passes horizontally through a sheet of tall, columnar cells belonging to a curved mucosa. The microscopic view is a collection of close-packed polygons with apparent cell boundaries, but no central nuclei.
- **Adipose tissue** (fat) shows adipocytes in which the nucleus is very small, having been marginalized by fat that fills the cytoplasm (Fig 2.9c). If fats have been dissolved in the tissue processing, this leaves cells with empty-looking circles bounded by a thin, cytoplasmic border.

- **Myelinated nerves** cut in cross section also show processing changes where the myelin sheaths (which are rich in lipid) are extracted and appear as an empty ring surrounding the central axon. The ring is itself bordered by a thin rim of Schwann cell cytoplasm (Fig 2.9d).
- **Skeletal muscle fibers** (multiple myoblasts fused end-to-end) cut in longitudinal section show multiple elongated nuclei located along the edge of the fiber—with no cellular boundary between the nuclei—making up the edge of the fiber which, in three-dimensions, is a long cylinder. The fiber is an example of many skeletal muscle cells that fill their cytoplasm with their own synthetic products—the contractile proteins (Fig 2.9e).
- **Mitotic figures** lack a nucleus. It disappears at the end of prophase as the nuclear material condenses to form chromosomes. The nucleus reappears toward the end of telophase as the chromosomes unwind and take on the typical interphase nuclear morphology (Fig 2.9f).
- **Erythrocytes** have no nucleus. It is lost before the red cell is released into the circulation from the bone marrow. This "cell" is a membrane-bound bag of hemoglobin plus enzymes—a cell in which the cytoplasm is the cell product (Fig 2.9g).

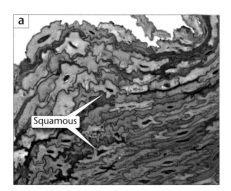

▲ **Fig 2.9a** Squamous epithelial cells, showing irregular flattened cells. × 600.

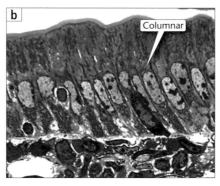

▲ **Fig 2.9b** Columnar epithelial cells. × 700.

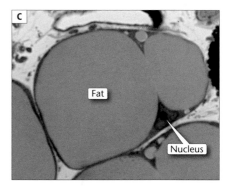

▲ **Fig 2.9c** Adipose (fat) cells show lipid occupying most of the cell. The cytoplasm is a thin rim and the nucleus is displaced peripherally. × 800.

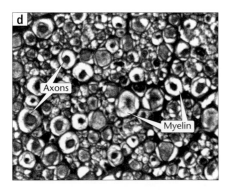

▲ **Fig 2.9d** Myelinated nerves with central axons surrounded by extracted myelin sheaths. × 400.

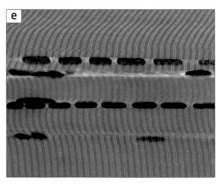

▲ **Fig 2.9e** Skeletal muscle cells showing multiple nuclei and cytoplasm filled with contractile filaments giving a striated appearance. × 275.

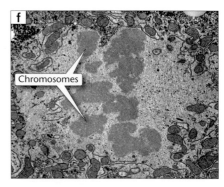

▲ **Fig 2.9f** Mitotic figure showing chromosomes. Note the absence of the nuclear envelope. × 4,000.

- **Mature lens fibers** of the eye have no nuclei. They are six-sided, elongated prisms (formerly epithelial cells) packed with high concentrations of proteins/crystallins making up the cytoplasm (Fig 2.9h).
- **Megakaryocytes** of the bone marrow are polyploid cells with central, multilobulated nuclei, the result of nuclear replication but no cell division (Fig 2.9i).
- **Hepatocytes** often show two nuclei within one cell (Fig 2.9j).
- **Platelets** of the blood are fragments of cytoplasm (from megakaryocytes), which are biconcave discs lacking a nucleus but containing granules and organelles (Fig 2.9k).

Extracellular material

Having discussed aspects of cell structure in histologic sections, can it now be concluded that all elements external to cells are therefore part of the extracellular material? No, unfortunately it is not quite as simple as that. For example, a particular cell located in, say, stratified epithelium, is immediately surrounded by other epithelial cells and not by extracellular material. Deep to the epithelium, however, there is always an extracellular matrix (i.e. intercellular substance on the opposite side of the basement membrane).

As a generalization, it is true that most cells (or associations of cells that make up an epithelium as noted above) are supported by extracellular tissue. The latter is defined as connective tissue and, depending on its type/location, can be hydrated with tissue fluid or, at the other extreme, solid such as the extracellular matrix that makes up bone.

A full understanding of what is or is not extracellular will be attained over the time spent studying how organs and tissues are made up of the four primary tissue types.

PRIMARY TISSUE TYPES

Perhaps the best kept "secrets of histology" with regard to the systematic study and understanding of tissue architecture and the detailed facts can be summarized in the following objectives:

- Understand and recognize what a cell is and how it differs from extracellular (non-living) material.
- Be familiar with the basic phenotypes of cells and the range of morphological appearances of all else that is clearly not cellular. In this approach the phenotypic patterns give strong clues to identifying individual cell types. This method ensures recognition of each and every one of the hundreds of different cell types of the body.
- Know the derivation and general fate of the embryonic germ layers.
- Be familiar with the basic histology of the four primary types, since this ensures correct identification (and therefore function) of any organ or tissue because all of them consist of several or all of the primary tissue types.

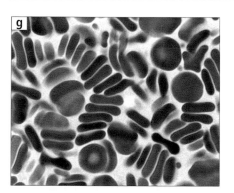

▲ **Fig 2.9g** Erythrocytes (red blood cells) lack nuclei. × 1,200.

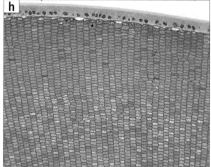

▲ **Fig 2.9h** Closely packed fibers of the lens. × 200.

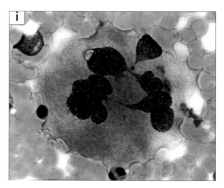

▲ **Fig 2.9i** Megakaryocyte of the bone marrow, showing a multilobulated nucleus. × 800.

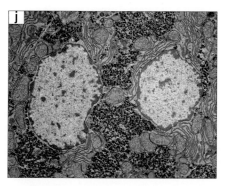

▲ **Fig 2.9j** Liver cell with double nuclei. × 3,000.

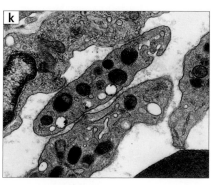

▲ **Fig 2.9k** Blood platelets are cytoplasmic fragments. × 17,000. (Courtesy P Cross, Stanford University, California, USA.)

- Develop pattern recognition skills (e.g. all pseudostratified epithelium looks the same, peripheral nerves have a unique pattern, elastic cartilage all looks the same).
- Be aware of morphological associations. Certain cell and tissue associations are always seen in normal organs and one expects to find one component occurring in association with another. If this rule is broken, variations of pattern recognition and structural associations = pathology.

To put a primary tissue review into perspective, it is worthwhile considering the big picture, that is to appreciate that all tissues and their cells are derivatives of the embryo, specifically of the embryonic germ layers. For example, the gastrointestinal tract and its derivative glands consist of a basic association of the four primary tissue types, which in turn are formed from the three embryonic germ layers. The differences in histology of the gut are merely regional variations on this basic theme.

It cannot be emphasized too strongly how important it is to learn about the primary tissues. Why so? Because a good understanding of primary tissue biology and the ability to recognize primary tissues in a microscope/book picture/displayed image will virtually guarantee that you will be a "card-carrying" histologist.

How can such a bold statement be justified? Thorough knowledge of the four primary tissue types will allow identification of *any* normal organ or tissue, because all organs and their various components are composed of at least one and usually of several or all of the primary tissue types. Consequently, it is not necessary to master histology by memorizing all the different cell types and specific tissue morphologies that present themselves in each and every specimen found in textbooks, the slide box, or the image bank. This does not mean that this secret to success can be acquired two days before an exam. What it does lead to is pattern recognition.

Pattern recognition (together with functional attributes) is the secret to learning about primary tissue types. For example, all hyaline cartilage looks the same wherever it is found; pseudostratified epithelium is always the same; smooth muscle all looks the same but has certain features that set it apart from similar-looking fibroblasts.

Another tip about pattern recognition is morphological association(s): that is, in normal tissues—but not in many pathologic tissues—certain cell and tissue associations are always seen and are invariant in the sense that one expects to see one component always occurring together with another. For example, ganglion cells (neuron cell bodies outside the central nervous system) may look similar to ovarian primary follicles, but ganglia are not found in the ovary and ovarian follicles are not found at sites containing ganglia (the gut, glands, and sites associated with spinal cord nerve roots). The ganglia and the follicles are associated with other characteristic surrounding tissues; the former perhaps with smooth muscle, connective tissue, and glandular cells, and nerve fibers; the latter with the ovarian connective tissue stroma.

The four primary human tissue types

Time spent studying the similarities of and differences between the basic tissue types will be rewarded when analyzing how organs are assembled from tissues. Most, if not all, of the guesswork will have been eliminated. The benefits are numerous:

- An ability to identify and discuss the functions of previously unseen normal histologic preparations

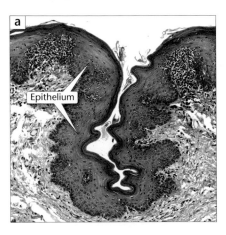

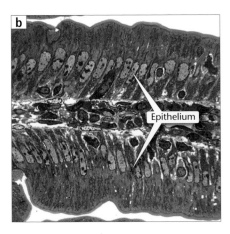

◀ **Fig 2.10b Epithelium**, showing tall columnar cells of the intestinal mucosa. Both upper and lower epithelia rest on a basal lamina. Toluidine blue, araldite, × 480.

▲ **Fig 2.10a Epithelium**, showing a multilayered arrangement of cells forming a protective barrier. The deep aspect of the epithelium rests upon a basal lamina that separates the layer from supporting tissue. Hematoxylin and eosin (H&E), paraffin, × 80.

- Confidence in recognizing the component parts of organs and tissues in studies of development and embryology.
- Skill in the interpretation of dysfunctional or unusual presentations of organ or tissue morphology in, for example, transgenic, mutant, or knock-out or knock-in–derived cases
- A solid foundation for interpretation of histopathological specimens.

An introduction is presented here. Detailed discussion of the primary tissues is found in following chapters.

Epithelial tissue

This consists of one or multiple cell layers that form a continuous sheet or lining "mucosa" covering an external surface or lining an internal cavity (Fig 2.10a & b). Epithelial cells are often closely packed together and joined by specialized junctions that provide adhesion and intercellular communication. Glandular tissue is often derived from epithelium (Fig 2.10c). Simple or complex invagination of the surface layer forms certain types of *exocrine glands*, which secrete onto the surface via a duct (e.g. sweat glands, seromucous glands of the tongue or glands of the respiratory tract and the pancreas) (Fig 2.10d & e). The secretory part of exocrine glands is called parenchyma and, when present, the mesodermal tissue surrounding parenchyma may form a capsule and septa (the stroma). *Endocrine glands* release their products into blood and/or lymph, and may also arise as epithelial outgrowths that eventually lose their connection with the surface. Epithelial tissues often form a boundary that may, for example, regulate absorption and secretion or act as a barrier.

Epithelia contain no blood vessels and are attached to and supported by a basement membrane consisting of various layers of connective tissue. Epithelia are usually dynamic, such that cells are constantly shed and replaced.

Connective tissue

This tissue is composed of cells in an abundant extracellular matrix that consists of fibers and an amorphous or gel-like ground substance. Connective tissues occur throughout the body, supporting and binding together all other tissues. Vessels and nerves often, but not always, travel within connective tissues. Bone, cartilage, tendons, ligaments, organ capsules, and fat are specialized connective tissues. Blood as a liquid with free-floating cells, and bone marrow as a blood-forming tissue, are also special forms of connective tissue. Much of the connective tissue consists of fibroblast cells, collagen, and elastic fibers, and a "gap-filling" matrix of macromolecules, such as polysaccharides, proteins, and water. Depending on their composition, connective tissues provide strength, elasticity, or a packing material allowing for diffusion of nutrients or waste products between blood and adjacent tissues.

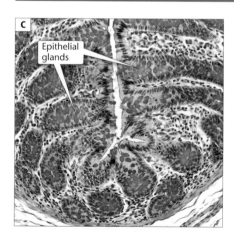

▲ **Fig 2.10c Epithelial lining of the colon,** showing glandular specializations that form deep crypts containing many individual mucus-secreting goblet cells (green). Alcian blue/van Gieson, paraffin, × 80.

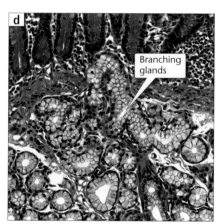

▲ **Fig 2.10d Duodenum,** showing branching glandular tissue derived from the upper surface epithelium. Glandular secretions are released into the deep crypts of the epithelium. H&E, paraffin, × 130.

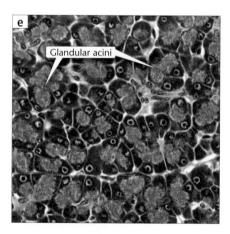

▲ **Fig 2.10e Multiple glandular secretory acini of the pancreas,** which release their secretory products into a series of branched ducts leading to the duodenum. H&E, paraffin, × 200.

Thus, the connective tissues show a wide range of morphological variation, a fact that students often find difficult to comprehend. The solution to this problem is a systematic study of the major histologic appearances, keeping in mind the broad generalization that in connective tissues the cells usually occupy a minor proportion of the tissue, with intercellular matrix predominating.

The basic forms are loose and dense connective tissue (Fig 2.11a–c). *Loose connective tissue* has few cells and much extracellular material not tightly packed together. Gaps, holes/spaces of areolar tissues contain transparent material forming a semi-fluid gel, supported by various types of fibers, notably collagen and elastin. Fat/adipose tissues and reticular tissues often forming a meshwork of fibers also belong to this class.

Dense connective tissue (Fig 2.11d–f) contains variable proportions of cells, but the intercellular materials are plentiful with few, if any, spaces. This tissue is characterized by masses of collagen/elastin/ground substance or, in the case of bone, crystalline matrix. This type of connective tissue thus confers strength and/or variable degrees of elasticity or plasticity.

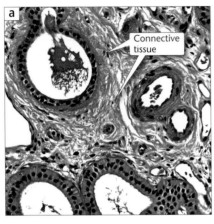

▲ **Fig 2.11a Loose connective tissue** surrounding ducts and blood vessels, consisting of scattered fibroblast nuclei, and collagen fibers mixed with amorphous extracellular materials. H&E, paraffin, × 150.

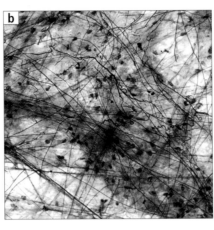

▲ **Fig 2.11b A spread of mesentery**, showing randomly oriented elastin fibers. H&E, × 120.

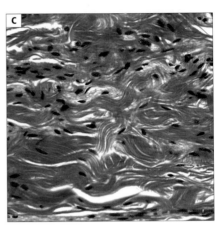

▲ **Fig 2.11c A meshwork of reticular fibers** providing support for the parenchyma of a lymph node. Reticulin method, paraffin, × 180.

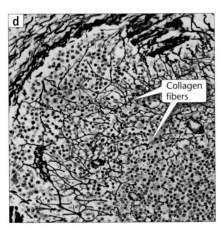

▲ **Fig 2.11d Dense connective tissue**, showing bundles of collagen fibers with irregular orientations. Scattered cell nuclei are fibroblasts. H&E, paraffin, × 300.

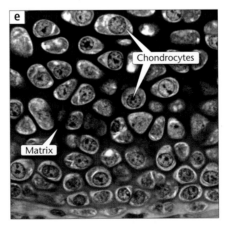

▲ **Fig 2.11e Dense connective tissue of cartilage surrounding many chondrocytes.** Cartilage is a dense matrix of collagen and proteoglycans. H&E, acrylic resin, × 350.

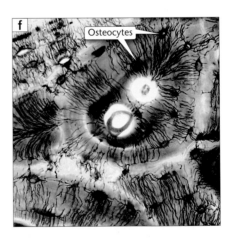

▲ **Fig 2.11f Dense connective tissue of bone**, showing osteocytes with many extending processes. The surrounding matrix of organic and inorganic elements contains collagen and calcium, and phosphate in a mineralized form. Silver stain, paraffin, × 250.

Muscle tissue

Muscle is composed of muscle cells called muscle fibers because of their elongated shape. The types of muscle are skeletal, cardiac, and smooth muscle (Fig 2.12a–c). In the cytoplasm of muscle cells, special contractile proteins—actin and myosin—are arranged such that, in response to an appropriate stimulus (generated intrinsically or via innervation), these proteins interact to produce relative movement between them (i.e. contraction of the cells, fibers, and whole muscle). *Skeletal muscle* is the most abundant type and is striated (dark and light bands), owing to segregation or interdigitation of actin–myosin; chiefly, it moves bones relative to one another. *Cardiac muscle* (the heart) is also striated but, unlike skeletal muscle, which is largely under voluntary neural control, it has an inherent contractile rhythm that can be modified by the autonomic nervous system. *Smooth muscle* is not striated and may have intrinsic motility, or contract in response to neural stimulation. Smooth muscle forms the walls of most arteries, veins and many hollow organs of the gut, respiratory, and urogenital systems. Exocrine glands are often surrounded by modified smooth muscle cells (myoid cells).

Nerve tissue

Nerve tissue forms the brain, spinal cord, peripheral nerves (including 12 pairs of cranial nerves), ganglia (clusters of neurons located outside the central nervous system) and special receptors. The *nerve cell or neuron* consists of a cell body (nucleus and cytoplasm) and

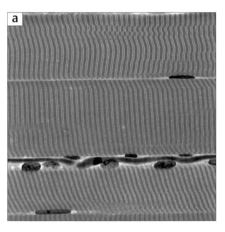

▲ **Fig 2.12a Skeletal muscle**, showing typical striations and multiple peripheral nuclei. H&E, acrylic resin, × 250.

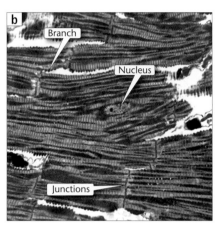

▲ **Fig 2.12b Cardiac muscle cells**, showing branching, a centrally located nucleus, striations, and intercellular junctions. Toluidine blue, araldite, × 500.

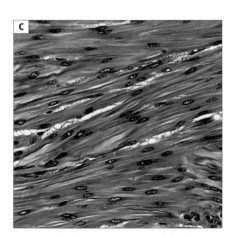

▲ **Fig 2.12c Smooth muscle cells**, showing central nuclei and lack of striations. H&E, paraffin, × 250.

73

extending nerve fibers composed of many dendrites and one axon (Fig 2.13a & b). Dendrites conduct impulses toward, and axons transmit signals away from, the cell body. Nerve tissue is fragile and soft, and its complex structure often makes it difficult to reconcile the fact that it is composed of cells and supporting material. Axons connect nerve cells via synapses (junctions) between neurons; thus the nervous system is made up of billions of individual cells, just like other tissues.

Neuroglia, or glial cells, are non-excitable supporting cells present in great numbers (5–10 times more numerous than neurons) in the central nervous system (Fig 2.13c). They provide structural and functional support, but they are the most common

source of central nervous system tumors (gliomas, astrocytomas).

Peripheral nerves may be myelinated or unmyelinated (Fig 2.13d). In both types, the axons are ensheathed by associated Schwann cell cytoplasm (analogous to a glial cell, but of neural crest origin). In myelinated nerves, Schwann cell cytoplasm winds spirally around the axon, forming the myelin sheath. In unmyelinated nerves, the axons are embedded in recesses of Schwann cell cytoplasm, but myelin is absent.

Ganglia (Fig 2.13e) are thickenings of bundled nerve fibers that contain encapsulated nerve cell bodies and glial cells in the peripheral nervous system. They function as relay stations for sensory or motor pathways. The equivalent structures in the

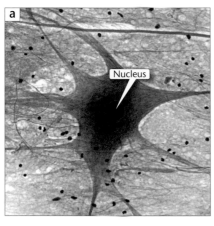

▲ **Fig 2.13a A motor neuron cell body,** showing numerous extensions consisting of dendrites and one axon. The nucleus is located centrally and is surrounded by dense materials that represent organelles and inclusions. H&E, spread prep, × 500.

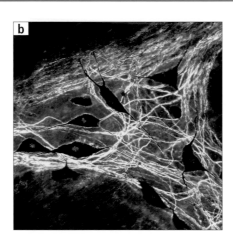

▲ **Fig 2.13b Cluster of nerve cell bodies in the muscle wall of the gut.** Note the dendritic extensions and many axons and dendrites of the neural network. Silver and gold stain, thick section, × 300.

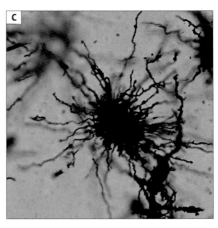

▲ **Fig 2.13c Glial cells of the brain,** typically showing many cytoplasmic extensions that provide attachment/ communication with adjacent cells. Golgi stain, paraffin, × 500.

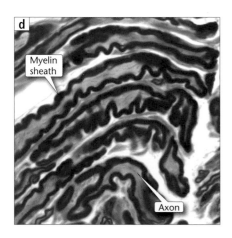

▲ **Fig 2.13d Longitudinal profile of myelinated nerves.** The myelin sheaths are stained blue and the axons stain weakly. Toluidine blue, araldite, × 500.

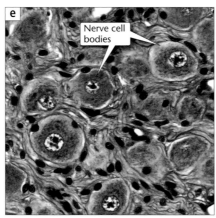

▲ **Fig 2.13e A cluster of nerve cell bodies within a ganglion.** Supporting cells and nerve fibers are located between the neurons. H&E, paraffin, × 350.

brain are the islands of gray matter called nuclei deep within the cerebrum and cerebellum.

Integration of tissues into the body plan

The reason why the origins of cell and tissue types have been reviewed as separate classifications is because it is a convenient method for discriminating differences or similarities in both morphology and function (Fig 2.14). In organs and the systems that they form during fetal and postnatal growth and development, however, many cell types and usually several or all of the primary tissue types are not separate but integrated into functional unions. These arrangements present a challenge—to recognize and understand the functions of the cells and tissues of normal organs during their development and when fully formed. If this challenge can be met, it provides a strong foundation for the interpretation

Tissue	Type	Structure	Examples	Embryonic origin
Epithelial	Simple	Squamous	Inner lining vessels, serous membranes	Mesoderm
		Cuboidal	Renal collecting tubules	Mesoderm
		Columnar	Sweat glands, secretory coil, lens epithelium	Ectoderm
			Inner lining gut	Endoderm
	Stratified	Squamous	Epidermis, cornea	Ectoderm
		Cuboidal	Excretory sweat ducts	Ectoderm
		Columnar	Large salivary gland ducts	Ectoderm
	Pseudostratified	Columnar	Trachea	Endoderm
	Transitional	Squamous + cuboidal + columnar	Urinary bladder	Endoderm
Connective	Loose	Areolar	Subcutaneous tissue	Mesoderm
		Adipose	Subcutaneous tissue, organ-associated fat	Mesoderm
		Reticular	Framework of lymph node, spleen, liver	Mesoderm
	Dense	Irregular	Dermis of skin	Mesoderm
		Regular	Tendon/ligament, cartilage, bone	Mesoderm
	Specialized	Cells and fluid	Blood	Mesoderm
Muscle	Smooth	Spindle	External wall of hollow viscera, many vessels	Mesoderm
	Cardiac	Branching cylinders	Wall of heart	Mesoderm
	Skeletal	Multinucleated cylinders	Skeletal muscle attaches to bone or cartilage or dense connective tissue	Mesoderm
Nerve	Cells	Neurons	CNS: gray matter of cerebral cortex, cerebellum, gray matter and nuclei of brain and spinal cord	Ectoderm
			PNS/ANS: ganglia	Ectoderm
		Neuroglia	Astrocytes	Ectoderm
			Oligodendrocytes	Ectoderm
			Microglia	Mesoderm
			Ependyma	Ectoderm
	Processes	Myelinated	CNS and PNS, most fibers of ANS	Ectoderm
		Unmyelinated		
	Receptors	Free, encapsulated	Skin, cornea, dermis	Ectoderm

ANS = autonomic nervous system; CNS = central nervous system; PNS = peripheral nervous system

▲ **Fig 2.14** Simplified classification of primary tissue types.

of histopathology, developmental biology, and the contributions to both made by the cell types found in the individual tissues, be they normal or otherwise modified. The specimen shown in Figure 2.15, a late-gestation rat embryo, is an example of such a challenge. Choose any component of the body and test your knowledge of (i) germ layer/s origin, (ii) primary tissue types present, (iii) definitive tissues types, and (iv) known or probable cell types.

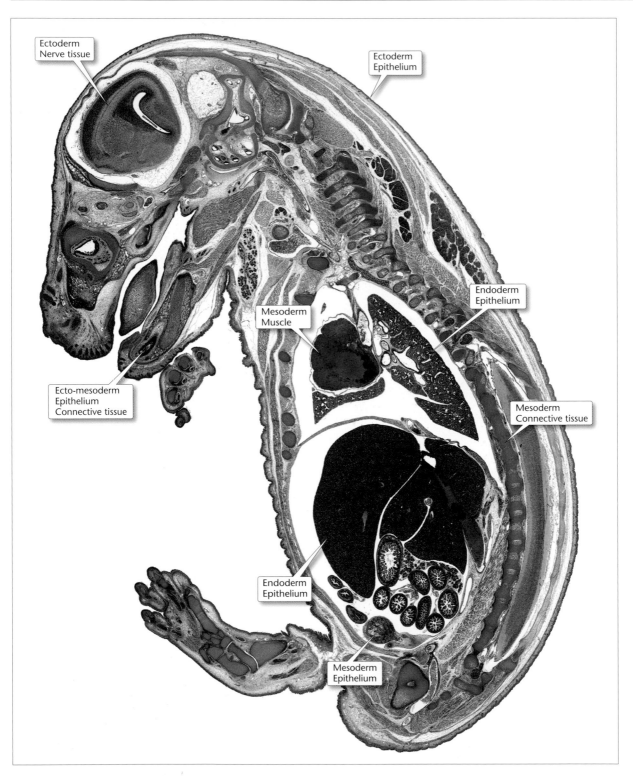

▲ **Fig 2.15 Rat embryo of 20 days' gestation.** Various organs or tissues are shown, indicating their origin from the embryonic germ layers and the primary tissue type(s) present. H&E/alcian blue, paraffin, × 12.

Blood

Blood is a special type of liquid connective tissue with a total volume of approximately 5 liters in an average human adult. The cellular elements comprise about 45% of blood volume, with the major fraction consisting of a protein-rich fluid called plasma. For diagnostic purposes the analysis of blood is performed more often than the analysis of any other tissue. The study of blood and blood-forming tissues encompasses basic, clinical, and laboratory sciences within the specialty of hematology; it is linked to other disciplines such as immunology, pathology, molecular genetics, and oncology with regard to the diagnosis and treatment of a wide range of disorders and diseases that either affect or are manifest in blood.

When learning about the histology of blood and bone marrow, the usual approach is to examine stained blood films and bone marrow smears, together with sections of the medullary cavity of bone that contains marrow. Although specimens of marrow reveal the highly cellular nature of this tissue, the histology of the blood film displays its formed elements but gives no indication of the true complexity of the tissue. More than 50 parameters may be measured in routine clinical laboratory tests on blood samples, excluding specific assays or assessments of microbial infection, antibodies, hormone levels, and special chemistry. Analysis of blood is also important for forensic investigation.

A basic understanding of the biology and medical significance of the blood and bone marrow requires consideration of the following topics:

- The formation of blood cells commences with bone marrow stem cells and is controlled by growth factors and/or hormones.
- Hemopoiesis differs between the embryo, fetus, and adult.
- The identification of various types of blood cells, and their normal proportions and functions.
- The function of hemoglobin (Hb) and coagulation and blood-group systems, particularly the ABO and Rhesus systems.
- Disorders of bone marrow and the formed elements of blood.

BONE MARROW

Bone marrow is a complex, highly cellular tissue which, in human adults, is restricted to the medullary cavities of selected bones. Approximately half of bone marrow mass is hemopoietically active red marrow, while the remainder is inactive yellow marrow and consists of adipose tissue (more predominant in yellow bone marrow) with clusters of hemopoietic cells (Fig 3.1a–d). Active marrow serves a number of functions, including:

- The formation and release of various types of blood cells (hemopoiesis).
- Steady-state renewal to replenish the loss of mature blood cells by continuous production of new cells.
- Phagocytosis of cellular debris and/or degenerating cells, and storage and recycling of iron essential for Hb synthesis.
- The production of immunoglobulins.
- Mobilization of cell reserves and/or acceleration of their development, and anatomic expansion of blood cell types into medullary cavities.

Morphology

The structure of bone marrow in histologic sections of normal human adults shows densely packed cords and islands of hemopoietic cells, between which are ramifying vascular sinuses (Fig 3.2). The marrow is supported by a connective tissue stroma of reticular cells and fibers that forms a delicate meshwork between islands or cords of hemopoietic cells together with fat cells. Macrophages are numerous and the vascular supply, derived from nutrient arteries, ramifies to form extensive plexuses of blood sinusoids; newly formed blood cells enter these from the bone marrow and exit the tissue through collecting veins.

In neonates and infants, the marrow cavities of bone are almost 100% red marrow, but during childhood and with increasing age red marrow is gradually, but incompletely, replaced by yellow marrow. In adults, red marrow persists in the sternum, ribs, vertebrae, clavicles, scapulae, pelvis, cranial bones, and proximal ends of the femur and humerus. Degeneration into gelatinous marrow may occur in the cranial bones in old age, or in cases of anorexia nervosa or starvation. Among the enormous numbers of nucleated marrow cells are stem cells, which are self-renewing and develop into various differentiating and/or proliferating blood-cell lineages. These cells account for about one per 10,000 to 100,000 marrow cells, the most primitive of which is the pluripotent hemopoietic stem cell (HSC).

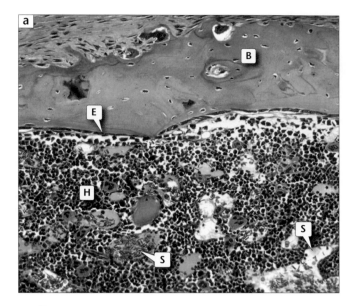

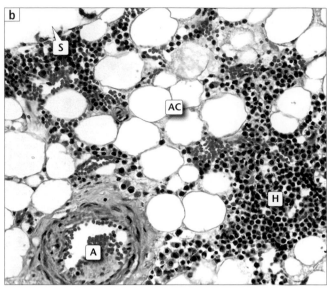

▲ **Fig 3.1a Red bone marrow.** Medullary cavity of a long bone that shows the highly cellular bone marrow deep to the endosteum (**E**) of compact bone (**B**). The cords of hemopoietic cells (**H**) are typical of red marrow (i.e. very little fat is present). Numerous vascular sinusoids (**S**) carry the newly formed blood cells to the venous system. The extent and organization of bone marrow is labile and alters rapidly in response to therapeutic agents, illnesses, and numerous stimuli. Hematoxylin and eosin (H&E), paraffin, × 150.

▲ **Fig 3.1b Yellow bone marrow.** This contains variable quantities of adipose cells (**AC**) and islands of hemopoietic tissue (**H**); both components are supported by a meshwork of connective tissue made of reticular cells and fibers. Vascular sinusoids (**S**) are derived from capillaries that are developed from nutrient arterioles (**A**). Intersinusoidal spaces are always filled with red or yellow marrow cells. H&E, paraffin, × 250.

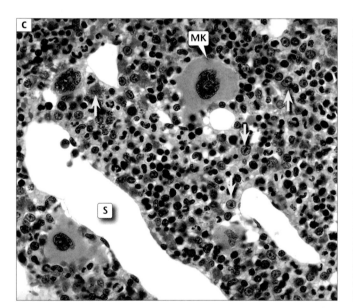

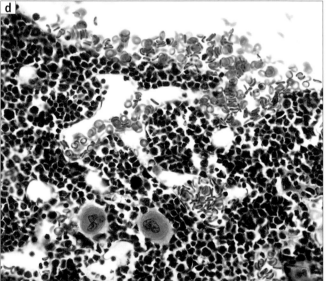

▲ **Fig 3.1c Hemopoietic tissue.** Megakaryocytes (**MK**), which enlarge and fragment to produce platelets, are the largest of the hemopoietic cells, usually 60 μm in diameter. The hemopoietic tissue is crowded with cells, some of which represent reticular cells and macrophages (**arrows**); the sinusoids (**S**) appear empty because of postmortem blood drainage. Hemopoietic stem cells are renewable and their myeloid and lymphoid progeny mature and proliferate to replace the more than 10^{11} blood cells normally lost each day. H&E, paraffin, × 350.

▲ **Fig 3.1d Bone marrow vascular sinusoids.** These contain many blood cells, mostly erythrocytes, that represent a mixture of circulating and newly formed cells. Release of the latter into the sinusoids is believed to take place across (transcellular) rather than between the endothelial cells. This event probably occurs by a combination of cell pressure and modification of the sinusoid walls by locally produced and circulating releasing factors. H&E, paraffin, × 300.

Origin

Traditionally, the origin and development of bone marrow in the embryo and fetus is considered first to involve the extraembryonic yolk sac, in which developing erythrocytes arise from mesodermal cells (erythropoiesis) at about 3 weeks' gestation. Thereafter, the fetal liver (Fig 3.3) and, to some extent, the spleen become the main hemopoietic sites during the second trimester, followed by the fetal bone marrow. However, recent studies in the fetal mouse, supported by immunohistochemical investigations of human embryo sections, show that founder cells for the blood system also arise from intraembryonic sites and colonize the liver; the bone marrow is later seeded and established as the principal hemopoietic tissue. The placenta is also believed to be a source of blood cells.

Multipotent blood cell progenitors (i.e. stem cells able to produce red and white blood cells) arise de novo from trunk mesoderm (para-aortic splanchnopleure, PAS), followed by the appearance of pluripotent HSCs in the region of the dorsal aorta, primitive gonads, and mesonephric tissue (AGM). In mice, there is evidence that blood-forming progenitor cells from the yolk sac can contribute to HSCs in adults. This suggests that HSCs within the AGM may at least in part originate from yolk sac progenitors. As the PAS–AGM region is transformed during organogenesis, the fetal liver is colonized by HSCs, which later in fetal life seed the bone marrow and thus establish it as the only normal site of hemopoietic tissue after birth. The factors that induce mesoderm and hemopoietic tissue formation are probably members of the transforming growth factor β superfamily and fibroblast growth factor family. Formation of erythrocytes and other blood cells in the yolk sac, PAS–AGM, and the liver is necessary because of the relatively slow development of the skeletal system and limited availability of cavities within the skeleton that can serve as a favorable environment for definitive hemopoiesis.

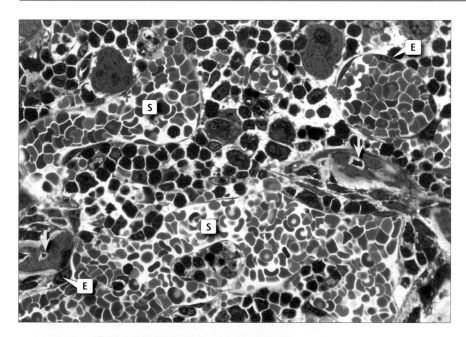

◀ **Fig 3.2 Bone marrow in situ**, showing detail of blood sinuses (**S**) containing many erythrocytes, and the cords of hemopoietic tissue with developing blood cells. The cords also contain bone cells (osteocytes, **arrows**) and are separated from the sinuses by endothelium (**E**). Toluidine blue, araldite, × 600.

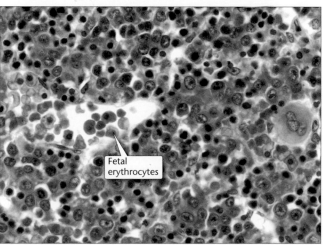

◀ **Fig 3.3 Fetal liver showing hemopoiesis.** The formation of blood cells in the human embryonic liver begins in week 6 and soon thereafter is responsible for the relatively large size of the liver in the fetal period. Liver hemopoiesis in humans peaks during fetal months 4–6. H&E, paraffin, × 400.

Hemopoiesis

The pluripotent or long-term HSC is self-renewing and is required for lifelong persistence of the whole hemopoietic system. This pool of relatively rare HSCs produces short-term HSCs that, in turn, give rise to two types of lineage-committed stem cells—the myeloid stem cells and the lymphoid stem cells. Both of these are thought not to self-renew, but are directed toward the proliferation and differentiation of progressively more specialized cells that belong to their particular lineages. Thus the differentiation of HSCs is characterized by HSCs at the top of a blood-cell hierarchy that extends to cell lineages with progressive loss of self-renewing ability and an increase of mitotic activity. Stem cells cannot readily be identified with certainty in vivo, but in culture these cells and their immediate descendants (i.e. committed progenitor cells) show large nuclei and cytoplasm rich in polyribosomes. All HSCs (pluripotent or committed progenitors) express the cluster of designation (CD) 34 surface antigen (a group of monoclonal antibodies that recognize cell surface antigens), but this marker is not expressed on normal mature white cells of blood and marrow.

In vitro, stem cells can be characterized on the basis of their ability to produce colonies of differentiating cells from which one or more types of blood cells arise. These colony-forming units (CFUs) are proliferative. Under the influence of various growth factors, CFUs produce irreversibly committed immature cells (or blast cells) of particular types, which proliferate and mature into blood cells. In bone marrow smears, blast cells are histologically distinct and show a morphology that resembles the cells that they form.

A general scheme of hemopoiesis (Fig 3.4) indicates the myeloid and lymphoid lineages and includes three cell types known to derive from bone marrow (dendritic cells [but not all types], mast cells, and natural killer lymphocytes), but the precise development of each of these is unclear. All the cells of the myeloid lineage are released into the blood sinusoids of the bone marrow. For the lymphoid pathway, this also applies to the natural killer cells, but the B and T lymphocytes enter the circulation as mature and/or naïve cells, in the sense that their further maturation into antibody-forming plasma cells, or functional T cells, occurs in the secondary lymphoid organs and in the thymus, respectively. Stem cells and CFU cells may occur in blood, but only in very small numbers (usually less than one in 1,000 leukocytes).

Regulation

Regulation of hemopoiesis relies upon surface interactions between stem cells and the bone marrow stroma, as well as on the action of numerous growth factors, mostly glycoproteins, which have broad multilineage or lineage-specific, hormone-like effects on hemopoietic tissue. The extracellular environment is critically important for the maintenance of marrow niches in which stem cells grow and mature. Many of the growth factors are produced locally in the marrow from reticular and endothelial cells, macrophages, and T cells; an exception is erythropoietin, which is produced mainly in the renal cortex.

Hemopoietic growth factors include interleukins, stem-cell factor, and a range of colony-stimulating factors (CSFs) that promote the development of one or more CFUs (e.g. GM-CSF [granulocytes, macrophages and dendritic cells in culture], M-CSF [macrophages], and G-CSF [granulocytes]). These growth factors may act synergistically, or one type may stimulate or inhibit the production and/or activity of another, and all seem to inhibit apoptosis, and thus allow further cell proliferation and/or maturation.

The biology of hemopoietic growth factors is complex and details are available in hematology texts. In clinical medicine, these factors have considerable importance in therapeutic approaches to bone marrow disorders. Preparations of G-CSF and GM-CSF may be used to stimulate hemopoiesis after radio- or chemotherapy, and to harvest HSCs and their progenitors from blood; these are used later in stem-cell transplantation.

Histologic study

Histologic study of marrow is best performed on smears, since cellular details are revealed clearly; however, tissue sections are required for the pathologic investigation of marrow in situ. A thorough discussion of the morphology of the many different cell types of the hemopoietic process is beyond the scope of this book, and therefore the basic features are summarized here.

> **Tip:** A bone marrow sample may be obtained by (i) aspiration using a needle inserted into a marrow cavity (often sternum or pelvis), which yields a "gritty" fluid used to make a smear; or (ii) trephine, in which a long, hollow wide-bore needle is used to extract a core of bone including marrow (often from the iliac crest). The sample is formalin fixed, decalcified, and sectioned, allowing a panoramic view of marrow architecture.

Erythropoiesis

Erythropoiesis, or red blood cell development, is recognized by the appearance of the pronormoblast (or proerythroblast), which proliferates and matures into a series of erythroblasts (Fig 3.5a). Red cells mature within erythroblast islands in which a central macrophage extends cytoplasmic protrusions to a ring of surrounding nucleated erythroblasts. These islands

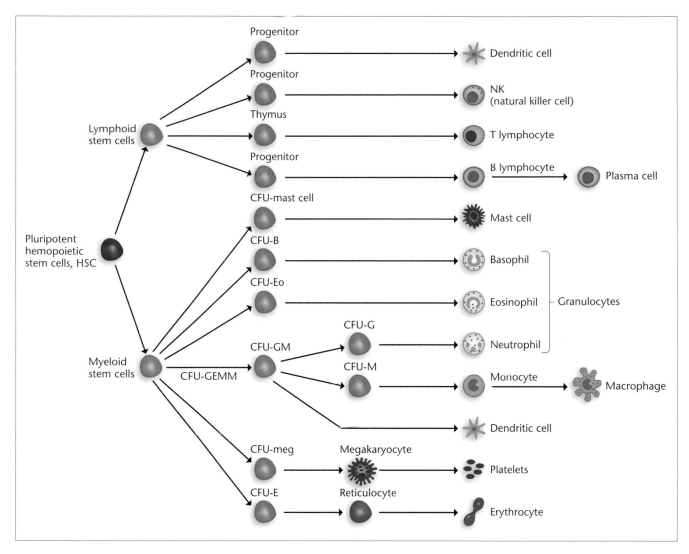

▲ **Fig 3.4 Hemopoiesis.** Pluripotent hemopoietic stem cells give rise to stem cells of the myeloid and lymphoid blood cell lineages; this activity is stimulated by various growth factors that act either broadly or upon specific lineages. The divisions within the myeloid pathways are indicative only, and similar hierarchical models vary between authoritative works on hematology. The myeloid lineage, possibly including the mast cells, arises from a colony-forming unit, CFU-GEMM (granulocytes, erythrocytes, monocytes, megakaryocytes), which is a multipotent stem cell that gives rise to the various committed progenitors designated as CFUs. Dendritic cells (i.e. antigen-presenting cells) are known to arise from either common myeloid or lymphoid progenitors. Mast cells are postulated to arise from a CFU mast cell, and this progenitor, or a promastocyte, enters the circulation and forms mast cells in the appropriate tissues.

also occur in the fetal liver. Erythroblasts synthesize Hb and finally extrude their nuclei to become marrow reticulocytes. These cells contain ribonucleic acid (RNA), which appears as granules (with cresyl blue staining), from which the final 35% of Hb is produced as the reticulocytes circulate in blood for 1–2 days before becoming mature erythrocytes. In mammals, fetal erythrocytes contain a nucleus (Fig 3.5b). Red cells of adult amphibians, reptiles, fish, and birds also have nuclei.

Erythropoietin (EPO) growth factor is derived mainly from the kidney and in minor amounts from the liver, and stimulates erythropoiesis and Hb synthesis. The three forms of Hb are embryonic, fetal (HbF), and adult (HbA); HbA predominates from 6–12 months after birth and accounts for 99% of adult blood Hb. The higher affinity of HbF for oxygen (compared with that of HbA) possibly facilitates the transfer of oxygen from the maternal to the fetal circulation.

Tip: In adults about 10 billion red cells are made each hour, producing over 400 mL per week (just under 1 pint). Red cell production is controlled by erythropoietin. To counterbalance this production, aging red cells are destroyed in the spleen and liver by macrophages. Hemoglobin is metabolized to (i) iron and amino acids that are recycled; (ii) other products of heme breakdown that become bile pigments excreted by the liver, gut, and kidneys.

Granulocytopoiesis

Granulocytopoiesis generates the granular leukocytes or polymorphonuclear leukocytes (irregular or multilobed nuclei) that comprise the neutrophils, eosinophils, and basophils; of these, the development of neutrophils is the best understood. The appropriate CFU forms myeloblasts, which proliferate into promyelocytes with granule formation, then into myelocytes, followed by a stage with horseshoe-shaped

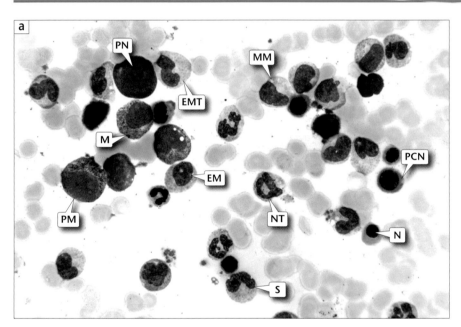

▲ **Fig 3.5a Erythroblast series:** The pronormoblast (**PN**, large nucleus, small cytoplasm) produces 8–32 erythrocytes; polychromatic normoblasts (**PCN**, round nuclei, moderate cytoplasm) synthesize much hemoglobin, the last stage of mitosis; normoblasts (**N**, smaller nucleus) carry out no DNA synthesis, prenuclear extrusion stage.
Neutrophilic series: Promyelocyte (**PM**, large cell, dark granules); myelocyte (**M**, round nucleus, small granules), the last stage of mitosis; metamyelocytes (**MM**, kidney-bean nuclei, mostly small secondary granules); stab cells (**S**, horseshoe-shaped nuclei), first stage that may appear in blood; neutrophils (**NT**, segmented, lobular nuclei).
Eosinophilic series: Myelocyte (**EM**, eosin-staining granules); metamyelocyte (**EMT**, plump S-shaped nucleus, eosinophilic granules). H&E, smear, × 750.

nuclei, indented nuclei ("band" or "stab'" cells), and finally mature neutrophils with extensively lobulated nuclei. Eosinophils and basophils show similar phases of development with respective coarse, red-staining granules or purple–black granules, but usually have only a bisegmented nucleus (Fig 3.5c).

Mast cells

Mast cells are related to basophils and probably develop from a CFU. Although this progenitor has yet to be identified, it is known that human mast cells arise from CD34-positive HSCs and possibly produce promastocytes similar to those identified in mouse fetal blood. Mature mast cells

are not normally seen in blood but complete their development typically in connective tissues.

Monocytopoiesis

Monocytopoiesis gives rise to the monocyte–macrophage lineage via monoblasts and promonocytes, which derive from the CFU granulocyte–macrophage (GM) progenitor. During their maturation the nuclei are often indented, bean-shaped, and finally horseshoe-shaped or slightly lobulated within a cell. The monocyte cell is among the largest (about 20 μm diameter) in the marrow. Granules are uncommon, and when monocytes leave the blood they mature into macrophages.

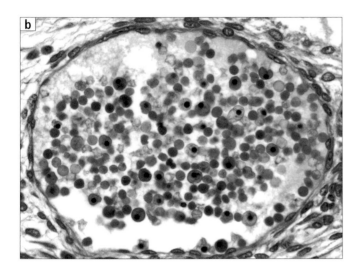

◀ Fig 3.5b Embryonic and fetal red blood cells may be nucleated with 5–10% showing a nucleus in week 12, then declining rapidly thereafter. At birth about 0.1% red cells are nucleated, but this feature is uncommon 4 days after birth. Persistence of nucleated red cells is associated with disorders such as hemolytic disease, hemorrhage, or hypoxia. H&E, paraffin, × 450.

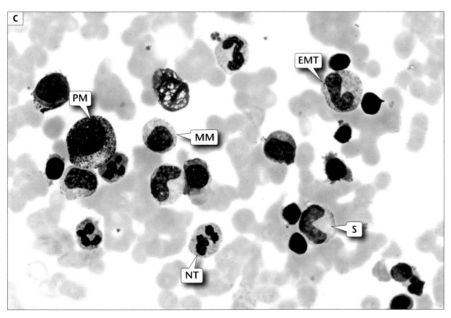

◀ Fig 3.5c Eosinophilic series: This shows maturational changes similar to neutrophilic development, but differs in that eosinophils form reddish-orange granules: promyelocyte (**PM**, large cell, many granules); eosinophil metamyelocyte (**EMT**, large sausage-shaped nucleus, eosinophilic granules). **Neutrophilic series:** Metamyelocytes (**MM**, ovoid–elliptical nuclei, small granules); stab cells (**S**, horseshoe- or hook-shaped nuclei); neutrophils (**NT**, segmented, lobular nuclei, small granules). H&E, smear, × 750.

Dendritic cells

Dendritic, or antigen-presenting, cells also arise (in vitro) from the CFU-GM, and leave the marrow to populate peripheral lymphoid tissues by vascular distribution (Fig 3.6). These cells may also arise from a lymphoid lineage, but little is known about their precise hemopoietic origin (for more information, see Ch 11).

Lymphocytopoiesis

Lymphocytopoiesis gives rise to the agranular leukocytes, or lymphocytes, that form into two main classes, the T and B lymphocytes, together with a third population of large, granular lymphocytes (natural killer cells). In bone marrow, histologic maturation is recognized by the presence of lymphoblasts, prolymphocytes, and lymphocytes, and is characterized by a high nucleus:cytoplasm ratio. The B cells emerge from the marrow to populate secondary lymphoid tissues, whereas T cells home in on the thymus during fetal and postnatal life, where they are processed to form immunocompetent T lymphocytes; these events are discussed in Chapter 11.

Platelet production

Platelet production, or megakaryocytopoiesis, commences with a CFU-GEMM (granulocyte, erythrocyte, monocyte, megakaryocyte) forming a CFU-meg, from which arises the megakaryoblast.

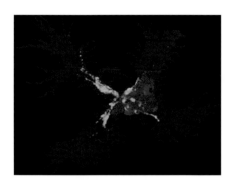

◀ **Fig 3.6 An isolated dendritic cell viewed with fluorescence microscopy.** Present in skin and throughout the body, dendritic cells are antigen-presenting cells. They capture antigen and via the vascular system travel to lymph nodes to interact with T lymphocytes. × 1,700. (Courtesy J Villadangos, Walter & Eliza Hall Institute, Melbourne, Australia.)

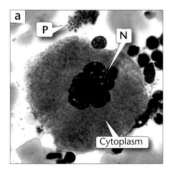

◀ **Fig 3.7a Mature megakaryocytes** have a multilobulated, polyploid nucleus (**N**, with 8–32n sets of chromosomes) and a huge cytoplasm that results from endomitotic maturation. Cytoplasmic particles are separated by membranous channels that form partitions between future platelets. At release, proplatelet clumps (**P**) are seen and at times form ribbons or sheets, like postage stamps, which disperse to enter marrow sinusoids. Early stages of development (CFU-meg, megakaryoblast) respond to marrow growth factors; thrombopoietin regulates megakaryocyte development. H&E, smear, × 700.

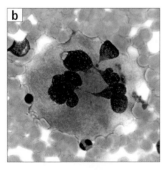

◀ **Fig 3.7b Advanced lobulation of megakaryocyte nucleus**, showing attenuated linkages between interconnected nuclear components. The atypical nuclear morphology is a result of duplicated chromosomes becoming incorporated into a single growing nucleus with numerous lobes, but cytokinesis is not completed. H&E, smear, × 600.

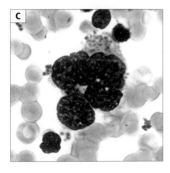

◀ **Fig 3.7c Fragmentation of the megakaryocyte** and discharge of thousands of platelets leaves the nucleus surrounded by a thin cytoplasmic rim. These cells degenerate and are eliminated by bone marrow macrophages. The period from the megakaryoblast stage until the platelets are shed into the marrow sinuses is about 1 week. H&E, smear, × 650.

This cell matures into a megakaryocyte by a process termed endomitosis, in which deoxyribonucleic acid (DNA) content is repeatedly doubled without nuclear or cytoplasmic division; this results in the formation of very large cells up to 60 µm or more in diameter with multilobulated nuclei that contain 4–32N or more sets of chromosomes (Fig 3.7a–c). The finely granular cytoplasm (Fig 3.8) fragments into platelets about 2–3 µm in diameter and numbering in the thousands per cell. Discharged into the marrow sinusoids, the platelets (Fig 3.9) circulate in blood, where they become available to form hemostatic plugs at sites of damage to vascular endothelium. Platelet production is stimulated by thrombopoietin growth factor, produced mainly by the liver, but also by the kidney and bone marrow.

BLOOD

Blood is composed of formed cellular elements, the red and white blood cells and the platelets suspended in a clear, slightly yellow fluid called plasma. In normal adults, blood volume is in the range 4.5–6.0 L (about 1–1.3 gallons), of which 55% by volume is plasma, about 45% is erythrocytes (i.e. the blood fraction or hematocrit), and 1% or less contains the leukocytes (white cells) and platelets.

The functions of blood are numerous and complex, and involve not only the formed elements, but also the very many substances dissolved in the plasma that reflect the metabolic activities of the tissues, connected via the blood circulation. Some main functions include:

- Distribution of oxygen to all tissues, and waste carbon dioxide and nitrogenous products, respectively, to the lungs and kidneys
- Transportation of nutrients processed by the gut and liver
- Regulation of body temperature, pH, electrolytes, glucose and cholesterol levels
- Maintenance of vascular fluid volume
- Protection against infection and prevention of blood loss following injury.

Plasma is about 90% water; if the clotting proteins it contains are removed, the fluid is called serum. The main dissolved substances in plasma are proteins (mostly albumin, along with immunoglobulins, clotting proteins and enzymes of metabolism, as well as many other proteins related to metabolism), respiratory gases, organic nutrients, waste products of metabolism, and numerous electrolytes.

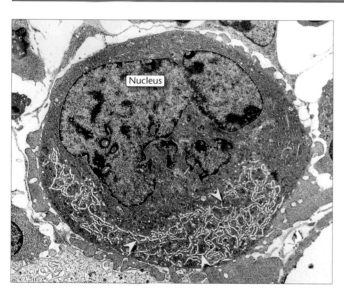

▲ **Fig 3.8 Ultrastructure of a megakaryocyte**, showing many cytoplasmic channels (**arrowheads**), the result of invagination of the cell membrane. With further development, the cell extends many pseudopodia, which use microtubules to elongate and form thin proplatelet processes with bulbous ends. These are dynamic structures that bend and bifurcate to greatly increase the numbers of free tips. Packets of platelet material are delivered to the tips, which disengage to release proplatelets from the megakaryocyte body. × 3,800. (Courtesy P Cross, Stanford University, California, USA.)

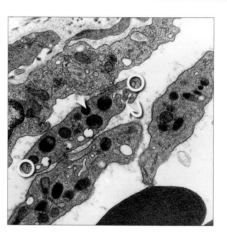

▲ **Fig 3.9** Ultrastructure of platelets showing their discoid shape. Platelets circulate for about 10 days before they are removed, mainly by splenic macrophages. They contain several types of granules (**arrowhead**), among which are lysosomes and others containing fibrinogen or platelet-derived growth factor (PDGF), the latter stimulating repair of blood vessels in wound healing. Coagulation factors from platelets may be released into the canalicular system (**curved arrow**). At the periphery of the platelet are microtubules (**circles**) forming a ring around the platelet to stabilize its shape. × 15,000. (Courtesy P Cross, Stanford University, California, USA.)

Formed elements

Each of the three main classes of formed elements (i.e. erythrocytes, leukocytes, and platelets) has some unusual features:

- Two of the three are not true cells—erythrocytes have no nuclei or organelles and the platelets are very small pieces of cytoplasm derived from fragmentation of bone marrow megakaryocytes.
- Leukocytes are complete cells.
- Some of the formed elements survive for only a few days and must be replaced, whereas others may survive for 20 years or possibly longer.
- Most blood cells do not divide and are replenished by hemopoiesis in the bone marrow.
- Some cells known to occur in blood may be seen rarely because of their low numbers and/or lack of distinctive histologic features.

In stained blood films, seven types of elements can be identified on the basis of shape, size, color, and nuclear–cytoplasmic morphology. Erythrocytes are by far the most abundant (about 99% of the total number), followed by platelets and then leukocytes. The very small size of platelets dictates that they are best identified with oil-immersion or high-dry objective lenses.

Leukocytes are composed of cells of five different types, often classified into two groups. Granulocytes display cytoplasmic granules (i.e. neutrophils, eosinophils, and basophils) and are cells mainly concerned with phagocytosis and inflammation. Granulocytes, particularly the neutrophils, may sometimes be called polymorphonuclear leukocytes because of their irregular, multilobulated nuclei. The second group of leukocytes lack prominent visible granules when examined in routine blood films and may be called agranular leukocytes, but are more commonly known by their definitive names— lymphocytes and monocytes. Lymphocytes are key elements concerned with humoral and cell-mediated immunity, and monocytes are a source of phagocytic cells.

Blood cell concentration or percentage values and the reference ranges of common hematologic values vary between textbooks, and in normal adults physiologic differences may occur according to age, sex, and geographic location. No fixed rule regarding individual blood cell size applies because of differences between living cells and stained, fixed preparations.

> **Tip:** A useful way to remember the relative proportions of leukocytes (in descending order) in normal blood is given by the mnemonic "never let monkeys eat bananas" (i.e. neutrophils, lymphocytes, monocytes, eosinophils, and basophils), as indicated in Fig 3.10.
>
> Blood films may be examined with or without a coverslip. With a low power objective lens, select a field towards the thinner end of the film in the mid region. Use an oil-immersion lens (60× or 100×) to examine the cell morphology in detail. Red blood cells heavily outnumber leukocytes (the white blood cells) by 500–1000:1.

Erythrocytes

Erythrocytes are biconcave in shape, anucleate, and may be likened to flexible (deformable) bags filled with Hb that transport oxygen from the lungs to tissues, and carbon dioxide from tissues to lungs (Fig 3.11a–c). A net of deformable, cytoskeletal proteins deep to the plasma membrane allows erythrocytes to change shape as they pass along the smallest capillaries and enter the splenic red pulp through capillary fenestrations that are 3 µm wide.

Properties of the main classes of formed elements in the blood							
	Erthrocytes	**Platelets**	**Neutrophils**	**Eosinophils**	**Basophils**	**Monocytes**	**Lymphocytes**
Size, µm	7	2–3	9–15	12–17	10–14	15–20	7–16
Lifespan in circulation	4 months	10 days	1–2 days	1–2 days	Hours–days	3 days	3 days–20 years
Differential leukocyte count	(99% of all elements)	–	60%	1–3%	0–1%	4–10%	20–30%
No. per µL	5×10^6	3×10^5			7×10^3		

▲ **Fig 3.10** Some properties of the main classes of formed elements of the blood.

When oxygen from lung alveoli diffuses into the blood and then into the erythrocytes, it combines reversibly with the heme iron pigment of Hb to form oxyhemoglobin with a characteristically bright-red color. Carbon dioxide taken up from the tissues is mainly (70%) dissolved and carried in blood plasma, but some carbon dioxide is loaded into the erythrocytes by reaction with the globin fraction of Hb. The red blood cell count is approximately 4–6 million/µL in adult males and 4–5.5 million/µL in females and children. Hb concentration in males is 13–16 g/dL (130–160 g/L or 80–99 mmol/L) and 12–15 g/dL in females (120–150 g/L or 74–93 mmol/L).

Aging erythrocytes are destroyed by macrophages, mainly in the spleen, but also in the liver and bone marrow; the Hb is degraded to yield globulins, which contribute amino acids to general metabolism. The iron is retrieved and recycled for new Hb synthesis or stored in the liver; the porphyrin fraction is converted into the yellow pigment bilirubin, which is processed in the liver and secreted into bile.

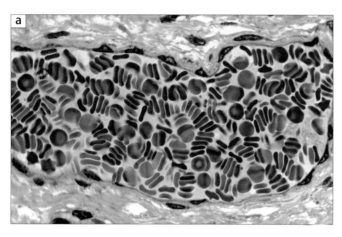

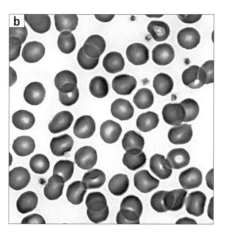

▲ **Fig 3.11a Erythrocytes.** Immobilized by the fixation of tissues, red blood cells are often found in sections of blood vessels, particularly veins, and venules. Note the variable shape of the erythrocytes, which reflects the plane of section and their capacity to reversibly deform. Flexibility of corpuscle shape allows the erythrocytes to squeeze along the narrowest capillaries (8–10 µm in diameter) and enter the red pulp of the spleen (3–4 µm wide fenestrations in sinusoids), where the most aged erythrocytes (4 months) are destroyed. H&E, acrylic resin, × 600.

▲ **Fig 3.11b In stained blood films, erythrocytes** are flattened and spheroid, and usually 7–7.5 µm in diameter. A central, pale-staining core is the thinnest aspect of the red blood cell, which reflects the biconcave disk shape (similar to a donut with a solid core). The pink staining with common Romanowsky-type stains results from the large amount of hemoglobin (90% of cell dry weight) that transports 97% of oxygen in the blood; most blood carbon dioxide is transported as bicarbonates in the plasma; this conversion occurs via carbonic anhydrase in erythrocytes. Romanowsky stains for blood or bone marrow smears contain dyes such as methylene blue or azure dyes, and eosin. Specific stains in common use are May-Grünwald-Giemsa (MGG), Wright's stain, or Leishman's stain. Depending on the technique the erythrocytes may be shades of pink or blue-gray. × 800.

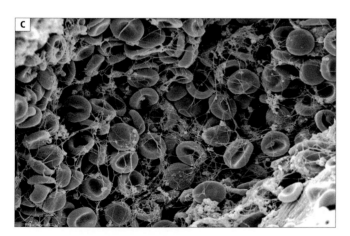

▲ **Fig 3.11c Scanning electron micrograph of erythrocytes**, showing their discoid biconcave shape, which gives a large surface-to-volume ratio for efficient gas exchange. The presence of fibrin strands indicates the early phase of blood coagulation. × 1,000. (Courtesy K Tiekotter, University of Portland, Oregon, USA.)

Platelets

Also known as thrombocytes, platelets prevent bleeding by aggregating to form a platelet plug at sites of vascular endothelial damage. Discoid in shape, they contain a highly organized cytoskeleton and a variety of secretory granules (see Fig 3.9). Platelets form a barrier to blood loss (hemostasis), referred to as a hemostatic plug. Platelets are thus responsible for blood coagulation; the factors involved and their regulation comprise a complex series of interactions between the platelets, injured endothelium, and numerous circulating enzymes and proteins within the plasma.

Following vessel injury, platelets adhere to subendothelial tissue, and convert from discoid to spheric shapes with projections or pseudopods that enhance aggregation. Next, the platelets are activated and, with continued aggregation, release the contents of their granules; the contents activate plasma and tissue-derived clotting factors that stimulate the production of the protein thrombin within plasma; in turn, thrombin converts plasma fibrinogen into a mesh of insoluble fibrin fibers, which encourages platelet fusion and the formation of stable hemostatic plugs (Fig 3.12). Some platelet granules release platelet-derived growth factor, which stimulates proliferation and repair of fibroblasts and smooth muscle cells to heal the vascular wall.

Blood coagulation is normally self-terminating in response to a range of specific circulating or local inhibitors (e.g. antithrombin, heparin) and by dilution of clotting factors with blood flow. In the inherited disorder hemophilia, clotting factors (e.g. factor VIII) are deficient, which results in spontaneous bleeding into joints or muscles.

> **Tip:** Hemophilias are of various types and are commonly an inherited deficiency of factor VIII or IX, the genes for which lie on the X-chromosome. Mutant forms cause the X-linked recessive traits hemophilia A and B and are usually expressed in males. Hemophilia affected the royal houses of Europe. In severe cases of hemophilia, many episodes of bleeding may occur after minor trauma involving muscles or joints. Advances in treatment options have included safer plasma-derived factors and recombinant antihemophilic factors.

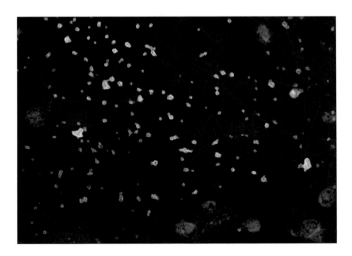

▲ **Fig 3.12 Hemostatic plug formation.** Human vascular endothelial cell culture coated with whole-blood-induced clotting in cell-free spaces. Fibrin is red; activated platelets, now stellate in shape, are yellow-green (DAPI). Coagulation of blood is a complex series of reactions in which a cascade of activating factors promote, in the final steps, the conversion of prothrombin to thrombin, the latter catalyzing the conversion of fibrinogen to a cross-linked network of fibrin fibers. In addition to adherence to injured vascular endothelium and aggregation, platelets accelerate the clotting process by providing a large surface area onto which clotting factors are adsorbed. Fibrin fiber clots entrap blood cells, platelets, and plasma. Vascular leaks are thus closed, preventing blood loss. × 1,700. (Courtesy J Zbaeren, Inselspital, Bern, Switzerland.)

Neutrophils

Neutrophils account for 50%–60% of all leukocytes and are phagocytes that engulf and kill bacteria or dead or damaged cells, usually at sites of tissue inflammation to which they are attracted. Neutrophils enter tissue compartments by adhesion or margination with vascular endothelium, followed by emigration from the blood by passing between endothelial cells. Their numerous, small, bluish-purple granules represent forms of lysosomes (Fig 3.13a & b). When an activated neutrophil has engulfed a pathogen by phagocytosis, the granules fuse with ingested microbes and/or particles to form a phagolysosome, within which oxidizing compounds kill or degrade their target. Neutrophil granules also contain many other antimicrobial substances, such as proteases, acid hydrolases, and lysozyme.

Neutrophils are important effector cells of the innate immune defense system. Following destruction of ingested foreign material, neutrophils die and, if their participation in acute inflammatory reactions is intense or prolonged, their enzymes may liquefy host cells and foreign material to form a viscous semi-fluid residue, pus. Neutrophils are terminally differentiated cells and cannot divide. Their short life span, limited to 1–2 days, demands their continual replacement from bone marrow hemopoietic tissue, which itself is substantially devoted to their production. Recent findings have shown that neutrophils can kill bacteria in the absence of phagocytosis by generating webs of extracellular fibers containing DNA, histones, and elastase. Designated as neutrophil extracellular traps (NETs), these fibers bind and trap bacteria and immobilize high concentrations of antibacterial proteins that kill bacteria and thus control infection.

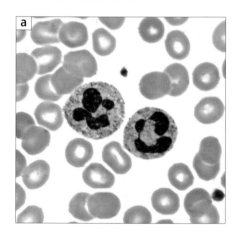

◀ **Fig 3.13a Neutrophils.** The most abundant of the leukocytes (about 60%), neutrophils (also called polymorphonuclear neutrophils or polys) contain a segmented nucleus with lobes connected by a thin, nuclear filament. Many small granules occur in the cytoplasm and contain dozens of proteins (hydrolases, proteases, oxidases, and other microbiocidal agents); these allow neutrophils to exercise their main function—phagocytosis and elimination of bacteria, dead cells, or foreign matter—particularly at sites of inflammation and infection, to which they are specifically attracted. Although neutrophils are often the first leukocytes to arrive at such sites, they are short-lived, and die having performed their phagocytic role; therefore, of all the types of leukocytes, the neutrophils are produced in relatively large numbers by bone marrow. May-Grünwald-Giemsa (MGG), × 1,000.

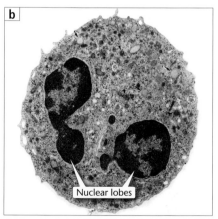

Nuclear lobes

◀ **Fig 3.13b Ultrastructure of a neutrophil,** showing two of the nuclear lobes and numerous cytoplasmic granules, such as azurophilic lysosome granules, specific neutrophilic granules, and tertiary granules. Azurophilic granules contain acid hydrolases and antibacterial agents; specific granules have lysozyme and degradative enzymes. Together these granules form phagolysosomes, which are involved with the phagocytosis and destruction of microorganisms and foreign matter. Tertiary granules have many proteolytic enzymes believed to be required for their migrations through connective tissues. Large amounts of glycogen in the cytoplasm supply energy for the neutrophil to function in anaerobic environments. × 8,000. (Courtesy M Pavelka and J Roth; from Functional ultrastructure. Vienna: Springer, 2005 with permission.)

Eosinophils

Slightly larger than neutrophils, but far less abundant, eosinophils perform several functions, including killing of parasites, a limited capacity to phagocytose bacteria, and modulation of allergic and inflammatory responses by phagocytosis of antigen–antibody complexes and by liberation of proteins that suppress the activity of other leukocytes. Their prominent cytoplasmic granules reflect storage of the eosinophil proteins, dark-red to crimson in color with appropriate stains (Fig 3.14). Most of the protein cytotoxic for parasites forms a crystalloid core visible only by electron microscopy (Fig 3.15). When bound to a parasite, the eosinophil releases its granules directly onto the parasite membrane, initiating membrane disruption.

Eosinophils may be found in connective tissues deep to mucosal surfaces that are exposed to the external environment.

Basophils

The smallest of the granulocytes, basophils are scarce in blood films, but their deep-violet, cytoplasmic granules, which often obscure the segmented cell nucleus, make them readily identifiable (Fig 3.16). The granules are relatively homogeneous (Fig 3.17) and contain histamine, which acts as a vasodilator, and heparin (an anticoagulant). Basophils complete their development in hemopoietic tissues, enter the blood, and are seen in peripheral tissues if recruited to sites of immune or inflammatory responses. Activated

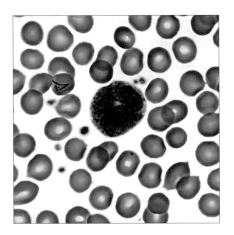

◀ **Fig 3.14 Eosinophils**. Slightly larger (12–17 μm diameter) than neutrophils, the eosinophils comprise 1–3% of the leukocytes and are recognized by their nucleus (usually two lobes) and cytoplasm filled with orange–red granules. These contain major basic and cationic proteins, specific neurotoxin, and peroxidase, which together are cytotoxic for protozoa and parasites, enable limited phagocytosis of bacteria, and are regulatory for several other immune cells such as T cells and mast cells. Eosinophils participate in inflammatory reactions (skin allergies, some forms of asthma), as they secrete factors that inactivate histamine and leukotrienes derived from basophils and/or mast cells and, thus, restrain the intensity of the inflammatory response. MGG, × 1,000.

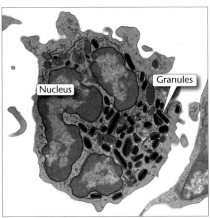

◀ **Fig 3.15 Ultrastructure of an eosinophil**, showing the characteristically large cytoplasmic granules and lobulated nucleus. The crystalloid body in granules is major basic protein and, with other proteins, is toxic for protozoa and helminthic parasites. Granules are directed to killing parasites following binding of the eosinophil. × 6,700.

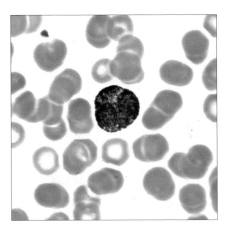

◀ **Fig 3.16 Basophils**. The smallest (10–14 μm in diameter) of the granular leukocytes and the least commonly encountered in blood films (0–1%), basophils exhibit violet or black granules that overlie the usually bilobular nucleus. Known to be a separate cell type to the tissue mast cell that they resemble, both cell types, when activated in inflammatory and hypersensitivity reactions, degranulate to release histamine, heparin, and slow-reacting substance of anaphylaxis. Allergens, in particular, bind to IgE receptors on basophils, which activates them and degranulation is initiated. This reaction results in vascular dilatation, bronchoconstriction, leakage of capillary fluid into tissues, and attraction of granulocytes to the reactive site. These allergic reactions result in various responses: hay fever, urticaria (hives), allergic asthma, and anaphylaxis (disseminated reaction). MGG, × 1,000.

particularly in allergic reactions through their surface IgE receptors, basophils degranulate and rupture, and the substances above (and others) cause local tissue reactions and symptoms associated with hay fever, urticaria (hives), and allergic asthma.

> **Tip:** Basophils and mast cells are often considered to be the "bad guys" of the blood system because of their roles in allergic reactions, hay fever, asthma, and anaphylaxis. But they may also qualify as "good guys" by immune reactions to parasites and innate immune responses to bacteria.

Monocytes

Usually larger than other leukocytes, monocytes show a central, ovoid, U-shaped, or indented nucleus, and the cytoplasm contains some small vacuoles and fine particulate granules (Fig 3.18). Although small in number and size (Fig 3.19), the granules store lysosomes used in the degradation of engulfed cells, microbes, or foreign matter (such as cellular debris and particulate matter). Circulating for up to several days, monocytes select and settle into many tissues, where they mature into macrophages; both cell types constitute the mononuclear phagocyte system.

In addition to phagocytosis, monocytes and/or macrophages capture antigens and present this to antigen-specific T lymphocytes, which in turn play key roles in directing cell-mediated and humoral immune responses. Monocytes and macrophages also synthesize and secrete interleukins for the stimulation of hemopoiesis in bone marrow; these growth factors have important biological effects on attraction and activation of leukocytes, especially lymphocytes, in numerous immune reactions.

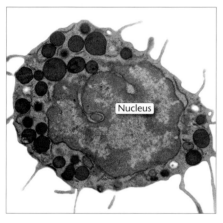

▲ **Fig 3.17 Ultrastructure of a basophil** from mouse connective tissue, with dense cytoplasmic granules (but fewer than in mast cells) and a typical lobulated nucleus. × 8,000.

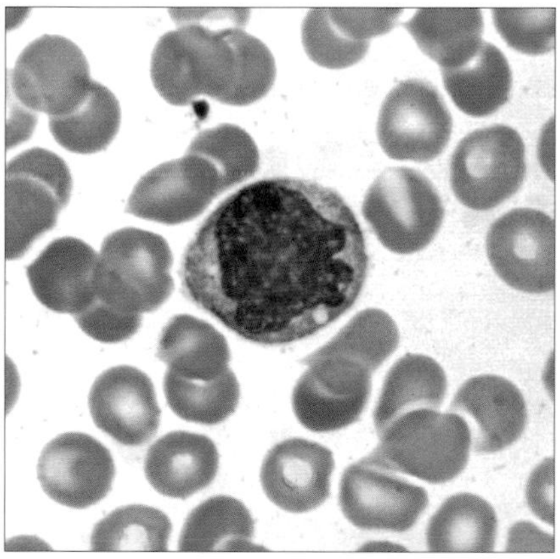

◀ **Fig 3.18 Monocytes.** The largest (15–20 μm diameter) of all cells seen in normal blood films, monocytes have irregular, slightly lobulated nuclei, often bean- or kidney-shaped, and a fine, particulate cytoplasm with occasional vacuoles. Monocytes contain lysosomes, the number of which increases as the monocytes leave the blood within a day of their appearance to mature into macrophages, which are extensively distributed in tissues that form the mononuclear phagocyte system. Monocytes (and macrophages) are vigorous phagocytic cells that engulf and destroy bacteria, as well as those cells and many types of materials recognized as foreign. Monocytes (and macrophages) are secretory, activating other immune cells and, importantly, they capture, process, and present antigens to specialized T lymphocytes and thereby activate a wide range of immune responses. MGG, × 1,000.

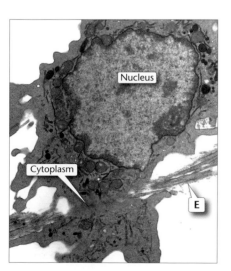

◀ **Fig 3.19 Ultrastructure of a monocyte** migrating across the endothelium (**E**) of a blood vessel, where it will differentiate into a tissue macrophage. The few lysosomes in the monocyte cytoplasm increase in number and size as the cell transforms into a macrophage, thereby conferring phagocytic capability. × 5,200.

Lymphocytes

Lymphocytes account for about one-third of all leukocytes. Although in blood smears they all look similar (Fig 3.20: round nucleus, thin-to-moderate cytoplasmic rim, no visible granules), functionally they comprise many millions of different clones of lymphocytes, broadly designated as B cells (from the bone marrow) and T cells (immature lymphocytes that originate in the bone marrow, but differentiate in the thymus).

Small- (7–10 μm) and large-diameter (11–16 μm) lymphocytes are noted in blood smears, but their size and morphology do not represent distinct classes or functionally different lymphocytes; identification of lymphocyte type requires the use of monoclonal antibodies. B cells give rise to antibody-secreting plasma cells, whereas T cells form subtypes that help other cells in immune reactions or produce cytotoxic lymphocytes that kill targeted cells. The role of lymphocytes in the immune system is considered in Chapter 11.

DISORDERS AND CLINICAL COMMENTS
Anemias

Anemia occurs when the Hb concentration is below the normal range associated with the age and sex of the individual, and is a symptom of some disorder in which oxygen-carrying capacity is abnormally low. Disorders that result in anemia include excessive blood loss, shortened erythrocyte survival, impaired erythrocyte function, inadequate nutrition, or increased plasma volume.

Iron-deficiency anemia is the most common blood abnormality, and perhaps the commonest non-infectious disorder worldwide. Inadequate supply of iron may occur because of inadequate diet, malabsorption, chronic or excessive hemorrhage (gastrointestinal, occasionally uterine), and normal menstruation.

Bone marrow also requires sufficient vitamins, such as folic acid and vitamin B_{12}, to maintain adequate DNA synthesis during erythropoiesis. In pernicious anemia, the gut fails to absorb sufficient B_{12}, which results in enlarged cells of the erythroblastic lineage in bone marrow and blood.

Hereditary anemias associated with abnormal Hb synthesis may be associated with serious illnesses (not necessarily a direct consequence of the anemia), and bone marrow transplantation may be an effective treatment. Abnormal variants of Hb structure (hemoglobinopathies) include sickle-cell anemias, whereas depression of the rate of Hb synthesis constitutes the thalassemia syndromes. In the former, the erythrocytes are distorted when they carry little oxygen, which results in vascular occlusion/hypoxia and causes pain (called sickle cell crises); the cells are short-lived, which results in anemia. In thalassemic disorders, one of the globin chains of Hb is absent or inadequately produced and the erythrocytes are typically pale and small, with reduced life expectancy.

Leukemias

Leukemias arise as bone marrow neoplasms, which form many abnormal white cells that normally enter the circulation and infiltrate the tissues. The disease includes a wide range of conditions from the severe and rapidly fatal to mild forms with good prognosis that require intermittent treatment. Leukemic cells are produced from transformed HSCs or CFUs that proliferate uncontrollably to form expanding clones of neoplastic cells. Leukemias are associated with decreased erythrocytes (anemia), decreased functional white blood cells (infections), and decreased platelets (bleeding disorders).

The etiology of leukemia is not well understood and, although several factors are known to be involved, it is likely that multiple mechanisms contribute to leukemogenesis. Among the etiological factors are radiation (e.g. from nuclear explosions), chemicals (e.g. benzene, alkylating agents), viruses

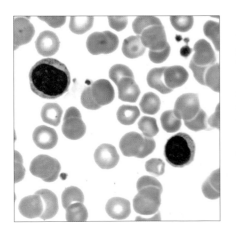

◀ **Fig 3.20 Lymphocytes.** The main function of lymphocytes is to react with specific antigens, which activate these cells to produce antibodies, or to stimulate other leukocytes, including other lymphocytes, to directly attack microbes, infected tissue, or foreign material recognized as antigenic. Circulating lymphocytes are of variable sizes (7–16 μm in diameter), mainly because of cytoplasmic volume, but the two main subtypes, T cells and B cells, cannot be identified with routine histology. The life span of lymphocytes ranges from a few hours to 20 years or more, and they often recirculate between lymphoid tissues, lymphatics, and blood. Together with macrophages and other antigen-presenting cells, they form the basis of the immune system (discussed in Ch 11). MGG, × 1,000.

(e.g. human T cell leukemia virus), genetic disorders (syndromes with chromosomal abnormalities), and environmental factors (as yet unclear).

Acute or chronic leukemias refer to the clinical progress in untreated patients, associated with short-term (weeks or months) or long-term (years) survival. Acute leukemias are associated with immature or abnormal leukemic cells of high malignancy and occur at any age. Acute lymphoblastic leukemia (ALL) is the common form of acute leukemia in children; acute myeloid leukemia (AML) is more common in adults. Many affected children who have ALL are cured by chemotherapy alone or in combination with bone marrow transplant (BMT), but these treatments are less successful in adults who have ALL. Most cases of AML have a poor, 5-year survival rate.

Chronic lymphoblastic leukemia (CLL) is the most common form of chronic leukemia; it is rarely found in children, and is usually associated with increased lymphocyte counts. With respect to the accumulation of abnormal lymphocytes and peripheral organ involvement, CLL is progressive; survival rates are in the range 1–20 years and chemotherapy is the usual treatment.

The white cell count is elevated in chronic myeloid leukemia (CML), which is less frequently encountered in adults than is CLL, and is rare in children. Gradually, CML transforms from a chronic or "stable" phase to advanced or accelerated phases, with an average survival of 5–6 years, but the range is wide. Treatments include interferon-g (interferon gamma—antiproliferative), hydroxyurea (impairs DNA synthesis), busulfan (alkylating agent), or BMT.

> **Tip:** With automated blood cell analyzers, the necessity for examining a blood smear (film) has declined and may only represent 10% of blood samples. Often, smears are needed when the blood count is abnormal, the autoanalyzer detects an unusual profile, or the clinical features suggest a thorough definitive diagnosis. Smears may be important in cases of specific infections and for diagnoses of thrombocytopenia (low platelet count), anemia, leukemia, lymphoma or bone marrow failure.

Human blood groups

Erythrocyte plasma membranes bear specialized proteins (antigens), the presence or absence of which allows blood cells to be classified into several major groups. Antigens that determine ABO and Rhesus factor (Rh) groups cause adverse transfusion reactions if one type is recognized as foreign by another; this results in agglutination and destruction of erythrocytes. Blood typing is always performed before transfusion.

The antigens that promote agglutination, type A and type B, form the basis of the ABO system; the frequency of ABO groups varies in different populations. In Caucasians nearly half the population have group O (i.e. neither A nor B antigens, or agglutinogens), about 40% have group A, around 10% have group B, and 3%–4% have group AB. Group O individuals were known as "universal donors," but this is a misleading concept as this group carries preformed antibodies in plasma (anti-A, anti-B), called agglutinins. Agglutinins are thought to arise from the absorption of substances by the gut. They have very similar antigenic properties to A and B groups, but are not present on the red cells. Very occasionally, donor O blood may contain sufficiently potent anti-A or anti-B to react with recipient blood and cause erythrocyte destruction. In practice, only matched blood types are used for transfusions.

The Rh system, first discovered in rhesus monkeys, encompasses a range of erythrocyte antigens, of which the D antigen is clinically the most important; it occurs in about 85% of individuals, who are termed Rh-positive (Rh+). The remainder are Rh-negative (Rh−). Transfusion of Rh+ blood into an Rh− recipient is not harmful, although antibodies against the Rh+ blood are formed. A subsequent, similar transfusion (perhaps several months) later may induce a reaction, as the newly formed antibodies agglutinate the Rh+ erythrocytes.

Similar problems arise in pregnant Rh− women who carry Rh+ babies; the first pregnancy is usually uneventful, but anti-Rh antibodies may be formed in the mother's circulation. If an Rh+ baby occurs in a subsequent pregnancy, maternal antibodies destroy the baby's erythrocytes, a condition termed hemolytic disease of the newborn, which is associated with anemia and hypoxia, and may be fatal. Protection against this outcome is achieved by treatment of these women at delivery during pregnancy, and again (if the newborn is Rh+) at delivery, with RhoGAM (anti-Rh gamma globulin), which prevents the production of anti-Rh antibodies.

Bone marrow transplants (BMT)

Intravenous infusions of whole marrow BMTs have been used for over 50 years to treat disorders of the blood and immune systems. Originally used as unfractionated tissue, in more recent years hemopoietic stem cell transplantation techniques have improved with cell purification and appropriate patient preparation. Apart from autologous transplants, success of BMT is limited by histocompatible donors, which is only around one-third of a given patient's family members. Half-matched donors for BMT (parents and children) may be a source of highly purified hemopoietic stem cells but are associated with unacceptably high rates of recipient mortality. Gene therapies for hemopoietic stem cell transplants have been used successfully in selected patients but, at present, the wider use of this approach is at the experimental stage.

Epithelium

Epithelial tissues cover inner and outer surfaces of the body and, in forming glands, fulfill a secretory function. Epithelial cells form continuous sheets that act as boundaries between the environment facing the free surface and the underlying tissues. Epithelia may consist of single or multiple layers of cells (with multiple functions), and the cells may vary in shape, size, and orientation. Terminology is therefore based on morphological description.

The recognition and classification of epithelia are based on a systematic appraisal of all the individual components. Having become familiar with the identification of the various types of epithelia, it is not always necessary to memorize their functions, because the size, shape, location, and organization will often provide a strong clue. As a surface layer covering the body or lining the inner surfaces of hollow structures, such as tubes or body cavities, epithelial cells serve many functions—protection, selective permeability, secretion, absorption, transport along their surface, and sensory perception. Epithelial cells are closely associated with each other, with very little material between apposing cells.

DIVERSITY OF EPITHELIAL CELLS
Development and homeostasis

The range of phenotypes and subdivisions into physiologically distinct compartments of epithelial tissues reflects their widespread distribution throughout the body. Most reviews of the biology of epithelial cells in the context of histology are concerned with their structure and functions in adult tissues relating to homeostasis. Epithelial cells also have fundamental roles, however, in the morphogenesis and growth of the embryo and fetus, as well as in postnatal organ and tissue development. Because epithelia are derived from all three embryonic germ layers (ectoderm, mesoderm, and endoderm), they are defining features of organ design, with an impressive repertoire of activities and characteristics.

Embryologic origins and diversity

Epithelia may be derived from any one of the three germ layers:
- Endoderm (an epithelial tissue) gives rise to epithelia of the gut, respiratory system, urinary bladder, liver, gall bladder, pancreas and other epithelial glands associated with the gut.
- Ectoderm (also an epithelial tissue) forms the epithelia of the skin and its glandular derivatives, as well as oral, nasal, and anal passages.
- Mesoderm (mesenchymal tissue) gives rise to epithelial linings of the cardiovascular system (i.e. endothelium) and to mesothelium lining the peritoneal, pleural, and pericardial cavities and various tubules, ducts, and accessory glands of the urogenital system.

Epithelial architecture

A distinctive phenotype of multicellular organisms (the metazoa) is epithelial tissue organization, and even the simplest animals such as *Hydra* consist of two concentric cylinders of epithelial cells. The ability to form sheets and layers of cells that are molded, folded, and grown into organ systems in higher animals is a hallmark of epithelia. Figure 4.1 lists some of the characteristics that allow epithelial cells to build

Epithelial characteristic	Function or role
Cell–cell adhesion	Critical for multicellular tissues and organs, between cells and at their base
Cells are polarized	Defines three surfaces (apical/free, lateral and basal) with corresponding asymmetric internal organization
Cells form sheets	With growth and modeling, this is the forerunner of geometric tissue and organ shapes
Anchored to an extracellular matrix	Essential for epithelial organization and interactions with adjacent tissues
Cell proliferation	For repair and renewal of most epithelia
Avascular	Does not have own blood or lymphatic supply
Barrier function	Protection, absorption, secretion, sensory
Forms glands	Most glands are derived from epithelial cells

▲ **Fig 4.1** Characteristics of epithelial cells and their functional attributes.

and maintain complex organs. All of these features are operative during the development of epithelial tissues either pre- or postnatally, and collectively they maintain homeostasis in epithelial-derived adult organs, particularly in relation to controlling what enters and exits such organs.

Descriptions of the different types of epithelial tissues and their associated functions in adults usually follow a familiar and systematic theme. Although this approach is important for the purpose of learning histology, the role of epithelia in organs will make more sense if the biology of epithelial cells is first reviewed before describing how they are classified and recognized in the organs to which they contribute.

Changing shape and pattern

Epithelial cells often form single or multilayered sheets, but this simple arrangement is obviously different for internal organs and the many glands within them or those existing independently. How does a sheet of cells alter shape to bend, twist, and fold? Molecular signals are not the exclusive forces that cause shape change in communities of cells. The creation of non-linear epithelial layers can be associated with simple mechanical stress resulting from widespread cellular movements, for example

during embryogenesis. Physical pressure applied to epithelial sheets is followed by activation of genes, such as *TWIST*, which regulates invagination to form tubules or cylinders. Mechanical compression causes movement of β-catenin proteins from some epithelial cell membranes into the nucleus where shape-changing genes are thought to be activated. How do such genes bring about "shape change"? A fundamental property of epithelial cells is their polarity (i.e. not all regions of an epithelial cell are necessarily created equal), an essential feature for their development and function that includes generation of a range of cell shapes.

Cell polarity

Epithelia are polarized. The orientation and shape of the cells, their organelles, and inclusions, and the composition of their membranes enable them to sequester specialized functions to different domains within each cell. Almost all cells show polarity, a property conserved from yeast to humans.

As a hallmark of epithelia, polarity is expressed in cell shape, contents, surface specializations, associations with adjacent cells, and, perhaps above all, spatial distribution of functional duties (Fig 4.2, Fig 4.3). Epithelial cells are genetically programmed to become polarized, but environment also exerts a major influence through external interactions

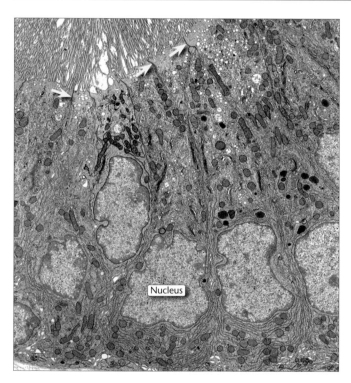

▲ **Fig 4.2 Ultrastructure of columnar epithelial cells,** showing polarized distribution of organelles. The rough endoplasmic reticulum is concentrated in the basal regions, and the Golgi membranes, lysosomes, and endocytic vesicles are found in the apical domains. Note plasma membrane densities (**arrows**) subjacent to the apical surface. These represent intercellular junctions. × 4,000.

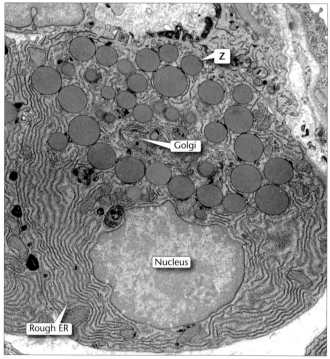

▲ **Fig 4.3 Ultrastructure of an epithelial glandular cell from the pancreas.** The basolateral regions of cytoplasm are dominated by rough endoplasmic reticulum. Golgi membranes are found in the central cytoplasm and the zymogen secretory granules (**Z**) are located in the mid-to-apical domains of the cell. × 10,000.

with other cells or the extracellular matrix. A good example is the response of epithelial cells to dissociation when isolated and grown in culture: The cells may lose much of their polarity (especially surface characteristics), but this is reversed when the cells are grown on a suitable collagen gel or extracellular matrix.

Three surfaces are the norm

Although epithelial cells differ in their morphology and function, their cell membranes share a common property—an asymmetric organization of their lipids and proteins giving apical/basal polarity. The cell membranes are organized into three domains: an *apical* surface (often facing a lumen), a *lateral* surface adherent to adjacent cells, and a *basal* surface facing the extracellular matrix, comprising the basal lamina and the vascular supply (Fig 4.4). Importantly, an adherens tight junction separates apical from basolateral membranes, creating surface polarity and, in accompaniment, internal cell polarity generated by membrane trafficking.

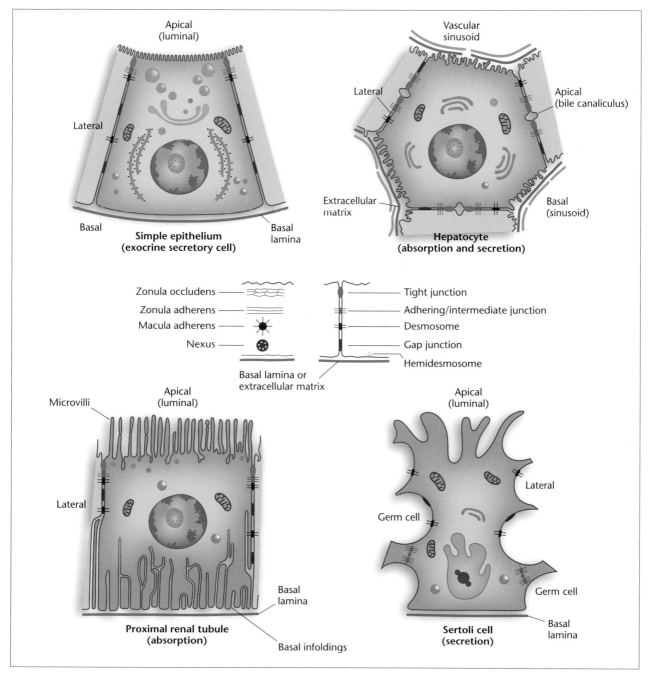

▲ **Fig 4.4 Polarity in epithelial cells.** Vectorial functions of epithelial cells are reflected in the polar organization of their surface plasma membranes and distribution of their organelles. Typically, the cell surface shows structural and functional specializations on the apical, lateral, and basal domains, as indicated by the four examples. Domains are separated by junctional complexes, which also provide intercellular attachment. Hemidesmosomes anchor to the basal lamina. Gap junctions allow electrical and metabolic coupling. Folding of surface membranes increases surface area for absorption or secretion. (Modified from Simons K, Fuller SD. Ann Rev Cell Biol 1985; 1:243–88.)

Apical and basolateral epithelial cell membranes regulate the movement of water, electrolytes, molecules, microorganisms, subcellular components, or whole cells across the epithelium. The processes involved include transcellular and intercellular diffusion, transcytosis of macromolecules within vesicles, endocytosis (inward transport) of membrane for subsequent recycling or degradation of unwanted substances by phagocytosis (engulfment of whole cells or parts thereof), pinocytosis (inward transport of small vacuoles) of fluids or regulatory molecules, and exocytosis (outward transport) or release of substances synthesized within the epithelial cell.

These properties have led to the hypothesis that the attainment of three surface types drives epithelial morphogenesis, in which each surface domain "fits" or "does not fit" into a specific location unique to that epithelial tissue.

Surface specializations

Modifications to plasma membrane surfaces are a striking example of epithelial cell polarity. Microvilli are short (about 1 μm in length) finger-like projections found on the surface of many epithelial cells. They are particularly abundant in the apical membrane of absorptive epithelia such as the intestinal mucosa (Fig 4.5) and proximal tubules of the kidney. Microvilli greatly increase the surface area of the apical membrane and thereby enhance the rate of absorption into cells. Very long microvilli are called stereocilia because they resemble true cilia in terms of size and shape but, in fact, they are not motile (Fig 4.6a & b).

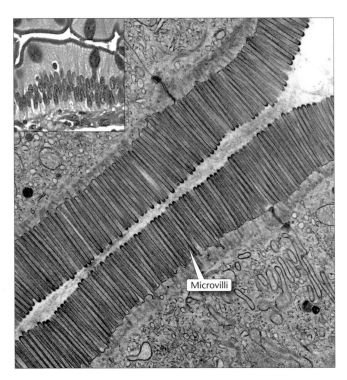

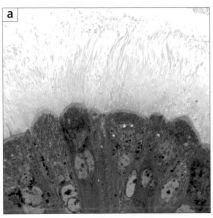
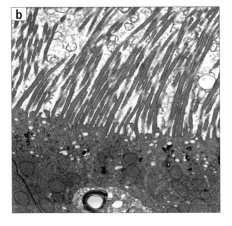

◀ **Fig 4.5 Microvilli (inset)** With light microscopy, the apical surface of this epithelium is bordered by a strip of magenta-colored material (polysaccharide-rich) following PAS stain. × 280.
At the ultrastructural level (main image), this border is resolved into many slender microvilli that are extensions of the apical epithelial plasma membrane. The membrane-bounded microvilli greatly amplify the surface area of the apical cell plasma membrane that faces the intestinal lumen. ×15,000.

◀ **Fig 4.6b Ultrastructure of stereocilia,** showing how the apical cell membrane is organized into many long extensions. These contain actin filaments giving flexibility. Thus stereocilia are not modified cilia but resemble microvilli. Their function is believed to be absorptive. × 6,000.

▲ **Fig 4.6a Stereocilia** are very thin, elongated projections of the apical surface of these epithelial cells. Toluidine blue, araldite × 1,000.

They occur in the epididymis and vas deferens (to increase surface area for fluid absorption) and in hair cells of the inner ear, acting as sensory receptors for balance and auditory function.

Cilia are motile processes up to 10 µm in length that project from the apical surface of epithelia involved with surface movement of particles, mucus, or cells (Fig 4.7). Ciliated epithelial cells are found in parts of the respiratory tract and in the uterine tubes. The core of each cilium contains an axoneme of precisely arranged sets of microtubules and associated proteins, forming a ring of nine doublets around a central pair of microtubules (9 + 2 pattern). A whip-like movement (frequency about 22 Hz) is generated by coordinated sliding of these structures (see Ch 1).

Notable specializations of basolateral membranes in epithelia include desmosomes (which, in large numbers, bind epidermal cells together) and the complex, extensive in-foldings of the plasma membranes of cells in proximal and distal renal tubules and in ducts of sweat and salivary glands. This amplification of the surface area facilitates transport of ions and fluids and, ultimately, is involved in the regulation of the composition of the secretory products or luminal contents.

The basal lamina

Epithelia rest upon connective tissue. Parallel to the basal epithelial cell membrane is a thin, mat-type layer of extracellular proteins called the basal lamina. As the lamina is normally only 100–150 nm wide, it is visible only with electron microscopy (Fig 4.8). External to the basal lamina is another layer of connective tissues, mainly collagen. The basement membrane of epithelia consists of the basal lamina and this collagen-rich layer. It is visible with light microscopy and may be ≥1 µm in width (Fig 4.9a & b). The basal lamina provides support, adhesion via hemidesmosomes, and selective permeability, and influences epithelial organization and survival. Details of these layers and their protein composition are given in Chapter 5.

> **Tip:** The terms basal lamina and basement membrane are often used interchangeably. Strictly speaking they are different structures, but as long as you remember that the former is a component of the latter this practice is acceptable in the context of histology.

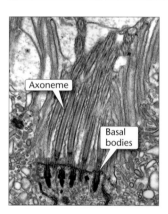

◀ **Fig 4.7 Ultrastructure of cilia projecting from the apical surface membrane.** Note the longitudinal microtubules in the core of each cilium, forming an axoneme. This is anchored to the cell via a basal body, which is a centriole. Cilia bend rhythmically to stir or move liquids, particles, or mucus across the surface of the epithelial cell. × 13,000.

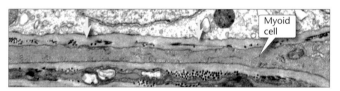

▲ **Fig 4.8 Ultrastructure of the basal lamina** seen as a thin opaque layer of extracellular material (**arrows**) adjacent to the plasma membrane of the overlying epithelial cell. Collagen fibers are found next to the basal lamina, external to which are attenuated layers of myoid cell and fibroblast. ×12,000.

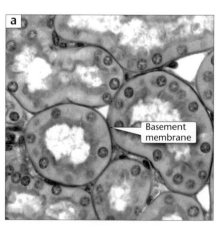

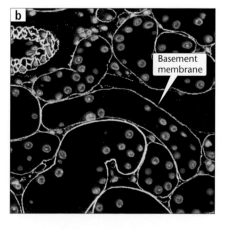

◀ **Fig 4.9b Basement membrane around renal tubules.** An immunofluorescence preparation shows laminin protein, which sharply defines the basement membrane surrounding renal tubules. Laminin provides adhesive properties to the extracellular matrix and resists tensile forces. Epithelial nuclei are blue. (Courtesy J Zbaeren, Inselspital Bern, Switzerland.) × 200.

▲ **Fig 4.9a Basement membrane around kidney epithelial cells.** Basement membrane forms a sharp border surrounding these tubules of epithelial cells in the kidney. The strong magenta color represents complex carbohydrates (especially proteoglycans) and many proteins. PAS stain, paraffin, × 350.

Proliferative capacity

For normal epithelia, their cells may be permanent for life, or constantly renewed to replace those lost naturally, or they may retain the capacity for renewal if damaged or otherwise stimulated to regenerate. Abnormalities of epithelial cell proliferation may result in a neoplasm (benign or malignant) or metaplastic changes involving transformation from one epithelial cell type to another.

Most epithelia are capable of renewal by mitosis and exercise this property continuously. Other epithelia can be stimulated to proliferate. In a few epithelia, the cells never proliferate. Thus, in the adult organism, epithelia can usefully be divided into three groups according to their proliferative capacity.

Permanent (non-renewable) and stable epithelial tissues

Permanent epithelial tissues are those in which cell division does not occur in adult life, such as the cells in the core of the lens and the auditory hair cells in the inner ear. Stable (conditionally renewable) tissues contain cells that do not normally divide in adult life; however, cell proliferation may occur if the tissue is damaged or if the physiologic needs of the organism change. An example is the liver in which hepatocytes are long-lived and very few cells are proliferating. If cells are destroyed (by a disease) or removed (following partial hepatectomy), new hepatocytes are formed by mitosis of existing hepatocytes.

Labile (steady-state renewable) epithelial tissues

In these tissues, cell proliferation normally occurs to replace cells as they are continually lost from the organ. This type of cell renewal often occurs through stem cells, a population of relatively undifferentiated cells that divide to replenish themselves and to yield progeny that will become specialized to perform the functions of the given epithelium. Examples of labile epithelia are the intestinal (Fig 4.10, Fig 4.11), epidermal, and seminiferous epithelia. Typically, the stem cells are located at the base of the epithelium, away from the luminal surface.

In a healthy organism, cell proliferation or its cessation is tightly regulated so that the number of cells produced matches the number needed for growth of the organism and replacement of worn-out cells. If cell proliferation is not properly controlled, too many or too few cells are produced or, in some cases, the new cells transform into other types of epithelium. All these abnormalities are of pathologic and clinical significance and are briefly discussed at the conclusion of this chapter.

The building blocks of epithelia

The combinations of cell proliferation, polarization, migration, and shape change are among the mechanisms by which epithelia create geometric structures—typically cysts, tubules, and cavities. In adults, these structures are commonly recognized as glands and tubular organs. Cyst-type structures of epithelial monolayers are recognized as acini in mammary glands, follicles in the thyroid, and alveoli in the lungs. When united with tubules made of cells, complex branching networks, such as the bronchial tree, terminate in alveolar cysts (Fig 4.12a & b). Tubes of epithelial cells with or without branching are very commonly found in organs. How then do epithelial cells form tubes and cavities? There are five general categories (Fig 4.13).

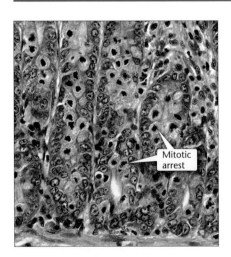

▲ **Fig 4.10 Epithelial cell proliferation.** Epithelium lining the small intestine shows many mitotically arrested cells following colchicine treatment. Colchicine arrests cell division at metaphase. This shows the location of stem cells and their dividing progeny at the base of the intestinal crypts. H&E, paraffin, × 200.

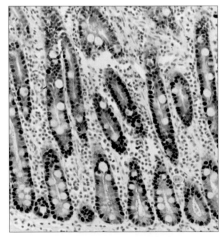

▲ **Fig 4.11 Immunocytochemistry of cell proliferation.** Epithelial cells at the S phase of the cell cycle, showing densely staining cells labeled with proliferating cell nuclear antigen (PCNA). The positively labeled cells are dividing stem cells and their progeny in the intestinal epithelium. Hematoxylin, paraffin, × 90.

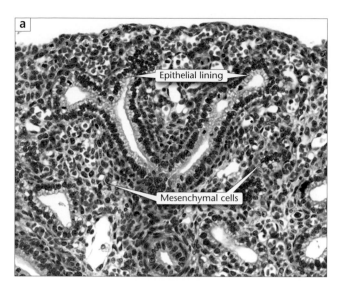

a

Epithelial lining

Mesenchymal cells

▲ **Fig 4.12a Epithelial morphogenesis.** Epithelial cells in the fetal lung organized into tubules and cyst-type structures. The developing epithelial cells are polarized and face a basal lamina, and the surrounding mesodermal tissue into which they grow controls the development of branches. H&E, paraffin, × 250.

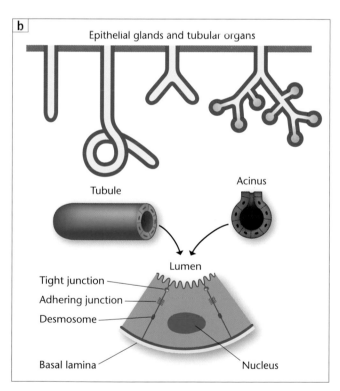

b

Epithelial glands and tubular organs

Tubule

Acinus

Lumen

Tight junction

Adhering junction

Desmosome

Basal lamina

Nucleus

▲ **Fig 4.12b Growth of epithelial tissues from two basic structures—tubules and acini.** The association of the cells is dependent upon the formation of cell polarity involving apical and basal surfaces and various intercellular junctions between them. As the epithelial cells proliferate during development, it is the surrounding mesenchymal cells in the connective tissue that regulates epithelial cell differentiation and phenotype.

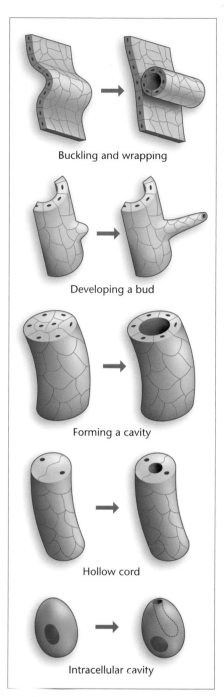

Buckling and wrapping

Developing a bud

Forming a cavity

Hollow cord

Intracellular cavity

▲ **Fig 4.13 Development of epithelial tubes.** Generalized scheme of epithelial tubulogenesis showing five processes—buckling/wrapping as in the formation of a neural tube; budding as in many organs such as lung, kidney, exocrine glands; cavity formation as in the vagina and uterus; hollowing out as for some invertebrate gut and heart; intracellular cavities may form in developing brain capillaries and in gastric parietal cells. (Modified from Lubarsky B and Krasnow MA. Tube morphogenesis: making and shaping biological tubes. Cell 2003; 112:19–28.)

1. **Wrapping** occurs as an epithelial sheet curls, making a crevice or groove, of which the edges meet and seal, forming a tube parallel to the cellular sheet.
2. **Budding** involves migration/proliferation from an existing sheet or tube, creating a tubular branch that, in turn, may generate additional buds all linked by a continuous internal lumen.
3. **Cavitation** requires elimination of cells in the center of a solid cylindrical mass.
4. **Cord hollowing** occurs when a lumen is created in a cylindrical cord of cells.
5. **Cell hollowing** requires that an inner membrane-bound lumen is formed inside a single cell.

Among the mechanisms required to bring about epithelial tissue modeling, the biogenesis of apical membranes (at future free surfaces), fusion of cytoplasmic vesicles (creates minicavities), and cell secretion (to keep lumina open) are believed to be especially important.

Additional mechanisms that play vital roles in epithelial construction include dynamic changes in the cell cytoskeleton and the associated intercellular junctions, production of anti-adhesive factors and membrane ion pumps, and the organizing effects of the extracellular matrix in specifying the basal cell surface.

Epithelial stem cells

Continual cell replacement is a necessity for most epithelia in order to replenish natural cell aging and death. The time frames for replacement vary widely. For example, intestinal epithelium self-renews about every 5–6 days, epidermal keratinocytes in 4 weeks, and lung epithelium perhaps every 6 months. Stem cells provide a lifelong supply of the necessary new cells by renewing themselves and by differentiating into the cell lineage/s specific for the epithelium. Stem cells usually enable repair of epithelial tissues following injury.

The generation of cell progeny by epithelial stem cells is of considerable interest, particularly for the prospect of repairing or replacing tissues post trauma or affected by disease.

Some well-characterized stem cells of epithelia include:

- Intestinal crypts where stem cells move upward, differentiating into a variety of villus epithelial cells, and downward forming Paneth cells
- The corneal epithelium is attached peripherally to the sclera at the limbus, a region where stem cells supply new epithelial cells by central migration
- Mammary gland terminal end buds (alveoli) that have stem cells capable of forming many new ducts or alveoli—for example, during pregnancy
- Hair follicles in which the stem cells found in the tube-like epithelium surrounding the hair follicle can differentiate into skin, hair, and sebaceous glands.

Although our knowledge of the factors that control the behavior of epithelial stem cells is far from complete, it is known that the evolutionarily ancient Wnt/β-catenin, Notch, and BMP signaling pathways each influence the specification, maintenance, and activation of these stem cells. (Wnt = wingless *Drosophila* + gene in mice causing breast cancer when activated by integration of a virus; β-catenin = protein linking cell junction with actin; Notch = *Drosophila* mutant with "notched" wings; BMP = bone morphogenetic protein.)

> **Tip:** If an acronym is unfamiliar, find out why it is used. This may not be easy, but it is better to know the derivation rather than to have to guess the meaning of DNA, FGF, LacZ, MHC, p53, Shh, TGF, and so on.

Epithelial–mesenchyme interactions

For their normal development and maintained function, epithelial tissues often depend upon interactions with associated connective tissue generally referred to as mesenchyme. The mesenchyme usually provides an inductive stimulus to the epithelium and may itself be altered by the encounter. Changes to epithelial type under the influence of mesenchyme have been shown by tissue recombination experiments and transplantation studies. Primitive lung buds develop into gastric glands when combined with stomach mesenchyme, into intestinal epithelium if combined with gut mesenchyme, and into liver cells if placed in contact with liver mesenchyme.

A reciprocal action of epithelial growth upon mesenchyme is observed when mouse, chicken, or lizard skin epithelium is cultured with mouse mesenchyme. The mesenchyme induces primordia of epithelial hair follicles, feathers, or scales, but each is arrested in development owing to the lack of specific, local mesenchymal cell support. It is thought that the epithelium produces its own signals necessary for organization of the mesenchyme. It is not known if similar interactions are normally operative in some or all adult epithelial stem cells.

CELL ADHESION AND COMMUNICATION

Epithelial cells are linked by cell junctions, which provide structural support, regulation of cell shape, adhesion and intercellular exchange of small molecules. Epithelial tissues rest on an extracellular connective tissue matrix, organized into a basal lamina or basement membrane. Blood vessels within the deeper underlying supporting tissue supply nutrients and humoral factors to the epithelium by diffusion across the basal lamina, because epithelial tissues are avascular.

In addition to the adhesive-type properties shown by almost all cells with neighboring cells, epithelia contain specialized cell junctions. These junctions, usually visualized with electron microscopy, allow intercellular attachment or anchoring sites, permit changes in cell shape, restrict transepithelial transport of selected (macro) molecules, and provide for exchange of signals from one cell to another. In a functional sense, cell junctions are one important factor contributing to cell polarity (discussed below) and form three major groups:

- Tight junctions
- Adhering junctions
- Communicating junctions.

The structure and function of junctions is presented in Chapter 1 and is briefly revisited here in the context of epithelial tissues (Fig 4.14a–c).

Tight junctions

Tight junctions make an epithelium leakproof. Also called occluding junctions, these are areas where fusion of lateral membranes of adjacent epithelial cells has occurred, usually located just below the apical surface. Also known as a zonula occludens, the tight junction is one of a triumvirate of cell junctions commonly referred to as a junctional complex. Tight junctions provide adhesion and control the intercellular passage of molecules (apex to base, base to apex) in the narrow space between epithelial cells (usually a barrier effect), and thus act as a type of gate, allowing the movement of some but not all ions or small molecules in the intercellular space. These junctions also act as a type of fence, in the sense that they segregate the various unique membrane proteins (receptors, transport complexes, anchoring domains) found in the apical and lateral plasma membranes. In Sertoli cells, junctional complexes are located toward the base of adjacent cells, forming the blood–testis barrier.

Adhering junctions

Adhering junctions make epithelial cells stick together. These serve to glue or anchor cells to each other or to the underlying basal lamina and show distinctive morphological features. The adherens junction (zonula adherens or intermediate junction) and the desmosome (macula adherens) are the second and third components respectively of the junctional complex. The adherens junction occurs as a thin band or belt (hence the name zonula) coursing around the cell's circumference and provides attachment for a strip of contractile filaments rich in actin. These filaments are capable of changing cell shape and, because epithelial

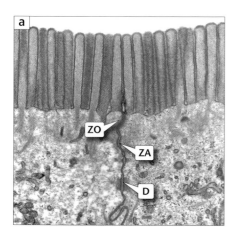

▲ **Fig 4.14a Junctional complex.** The zonula occludens (**ZO**), or tight junction, regulates the flow of molecules and ions into and out of the epithelium. The zonula adherens (**ZA**) forms an anchoring belt around the cell, apposed to a similar belt on the adjacent cell, and provides attachment for bundles of cytoplasmic actin filaments. The desmosome (**D**), or macula adherens, is an anchoring, spot-like junction of intercellular contact acting like a rivet, to which cytoplasmic intermediate filaments attach and extend throughout the cell as part of the cytoskeleton. × 17,000.

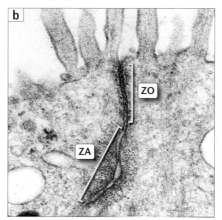

▲ **Fig 4.14b Detail of zonula occludens (ZO)**, showing fusion points between adjoining plasma membranes and zonula adherens (**ZA**); the gap between the membranes is occupied by cadherin receptor proteins, which bind the membranes closely. The ZA is associated with bundles of actin filaments, which link to the cadherins. × 60,000. (Courtesy P Cross, Stanford University, California, USA.)

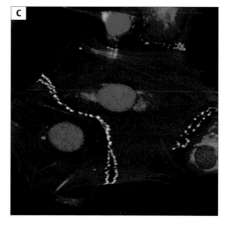

▲ **Fig 4.14c Cadherin proteins.** Immunofluorescence of epithelial cells cultured from mouse skin showing location of cadherin proteins (yellow puncta), which initiate the formation of adherens junctions. These are referred to as "adhesion zippers," which will merge to form junctions, thus sealing the cell borders. Actin filaments are stained red and nuclei are blue. × 600. (Courtesy E Fuchs, Rockefeller University, New York, USA; from Vasioukhin V, et al. Directed actin polymerization is the driving force for epithelial cell–cell adhesion. Cell 2000; 100:209–19.)

cells are cohesive, this activity can convert a flat sheet of cells into folds, grooves, and, ultimately, a hollow tube of epithelial cells fundamentally important in tissue growth, particularly during organogenesis. Desmosomes are analogous to rivets or spot welds and attach intermediate filaments that contribute to the internal cytoskeletal support of the cell. At sites of adherens junctions and desmosomes, the apposing membranes are not fused but are separated by a small intercellular space that contains linkage proteins serving to ensure cell-to-cell adherence. Hemidesmosomes are essentially half-desmosomes facing the basal lamina; cell-matrix adhesion plaques or focal contacts occur also in the basal cell membrane and provide a link between actin filaments within the cell and the extracellular connective tissue matrix.

Communicating junctions

Communicating junctions allow cell-to-cell transport. Nexuses or gap junctions are common in most cells and epithelia, and are sites of very close but not fused apposition of adjacent cell membranes—up to 1 μm in size. Gap junctions are discrete patches between cells where intercellular communication is available via minute pores or channels spanning the junction. These passageways allow chemical and electrical coupling between adjacent epithelial cells.

TYPES OF EPITHELIA
Simple epithelium

Simple squamous epithelium (Fig 4.15a–c) consists of a single layer of cells, the cytoplasm of each cell often being too thin to be clearly visible in histologic section, but the nucleus of each cell may bulge toward the surface. Examples are the epithelium of blood vessels (known as endothelium), the epithelium of lung alveoli, and the epithelium of the peritoneal, pleural, and pericardial cavities (known as mesothelium). Simple cuboidal epithelium (Fig 4.16a–c) consists of a single layer of cells whose height is about the same as their width; the cells

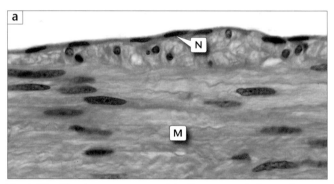

Fig 4.15a Simple squamous epithelium. A single layer of squamous cells forms a mesothelium, lining the external surface of the gut. Nuclei (**N**) are visible but the cytoplasm is flattened and barely apparent. Smooth muscle (**M**) lies deeper. This epithelium is kept moist, assisting with frictionless gut movements. H&E, paraffin, × 450.

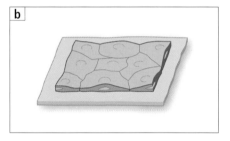

▲ **Fig 4.15b Representation of simple squamous cells** arranged like paving stones, resting on a supporting basal lamina. Nuclei tend to be thicker than the cytoplasm, hence their bulging appearance.

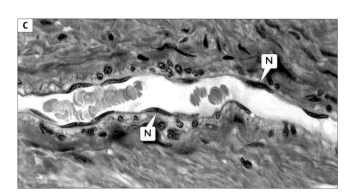

◀ **Fig 4.15c Endothelium.** All vascular elements (arterial, venous, capillary, lymphatics) are lined internally by a simple squamous epithelium, termed endothelium. Note the flat nuclei (**N**) and attenuated cytoplasm. The epithelium may allow gas and metabolic exchange, produce vasoactive factors, enable cell migration, and regulate platelet coagulation. H&E, paraffin, × 400.

appear polygonal in sections cut horizontal to the surface. Examples are the epithelium covering the outer surface of the ovary, the capsule of the lens, the lining of the collecting tubules of the kidney, and the ducts draining exocrine glands, although these may also show columnar cell types. Simple columnar

epithelium (Fig 4.17a–f, see p 106) is often seen in secretory and absorptive tissues such as the lining of the gut (stomach, small and large intestine), and in the larger caliber ducts of exocrine glands, such as salivary glands. Ciliated columnar epithelium lines the uterine tubes and the uterine cavity.

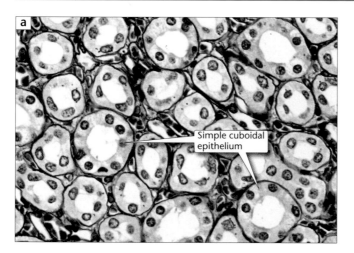

◀ **Fig 4.16a Simple cuboidal epithelium.** Renal tubules show a single layer of cuboidal epithelium in which cell width is similar to height. Functionally, this epithelium may be absorptive or secretory, thus modifying the internal luminal environment. Silver stain, paraffin, × 330.

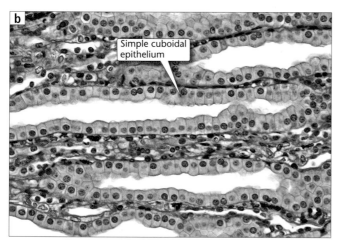

◀ **Fig 4.16b Simple cuboidal epithelium lining tubules in the kidney.** These tubules carry the urinary filtrate and serve to absorb water to concentrate the urine. The cells also play important roles in acid–base balance by absorption of sodium ions and secretion of potassium and bicarbonate ions. H&E, paraffin, × 250.

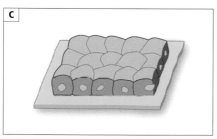

▲ **Fig 4.16c Simple cuboidal epithelium.** Cells of cuboidal epithelium are of similar size and shape, resembling cubes in vertical section or polygons in horizontal section. They are found in parts of ducts of many exocrine glands, ovarian surface, thyroid follicles, and the anterior capsule of the lens.

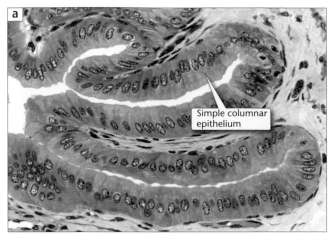

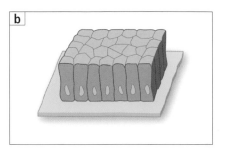

▲ **Fig 4.17a Simple columnar epithelium.** The tall columnar cells of the gall bladder epithelium are shown, where most of the nuclei are at the same level in the cells. These cells are usually involved in secretion and/or absorption, the latter predominating in this specimen (absorption of water). H&E, paraffin, × 125.

▲ **Fig 4.17b Simple columnar epithelium.** Cells are usually the same height and are arranged in upright columns in vertical section. In transverse sections the cells appear hexagonal or polyhedral. Examples of location include the inner lining of the gut and the larger ducts of some exocrine glands.

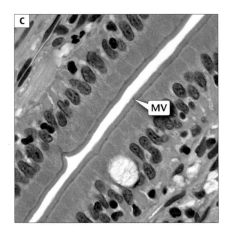

◀ **Fig 4.17c Simple columnar epithelium with microvilli.** The brush or striated border of the epithelium consists of microvilli (**MV**), slender extensions of the apical plasma membrane, which increase the surface area for absorption of luminal contents. Found chiefly in the intestine. H&E, paraffin, × 350.

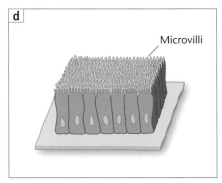

Fig 4.17d Simple columnar epithelium with microvilli. The microvilli of the brush border resemble the close packing of the hairs of a brush, numbering several thousand per cell. Microvilli are 1–1.3 μm in length and their core of filaments anchors them to the apical cell surface.

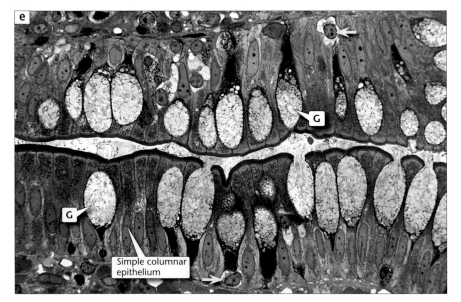

▲ **Fig 4.17e Simple columnar epithelium with goblet cells.** Goblet cells (**G**) secreting mucus occur in the intestinal mucosa. The numerous spherical cells (**arrows**) are wandering lymphocytes. Their transient nature but universal occurrence in the epithelium does not alter the classification of simple columnar epithelium. Toluidine blue, araldite, × 500.

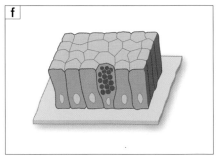

▲ **Fig 4.17f Simple columnar epithelium with goblet cells.** The presence of goblet cells in this simple epithelium represents a population of individual mucus-secreting cells, referred to as unicellular glands, among many other epithelial cells that are both secretory and absorptive.

Pseudostratified epithelium

The nuclei of the cells appear at different levels, giving the impression of strata when, in fact, only a single layer of cells is present (Fig 4.18a–d). All the cells rest on a basal lamina, but not every cell reaches the free surface (Fig 4.19). Pseudostratified columnar epithelium occurs in the upper respiratory tract (trachea and bronchi), the basal cells serving as stem cells, whereas

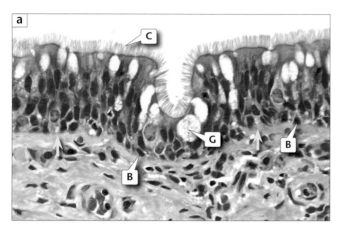

▲ **Fig 4.18a Pseudostratified epithelium.** A columnar epithelium with one or more rows of basal cells (**B**) suggesting layers of cells. In fact, all cells contact the basal lamina (**arrows**), but not all reach the surface. Goblet cells (**G**) and cilia (**C**) are present. Full classification: ciliated, pseudostratified columnar epithelium with goblet cells. Typical of trachea and bronchi. H&E, acrylic resin, × 250.

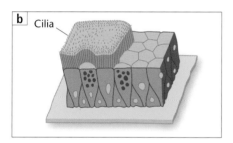

▲ **Fig 4.18b Pseudostratified epithelium.** All cells rest on the basal lamina, but only the columnar cells reach the surface; i.e. it is a simple epithelium with cell nuclei at different levels.

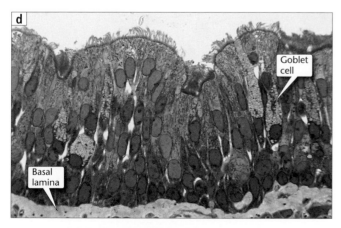

▲ **Fig 4.18d Tracheal epithelium** is a pseudostratified columnar epithelium with cilia. Cell nuclei are at various levels in the epithelium, but the cytoplasm is very thin and in contact with the basal lamina. Goblet cells show numerous pale-staining mucus granules. Toluidine blue, araldite, × 500.

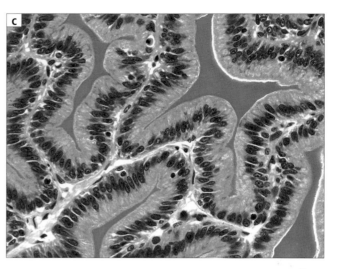

▲ **Fig 4.18c Pseudostratified columnar epithelium of the seminal vesicle,** showing mostly tall columnar secretory cells and basal cells, some of which are intraepithelial lymphocytes and others self-renewing stem cells. The apical surface defines a sharp border and consists of short microvilli similar to the brush border of the intestinal epithelium. H&E, paraffin, × 200.

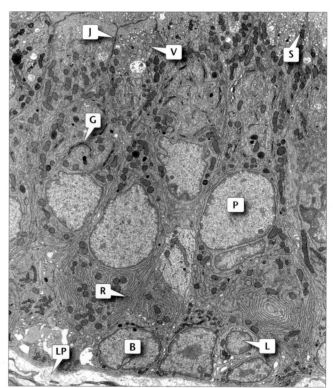

Fig 4.19 Epithelial ultrastructure. Pseudostratified columnar epithelium of the epididymis, showing principal cells (**P**) with apical stereocilia (**S**), basal cells (**B**), and an intraepithelial lymphocyte (**L**). Note the polarized distribution of rough endoplasmic reticulum (**R**), Golgi apparatus (**G**), and vesicles (**V**) called endosomes. Junctional complexes (**J**) join cells together in their apical regions, restricting entry of substances into the epithelium from the lumen. The lamina propria (**LP**) is also indicated. × 3,000.

many of the columnar cells exhibit cilia on their apical surface and others have become specialized to form goblet cells that secrete mucus. Hence, the full classification of the tracheal and bronchial epithelium is pseudostratified ciliated columnar epithelium with goblet cells. Other examples of pseudostratified columnar epithelium are found lining parts of the excretory passages of the male reproductive tract, such as the epididymis, vas deferens, and penile urethra.

Stratified epithelium

There are two or more layers of cells in this epithelium, and its main functions are to provide resistance to wear and tear and to form a physical barrier to deeper tissues. Where secretion is required, this is often met by underlying secretory glands, whose ducts reach the surface via a passageway through the epithelium (e.g. sweat glands of the skin).

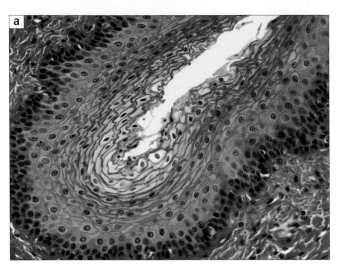

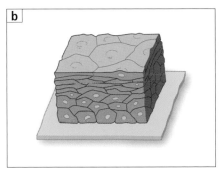

▲ **Fig 4.20b Stratified squamous epithelium.** Note the layered appearance, the superficial squamous cells giving the characteristic classification; this epithelium is kept moist. Examples occur in the buccal mucosa, parts of pharynx and larynx, esophagus, cornea, and portions of the anal canal and in the vagina.

▲ **Fig 4.20a Stratified squamous epithelium.** Cells are arranged in many layers, cuboidal in the base (and proliferative) but squamous at the luminal surface, in this case not showing a keratin layer. These deep layers act as a barrier and partly mitigate abrasion, the cells migrating steadily toward the surface, where they are shed. H&E, paraffin, × 250.

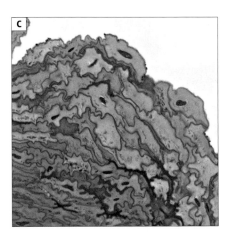

◀ **Fig 4.20c In non-keratinized stratified squamous epithelia**, the superficial epithelial cells are irregular or polygonal in shape, becoming more elongated and finally squamous at the surface. The cells do not lose their nuclei and do not become filled with excessive keratin; hence the surface is relatively smooth, not subject to strong abrasive forces. This specimen is from the tongue. Toluidine blue, araldite, × 600.

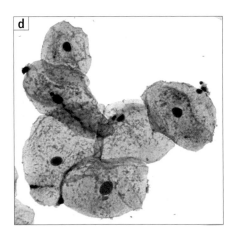

▲ **Fig 4.20d Isolated squamous epithelial cells** obtained from the buccal mucosa, showing a large cytoplasmic area consistent with a flat morphology. H&E, cytology preparation, × 650.

Stratified squamous epithelium is the chief protective epithelium of the body and is of two types: non-keratinized or keratinized. Stratified squamous non-keratinized epithelium (Fig 4.20a–d) is found lining much of the oral cavity, the esophagus, part of the anal canal, and vagina. The skin is an example of stratified squamous keratinized epithelium in which a thick, superficial, dead layer of keratin is strongly attached to the deeper, living cells (Fig 4.21a & b). The deepest cells in the epithelium are cuboidal-shaped cells, which migrate up through the epithelium, become flattened and squamous, lose their nuclei, and become entirely composed of keratin.

Stratified columnar (Fig 4.22) and stratified cuboidal epithelia are relatively uncommon. In the former, columnar cells overlie one or more deeper layers of cuboidal or polyhedral cells. This epithelium occurs in the larger ducts of some glands and in the pharynx. Occasionally, the surface cells are ciliated, such as those found on parts of the epiglottis and the nasal part of the soft palate. Some ducts of salivary glands show a stratified cuboidal epithelium; part of the lactiferous sinus in the mammary gland adopts this arrangement. Highly specialized examples of stratified cuboidal epithelium are shown in the granulosa cells of developing ovarian follicles and germ cells which form the seminiferous epithelium of the testis (Fig 4.23). The stria vascularis, which forms part of the wall of the cochlea, is a stratified epithelium with an unusual feature—it has a plexus of intraepithelial capillaries and associated basal lamina.

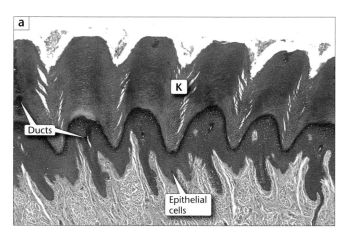

▲ **Fig 4.21a Keratinized stratified squamous epithelium** from the palmar surface of the hand, showing a thick keratin layer (**K**) of dead, flattened plaques that flake from the surface. Ducts from sweat glands traverse the protective keratin layer. H&E, paraffin, × 50.

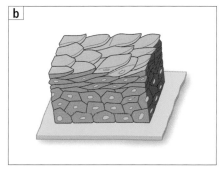

▲ **Fig 4.21b Keratinized stratified squamous epithelium.** Epidermis of thick skin, showing loss of epithelial nuclei, leaving multiple layers of keratin, or squames, which prevent desiccation and resist wear and tear. Found in skin, other examples are the gingival epithelium, filiform papillae of tongue, and nasal and anal epithelium.

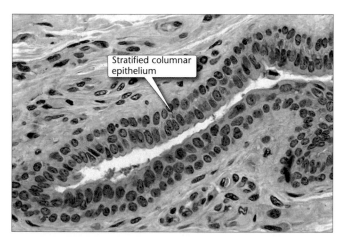

▲ **Fig 4.22 Stratified columnar epithelium.** Mainly lining large-caliber ducts from exocrine glands such as salivary glands, pancreas, sweat glands, and part of the urethra, this epithelium may show regions of stratified cuboidal cells. The superficial cells do not contact the basal lamina. Functions may include modification of luminal contents (absorption) and maintenance of duct integrity. H&E, paraffin, × 200.

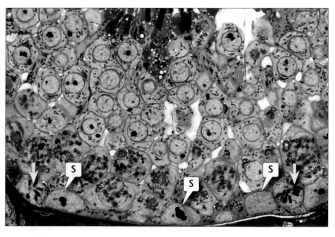

▲ **Fig 4.23 Complex epithelium of the testis called seminiferous epithelium.** Note multiple cell layers of different types of germ cells, two of which are in mitosis (**arrows**). The non-proliferative Sertoli cells (**S**) rest on the basal lamina. Toluidine blue, araldite, × 600.

Transitional epithelium

This epithelial type is so named because it represents a transition between stratified squamous and stratified columnar epithelium (Fig 4.24a & b). It is found lining the renal calyces, the ureters, the urinary bladder, and a portion of the urethra. In a contracted or resting condition, the epithelium is multilayered and the cells are polyhedral and/or columnar, but, with stretching, the epithelium may be only two to three cells thick with a mixture of cuboidal and squamous-type surface cells.

> **Tip:** An epithelial surface may be called a "mucosa" or "mucous membrane." This usually refers to the epithelial lining of the gastrointestinal tract but can be used to describe epithelia lining other hollow organs, cavities, or passageways. It includes the epithelium, its associated connective tissue, and frequently (in the gut), but not always, a layer of smooth muscle. Examples include the oral/nasal mucosa, bladder/urethral mucosa, uterine mucosa. A "serous membrane" is simple squamous epithelium and its connective tissue. It lines body cavities such as peritoneal, pleural, and pericardial cavities, and the exterior of organs within them (thoracic and abdominal viscera).

GLANDS AND SECRETION

Epithelia are often specialized to form glands for secretion of products to a surface (either external or internal cavity, or tubule) via ducts; these are named exocrine glands. Some epithelial cells (e.g. goblet cells) are specialized for secretion and can be considered to be unicellular glands. Endocrine glands may be derived from epithelia, but they do not have ducts and secrete directly into the vascular system.

Most glands are derived from epithelium. Glands are collections of secretory cells specialized to synthesize and to secrete specific products (Fig 4.25a & b). During their development from epithelium (or mesoderm or neuroectoderm), endocrine glands lose their connections with the epithelium or free surfaces (hence no duct), but retain a rich vascular supply that enables their products—hormones—to be distributed to local or distant target tissues elsewhere in the body. The major endocrine glands are the pituitary gland, adrenal glands, gonads, thyroid and parathyroid glands, pancreatic islets of Langerhans, and the pineal gland. Their histology and function are reviewed in Chapter 17.

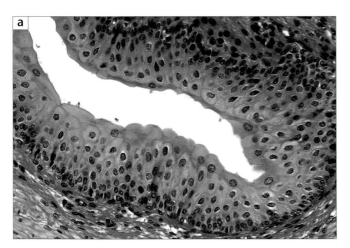

◀ **Fig 4.24a Transitional epithelium.** Also called urothelium, this epithelium occurs in the urinary tract from renal calyces to urethra and is commonly studied in the bladder, shown here. The epithelium is multilayered and folded when relaxed (not distended with urine) but stretched thinly as bladder volume increases. The surface cells change from cuboidal to squamous type shape. Transitional epithelium acts as a barrier to urine leakage. H&E, paraffin, × 200.

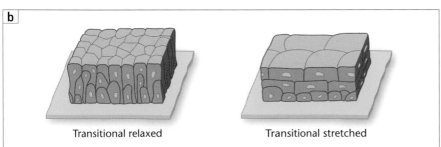

Transitional relaxed   Transitional stretched

▲ **Fig 4.24b Transitional epithelium.** Variation in histologic appearance of transitional epithelium when contracted (e.g. empty bladder) and stretched (e.g. full bladder). Superficial cells become very thin but junctional complexes remain to prevent paracellular leakage into the epithelium.

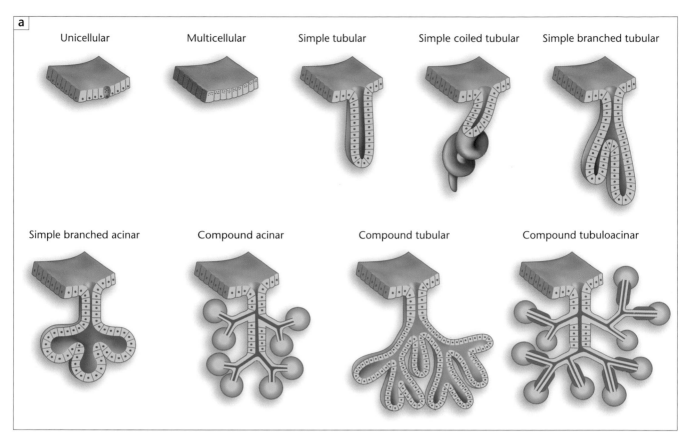

▲ **Fig 4.25a Classification of glands.** Secretory portion is green, and ducts or non-secretory structures are blue. *Unicellular* glands are typically represented by goblet cells of the intestinal and respiratory tract. *Multicellular* types occur in the epithelial lining of mucus cells of the stomach. *Simple tubular* glands are without ducts, such as those of the large intestine. *Simple coiled tubular* glands with ducts occur in sweat glands. *Simple branched tubular* glands with/without short ducts occur in gastric glands and minor salivary glands. *Simple branched acinar* glands occur in sebaceous glands. *Compound acinar* (alveolar) glands occur in exocrine pancreas glands. *Compound tubular* glands with multiple branching occur in Brunner's glands of the duodenum. *Compound tubuloacinar* glands occur in submandibular salivary glands.

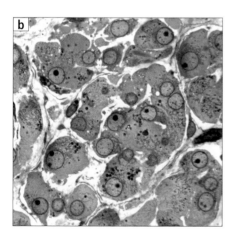

Fig 4.25b Endocrine cells. Cells of endocrine tissues or glands secrete their products (hormones) directly into the vascular system, and this may require diffusion of the hormones through the extracellular space before reaching a blood vessel. Endocrine cells are often epithelioid in appearance (but not always derived from epithelium) and may be singular or collected together in large numbers, as seen here for Leydig cells in the intertubular tissue of the testis. Toluidine blue, araldite, × 600.

There are various ways in which exocrine glands may be classified and, of these, the functional classifications rather than the histologic descriptions are of greater importance.

- Glands can be classified as unicellular or multicellular. Unicellular glands such as mucus-secreting goblet cells are single secretory cells among many other non-mucus-secreting epithelial cells (Fig 4.26). Multicellular glands are described by the arrangements of cells

and the branching pattern of their ducts. The simplest multicellular gland or glandular epithelium consists of a sheet or layer of secretory cells, such as the secretory cells facing the lumen of the stomach (Fig 4.27).

- Glands can be classified according to their duct morphology, being described as simple (i.e. unbranched ducts that may also be coiled; Fig 4.28a & b) or compound, with a branching duct system (Fig 4.29a & b).

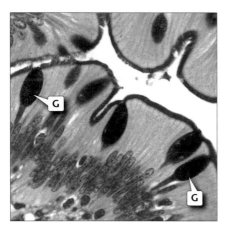

▲ **Fig 4.26 Unicellular gland.** Paraffin section of small intestine stained with the PAS reaction to show mucus-rich structures, seen here as goblet cells (**G**) of magenta color. Each of these epithelial cells is an example of a unicellular gland, although a gland is usually considered to be a larger structure containing many individual secretory cells. PAS stain, paraffin, × 400.

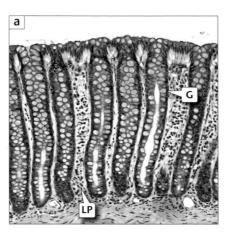

▲ **Fig 4.28a Simple tubular glands.** Deep invaginations of the epithelium into the lamina propria (**LP**) of the large intestine form simple tubular glands termed intestinal glands, or colonic crypts. Crypts contain goblet cells (**G**) and epithelial absorptive cells. Secretion into or absorption from the lumen is achieved by narrow passageways within the crypts, which are not always seen in continuity in a single section. H&E, acrylic resin, × 100.

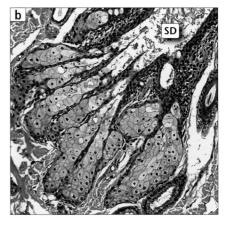

▲ **Fig 4.28b Simple coiled tubular glands** are typical of the sweat glands, which show a cuboidal epithelium. The lumen appears disconnected in sections because of the coiled nature of the tubular gland, which via a single duct (more heavily stained) reaches and opens on to the surface of the skin. H&E, paraffin, × 100.

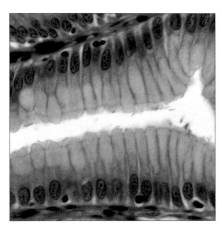

▲ **Fig 4.27 Multicellular gland.** Mucus-secreting columnar epithelial cells lining the gastric pits of the stomach. Nuclei are basally located and the tall columnar cytoplasm is filled with secretory vesicles. All of these epithelial cells are short-lived, being replaced with new cells every 4–5 days. H&E, paraffin, × 600.

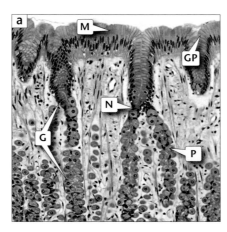

▲ **Fig 4.29a Simple with branching tubular glands.** Gastric glands (**G**) of the stomach show branching from the neck region (**N**) with a gastric pit (**GP**) at the surface. Acid-secreting parietal cells (**P**) and surface mucous cells (**M**) are indicated. H&E, paraffin, × 125.

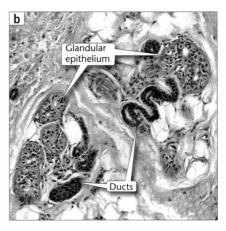

▲ **Fig 4.29b Simple with branching acinar-type glands.** Sebaceous glands show multiple elongated or lobular alveolar-type secretory units all emptying into a single sebaceous duct (**SD**) associated with a hair follicle. Whole cells are discharged, an example of holocrine secretion. H&E, paraffin, × 150.

- Depending on the arrangement of the secretory cells, glands may be classified as tubular (shaped like a tube), alveolar or acinar (flask-shaped), or tubuloalveolar/acinar (the tube ends in a sac-type dilatation). However, in two-dimensional histologic sections, it may be difficult to distinguish between some of these different types.
- Examples of simple glands include those showing tubular, coiled, and bifurcating secretory structures. Compound gland types with branched duct systems show acinar, tubular, and tubuloacinar secretory units (Fig 4.30, Fig 4.31, Fig 4.32).
- Also important is the classification of glands by the nature of their secretions. Mucous, serous, and mixed (or seromucous) glands are identified respectively by their mucoid secretion (e.g. some of the lingual glands), their serous or watery secretion (e.g. parotid gland), or a combination of both from aggregations of different secretory cells (e.g. submandibular gland).

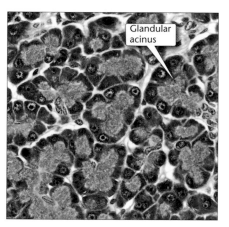

▲ **Fig 4.30 Compound acinar gland.**
The exocrine pancreas here shows multiple acini supported by loose connective tissue. The pancreatic acinar cells, pyramidal in shape, contain a heavily stained basal cytoplasm and eosinophilic zymogen granules in the apical cytoplasm. These granules are released into a duct system that is branched to join with acini, and united to form larger ducts that ultimately converge into the accessory, or main, pancreatic duct. H&E, paraffin, × 225.

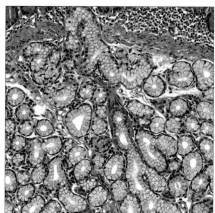

▲ **Fig 4.31 Compound tubular gland.**
Mucus-secreting Brunner's glands of the duodenum show tubular morphology with numerous branchings. The mucus secreted is transported within the tubular glands that empty into the base of an intestinal crypt. H&E, paraffin, × 100.

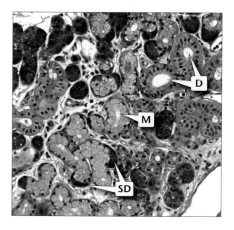

◀ **Fig 4.32 Compound tubuloacinar gland.** The submandibular gland is a mixed seromucous exocrine gland exhibiting mucus cells (**M**) and serous cells, here organized into serous demilunes (**SD**). The morphology is sometimes tubular, sometimes alveolar, with numerous branchings, which are continuous with a complex duct system (**D**), leading to a primary duct emptying into the oral cavity. A similar arrangement applies to the sublingual gland. H&E, paraffin, × 150.

- Finally, exocrine glands may be classified according to the mechanism by which the secretory product is released (Fig 4.33). Merocrine (or eccrine) secretion occurs when secretory granules discharge their contents by fusion with the plasma membrane (e.g. sweat glands, pancreas). Apocrine secretion involves release of secretory granules together with a small amount of attached cytoplasm (e.g. from mammary glands), and holocrine secretion involves the discharge of whole cells together with their internal secretory products (e.g. from sebaceous glands).

Tip: Common types of secretions from exocrine glands are mucus (thick and viscous), serous-types (water-like but with abundant proteins), sweat, sebum (lipid-rich oily secretion of the skin), milk (from lactating breast), and cerumen (modified sebum, also known as earwax). Endocrine gland secretions are biochemically diverse, but proteins or steroids are common types.

ABNORMAL CONDITIONS AND PATHOLOGIC FEATURES

Epithelia and the glands derived from them are diverse and are situated in most organs. Consequently, the range of disorders affecting phenotype, cell numbers, and/or cell size is considerable. Some of the more common abnormalities associated with particular epithelial tissues are noted in the relevant chapters.

In general terms, disturbances of epithelial cell function result in alterations of cell size, proliferation, and differentiation. Cells reduced in size or volume are atrophic, and the tissue or organ to which they belong is said to atrophy if sufficient numbers of epithelial cells shrink in size. This phenomenon may be physiologic (e.g. during epithelial growth in the embryo or fetus, or the shrinkage of endometrial glands after the menopause) or pathologic (e.g. a variety of disease states affecting the epithelium of the gut). Atrophy may be reversible: Some glandular epithelia return toward normal size if appropriately stimulated after previous withdrawal of hormonal or growth factor support. Hypertrophy is a reversible increase in cell size, related to a specific stimulus, and is well demonstrated by hormone-responsive epithelial tissues such as the thyroid gland (goiter) and accessory sex glands in the male (seminal vesicles).

Epithelial tissues that fail to reach an expected overall mass usually lack the numbers of cells normally seen in the organ. During development, when an organ completely fails to form, the phenomenon is termed *agenesis* (e.g. the development of only one kidney). In the condition referred to as *aplasia*, the organ commences growth by cell proliferation but is arrested early in development, and ultimately forms a rudimentary tissue. If the epithelium continues to grow but fails to attain normal size because of insufficient cell proliferation, the organ or tissue is classified as *hypoplastic*. Conversely, if an ongoing stimulus produces an increase in the number of epithelial cells in a particular population, this condition is known as *hyperplasia*. Physiologic examples of hyperplasia are the enlargement of mammary glands (proliferation of glands and their ducts) during pregnancy and postpartum lactation, and increased epidermal cell proliferation in conditions such as psoriasis and eczema. Pathologic forms of hyperplasia are common, examples being prostatic gland hyperplasia and several conditions that cause excessive growth of the thyroid gland.

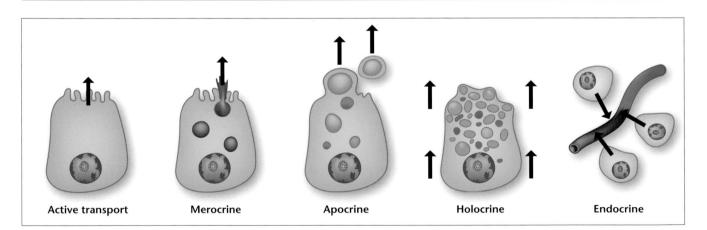

| Active transport | Merocrine | Apocrine | Holocrine | Endocrine |

▲ **Fig 4.33 Modes of secretion by cells of glands.**
Active transport occurs for ions (such as Na^+, K^+) and maintenance of osmotic pressure; *merocrine* secretion (or exocytosis) occurs where, after plasma membrane fusion, secretory granules discharge their contents; *apocrine* secretion occurs when part of the cytoplasm is released together with the secretory products; *holocrine* secretion involves release of the whole cell as the secretory product; *endocrine* secretion involves release of secretory products directly into blood vessels.

When epithelia differentiate to produce progeny that are structurally and functionally specialized to perform specific tasks, it is possible that the cell types produced are not normally found in that particular epithelium. This change is termed *metaplasia*. It is associated with an abnormal stimulus of tissue growth or tissue damage that originates with the precursor epithelial cells; however, the new type(s) of epithelial cells produced may be simply a normal cell lineage in an abnormal location (i.e. these cells are not necessarily abnormal or uncontrollable as in the case of cancers). Metaplasia of the squamous type is commonly found in the bronchi, particularly of cigarette smokers. The normal ciliated pseudostratified epithelium with goblet cells is replaced by an epithelium that closely resembles the epidermis of skin. Glandular metaplasia may occur in the gut—for example, in ulcers or chronic inflammation of the gastric epithelium (gastritis), where the mucosa may form intestinal crypts.

Dysplasia of epithelium occurs when abnormal differentiation results in altered size, shape, and organization of mature cells. This may be a prelude to neoplastic change. Sometimes referred to as atypical hyperplasia, this phenomenon has been extensively studied in the uterine cervix and is histologically graded as mild, moderate, or severe, the latter of which is strongly associated with preinvasive cancer, otherwise known as carcinoma in situ.

Neoplasia (i.e. cancer) occurs if cell proliferation is not controlled and results in an abnormal mass of proliferating cells (a tumor). The biology of neoplasms is beyond the scope of this commentary, but they are of two types—benign (non-cancerous) and malignant (cancerous). The former is a localized growth or tumor that does not spread or metastasize to a distant site and is often confined by a layer of connective tissue. Malignant neoplasms invade or infiltrate their surroundings (a primary cancer) and may spread or metastasize to grow in other organs, forming secondary cancers, or secondaries. Cancer of epithelial tissues is referred to as carcinoma.

Epithelia and regenerative medicine

Skin epithelial tissues are well known for their applications as transplants for burn patients. Cultures and colonies of epithelial cells grown on fibrin matrices can form sheets of skin epithelium, which are grafted with high success. The prospect of gene therapy applied to cultures may in the future obviate a range of debilitating skin disorders, and the isolation of epithelial stem cells from primitive hair follicles may lead to methods for regrowth of hair. Similar success has been achieved in the treatment of disorders or damage to the cornea, often accompanied by blindness. Transplants of the limbus-containing corneal epithelial stem cells have been used to regenerate the tissue and restore sight. Culturing limbal stem cells and transplanting corneal epithelial sheets have also been used to treat eye damage.

115

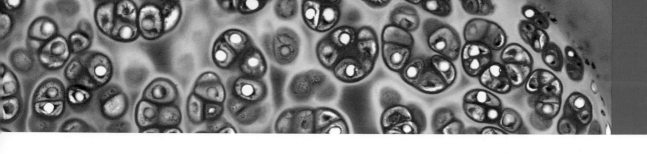

Connective tissue

Connective tissue is found throughout the body providing support for all organs, both externally and internally. However, the function of connective tissue extends far beyond a simple role as a framework or chassis. In recognition of its complex interactions with other tissue types, it may be designated as supporting tissue, indicating that it not only fulfils an architectural role but also has a dynamic function in the development, growth and homeostasis of adjacent and different tissue types.

An understanding of the biology of connective tissue provides an important foundation for an understanding of relevant medical science and clinical practice, including bone growth and repair, tendon and ligament injuries, emphysema, atheroma, hypertension, wound healing, aging of skin, joint disease, and certain tumor formations.

The three major problems challenging students when introduced to the concept of supporting or connective tissue are:

- Textbooks of histology may present different classification systems.

- The sheer volume and complexity of structure–function relationships is considerable and is, at times, magnified by a seemingly bewildering array of molecular biology.
- The difficulty comprehending that connective tissues range from fluid-like components (blood and liquid plasma is sometimes considered to be connective tissue) to those that are rock-hard (bone).

Connective tissue consists of cells and a surrounding matrix. The relative proportions and individual make-up of each component vary greatly. The matrix, or extracellular matrix (ECM), may be watery, rigid, or somewhere in between. This diversity is attributable to the way the matrix is constructed and to the duties it serves. Essentially the ECM is a mixture of fibers or a sol–gel-type substance consisting of carbohydrates, proteins, and water with dissolved mineral salts, nutrients, and hormones. Matrix is the dominating component of supporting tissue (Fig 5.1). One unusual example is blood plasma; some texts classify blood as fluid connective tissue in which a number of dissolved proteins come from non-connective tissue sources, such

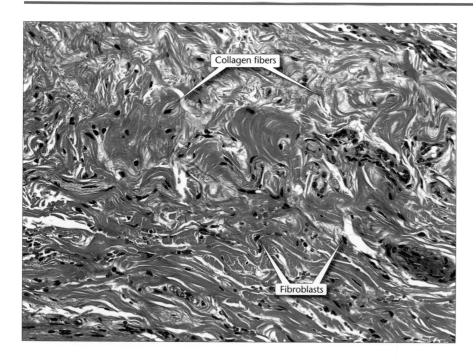

◀ **Fig 5.1 Typical connective tissue.** The tissue is dominated by irregular bundles of collagen fibers, between which are gaps or empty-looking spaces that are largely artifacts of tissue preparation caused by mechanical stress and extraction of the gel-type extracellular matrix. Fibroblasts are scattered throughout. Hematoxylin and eosin (H&E), paraffin, × 300.

as the liver. It is also relevant to note that the wetness of organs is due to interstitial fluid or extracellular fluid, which may be either a product of connective tissue or epithelial tissue, or a natural exudate from blood.

Broadly speaking, connective tissues contain the following:

- Variable amounts and types of cells
- Insoluble fibers, usually in a network or matrix
- Protein-rich polymers that inflate the fibrous network
- Adhesive proteins that may bridge the cells and the matrix
- Water, giving a fluid or gel-like consistency to the interstitial tissues with electrolytes and escaped plasma proteins.

Tip: Connective tissues of many organs consist of two components: parenchyma, which is the cellular population responsible for specific organ function; and stroma, which supports the parenchyma. Connective tissue is continuous throughout the body.

CELL TYPES

Although the various types of definitive connective tissue cells may exhibit quite different morphology and function, they all arise from mesenchymal cells, which are developed from the embryonic mesoderm (Fig 5.2):

- Fibroblasts. Chief among these connective tissue cells is the fibroblast (Fig 5.3), best known for its widespread occurrence in those supporting tissues that "fill in the spaces" and form organ capsules, tendons, and ligaments.
- Adipose cells. Fat or adipose cells appear to develop from mesenchymal-type cells, with a lipoblast being an intermediate cell type (Fig 5.4).
- Other supporting tissue cells. Other members of the group are chondroblasts (produce cartilage) (Fig 5.5), osteoblasts (lay down bone), and myoblasts (form muscle cells). Other tissues for which mesoderm or mesenchyme are the precursors include blood and hematopoietic elements, vessels, gonads, adrenal cortex, spleen, and kidney. These tissues are not discussed here in the context of introducing the histology of connective tissue.

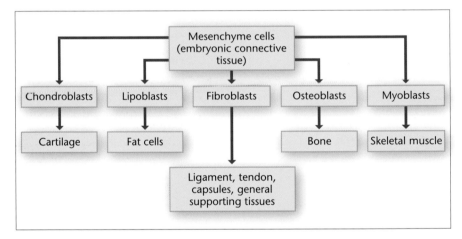

◀ **Fig 5.2 Cell lines derived from mesenchyme cells.** Mesenchyme cells can potentially develop into a variety of cells that make up different tissue types.

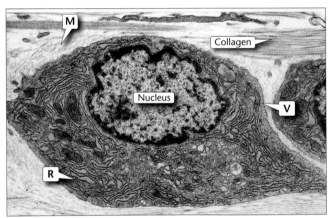

◀ **Fig 5.3 Fibroblasts and collagen.** Fibroblasts that are actively synthesizing collagen molecules contain much rough endoplasmic reticulum (**R**). The intracellular precursor form of collagen, procollagen, is secreted into the extracellular space via vesicles (**V**). The matrix (**M**) shows regions of fibrous aggregations—probably tropocollagen molecules derived from procollagen, which self-assemble into collagen fibrils. × 8,000.

- Migratory, transient and resident cells. Connective tissues often show one or more varieties of cells derived from blood. This is not surprising, as the connective tissue is the compartment between the vascular system and the tissue it supplies. Examples are leukocytes, often as plasma cells, as well as macrophages and mast cells. The latter two cell types may be temporary or long-term residents (Fig 5.6a–c).
- Mesenchymal cells. These are fundamentally important in the overall classification of supporting tissue (Fig 5.7a–c). In addition to self-replication, they are capable of differentiating into all the cell types described above either during embryonic and fetal development, or during adult life by regeneration, or both. Therefore, they may be regarded as stem cells or pluripotent cells—the term mesenchymal cell implies a type of immature or precursor fibroblast awaiting a specific stimulus to differentiate itself. All of the blast-type cells mentioned above are capable of division and development into more specialized cells (e.g. a fibroblast contributing to tendon formation becomes a mature fibrocyte within the tendon).

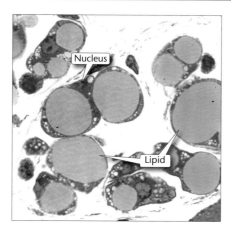

▲ **Fig 5.4 Adipose cells.** Occurring singly but more often in aggregations, adipocytes assemble and store fat droplets, which grow in size to displace the cell nucleus to one pole of the cell with the cytoplasm also confined to a thin rim. In addition to fat storage and mobilization, adipose tissue has insulating properties and is a source of several hormones affecting metabolism. Toluidine blue, araldite, × 480.

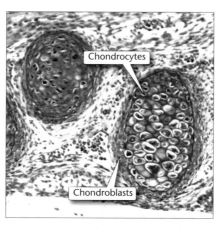

▲ **Fig 5.5 Chondroblasts.** Islands of chondrocytes (blue) that have formed from a peripheral layer of chondroblasts. The blue matrix is cartilage. These particular cartilaginous structures are the precursor tissues of bone and the specimen was taken from the early vertebral column of a fetus. H&E–Alcian blue, paraffin, × 90.

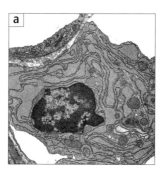

▲ **Fig 5.6a A plasma cell within connective tissue.** Derived from an activated B lymphocyte, a member of the leukocyte family, plasma cells are transient residents in tissue and are widely found throughout the loose connective tissues. Their role is to produce antibodies in response to foreign antigens. × 2,200.

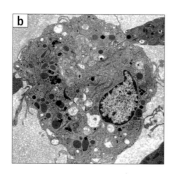

◀ **Fig 5.6b Macrophages** are very common in most connective tissues. These cells are phagocytic and act as antigen-presenting cells as part of the immune surveillance system. They are derived from blood monocytes that enter the connective tissue and mature into macrophages. Macrophages may be temporary or longer-term residents in connective tissues. × 1,600.

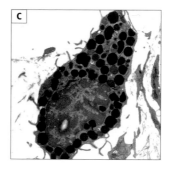

◀ **Fig 5.6c Mast cells** are not abundant in connective tissues but are usually found in proximity to blood vessels being derived from bone marrow precursors. Their many dense granules are discharged, particularly in allergic and inflammatory reactions, to regulate vascular tone and vessel permeability. × 5,200.

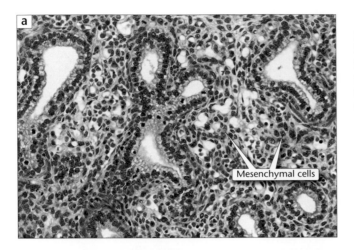

◀ **Fig 5.7a Mesenchymal cells** are derived from embryonic mesoderm and play many essential roles in organogenesis. In this example of the embryonic lung, mesenchymal cells surround the growing endodermally derived epithelial cells of the primitive respiratory tube. Mesenchymal cells are inductive for many epithelial tissues during embryonic and fetal development, a process referred to as epithelial–mesenchyme interaction. H&E, paraffin, × 250.

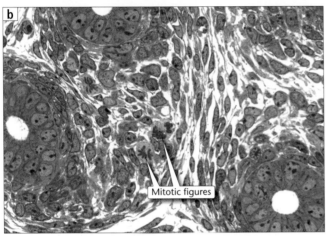

◀ **Fig 5.7b Mesenchymal cells in the developing intertubular connective tissue of the fetal epididymis.** These cells show typical stellate and fusiform morphology and mitotic activity. They are variously capable of many pathways of differentiation, including fibroblasts, muscle, or myoid cells, or other cell lineages depending on the type of organ or tissue. Toluidine blue, araldite, × 650.

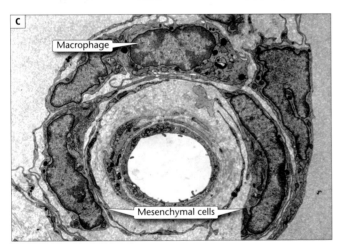

◀ **Fig 5.7c Ultrastructure of mesenchymal cells in adult connective tissue**, showing their association with a postcapillary venule. Although these cells resemble fibroblasts, collagen is scarcely evident. Depending on the specific tissue and local stimuli, mesenchymal cells may give rise to a wide range of differentiated cell types. A macrophage is indicated. × 2,900.

MATRIX

The components of the matrix are represented by fibers, proteoglycans, structural glycoproteins, water and dissolved substances such as electrolytes, hormones, and gases. Fibers have a more or less definitive structure, while the protein macromolecules, polysaccharides, and water lack this feature and appear amorphous or lacking structure. Coexistence of both is often the basis for confusion, since it is difficult to come to terms with a tissue component that has little or no microscopic structure.

Matrix components with a definitive structure are the histologically visible fibrous proteins or fibers for structural support: collagen (including reticular fibers) and elastic fibers.

The amorphous, gel-like appearance of the matrix, formerly known as "ground substance," consists of large complexes of polysaccharides and proteins called proteoglycans, which are composed of smaller molecules called glycoproteins (formerly referred to as mucoproteins).

All of these aggregations of macromolecules are associated with significant amounts of water because of their high negative charge. The total volume of extracellular or interstitial water, excluding the blood plasma, in an average adult is about 11 liters (i.e. 25% of total body water volume or 15% of total body weight).

The primary function of the fibrous elements is to provide strength and resistance to deformation and stretching; the primary function of the hydrated matrix proteins is to provide nutrient supply and mechanical support dependent upon the density of the sol–gel complex. The mechanical and physical properties of supporting tissues are dependent upon their mixture of fibrous and matrix components and the dominance of any single type.

Matrix fibers

Collagen fibers are synthesized by fibroblasts and occur in at least 20 variants designated I–XX (Fig 5.8a & b). Type I is the most common form. Their high tensile strength (some are equivalent to mild steel on a weight-for-strength basis) derives from their rope- or cable-type organization of three primary protein

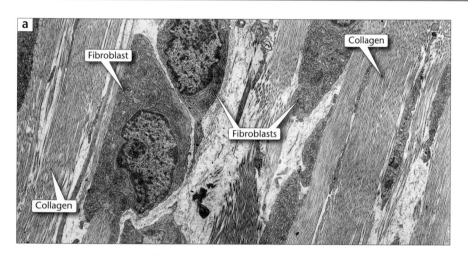

◀ Fig 5.8a Collagen and fibroblasts. Fibroblasts are intimately associated with the collagen molecules they secrete. The collagen molecules become organized into many collagen fibrils. These are visible in histologic sections as collagen bundles or fibers. The orientation and stacking of collagen fibrils is directed by fibril-associated collagens (e.g. collagen type XII) and by proteoglycans such as decorin. The collagen molecules, as triple helix peptide precursors, are synthesized inside the fibroblast. With extension peptides cleaved off extracellularly, the protein is then called tropocollagen. Spontaneous aggregation and cross-linking then follows. × 4,000.

◀ Fig 5.8b Collagen fibrils from a tendon after incubation of the tissue with elastase. Note the distinctive banding pattern, which indicates the repetitive and orderly arrangement of collagen molecules that make up a fibril. Fibrils are stabilized by filamentous strands, probably collagen type XII and collagen type XIV. Aggregation of many fibrils forms collagen fibers, often 0.5–3 μm in diameter. Large clusters of fibers are visible with light microscopy as bundles. × 38,000.

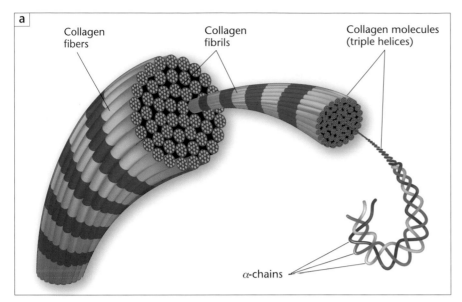

a

Collagen fibers

Collagen fibrils

Collagen molecules (triple helices)

α-chains

◀ **Fig 5.9a Collagen structure.** Diagram showing the structure of the superhelix of polypeptide chains forming a collagen molecule. The composition of the chain determines the type of collagen formed. Procollagen molecules inside the fibroblast assemble as triple helix "coiled coils" 1.5 nm in diameter and 300 nm in length. Following release within secretory vesicles, peptidases cleave propeptide ends to form tropocollagen molecules, many of which associate to form fibrils 10–300 nm in diameter. Many fibrils aggregate into larger fibers (diameter up to 3 μm), and ultimately into the collagen fiber bundles seen in histologic sections. Collagen types I–III, V, and XI make up fibrils, whereas type IV forms a fine meshwork within basement membranes.

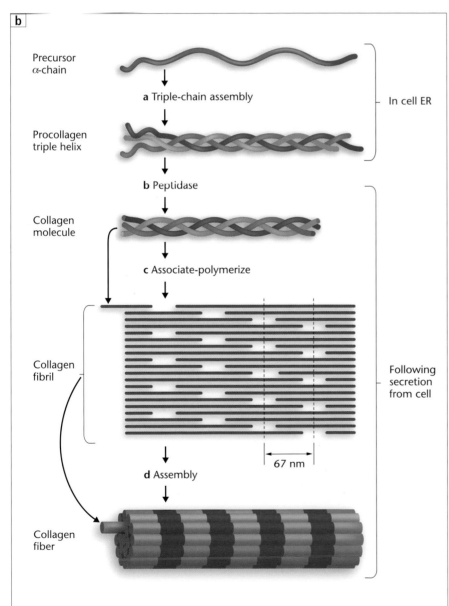

b

Precursor α-chain

a Triple-chain assembly

Procollagen triple helix

b Peptidase

Collagen molecule

c Associate-polymerize

In cell ER

Collagen fibril

67 nm

d Assembly

Following secretion from cell

Collagen fiber

◀ **Fig 5.9b Collagen assembly.** Fibers of collagen are often 0.5–3 μm in diameter, depending on the type. They are organized as many smaller fibrils up to 300 nm each in diameter. The actual collagen proteins are triple helices comprising coiled chains. The repeating dark and light striations are due to a 67 nm gap between the aggregated and staggered arrangements of collagen molecules within the fibrils. Collagen has considerable physical strength and accounts for the robust properties of tissues such as tendons, ligaments, cartilage, and bone.

chains wound into a superhelix (Fig 5.9a & b). They make up about 25% of the total protein of the body, and individual fibrils aggregate together to form large bundles or fibers that are visible microscopically.

Collagen types

Collagen is the most abundant protein of the body. Bone, ligament, tendon, fasciae, and joint capsules contain type I collagen. Types II and III have also been intensely studied. Type II occurs in cartilage and the vitreous of the eye, and type III occurs as a mesh or reticular framework in numerous glands, skin, and, in particular, large blood vessels. Collagen types I, II, and III make up about 90% of all the collagen in the body. Collagen fibers are relatively stable, long-lasting proteins, with type II having a turnover time of almost 1 year. Type IV lacks distinct fibrils and occurs in basal laminae.

Bone is discussed separately, but tendons and ligaments are considered here because of their high content of collagen (>80%). Tendons have great tensile strength and, in humans, this ranges from about 280 to 1,260 kg/cm^2 (4,000 to 18,000 lb/in^2). Muscle can withstand forces up to only 5 kg/cm^2 (75 lb/in^2). In cross section, the ultrastructure of tendons and ligaments shows large- and small-caliber collagen fibers. Physiologically, tendons and ligaments may undergo strains up to 3–4% of their initial length without

irreversible damage. Mild-to-moderate tearing (greater than 4% strain) is associated with fiber disruption and usually presents clinically as joint laxity on stress testing. This clinical picture represents rupture of about 50% of fibers. Complete rupture of fibers (10–20% strain) and ligament–tendon failure can be perilous, since pain may be only momentary and further load bearing may provoke multiple injuries.

Elastin, elastic fibers, and reticular fibers

Elastin and elastic fibers consist of a microfibril called fibrillin, together with elastin, a biopolymer; with water, these two components confer elasticity to the fibers. The fibers may branch and may form concentric or flat sheets, as seen in arterial walls, the mesenteries, and where muscle aponeuroses require elasticity (Fig 5.10a–e). The elasticity of skin, larger blood vessels, large ligaments, and the lung depends upon the rubber-like properties of elastic fibers.

Extensive patterns are seen in the dermis, where elastin content is less than 5% by weight yet is very important for skin elasticity. They are also seen in the external ear, and in the elastic ligamentum nuchae and flavum of the vertebral column.

The ligamentum nuchae contains 80% elastin and 20% collagen, and allows flexion and extension of the vertebral column without buckling of the ligament, which otherwise would injure the spinal

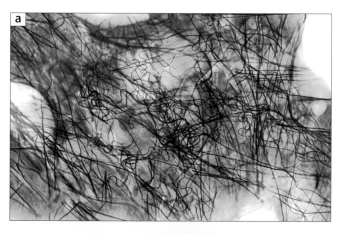

◀ **Fig 5.10a Elastic fibers in ligament.** Section through a retaining ligament of the zygomatic major muscle showing the high content of elastic fibers. Because the tissue has contracted when excised and fixed in formalin, the elastic fibers are lax and very tightly recoiled, similar to a non-stretched rubber band. The elastic property of this ligament acts against sagging of connective tissue with increasing age. Gomori trichrome, paraffin, × 120.

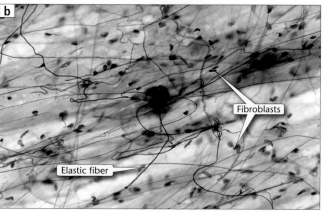

Fibroblasts

Elastic fiber

◀ **Fig 5.10b Elastic fibers in mesentery.** Whole-mount spread of mesentery stained to show elastic fibers, which bend and turn within this loose connective tissue. These fibers permit stretching and mobility, which is important for the distension and the peristaltic movements associated with the gastrointestinal tract. Cell nuclei seen in a different plane of focus represent, among other cells, numerous fibroblasts. These fibroblasts synthesize the elastic fibers and the extracellular matrix that provides their support. Gomori, × 250.

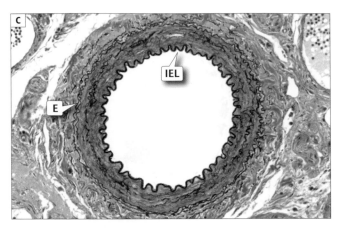

▲ **Fig 5.10c Elastic fibers in arterial walls.** The walls of arterial vessels and, to a lesser extent, those of muscular venules and larger venous vessels, show distinctive arrangements of elastic fibers, synthesized by smooth muscle cells. In this arteriole, an undulating sheet of elastic material—the internal elastic lamina (**IEL**)—is shown, and thinner sheets of elastin (**E**) can be seen within the tunica media and the outer connective tissue of the tunica adventitia. Following dilatation of the vessel, the elastic laminae recoil and assist with blood flow. Gomori trichrome, paraffin, × 150.

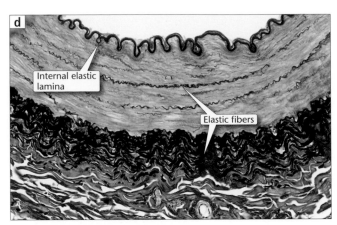

▲ **Fig 5.10d Muscular arteries** are commonplace and have thick walls designed to resist excessive blood pressure. Following fixation, the vessel has partly contracted giving a scalloped appearance to the internal elastic lamina. Few elastic lamellae are noted in the smooth muscle of the vessel wall (stained black), but many more are in the tunica adventitia, which blend with peripheral connective tissue. The elastic fibers allow vascular distension followed by recoil. Verhoeff's/H&E, paraffin, × 300.

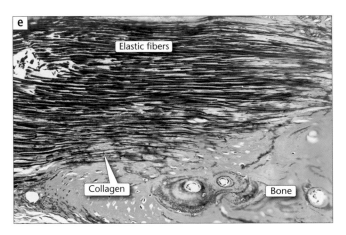

▲ **Fig 5.10e Vertebral ligaments.** The ligaments between vertebral bodies maintain strong attachments within the vertebral column, but they contain abundant elastic fibers that allow for flexion and extension. The extent of the flexion and extension is limited by collagen fibers intermixed with the elastic fibers. Other ligaments rich in elastic content are the ligamentum nuchae of cervical vertebrae, the vocal ligaments, and the suspensory ligament of the ocular lens. Gomori trichrome, paraffin, × 100.

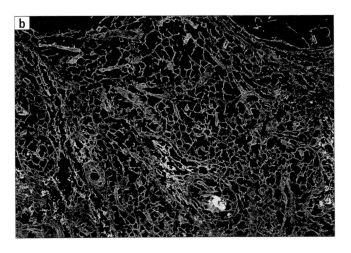

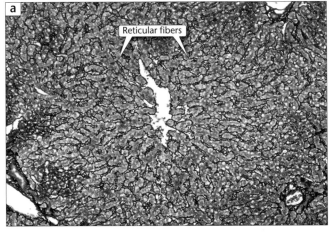

▲ **Fig 5.11a Reticular fibers in liver.** In this liver specimen, reticular fibers occur in the margins of the vascular sinusoids (i.e. in the spaces of Disse between the endothelial cells and the hepatocytes). Reticular fibers are type III collagen and provide structural support to the cells of the liver lobules. These fibers are synthesized by specialized types of fat-storing (Ito) cells, which also produce collagen types I, IV, V, and VI, glycoproteins, and proteoglycans. However, no visible basal lamina can be observed by electron microscopy. Gordon & Sweet–H&E, paraffin, × 80.

◀ **Fig 5.11b Reticular fibers in lymph nodes.** Lymphoid organs such as lymph nodes rely upon an internal framework of reticular fibers to accommodate their large cellular populations of lymphocytes, macrophages, and other immunocompetent cells. In this section, the complex and dense fiber network is clearly seen using darkfield microscopy. A similar arrangement occurs in the spleen. Reticular cells (fibroblasts) produce the fibers. Gordon and Sweet, paraffin, × 150.

cord. In humans this ligament is rudimentary, but in quadrupeds it helps hold the head upright. Elastic fibers may be synthesized by fibroblasts, smooth muscle cells, or chondrocytes, and are capable of extending to 120% strain without irreversible damage.

Dysfunctional states include:
- Emphysema (loss of elastin)
- Reduction in skin elasticity by exposure to ultraviolet light (e.g. excessive sunlight)
- Inadequate elasticity in arterial walls, which may cause stiffness and high blood pressure.

Reticular fibers (type III collagen) form a mesh or framework in a wide variety of tissues, including numerous glands and around smooth muscle, blood vessels, within lymphoid organs, and in less compacted forms of supporting tissue (Fig 5.11a & b).

Microfibrils

Microfibrils are apparently tubular proteins, about 10–12 nm in diameter, the most abundant of which is fibrillin. It is thought to provide a scaffold on which elastin is formed to make elastic fibers.

Matrix: macromolecules

The matrix surrounds and supports the cells and fibers, as mentioned above, and is also a secretory product of fibroblasts or, in the case of cartilage and bone, of chondroblasts and osteoblasts. Under microscopic examination, the matrix component can appear translucent or empty, or presents an amorphous appearance of variable density, depending on the tissue type and the stain. Basically, the matrix contains mixtures of proteoglycans and glycoproteins. The distributions and functions of some major proteins in the extracellular matrix are shown in Fig 5.12.

Proteoglycans

The proteoglycans are predominantly, but not exclusively, made by fibroblasts (chondroblasts

Some major proteins in the extracellular matrix			
Molecule	**Type**	**Common distribution**	**Function**
Aggrecan	Proteoglycan	Cartilage	Hydration, swelling of collagen (type II) framework
Cartilage matrix protein	Glycoprotein	Nonarticular cartilage	Bridging for collagen
Collagen type I	Fibrils	Bone, tendon, ligament, skin	Tensile strength
Collagen type II	Fibrils	Cartilage, vitreous humor	Tensile strength, resists compression
Collagen type III	'Reticular' fibrils	Numerous glands, immune tissues, skin, blood vessels	Mesh-like support, compliance
Collagen type IV	Network mesh	Basal laminae	Support, cell behavior
Collagen type VIII	Lattice	Descemet's membrane	Tensile strength
Collagen type X	Lattice	Fetal cartilage	Early bone formation
Decorin	Proteoglycan	Bone, tendon, ligament, skin	Bridging for collagen
Elastin	Fibrillar network	Many supporting tissues	Elasticity, resilience
Fibrillins	Microfibils, glycoprotein	With elastic fibers	Scaffolding
Fibrinogen	Plasma protein	Plasma	Fibrin clot
Fibronectin	Glycoprotein	Widespread in extracellular matrix	Adhesion, cell migration
Laminins	Glycoprotein	Basal laminae	Development, differentiation
Osteocalcin	Matrix, protein, glycoprotein	Bone, teeth	Regulates crystal growth
von Willebrand factor	Glycoprotein	Plasma	Platelet–vascular adhesion

▲ **Fig 5.12 Some major proteins in the extracellular matrix.** The common distributions and functions of some of the major proteins in the extracellular matrix. (Based on data from Ayad S, et al. The extracellular matrix facts book. London: Academic Press, 1994.)

in cartilage and osteoblasts of bone also secrete proteoglycans), and are large complexes of highly negatively charged carbohydrate-rich chains called glycosaminoglycans (GAGs) anchored to a central protein core—the whole macromolecule is not unlike a bristle brush (Fig 5.13). GAGs are polymers of amino sugars, most of which are sulfated, like chondroitin, keratan, dermatan, and heparan sulfate. Multiple proteoglycans in turn may attach to a giant non-sulfated GAG called hyaluronan, which may be 5 μm in length. The whole complex weaves its way through the fibers (collagen, elastin, and microfibrils) of the connective tissue. The proteoglycans are constantly being degraded and synthesized, and have a turnover time of 2–3 weeks.

When many proteoglycans link together, they form a proteoglycan aggregate (e.g. aggrecan in cartilage) that has high affinity for water because of the negatively charged amine and sulfate groups; hence the term porous hydrated shell. The clearest histologic example of this is seen in hyaline cartilage. Water occupies the tiny spaces, about 3 nm radius inside the GAG matrix of cartilage and about 300 nm in the vitreous body of the eye. Thus, resistance to flow is high, which is why some connective tissues are gel-like. Where the hydrated complexes are bound to the collagen, together they resist compressive deformation (e.g. under loading of articular cartilage).

In other tissues they serve a rigid support role, such as the hyaline cartilaginous rings of the trachea and respiratory tree.

Because proteoglycans are water soluble, they can be extracted from tissue sections during histologic preparation. This causes the washed-out appearance of some connective tissues, including hyaline cartilage, in which 95% of the volume is matrix and only 5% is occupied by the synthesizing and controlling cells, the chondrocytes.

Adhesive glycoproteins

Glycoproteins in the matrix include the following main groups:

- Adhesive types, such as fibronectin and laminin
- Skeletal forms, which influence calcium binding and calcification
- Others, such as fibrillin, that assist with elastic fiber formation
- Integrins, membrane proteins binding cells to the matrix.

Tip: Connective tissues have cells surrounded by an organic matrix. The cells may be very small as for fibroblasts, or large as for fat cells. All the cell types secrete and/or are embedded in a matrix of macromolecules, which appears amorphous in histologic sections. It is the fibers within the matrix that are usually visible, but this depends on the type of connective tissue.

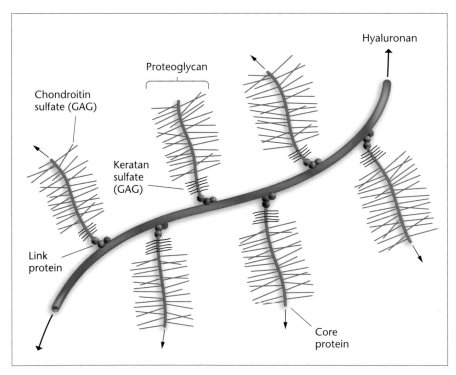

◀ **Fig 5.13 Cartilage matrix molecules.** Diagram of a glycosaminoglycan (GAG) megacomplex found in hyaline cartilage. These molecule complexes are visible with the electron microscope, are voluminous, and may be several micrometers in length. Hyaluronan is the backbone GAG protein to which the proteoglycan aggrecan attaches. The GAGs in aggrecan resemble a bristle brush and consist mainly of chondroitin sulfate and some keratan sulfate. Aggrecan binds to collagen, thus giving a degree of rigidity to the cartilage matrix. These complexes also attract and bind water, however, making cartilage swell and become turgid, an important property, for example, in weight-bearing articular cartilage of synovial joints.

BASEMENT MEMBRANE

The basement membrane is a special collection of connective tissue fibers and matrix that is found subjacent to the base of epithelia. It is also seen surrounding endothelia, muscle, fat, and peripheral nerve cells. The term applies to the thin, sheet-like structure observed with the light microscope (Fig 5.14a–c), but at the ultrastructural level it is seen as two components: a thin matrix layer called the basal lamina, external to which is the reticular lamina with collagen fibrils (Fig 5.15). Basement membranes provide anchorage and support to epithelial tissues and act as selective filters for diffusion. The combined width of these layers can be variable, up to several micrometers, depending on the epithelial tissue type and the presence of associated fibroblasts. The basal lamina is often in contact with the plasma membrane of the overlying cell that secretes it, although at times it is separated by another layer called the lamina rara or lucida. In these cases, the basal lamina is referred to as the lamina densa. The lamina lucida may contain integrins for bridging between intracellular actin and intermediate filaments and the lamina densa. Laminins are abundant in the lamina densa and form a structural network with the collagen fibrils (type IV) present in the lamina reticularis. Other structural proteins of the basal lamina include heparan sulfate (perlecan) and entactin. As a barrier protecting an epithelium, the basement membrane/basal lamina plays an important role in the invasion of cancerous cells into the underlying connective tissue.

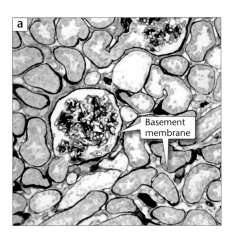

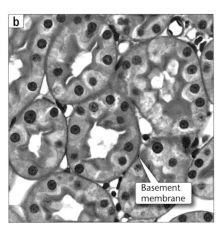

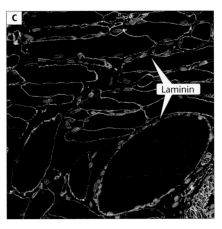

▲ **Fig 5.14a Basement membrane in kidney.** Kidney tissue stained with a silver method highlights basement membranes of a glomerulus and renal tubules, which stain black–brown. Basal laminae underlie epithelium and endothelium, and surround most muscle cells, fat cells, and peripheral nerve axons. They consist of collagen type IV and the structural glycoprotein, laminin, which together form irregular networks by self-assembly. Silver stain, paraffin, × 100.

▲ **Fig 5.14b Basement membrane.** With periodic acid–Schiff (PAS) staining for carbohydrates, the basement membrane is positively stained owing to its content of perlecan (proteoglycan), laminin, and a structural glycoprotein (either entactin or nidogen). Basal laminae have many functions, including support, selective cellular or molecular filtration, and interactions with cells to assist with tissue architecture and growth. PAS, paraffin, × 250.

▲ **Fig 5.14c Basal lamina.** Immunofluorescence method for laminin in the basal lamina. Laminin is detected around skeletal muscle fibers (with blue nuclei) and the thin wall of smooth muscle of a venule. Thus basal laminae are not restricted to epithelial tissues but are found in many other tissues. × 200. (Courtesy J Zbaeren, Inselspital, Bern, Switzerland.)

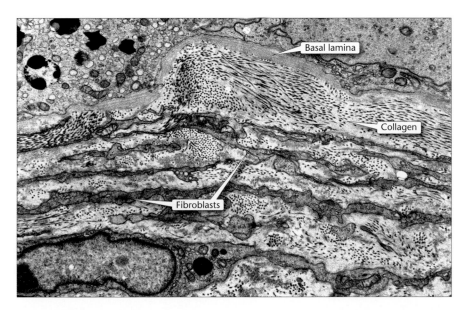

◀ **Fig 5.15 Fine structure of basement membrane.** Ultrastructure of the supporting layers associated with epithelia, showing the basal lamina, several layers of thin fibroblast cytoplasm, and collagen fibers embedded in extracellular matrix. Depending upon the epithelial type, these layers vary in number and width. They provide support, flexibility for the tissue, and attachment for the basal epithelial cells. × 7,000.

CLASSIFICATION

Although it is apparent that the various histologic types of supporting (or connective) tissue are significantly different from one another, they may be allocated to major and minor groupings based upon their morphology. The basic term connective tissue is used because it remains a common expression in anatomy, pathology, and clinical research.

Loose connective tissue

Basic loose connective tissue, or areolar tissue (i.e. spaces or gaps in the matrix formed during tissue preparation), is the most widespread.

Loosely packed fibers are separated by abundant amorphous matrix (Fig 5.16a–c). It also provides a deformable and space-occupying "packing" framework for organ support.

Adipose tissue

Adipose tissue consists of two types of adipose cells (Fig 5.17a–c): white adipose cells in adults; and brown adipose cells, which are abundant in neonates but diminished in postnatal life. The traditional functions of adipose tissues are:
- Synthesizing and storing fat
- Acting as a reserve energy source
- An insulating material under the skin

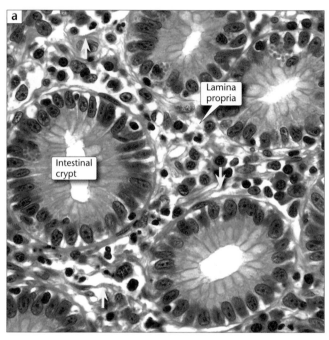

▲ **Fig 5.16a Loose connective tissue.** Transverse section of intestinal crypts surrounded by loose (or areolar) connective tissue termed the lamina propria, which allows cell migration. Here, the fibrous protein component is minimal, with much of the interglandular tissues containing neurovascular elements and wandering cells of the immune system. The structural framework of collagen (**arrows**) is a delicate mesh of fibers. Empty spaces are, in part, artifacts of preparation but, in vivo, are filled with a sol-gel matrix. H&E, paraffin, × 400.

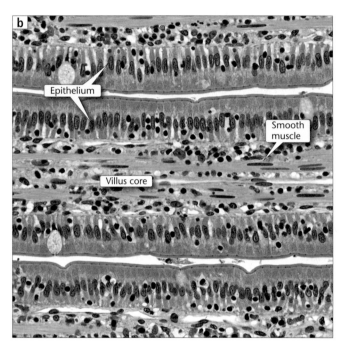

▲ **Fig 5.16b Vertical section through the gut mucosa,** showing three villi, the cores of which contain loose connective tissue. It is highly cellular with fibroblasts, leukocytes, macrophages, and mast cells, together with blood vessels and spindle-shaped smooth muscle cells. All of these are supported by the extracellular matrix, which contains fibrous proteins (collagen, elastin) embedded in hydrated polysaccharide–protein polymers. H&E, paraffin, × 300.

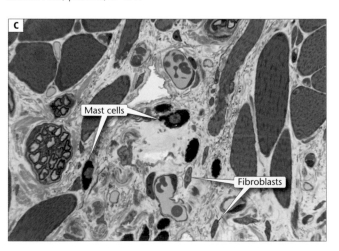

◀ **Fig 5.16c Loose connective tissue providing support for muscle, nerve, and vascular elements.** Mast cells show densely stained granules, and numerous fibroblasts are scattered throughout. Small collagen bundles and other microfibrils separated by matrix are typical of this type of connective tissue. Exchange of nutrients between the vascular system and the tissues occurs by diffusion through the connective tissue matrix. Toluidine blue, araldite, × 490.

- A shock absorber around many joints.

Fat tissue is, however, a complex and very active metabolic and endocrine organ. White adipose tissue secretes bioactive peptides called adipokines, such as leptin, tumor necrosis factor α and adiponectin. The endocrine roles played by these peptides is noted in situations of excess or deficiency of adipose tissue because of the associated adverse effects upon general metabolism, including disturbances in insulin actions and inflammatory reactions.

Reticular tissue

Exhibiting fine fibers that form extensive branching networks, reticular tissue is seen, for example, in some lymphoid tissues, in the liver, and in numerous glands (Fig 5.18).

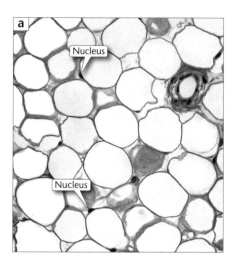

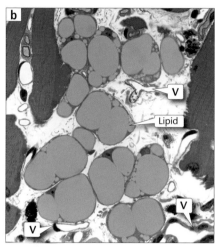

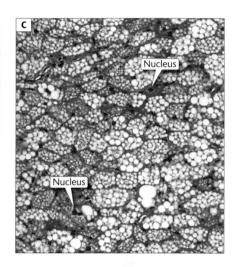

▲ **Fig 5.17a Adipose tissue.**
Adipocytes (fat-storing cells) in histologic section often show only a thin rim of cytoplasm and a peripheral nucleus because their lipid content is usually dissolved by the organic solvents used in tissue preparation. Most adipose tissue is white fat (in which there is a single fat droplet per cell). Brown fat (in which there are multiple lipid inclusions in each cell) is found in association with the scapula, the sternum, and the axillae, notably in the newborn. Adipose cells are supported by loose connective tissue. H&E, paraffin, × 300.

▲ **Fig 5.17b Fat droplets in adipocytes** contain fatty acids, stored as triglycerides. These are well preserved in this specimen fixed in glutaraldehyde–osmium. Fatty acids from the liver and gut circulate via blood vessels (**V**) as lipoproteins. These lipoproteins are converted to free fatty acids at the adipocyte surface and are subsequently re-esterified to form triglycerides within the cell. Fatty acids released from adipose tissue provide fuel for other tissues. Fat also provides thermal insulation and mechanical protection for underlying tissues. Toluidine blue, araldite, × 350.

▲ **Fig 5.17c Brown fat cells**
(or multilocular adipose tissue) contain many lipid droplets with a central nucleus. The brown color is due to a rich vascular supply and abundant mitochondria, providing high respiratory capacity and thus generating heat. Brown adipocytes are smaller than white adipose cells; they are highly innervated and controlled by sympathetic nerves. Norepinephrine (noradrenaline) release results in the oxidation of fatty acids within the mitochondria to produce heat. This energy source is important in neonates and is known as non-shivering thermogenesis. Beginning with a multipotential mesenchymal stem cell, white or brown adipose cells are thought to differentiate along initially common but ultimately divergent pathways. Beyond childhood, brown fat gradually diminishes but can persist around the adrenal glands, kidneys, and aorta throughout adult life. H&E, paraffin, × 250.

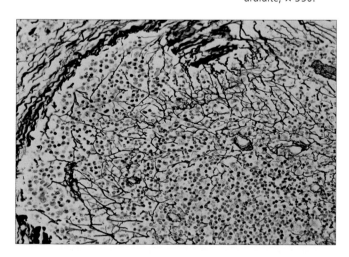

◀ **Fig 5.18 Reticular fibers.** Lymphoid tissues such as lymph nodes are supported by a delicate network of reticular fibers of type III collagen. Fibers originate from the organ capsule, extending into and arborizing throughout the parenchyma of the node. At the lymphoid follicle, the reticular fibers encircle and penetrate the follicle to provide a framework for the lymphocytes, seen here as many small dense nuclei. Reticulin method, paraffin, × 180.

Mucous connective tissue and mesentery

Mucous connective tissue occurs mainly in the embryo, showing much matrix with few cells or fibers (Fig 5.19). The umbilical cord is an example, where hyaluronic acid (hyaluronan) predominates.

Mesenteries and mucous and synovial membranes are examples of loose connective tissue associated with a covering epithelium; their major function is to provide support, nutrients, or fluid secretion (Fig 5.20).

Dense connective tissue

In dense irregular connective tissue, the collagen bundles are oriented in various three-dimensional arrays, enabling the tissue to withstand tension from different directions. Examples include dermis, sheaths surrounding nerves and tendons, organ capsules, and deep fascia (Fig 5.21a–d).

> **Tip:** Loose, or areolar, connective tissue has variable fiber content, but the ECM is always prominent. Dense connective tissue is dominated by fibers (usually collagen) with little ECM.

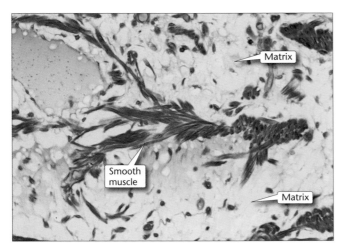

◀ **Fig 5.19 Mucous connective tissue.** In the embryo and fetus, the loose connective tissue is characterized by a high proportion of gelatinous-type matrix with scattered mesenchymal cells. In this specimen, the twisting cell fibers are developing smooth muscle cells. The matrix appears empty because it is rich with proteoglycans that attract and retain water, hence the gel-like morphology. Toluidine blue, araldite, × 100.

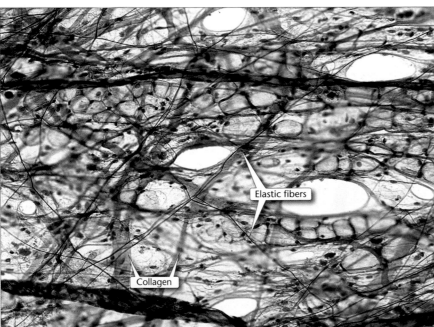

◀ **Fig 5.20 Mesentery.** A whole mount (i.e. not a section) of mesentery, which is a semi-transparent, double layer of peritoneum attached to the abdominal wall and most of the abdominal viscera. It consists of loose networks of collagen fibers and very fine elastic fibers, which support fat cells (empty spaces due to extraction of lipids) and the extracellular matrix. The numerous cells include fibroblasts, mast cells, macrophages, and leukocytes. Although this tissue has a squamous epithelial surface, the cells of these layers are not identifiable in this preparation. Reticulin method, × 150.

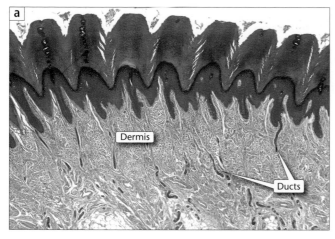

▲ **Fig 5.21a Dense irregular connective tissue of the dermis.** Section of thick skin showing an extensive subepithelial layer of dense irregular connective tissue referred to as the dermis. This layer has few spaces. A number of densely stained narrow ducts of sweat glands are noted in the dermis. This connective tissue supports the epithelium and, being deformable, allows for mobility and stretching of the skin. Attachment of the dermis to the superficial epidermis is enhanced by the many interdigitations at the interface between the two tissues. H&E, paraffin, × 40.

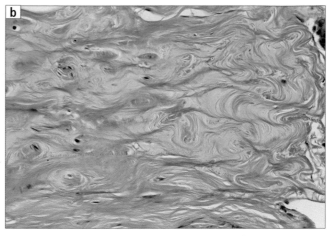

▲ **Fig 5.21b Dense irregular connective tissue of the dermis**, illustrating layers of collagen bundles in sheets and wave forms that characterize the irregular type of dense connective tissue. Occasional nuclei of fibroblasts are seen and extracellular matrix occupies the territories between the collagen fibers. The shape of the bundles and fibers indicates that the tissue is subject to mechanical forces from different directions, as is the case in this specimen of skin. Masson's trichrome, paraffin, × 300.

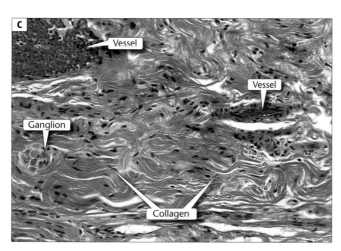

▲ **Fig 5.21c Submucosa of the gut** is shown. Bundles of collagen separated by areas of fewer collagen fibers but more extracellular matrix allow for a degree of plasticity, but resistance to tensile forces is the major function of this type of connective tissue. Lighter stained areas in the collagen bundles contains glycosaminoglycans or proteoglycans and glycoproteins. These matrix molecules are involved in hydration, adhesion, binding to collagen and elastin, and molecular organization of the fibrous and matrix components. Most of the cell nuclei represent fibroblasts. Blood vessels and a nerve ganglion are shown. H&E, paraffin, × 200.

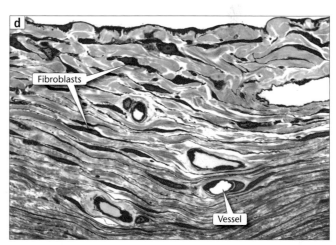

▲ **Fig 5.21d Capsules of some organs** consist of multiple layers of collagen bundles oriented in different directions, and elongated fibroblasts. The slender spaces between the collagen are filled with tissue-specific glycoconjugates and glycosaminoglycans. Capsules can be very resistant to stretch or tearing forces, but they also play an important role in preserving the contents and integrity of the tissues they surround (e.g. ovary, testis, spleen, joint space, prostate). Blood vessels are also indicated. Toluidine blue–basic fuchsin, araldite, × 400.

131

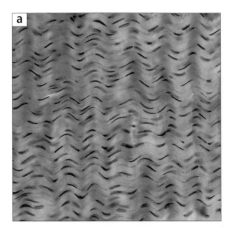

▲ **Fig 5.22a Dense regular connective tissue of a tendon.** Tendons may show a crimp pattern of the collagen fibers forming undulating ribbons, corresponding to the direction of the stress–strain force that occurs when the muscle exerts force through the tendon. Crimp angle and tendon strain decrease with age. The high proportion of collagen confers considerable strength to tendons, for example, the Achilles tendon. H&E, paraffin, × 250.

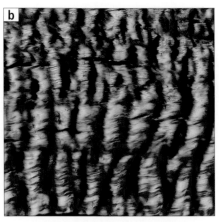

▲ **Fig 5.22b Tendon examined with circular polarized light** that emphasizes the crimp morphology of the collagen bundles. The regular, alternating light and dark bands are due to the periodic birefringent properties of the collagen proteins caused by their orientations with respect to the polarized light waves. It is believed that the crimp acts as a shock absorber during tension and release of the contractile forces transmitted from muscle to the tendon. Masson's trichrome, paraffin, × 250.

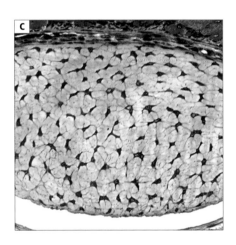

▲ **Fig 5.22c Cross section through a small-diameter tendon**, showing the regular arrangement of fibroblasts, which synthesize the intervening type I collagen. The fibroblasts are stellate in shape. Tendons may be confused with skeletal or smooth muscle. In skeletal muscle, the nuclei are peripheral in each muscle fiber; in smooth muscle the nuclei are central within each muscle cell. Toluidine blue, araldite, × 300.

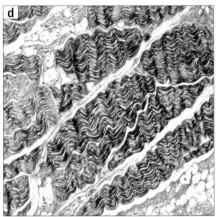

▲ **Fig 5.22d Section of a short ligament**, showing groups of undulating collagen bundles separated by loose connective tissue septa. Compared with a tendon, more matrix separates the collagen fibers, and these areas contain finer collagen and variable amounts of elastic fibers, both of which stain poorly. The smaller, shorter fascicles and extra matrix provide flexibility combined with strength for interosseous attachment, consistent with the role of ligaments in contributing to joint stability during normal ranges of movement. Masson's trichrome, paraffin, × 175.

In dense regular connective tissue, there are many collagen bundles aligned in one general direction with parallel or regular orientations in order to provide maximum tensile strength. Examples include tendons, ligaments, aponeuroses, and retinacula (Fig 5.22a–d).

Cartilage

Cartilage consists of an abundant ECM produced by scattered chondrocytes. The ECM consists of collagen fibrils in which aggregating proteoglycans are embedded. In adults, it does not contain nerves, blood, or lymphatic vessels. It is not as hard or as strong as bone, yet it may be resistant to crushing or stretching forces, hence its lay description as "gristle."

Hyaline cartilage

Transparent or glass-like, hyaline cartilage is the most widespread type of cartilage. Elastic cartilage and fibrocartilage may be considered as variants of hyaline cartilage, based upon their different matrix compositions.

Hyaline cartilage has a bluish, opalescent color, with chondrocytes surrounded by a matrix mainly of proteoglycans and non-collagenous proteins and collagen. The cells that mature into chondrocytes are called chondroblasts, but the morphological distinction between the two is arbitrary (Fig 5.23a & b). The collagen is not visible by light microscopy. Hyaline cartilage is rigid but not brittle, and it resists compression and shear forces. Examples are articular surfaces of synovial joints, costal and respiratory cartilages, and epiphyseal growth plates.

In articular hyaline cartilage, the hyaluronic acid–protein complexes give the cartilage a viscous, slippery property and a very low coefficient of friction—ideal for joint surfaces. Chondrocytes are surrounded by a thin rim of matrix that defines the space occupied

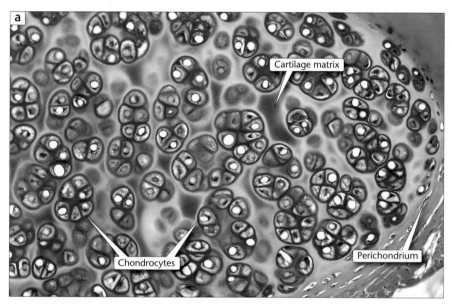

◄ **Fig 5.23a Growing hyaline cartilage**, showing large ovoid and polygonal chondrocytes, which secrete cartilage matrix of collagen and proteoglycans. The perichondrium is to the right and from this new chondrocytes are produced, in growing cartilage, by proliferation and assembling into multicellular groups, which later disperse. Note that the matrix is deeply stained, indicating the concentration of particular types of proteoglycans. Other types of cartilage are fibrous, elastic, and fetal types. Each may be subclassified (e.g. hyaline cartilage can be epiphyseal, articular, tracheal, or bronchial). H&E–Alcian blue, paraffin, × 250.

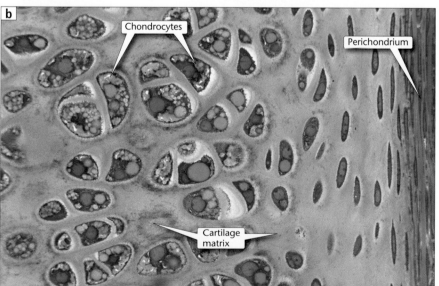

◄ **Fig 5.23b Hyaline cartilage.** The perichondrium of this specimen of hyaline cartilage shows a superficial fibrous layer, which blends with a deeper chondrogenic layer containing flat, newly formed chondrocytes. These newly formed chondrocytes secrete matrix, adding to appositional growth of cartilage. When the deeper chondrocytes divide, they form clusters called isogenous groups, which contribute to interstitial cartilage growth. Note the denser staining of matrix around mature chondrocytes, which indicates synthesis of matrix that is rich in proteoglycans. Toluidine blue, araldite, × 350.

by the cell as a lacuna (Fig 5.24). Sometimes two chondrocytes are found in a lacuna. The distribution of proteoglycans in the matrix may be revealed by metachromatic or basophilic stains such as toluidine blue. A zone of territorial matrix surrounds the lacuna and is thought to protect cells and regulate matrix assembly. A less dense interterritorial matrix occupies the spaces between chondrocytes. Its role is to provide mechanical strength to the tissue. Collagen fibrils in the inner territorial matrix are aligned parallel to the chondrocyte surface. When isolated by enzymatic digestion, this zone and its chondrocyte is called the chondron and is believed to be the basic functional unit of hyaline cartilage. If damaged or eroded by disease, hyaline cartilage has very poor regenerative properties. The biology of articular hyaline cartilage is reviewed in Chapter 10.

Elastic cartilage

Elastic cartilage tends to be yellowish. It contains many chondrocytes and the matrix is criss-crossed by a dense network of elastic fibers produced by the precursor cells of the mature chondrocytes (Fig 5.25). It exhibits great flexibility and elasticity. Examples include the external ear, epiglottis, and auditory tube.

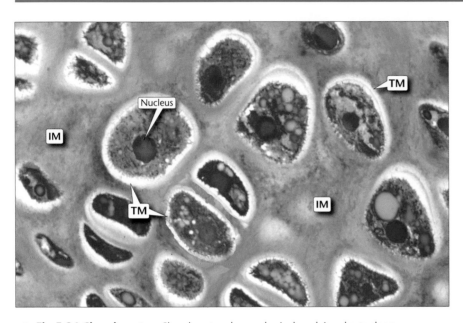

▲ **Fig 5.24 Chondrocytes.** Chondrocytes show spherical nuclei and cytoplasm with glycogen, rough endoplasmic reticulum, Golgi, and lipid (blue–green inclusions). A pericellular halo or lacuna is a shrinkage artifact but, in vivo, the lacuna is mainly aggrecan, a giant proteoglycan with a hyaluronan core that traps water. This layer blends with the territorial matrix (**TM**), and all components within this border form the chondron, the primary unit of cartilage homeostasis. The TM contains type II collagen (and some type XI) and chondroitin sulfate glycosaminoglycans in the proteoglycans. Keratan sulfate predominates in the proteoglycans amongst the type II collagen of the interterritorial matrix (**IM**). Toluidine blue, araldite, × 600.

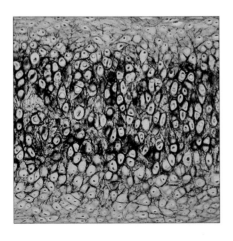

◄ **Fig 5.25 Elastic cartilage.** Tissue of the epiglottis, showing a core of elastic cartilage, with partial extraction of the chondrocytes, embedded in a matrix that comprises an abundant network of elastic fibers in the interterritorial matrix, which extends toward the perichondrium. The matrix also contains aggrecan and type II collagen. Elastic cartilage is found also in the external ear, Eustachian tube, and laryngeal cartilages. Gomori trichrome, paraffin, × 80.

Fibrocartilage

Fibrocartilage is white and marked by strong bundles of collagen and smaller amounts of amorphous matrix than other types of cartilage (Fig 5.26a & b). It is an intermediate type of tissue between hyaline cartilage and dense fibrous tissue. Fibrocartilage is not found alone. It blends with adjacent tissues and therefore has no definite perichondrium (Fig 5.27a & b). It possesses considerable tensile strength and resistance to compression. Examples include:

- Annulus fibrosus of intervertebral discs
- The link between tendon and bone
- The menisci of the knee joint, and coracoclavicular and temporomandibular joints.

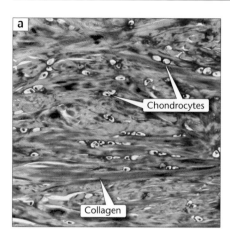

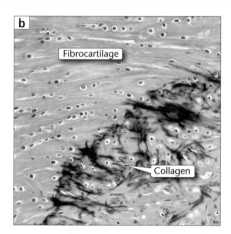

◀ **Fig 5.26a Fibrocartilage in knee joint.** Resembling a hybrid tissue of hyaline cartilage and dense fibrous connective tissue, fibrocartilage is a fiber-reinforced tissue containing abundant aligned collagen bundles and chondrocytes in pairs or isogenous groups surrounded by a matrix of proteoglycans. Fibrocartilage is strong and resists compression or stretching. It is found in the intervertebral discs, the symphysis pubis, the labra of the glenoid and acetabular fossae, and the articular disks of some joints, such as this specimen of the meniscus of the knee joint. Masson's trichrome, paraffin, × 180.

▲ **Fig 5.26b Specimen of fetal fibrocartilage,** merging into developing cartilage and bone. Chondrocytes in fibrocartilage are aligned in rows with collagen fibers interdigitated into the growing cartilage–bone tissue. This provides anchorage between the tissues. Masson's trichrome, paraffin, × 150.

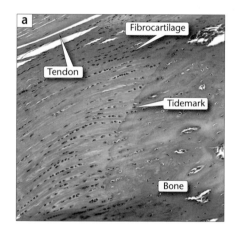

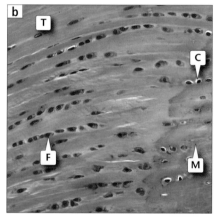

▲ **Fig 5.27a Fibrocartilage and the enthesis.** The enthesis is the attachment site for a ligament or tendon into bone. In the case of tendons there are four zones—tendon, fibrocartilage, mineralized cartilage, and bone. Together these form a tissue that is useful for comparison of these different connective tissues: tendon—scattered fibroblast nuclei; the fibrocartilage—rows of chondrocytes in pairs; mineralized cartilage—denser matrix; the bone—the largest proportion of matrix with scattered osteocytes. The attachment zone is marked by a tidemark or cement line. H&E, paraffin, × 100.

▲ **Fig 5.27b The tidemark of the enthesis.** The tidemark shown here represents a band of fine striations that correspond to aggregates of mineral (calcium) deposited by matrix vesicles produced by nearby chondrocytes (**C**). Calcium and hydroxyapatite crystals accumulate in the matrix vesicles, and their contents of a specific glycoprotein, abundant in the tidemark zone, induce calcium phosphate (hydroxyapatite) deposition in association with binding to matrix collagen. Thus the fibrocartilage (**F**) acts as a transitional tissue between the tendon (**T**) and the calcified matrix (**M**) peripheral to fully mineralized bone. H&E, paraffin, × 200.

Bone

Bone is discussed in Chapter 10, but it can be considered briefly here as an extremely rigid form of dense connective tissue, in which the ECM takes the form of needle-type crystalline mineral salts called hydroxyapatite. The mineral is calcium phosphate, which makes up about 65% of bone weight. Both the ground substance and the collagen fibers are mineralized. Recognizable cells in bone are the osteocytes, located within small spaces called lacunae. Dense, or compact, bone is a solid mass of calcified tissue. Cancellous, or spongy, bone is porous. It consists of slender beams (trabeculae) of mineralized tissue that form a meshwork pattern filled with bone marrow and fat.

Specialized connective tissue

Blood and bone marrow are discussed more extensively in Chapter 3; some histologists classify them as connective tissue.

Blood is derived from mesoderm and consists of formed cellular elements and plasma. It is a fluid connective tissue in which the plasma (the ground substance or matrix) consists mostly of water in which various substances are dissolved. The fibers of blood plasma are strands of fibrin, seen in clot formation.

Bone marrow is composed of the precursor cells of erythrocytes, leukocytes, and platelets. It is found in the medullary cavities of bone. Red marrow is so colored because of the hemoglobin in erythrocytes. Yellow marrow contains a high proportion of fat cells. The marrow is supported by a network of reticular fibers produced by reticular cells, a special type of supporting cell that lines the blood vessels externally as they penetrate through the islands of marrow.

DISORDERS
Marfan's syndrome

Marfan's syndrome is caused by mutations in the fibrillin gene, resulting in disorders of elastin. This leads to a widespread range of tissue irregularities, including lax joints, long extremities, fragile vascular walls, and dislocations of the lens of the eye.

People with Marfan's syndrome often die in their mid-40s owing to catastrophic rupture of the aortic wall. Current research efforts are aimed at characterizing the genetic basis and using transgenic models to study the basic biology and pathology before developing effective treatment.

Ehlers–Danlos syndrome

Ehlers–Danlos syndrome is an inherited disorder arising as a result of abnormalities in the collagen fibers of the dermis and tendons. It presents as joint dislocations and skin deformation. Future treatment is dependent upon additional genetic and molecular biological study.

Lipomas

Lipomas are generally superficial benign tumors of fatty tissue. They are usually encapsulated and may contain more fibrous tissue septa than normal tissue. Most occur on the trunk or upper limb.

Granulation tissue

Granulation tissue repairs disrupted connective tissue and is associated with wound healing. It contains layers of fibroblasts within a vascularized collagen matrix, type I collagen becoming the chief fiber type in mature wounds. Granulation tissue occurs in sites of resorption (where there is dead tissue), replacement (where there is a skin lesion), or limitation (where there is isolation of an abscess). It results in scar formation.

Scurvy

Vitamin C deficiency, or scurvy, results in the synthesis of abnormal collagen that lacks its usual strength. Scurvy is associated with an inability of wounds to heal, and, in the oral cavity, loss of teeth, and gum bleeding (caused by bone abnormalities and vascular fragility).

Fibromas

Fibromas are benign soft-tissue tumors that produce collagen. They present as a lump in dense supporting tissue. These tumors and their malignant variants are uncommon.

Rheumatoid arthritis

Rheumatoid arthritis is an inflammatory joint disease (see Chapter 10). It involves destruction of articular hyaline cartilage by synovial granulation tissue. Its cause is unknown, but local production of antibodies forming immune complexes can be associated with this condition.

Tendon sheath tumors

Tendon sheath tumors show accumulations of collagen, macrophages, and fibroblasts. They occur most commonly in the fingers and the feet. They are not malignant.

Muscle

Three major categories of muscle are recognized in humans and other mammals (Fig 6.1):

- Skeletal muscle, most commonly attached to bone via tendons
- Cardiac muscle in the heart
- Smooth muscle in the walls of hollow tubes and visceral organs.

Although each type generates movement by way of mechanical forces associated with contraction, each shows structural specializations pertaining to its particular anatomic location and function. All muscle cells rely on the interaction of cytoplasmic actin and myosin filaments—actin slides along closely aligned and parallel myosin filaments. Muscle tissue is a good example of why an understanding of cellular mechanisms is dependent on knowledge of ultrastructural organization and molecular biology.

In addition to contraction, muscle cells also have the following abilities:

- To stretch beyond their resting length
- To return to the resting state (elasticity)
- To increase in size (hypertrophy) or number (hyperplasia), or both.

Various subclassifications of each of the three types of muscle are based on special physiologic functions or locations within organs and tissues.

SKELETAL MUSCLE

Skeletal muscle is striated. Skeletal muscle, also known as striated or voluntary muscle, is readily recognized in stained teased preparations or sections. Individual cells are cylindrical with multiple elliptical nuclei (hundreds or more nuclei per cell) located peripherally, and the cytoplasm shows alternating dark and light cross-striations in longitudinal sections (Fig 6.2a–c). These striations represent overlapping bands of contractile filaments, and they may be made to appear more distinct by closing down the microscope condenser diaphragm to increase contrast.

Skeletal muscle cells are commonly referred to as muscle fibers—a term used to describe all types of muscle cells. Their long length is a result of the fusion of many myoblasts during embryonic and fetal growth. In transverse sections they present as polygonal profiles and, with high magnification, they may show a stippled appearance, outlined by one or more peripherally located nuclei (Fig 6.3a–c).

Characteristics of the three major categories of muscle			
	Skeletal	**Cardiac**	**Smooth**
Cell length	Wide range: 1 mm–20 cm	50–100 µm	50–100 µm (up to 0.5 mm in uterus)
Cell diameter	10–100 µm	10–20 µm	5–10 µm
Morphology	Long parallel cylinders, multiple peripheral nuclei, striations	Short branched cylinders, single central nucleus, striations	Spindle-shaped, tapering ends, single central nucleus, no striations
Connections	Fascicle bundles, tendons	Junctions join cells end to end	Connective tissue, gap and desmosome-type junctions
Control	Somatic motor neurons, voluntary control	Intrinsic rhythm, involuntary autonomic modulation	Involuntary, autonomic, intrinsic activity, local stimuli
Power	Rapid, forceful	Lifelong variable rhythm	Slow, sustained or rhythmic

▲ **Fig 6.1 Characteristics of the three major categories of muscle.** Various subclassifications of each type of muscle are based on special physiologic functions or locations within organs and tissues, particularly for skeletal and smooth muscle.

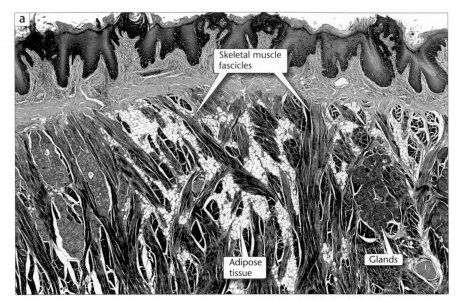

◄ **Fig 6.2a Skeletal muscle fibers of tongue.** Low magnification view of the skeletal muscle arrangement in the tongue showing interlacing muscle bundles called fascicles. Although most fibers are not attached to bone but blend with connective tissue, the muscle mass is regulated by motor neurons and the morphology is identical to skeletal muscle. Glands and adipose tissue are seen between fibers. Masson's trichrome, paraffin, × 10.

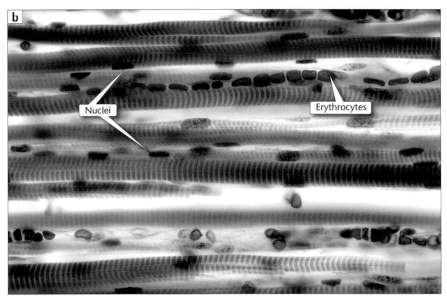

◄ **Fig 6.2b A thick section of skeletal muscle fibers**, showing their long cylindrical shape and prominent, highly ordered dark and light striations. Numerous flat nuclei are noted along the edge of some fibers. Regions between fibers show densely stained erythrocytes in capillaries. Heidenhain's iron hematoxylin, paraffin, × 500.

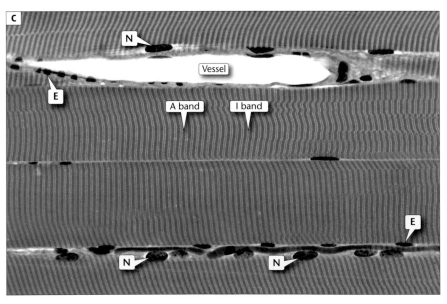

◄ **Fig 6.2c Several skeletal muscle fibers, shown at medium magnification**, are bordered by endomysium, which contains vessels such as capillaries and venules. Striations consisting of dark A bands and lighter I bands indicate the highly ordered pattern of sarcomeres—the region between the middle of each I band. Fibers contain peripheral nuclei (**N**), which slightly indent the striations. Other slender nuclei (**E**) in the endomysium are endothelial cells, pericytes, or fibroblasts. Hematoxylin and eosin (H&E), acrylic resin, × 240.

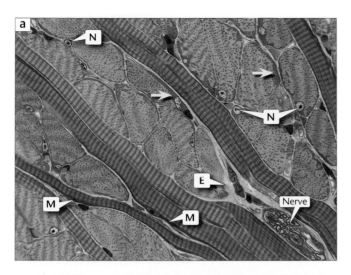

◀ **Fig 6.3a Fiber cytology.** Thin araldite resin section of longitudinal and transverse views of muscle fibers, separated by endomysium (**E**) containing a myelinated nerve. Note peripheral nuclei (**N**) in the transverse fibers and the sarcoplasm studded with mitochondria, which are also aggregated beneath the sarcolemma (**arrows**). Similar concentrations of mitochondria are shown in the longitudinal fibers (**M**) extending many micrometers along the subsarcolemmal cytoplasm. Toluidine blue, araldite, × 250.

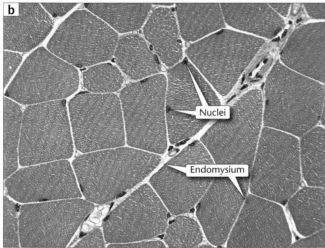

◀ **Fig 6.3b In cross section, skeletal muscle fibers** are polygonal in shape, characteristically showing one or more peripheral nuclei, which is indicative of their multinucleated nature. In stained paraffin sections, the fibers are mottled or stippled, often forming faint dark and light bands, which represent oblique sections through A and I bands of contractile filaments. A thin endomysium surrounds each fiber and contains blood vessels, with attendant endothelial cells and fibroblasts producing collagen, reticular fibers, and extracellular matrix. H&E, acrylic resin, × 300.

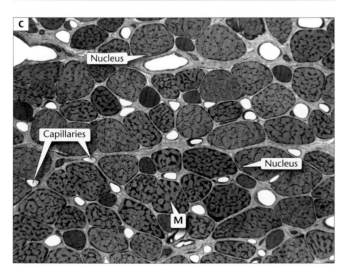

◀ **Fig 6.3c Extraocular muscles.** A transverse section through small-diameter extraocular muscles, which are specially adapted for rapid contractions and moderately resistant to fatigue. Some smaller fibers show abundant mitochondria (**M**) for aerobic metabolism (they burn oxygen to produce ATP) and are densely stained owing to moderate-to-high amounts of myoglobin (an auxiliary oxygen supply). Slightly larger fibers show fewer mitochondria and possibly less myoglobin, giving a lighter color. These are probably fast glycolytic fibers. The section illustrates the histologic heterogeneity of fibers, small for functional endurance, larger for fast twitch. Note peripheral nuclei and numerous capillaries. Toluidine blue, araldite, × 400.

Fascicles

A muscle has compartments. An individual muscle is surrounded by a sheath of connective tissue—the epimysium. The epimysium extends inward to form septa of the perimysium, which outlines subcomponents known as fascicles. Fascicles are bundles containing tens or hundreds of muscle fibers (Fig 6.4), each fiber being surrounded by connective tissue called the endomysium (Fig 6.5a & b).

All three connective tissue layers allow for the entry and exit of arteries, nerves, veins, and lymphatics, as well as freedom of motion between fascicles and muscle fibers. This organization applies to small muscles (e.g. the muscles of the inner ear, the extraocular muscles) and long muscles (e.g. the muscles of the lower limb).

Most skeletal muscles attach to bone via tendons—strong connective tissue that is continuous with the connective tissue sheaths mentioned above. Not all

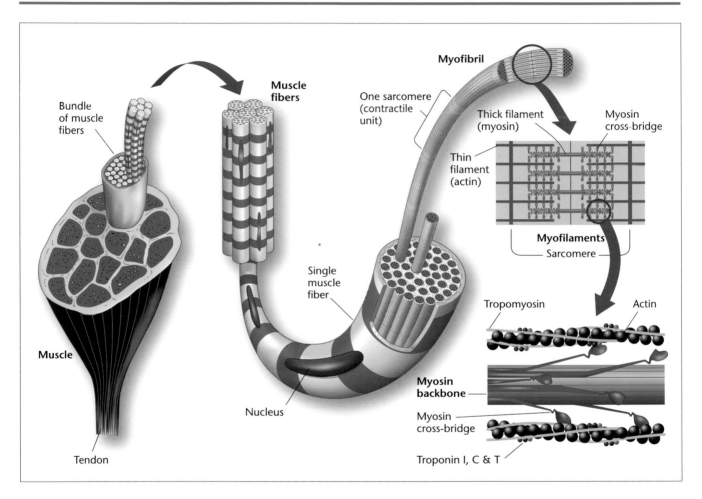

▲ **Fig 6.4 Macro, micro, and molecular organization of skeletal muscle.** Each muscle fiber is the product of multiple cell fusions and contains many rod-like myofibrils. These occupy most of the sarcoplasm, with smooth membranes and mitochondria intervening. The contractile filaments making up a myofibril are organized into units of contraction—the sarcomeres. Thin filaments of actin slide telescopically over the thicker myosin filaments, which causes muscle contraction. Proteins associated with actin (tropomyosin and the troponin complex) respond to fluctuating concentrations of calcium ions by acting as a switch to enable or disable the interaction and cross-bridging between myosin and actin.

skeletal muscles attach to bone; those of the tongue and some in the pharynx and esophagus exert contractile forces via connective tissue attachments. A similar arrangement applies to the fascicles (and their internal fibers) of long muscles (e.g. sartorius in the thigh) that may attain lengths up to 20 cm but still shorter than the whole muscle. Other muscles are composed of smaller, in-series fascicles/fibers with tapered endings occurring frequently in the middle of the muscle.

Fibers

A muscle fiber is a very long single cell. Skeletal muscle fibers are derived from the end-to-end fusion of many individual precursor myoblasts during embryogenesis (Fig 6.6). Myoblasts multiply by mitosis but, once formed into a developing muscle fiber (a myotube), they no longer divide. With continuous addition of myoblasts forming a syncitium of cells, the fiber grows in length and

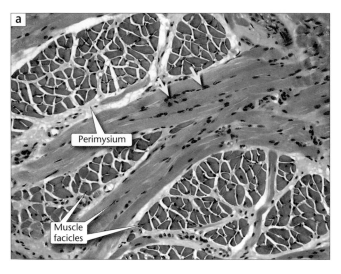

▲ **Fig 6.5a Fascicles and fibers.** Low-magnification view of skeletal muscle, showing bundles of muscle fibers grouped into fascicles running longitudinally or transversely through the section. Although striations are not apparent, the tissue is recognizable as skeletal muscle because (i) in cross section the nuclei are located peripherally and (ii) in longitudinal sections the slender nuclei tend to be aligned in defined rows (**arrows**) with eosinophilic fibers in between. Fascicles are supported by perimysium conveying nerves and blood vessels throughout the muscle. H&E, paraffin, × 80.

▲ **Fig 6.5b Laminin.** Immunofluoresence demonstration of laminin (green) surrounding skeletal muscle fibers, with their nuclei labelled in blue. Laminin is a component of the extracellular matrix of the muscle endomysium. × 200. (Courtesy J. Zbaeren, Inselspital, Bern, Switzerland.)

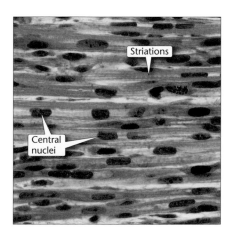

◄ **Fig 6.6 Skeletal muscle development.** Derived from mesenchymal cells, myoblasts proliferate and fuse end-on-end to form myotubes, with nuclei in series. Note the faint striations indicating synthesis and assembly of developing contractile filaments. The primitive muscle fibers grow in length by addition of myoblasts. H&E, paraffin, × 450.

begins to synthesize proteins that remain within the cell cytoplasm, eventually displacing the nuclei to the periphery of the fiber. The growing fiber thus becomes multinucleated, a structural hallmark of skeletal muscle (Fig 6.7a–c). Developing muscle fibers are biochemically and physiologically specialized, maturing into type I fibers (slow, red in color) and type II fibers (fast, white in color), determined by differentially expressed genes. At different times and locations in the embryo and fetus, fibers are formed in primary and secondary waves; the former generally become slow fibers and the latter, fast fibers.

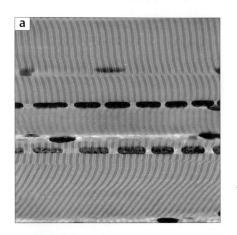

◀ Fig 6.7a Multinucleated muscle fibers. Skeletal muscle fibers have many nuclei located at the periphery of the fiber. The fiber is a multinucleated cell filled with proteins organized into dark and light striations, which represent overlapping and non-overlapping filaments. Production of these filaments during fiber maturation displaces nuclei to the edge of the cell. H&E, acrylic resin, × 320.

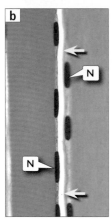

◀ Fig 6.7b Multinucleated muscle fiber. A muscle fiber showing its multinuclear nature (**N**), with nuclei just deep to the plasma membrane or sarcolemma (**arrows**). During embryogenesis and fetal growth, progenitor cells form myoblasts, which proliferate and then cease mitosis to fuse into multinucleated fibers that form internal myofibrils. Genes within the adult nuclei control the production of different isoforms of the contractile proteins, particularly myosin, giving rise to subtypes of fibers (e.g. fast- or slow-contracting). Exogenous electrical stimulations, exercise, or surgical transfer of fast fibers to a slow-fiber muscle or vice versa can alter expression of these proteins. H&E, acrylic resin, × 250.

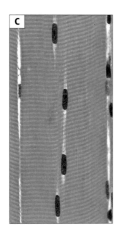

◀ Fig 6.7c Focus on the surface of a skeletal muscle fiber at high magnification, showing alignment of its nuclei enclosed by paler areas, which contain mitochondria. This section gives the false impression that the nuclei are centrally located within the fiber, making it appear to resemble cardiac muscle, which is also striated. This is because the section is fortuitous in passing through a plane that is slightly deep to the sarcolemma but parallel to the position of the nuclei that lie beneath it. H&E, acrylic resin, × 250.

Myofibrils

Fibers are filled with myofibrils. Each muscle fiber (i.e. a muscle cell) is filled with many longitudinal columns of myofibrils about 0.5–2 μm in diameter, each of which shows alternating light and dark bands (Fig 6.8a & b). A single muscle fiber may have more than 1,000 myofibrils. The striated pattern represents repetitive contractile units, or sarcomeres, consisting of segments of contractile cytoplasmic filaments. Sarcomeres are assembled as myotubes form muscle fibers. Continuity of the connective tissues throughout the muscle ensures that forces generated at the ends of fibers are transmitted to the tendon at the end of the whole muscle. In transverse sections, the stippled appearance of fibers represents the cut ends of myofibrils (Fig 6.9a & b). The plasma membrane of a fiber is called the sarcolemma, and is bordered externally by a basal lamina, and reticular and collagen fibers. Occasionally, slender satellite cells are located between the sarcolemma and basal lamina; these cells have myogenic potential—they may form new muscle fibers following tissue injury, and they contribute nuclear DNA during fiber hypertrophy.

The cytoplasm of muscle fibers is called the sarcoplasm. It chiefly contains myofibrils, with Golgi membranes and mitochondria concentrated near the nuclei and subjacent to the sarcolemma. Glycogen, lipid, other mitochondria, and networks of smooth membranous tubules called the sarcoplasmic reticulum (SR), and transverse tubular (TT) system occupy slender spaces between the myofibrils. The SR is analogous to smooth endoplasmic reticulum of other cell types, and the TT system represents invaginations of the sarcolemma extending inward to cross the myofibrils (Fig 6.10a & b).

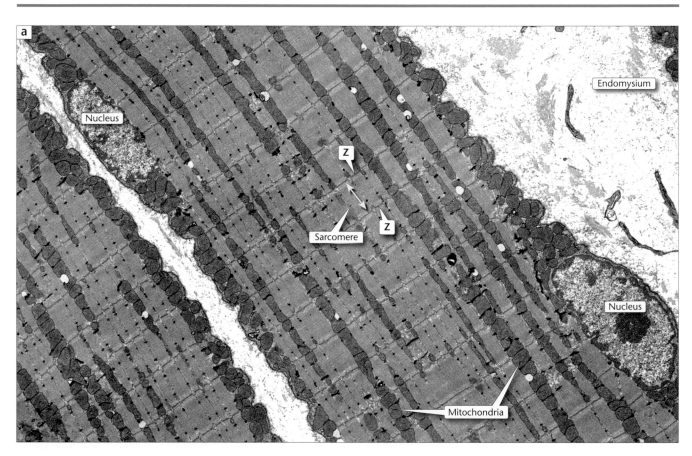

▲ **Fig 6.8a Skeletal muscle ultrastructure: longitudinal section.** Part of a fiber is illustrated, showing two nuclei just deep to the sarcolemma, together with numerous mitochondria, which are arranged in rows amongst the myofibrils. The units of contraction, the sarcomeres, extend in repetition between successive Z lines and appear in almost perfect register across the muscle fiber. The loose connective tissue of the endomysium provides passageways for vessels and nerves, and may allow movement of fibers during muscle contraction, stretching, and relaxation. × 5,600.

143

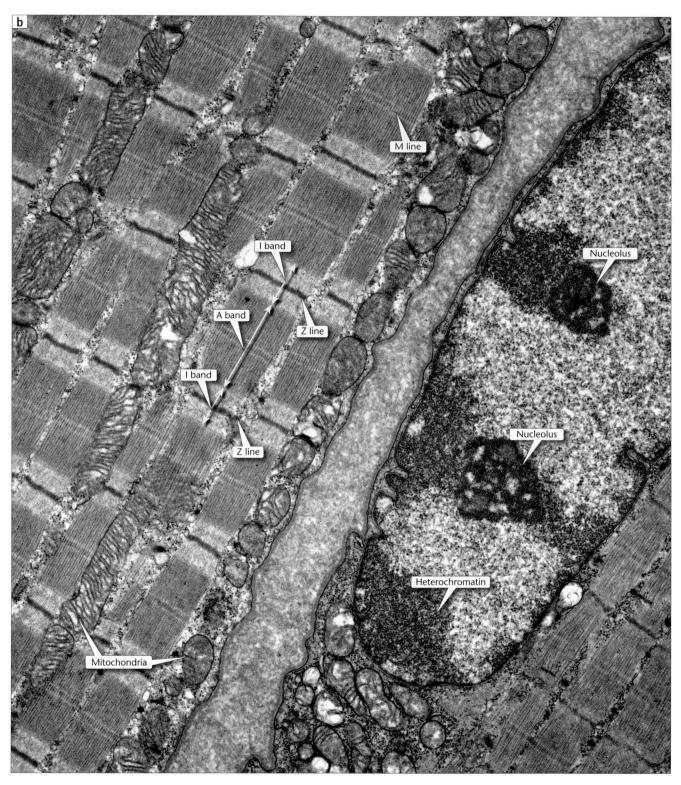

▲ **Fig 6.8b Two parallel fibers** are shown, bordered by the sarcolemma and a thin external lamina. The nucleus of one fiber contains nucleoli and heterochromatin. The sarcoplasm is filled with myofibrils and columns of mitochondria and glycogen particles. Sarcomeres show Z lines, A bands (which remain at constant length), and I bands (which shorten with muscle contraction). The M line situated within the lighter H band marks the middle of a sarcomere. The I bands contain thin filaments of actin, with associated proteins troponin and tropomyosin. A bands additionally contain thick filaments of myosin, consisting of two heavy chains in a long helix and two light chains associated with the globular head of the heavy chain. × 20,000.

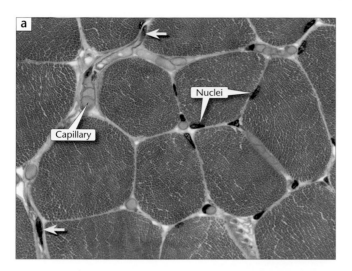

◄ **Fig 6.9a Muscle fibers: transverse section.** Section of large-diameter muscle fibers filled with very densely packed myofibrils, suggesting that the fibers are type IIB (i.e. white or fast-twitch fibers), in which mitochondria are not particularly abundant. The chief source of ATP (for energy) comes from anaerobic metabolism of glycogen into glucose, and the fibers contract rapidly but soon fatigue. Fiber nuclei are indicated, together with capillaries and fibroblasts (**arrows**) in the endomysium. H&E, acrylic resin, × 370.

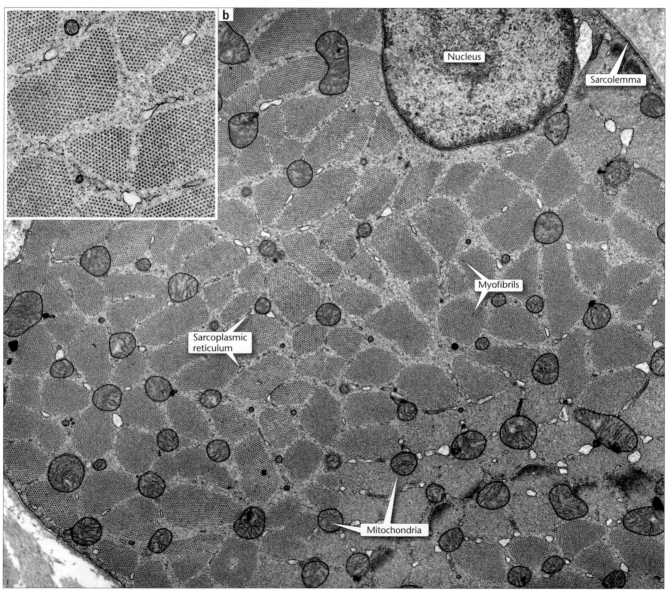

▲ **Fig 6.9b Ultrastructure of a cross section of a muscle fiber**, showing the nucleus and sarcolemma with external lamina. Columns of myofibrils are seen end on, each separated by sarcoplasm containing mitochondria and membranes of the sarcoplasmic reticulum. × 12,000. **Inset:** Higher magnification, showing the ordered arrangements of contractile filaments in each myofibril forming hexagonal arrays. The dense punctate structures are myosin filaments. × 25,000.

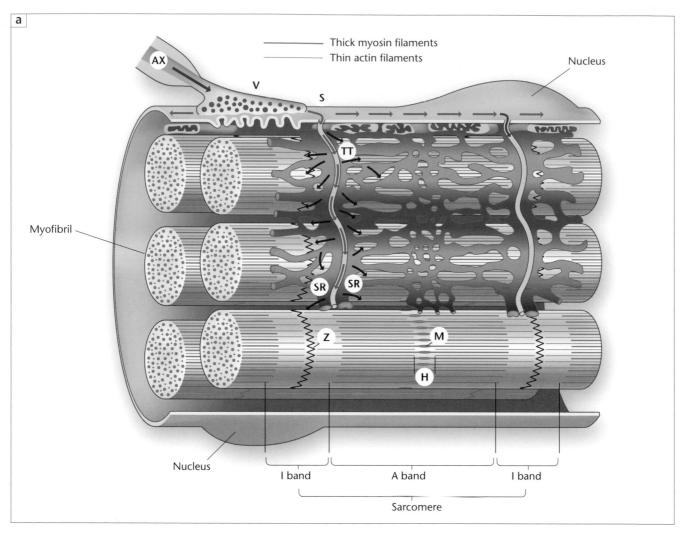

Thick myosin filaments
Thin actin filaments

Nucleus

AX

V

S

TT

Nucleus

Myofibril

SR   SR

Z   M

H

Nucleus

I band   A band   I band

Sarcomere

▲ **Fig 6.10a Neuromuscular junction, membranes, and myofibrils of skeletal muscle.** The axon (**AX**) from a motor neuron forms a motor end-plate with terminal swellings (one of which is shown here) containing many vesicles (**V**) of the neurotransmitter acetylcholine. Action potentials arrive at the terminals (**purple arrow**), which depolarize to allow acetylcholine to bind to receptors in the sarcolemma (**S**). The sarcolemma is itself depolarized, and action potentials spread along the muscle and down into the transverse tubular system (**TT, green arrows**), reaching all parts of the fiber within a few milliseconds. Membranes of the sarcoplasmic reticulum (**SR**) are closely associated with the transverse tubules, forming triads; the electrical impulse in the triads releases calcium from the sarcoplasmic reticulum (**red arrows**), which temporarily floods the myofibrils and their sarcomeres. Components of a sarcomere are indicated: A band, I band, M line (**M**), H band (**H**) and Z line (**Z**).

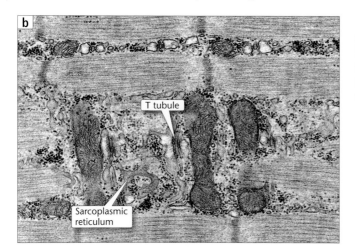

T tubule

Sarcoplasmic reticulum

◀ **Fig 6.10b Ultrastructure of sarcoplasm.** Membranes of sarcoplasmic reticulum are noted, extending between myofibrils and forming a triad structure with slender extensions originating from the plasma cell membrane. These invaginations are called T tubules and synchronize the depolarization of the T tubule and the release of calcium ions from within the sarcoplasmic reticulum. × 40,000.

Sarcomeres—the units of contraction

Contractile filaments in myofibrils are of two types:

- Thick filaments, composed of the protein myosin (Fig 6.11)
- Thin filaments, composed primarily of the protein actin.

Both types of filaments are arranged in regularly repeating segments delineated by transverse structures called Z lines, which anchor the actin filaments (Fig 6.12). A sarcomere is the region between and including two successive Z lines. The broad dark bands that are seen are A bands, where thick and thin filaments overlap. The less dense I bands are regions containing thin filaments. H bands and M lines within the A band are detected by electron microscopy.

Interdigitation of the myosin (A band) and actin (I band) filaments provides for sarcomere contraction, which is best explained by the sliding filament model in which actin filaments slide along the myosin filaments. ATP supplies the energy required. Filaments do not alter their length, but during sliding the Z lines move closer, the I bands shorten and the A band width is unchanged. Since sarcomeres are in series, the net effect of their shortening enables whole-muscle contraction. The force generated is considerable, owing to hundreds or more myofibrils in each fiber, and many fibers in the muscle fascicles. With muscle stretching, sarcomeres increase in length but can elastically recoil when returned to the resting state.

Positioning of filaments

Myosin and actin filaments are stabilized and kept aligned by accessory protein filaments. Actinin is an actin-binding protein that stabilizes actin by cross-links. Dystrophin is a cross-linking protein that stabilizes the cortical regions of muscle fibers. Defects in this protein may cause muscle weakness and atrophy (e.g. as in muscular dystrophy). Titin is a giant protein that attaches to Z lines and spans the A bands and the I bands. It centers the myosin filaments and, in I bands, acts as a type of spring between the end of a myosin filament and the Z line. Desmin is an intermediate filament protein essential for all muscle types. It extends between sarcomeres and acts to resist excessive stretching.

The molecular key to muscle contraction is the myosin molecule. In the A band, myosin filaments extend side arms similar to the shape of golf club ends. These form transient bridges with the actin, which flex (energy for which is generated by ATP hydrolysis) and cause sliding of the actin past the myosin. Disengagement and repetition of the cycle gives the impression that the globular end of the myosin "walks" along the actin—pulling the thin filaments over the thick filaments (see Fig 6.4).

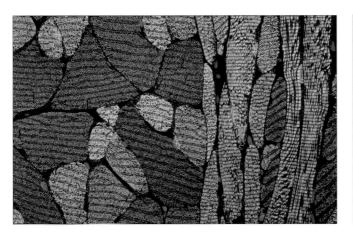

▲ **Fig 6.11 Myosin filaments.** Immunofluorescence image of skeletal muscle fibers, showing localization of myosin II protein. Myosin filaments are found in precisely ordered bands corresponding to the A bands of sarcomeres. Fiber nuclei nucleic acids are colored blue. × 350. (Courtesy J Zbaeren, Inselspital, Bern, Switzerland.)

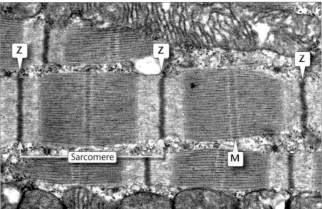

▲ **Fig 6.12 Sarcomere.** The sarcomere is the basic unit of contraction of a skeletal muscle fiber and extends between successive Z lines (**Z**). When contracted or stretched, the sarcomere length alters correspondingly, but the width of the A band, comprising thick myosin filaments, remains unaltered. The I band is less dense, comprising mainly of thin actin filaments that extend through the A band, thus contributing to its greater density with myosin filaments. The dense M band (**M**) anchors the myosin filaments. × 19,000.

The stimulus for contraction

About 98% of fibers are electrically independent, supplied by a single axon of a motor neuron. A motor neuron may innervate just one fiber, two or three fibers (extraocular muscles), or as many as several hundred fibers in major muscles of a limb. A single motor neuron, its axon, and all the fibers it supplies comprise a motor unit. The junction(s) between nerve endings and muscle that are formed midway along the fiber are called myoneural or neuromuscular junctions (Fig 6.13). About 2% of fibers have two such junctions. Motor end-plates are sites where axons terminate at the sarcolemma and excitatory nerve impulses initiate electrical impulses in the sarcolemma via release of acetylcholine from axon synaptic vesicles. Action potentials travel through the transverse tubular system (which penetrates into the myofibrils; see Fig 6.10), causing calcium ions to be released from the membranous sacs of the sarcoplasmic reticulum system. These then flow into the sarcoplasm and myofibrils in a fraction of a second. Calcium alters the molecular topography of special proteins bound to actin, allowing repeated cycles of cross-bridging with myosin (i.e. sarcomere contraction in association with energy made available by ATP). Cessation of action potentials returns calcium back to the sarcoplasmic reticulum, which terminates the interactions.

Sensing muscle length

Muscle spindles are small-diameter fibers inside capsules and are usually located in mid-regions of fascicles (Fig 6.14a & b). Spindles are important for the regulation of posture and movement. They act

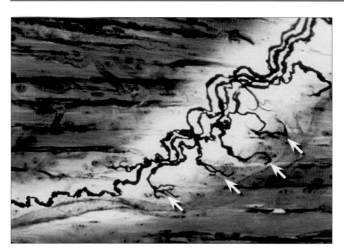

◀ Fig 6.13 Myoneural junction. Surface view showing branching of a motor nerve to supply nerve fibers ending as motor end-plates on the sarcolemma of skeletal muscle fibers (**arrows**). Motor end-plates are larger in fast-twitch fibers than in slow-twitch muscles. Small terminal swellings of the axon contain vesicles of the neurotransmitter acetylcholine. The efferent nerve impulse causes release of acetylcholine, which is then bound to receptors on the sarcolemma. This initiates an action potential propagated along the muscle. Motor end-plates occur in the middle of muscle fibers, allowing transmission of action potentials toward the two ends of the fibers. Silver impregnation, thick section, × 130.

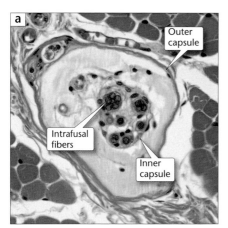

◀ Fig 6.14a Muscle spindles. Changes in muscle length and tension are detected by stretch receptors in muscle spindles. These are located on intrafusal (modified) muscle fibers, which are surrounded by inner capsules and outer capsules. Stretching activates the sensory receptors, sending signals to the spinal cord and then to efferent motor neurons that innervate the same muscle, causing contraction and relaxation of the spindle fibers. H&E, paraffin, × 250.

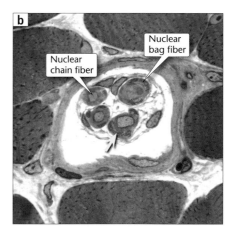

▲ Fig 6.14b Detail of a muscle spindle, showing large nuclear bag fibers and a nuclear chain fiber. The periphery of one fiber shows the sensory end-plate (**arrow**), which transmits signals via afferent fibers to the spinal cord. The spinal cord sends alpha motor neurons to the extrafusal muscle and gamma motor neurons to the intrafusal fibers, thus maintaining tension on the sensory receptors at a level close to their threshold for excitation. Toluidine blue, araldite, × 650.

as mechanoreceptors, detecting changes in muscle length via associated afferent nerve fibers linked to the spinal cord where they synapse with motor neurons, which innervate the muscle and its spindles. Contraction and stretching of spindles initiates and controls reflex muscle contractions (e.g. the "knee-jerk" reaction).

Skeletal muscle fiber types

Skeletal muscle fibers are designed for "fast" or "slow" contractions:

- Fast-contracting muscles such as gastrocnemius (superficial leg muscle) and extraocular muscles, have contractions of short duration and respectively show early fatigue or moderate resistance to fatigue.
- Slow-contracting muscles (e.g. soleus [deep muscle in the leg], the postural muscles of the back) are capable of repetitive, longer-lasting contractions and are resistant to fatigue.

Traditionally these types are said to be white or red fibers respectively (or the "fast whites" and the "slow reds"). There is also an intermediate type, and humans show a mixture of fast and slow fibers. Based upon oxidative or aerobic metabolic properties, slow fibers are termed type I, with rich vascularization and abundant myoglobin. Fast fibers are called type IIB, utilize anaerobic metabolism (i.e. they form ATP using glycolysis), and have fewer capillaries (Fig 6.15a–c). Fibers that use both aerobic and anaerobic metabolism are uncommon: they are fast and long-lasting (e.g. the vastus lateralis in the thigh).

Different versions of the myosin gene produce various isoforms of the globular part of myosin, and this is what determines the rate at which myosin interacts with actin. Different isoforms of myosin occur in embryos, newborns, and adults, and in response to different types of exercise.

> **Tip:** How fast can a muscle shorten? In about 1/10th or 1/100th of a second, a muscle can shorten by 10% of its length; this is equivalent to a maximum speed of 70 mph (110 km/h).

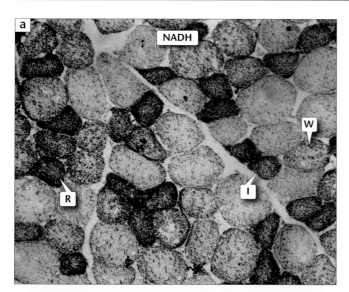

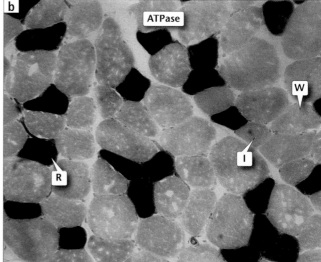

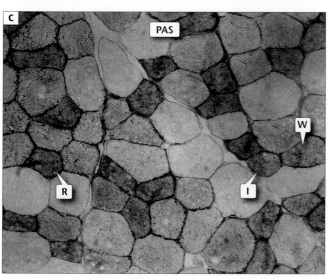

Fig 6.15 Fiber typing. Serial frozen sections of muscle fibers in cross section. **a** This panel (**NADH**) shows the histochemical reaction to NADH in mitochondria, which contribute to oxidative (aerobic) metabolism, using oxygen to make ATP. **b** In this panel (**ATPase**), the tissue shows the localization of ATPase (pH 4.3), indicating the degree of metabolic activity in the myofibrils. **c** The third panel (**PAS**) shows the PAS reaction for the distribution of glycogen, which is degraded via anaerobic (glycolytic) metabolism to produce ATP. The fiber marked (**I**) exhibits properties associated with intermediate, fast-twitch, or type IIA fibers. The fiber marked (**W**) shows reactions associated with white, fast-twitch, or type IIB fibers. Fibers marked (**R**) correspond to red, slow-twitch, or type I fibers. In sections stained with hematoxylin and eosin, all the fibers would appear similar except for their shape or size. Histochemical fiber-typing reveals structural and metabolic variations, emphasizing the heterogeneity of fibers in a single muscle. Histochemical reactions, frozen sections, × 200.

CARDIAC MUSCLE

Heart muscle consists of cardiac myocytes, traditionally described as fibers of the myocardium. These fibers are individual cells joined end to end by special intercellular junctions, called intercalated discs, which also provide electrical coupling. Myocytes have a single central nucleus. The fibers branch, forming further interconnections, and the sarcoplasm shows cross-striations and sarcomeres (Fig 6.16a–d, Fig 6.17a–c). These represent repeating regions of actin and myosin filaments, which slide along each other during contraction. Myofibrils of cardiac muscle are held in position by various filaments, one of which—desmin—is anchored to the plasma membrane by costameres. These are protein aggregates that form the rib-like structures seen along the boundary of each cell; they also attach the cell to the extracellular matrix.

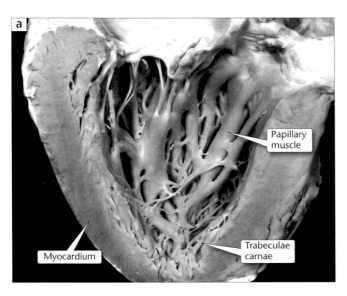

▲ **Fig 6.16a Heart muscle.** Vertical section through the right ventricle showing the thick walls of myocardium, which have numerous irregular and branched internal extensions. These are called trabeculae carnae and provide anchorage for the papillary muscles that attach via the chordae tendinae to the tricuspid valve to restrain eversion of the valve into the right atrium.

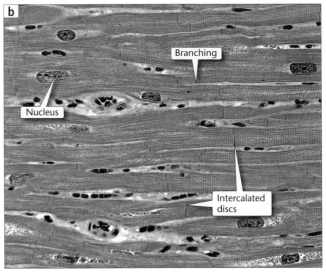

▲ **Fig 6.16b Cardiac muscle fibers in longitudinal section.** The identifying features are (i) faint striations in paraffin sections, (ii) central nuclei within clear areas that contain organelles, (iii) fiber branchings, which form extensive linkages throughout the muscle, and (iv) intercalated discs where adjacent cells attach for mechanical and electrical coupling. Endomysium contains the nuclei of fibroblasts and many blood vessels. H&E, acrylic resin, × 240.

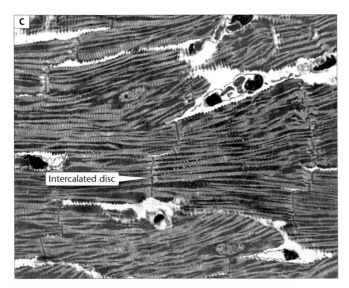

▲ **Fig 6.16c Thin epoxy resin section of cardiac muscle,** showing central nuclei surrounded by many columns of mitochondria, which reflect the oxidative or aerobic metabolism of fatty acids, lactate, and glucose. Striations representing A and I bands of sarcomeres occupy the remainder of the myocyte sarcoplasm. Intercalated discs are numerous between the terminal ends of adjacent cells. Serrated edges are the costameres for attachment to the connective tissue. Toluidine blue, araldite, × 400.

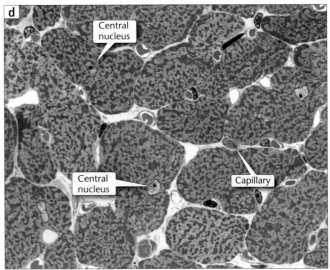

▲ **Fig 6.16d Cardiac muscle in transverse section,** illustrating dense packing of darkly stained mitochondria, and myofibrillar areas within the sarcoplasm, which surround the central nucleus. The lobular profiles of the myocytes represent end-on views of their branchings. Capillaries are noted in the endomysium. Toluidine blue, araldite, × 400.

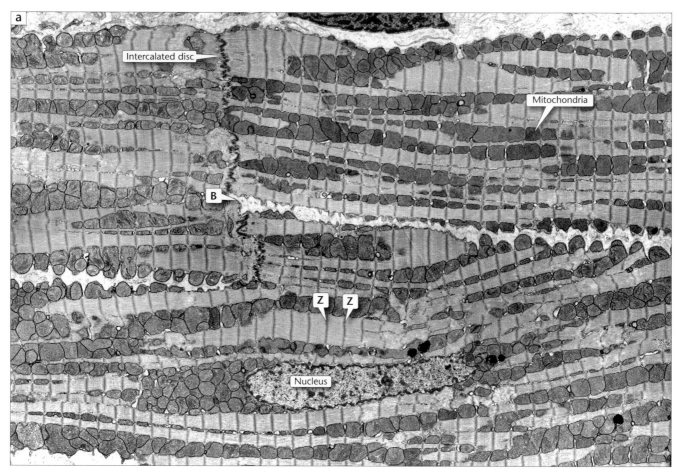

▲ **Fig 6.17a Cardiac muscle ultrastructure, longitudinal section.** Three myocytes are shown with branching (**B**) at the level of the intercalated disc. A central nucleus is indicated. The sarcoplasm is filled with many hundreds of mitochondria in columns, together with sarcomeres showing highly ordered Z lines (**Z**) with fainter A and I bands between them. × 3,800.

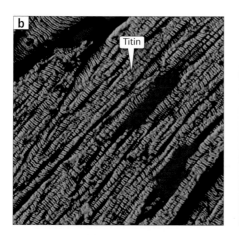

▲ **Fig 6.17b Titin.** Immunofluorescence preparation of cardiac muscle, showing periodic striations of titin, a filamentous protein between Z lines and the myosin filaments. Titin centers the myosin and counteracts overstretching of the sarcomeres. Cell nuclei are red. × 1,000. (Courtesy J Schaper, Max Planck Institute, Bad Nauheim, Germany.)

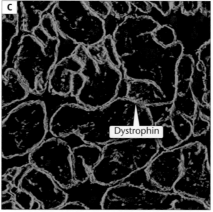

▲ **Fig 6.17c Dystrophin.** Immunofluorescence preparation of cardiac muscle showing location of dystrophin protein, an actin cross-linking protein. Dystrophin is seen at the periphery of the cells and links actin filaments to transmembrane proteins of the plasma membrane. × 350. (Courtesy J Schaper, Max Planck Institute, Bad Nauheim, Germany.)

The matrix is abundantly supplied with capillaries from the coronary arteries and these vessels are always noted between the myocytes.

Cardiac muscle fibers attach to the fibrous skeleton, a system of rings of connective tissue and elastic fibers separating atria from ventricles. The myocardium of these chambers is lined by supporting tissue of the inner endocardium and outer epicardium (see Ch 8). Cardiac muscle of the ventricles is organized in a circumferential and spiral pattern, ensuring that, with contraction, blood within the chamber is expelled in the direction of the great outlet vessels.

Cardiac muscle sarcomeres and contraction

Cardiac sarcomeres are morphologically similar, but not identical, to skeletal muscle sarcomeres. They have Z lines and A and I bands, but the myofilaments form a continuous mass within the cell that is interrupted by extensions of sarcoplasm containing mitochondria and sarcoplasmic reticulum (Fig 6.18a & b). Mitochondria are abundant, commensurate with a highly aerobic metabolism. The transverse tubular system is closely associated with the sarcoplasmic reticulum, which usually shows a single terminal sac apposed to the transverse tubular, forming a "dyad" (Fig 6.19). as opposed to the triads in skeletal muscle.

Calcium, which is required for contraction, is supplied from outside the cell. It enters through the sarcolemma in response to action potentials, and is also released into the sarcoplasm from stores within the sarcoplasmic reticulum. The former source triggers calcium release from the sarcoplasmic reticulum in a process known as calcium-induced calcium release. Calcium influx is counterbalanced by calcium exit mechanisms, which reverse the calcium movement described above. Synchronization of contraction is

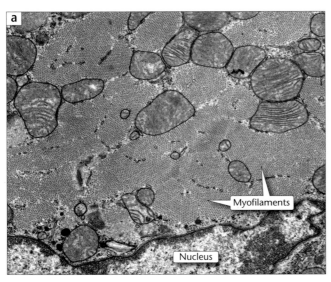

▲ **Fig 6.18a Myofilaments.** Cardiac muscle ultrastructure: transverse section. In contrast to skeletal muscle, distinct myofibrils are absent; instead the myofilaments of myosin and actin form continuous masses in the sarcoplasm. Mitochondria and sarcoplasmic reticulum penetrate through the sarcoplasm between the myofilaments. A myocyte nucleus is indicated. × 12,000.

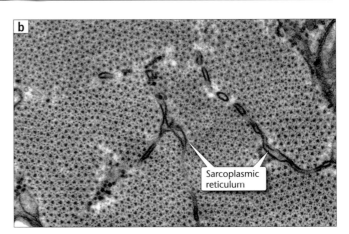

▲ **Fig 6.18b Ultrastructure of myofilaments**, showing thicker, denser myosin filaments surrounded by many thin filaments of actin, which are arranged in a hexagonal pattern. Release of calcium ions from membranes of sarcoplasmic reticulum is a stimulus for muscle contraction. × 40,000.

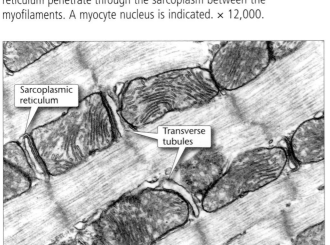

◀ **Fig 6.19 Sarcoplasmic reticulum.** During contraction, calcium is released from stores in the sarcoplasmic reticulum. This release of calcium is supplemented by an influx of calcium from the extracellular fluid into the transverse tubules, forming a pair of membrane sacs called dyads. Calcium inflow into the transverse tubules triggers the release of calcium in the sarcoplasmic reticulum, and the combined rise in intracellular calcium is sufficient to activate myosin–actin cross-bridging and muscle contraction. × 25,000.

achieved by the intercalated discs, which contain adherens-type junctions, desmosome junctions, and gap junctions (Fig 6.20a & b). These together ensure that cardiac muscle behaves as a functional syncitium. Because ions flow from cell to cell via the gap junctions, electrical excitation occurs through the heart muscle similar to an electrically continuous sheet of tissue.

Control of cardiac muscle

Action potentials generated in the sinoatrial node pass to the atrioventricular node and then on to the ventricles. These impulses are carried by specialized myocardial cells of the conducting system, which are organized into fibers. Cells of the nodes, the bundle of His, and the left and right bundle branches are smaller than usual myocytes, while cells of the Purkinje fibers (the distal conducting system to ventricles) are much larger, with fewer myofibrils and abundant glycogen (Fig 6.21).

SMOOTH MUSCLE

Smooth muscle cells are not striated and have no sarcomeres, but they still rely on actin–myosin interactions for contraction. The cells are long and

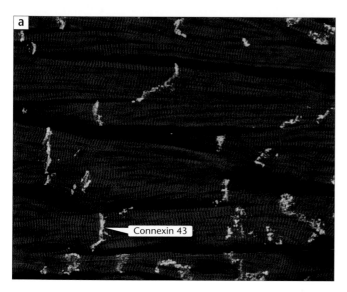

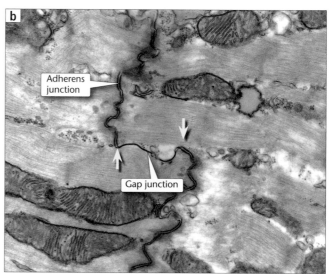

▲ **Fig 6.20a Intercalated disc.** Immunofluorescence view of cardiac muscle intercalated discs showing the localization of connexin 43 protein. This protein forms the gap junctions of the intercalated disc, and is responsible for ionic/electrical conduction between adjacent cells. Myosin filaments are red. × 400. (Courtesy J Schaper, Max Planck Institute, Bad Nauheim, Germany.)

▲ **Fig 6.20b Intercalated disc joining cardiac muscle cells**, showing a step-type arrangement (**arrows**) highlighted with an electron-dense dye. Discs occur as substitutes for Z lines where cells meet end to end. Discs show adherens-type junctions attaching cells and providing anchorage for actin filaments, together with gap junctions for electrical coupling. Desmosomes also occur between regions of adherens junctions. × 18,000.

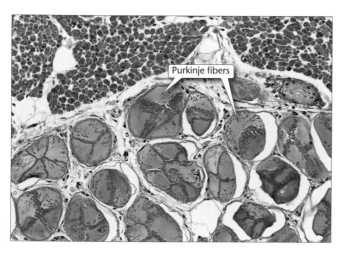

◀ **Fig 6.21 Purkinje fibers.** Actually cells, these are much larger than cardiac muscle cells. They show peripheral and central mitochondria and myofilaments, and clear regions that are filled with glycogen. Purkinje fibers are part of the cardiac conduction system and rapidly activate the endocardial surface of the ventricles. H&E, acrylic resin, × 200.

153

spindle-shaped with a central nucleus, and they often form sheets, bundles, or layers consisting of thousands or millions of cells (Fig 6.22a–e). Alternatively, they may occur as single cells such as myoid, myoepithelial, or myofibroblast cells.

Smooth muscle often forms contractile walls for hollow organs, passageways, or cavities serving to modify their volume. Examples are vascular structures and tubes or glands of the respiratory tract, the gut, and the genitourinary system. Therefore, smooth muscle function may be of clinical significance in disorders such as high blood pressure, dysmenorrhea, asthma, atherosclerosis, and abnormal intestinal motility.

Smooth muscle is slow to contract and relax—it may remain contracted for hours or days. It can undergo stretching and respond to stimuli such as nerve signals, hormones, drugs, or local concentrations of blood gases.

Ultrastructure and contractile mechanism

Smooth muscle cells are closely packed and show an external lamina with thin extracellular matrix. Gap junctions and collagen provide intercellular attachments, and the sarcoplasm contains a cytoskeleton plus actin and myosin contractile

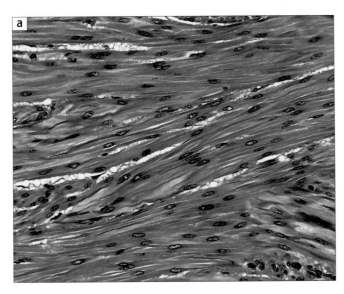

◀ **Fig 6.22a Smooth muscle.** Longitudinal section of bundles of smooth muscle cells characterized by a slender, fusiform cell shape with a single central nucleus. The cells are closely aggregated, often with no apparent separations, except where bundles of cells travel at different angles when thin connective tissue marks their borders. This thin connective tissue transmits the contractile forces that are generated when the cells and cell bundles shorten. H&E, paraffin, × 200.

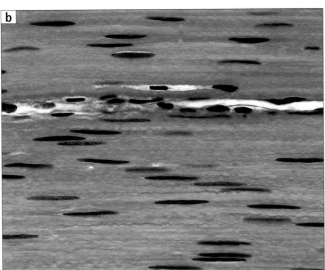

◀ **Fig 6.22b Relaxed smooth muscle.** When relaxed, smooth muscle cells may be very thin, forming multiple parallel profiles with squamous-type nuclei resembling a school of fish. The cell borders are faintly visible owing to the close apposition of the cells. No striations can be seen, but the homogeneously stained cytoplasm is filled with longitudinal arrays of actin and myosin (myosin content is only 20% of that found in skeletal muscle) that are not highly ordered into sarcomeres. × 480.

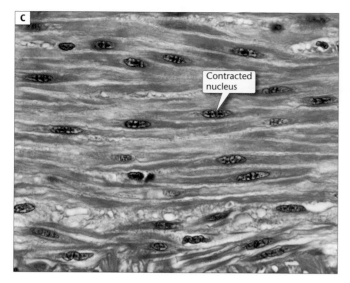

Contracted nucleus

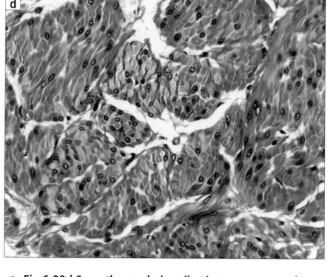

▲ **Fig 6.22c Contracted smooth muscle.** In the contracted state, smooth muscle cells may shorten to one-fifth of their resting length, causing the nucleus to twist and shorten into a characteristic corkscrew shape. Control of contraction may be complex and dependent on tissue location. Control may be by nerve impulses (neurogenic), spontaneously (myogenic tone) or by pharmacomechanical coupling (hormones, drugs, neurotransmitters)—the last mechanism occurring with no detectable change in membrane potential. Whatever the stimulus, calcium ions are necessary for the interaction of actin and myosin to cause the contraction. H&E, paraffin, × 480.

▲ **Fig 6.22d Smooth muscle bundles in transverse and oblique section.** Some cells are fusiform in shape if sectioned at an angle, and appear ovoid when seen end on. Note that in contrast to skeletal muscle, in which nuclei are located on the edges of the cell, the nuclei of smooth muscle are central in the cytoplasm. H&E, paraffin, × 200.

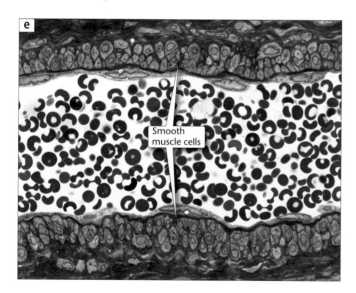

Smooth muscle cells

◀ **Fig 6.22e Smooth muscle in a small artery.** The walls of many blood vessels rely upon smooth muscle for control of vessel diameter. In this small artery, the tunica media comprises several layers of smooth muscle cells closely packed together. Toluidine blue, araldite, × 350.

filaments, which contract via a sliding mechanism (Fig 6.23a–c). The force generated is transmitted in the cell through contractile filaments, which form links between actin-binding dense plaques in the cytoplasm and the sarcolemma, equivalent to the Z lines of striated muscle. During contraction, the plaques move closer together, causing shortening of the cell. Plaques are also linked to intermediate cytoskeletal filaments, facilitating homogeneous contraction (Fig 6.24a & b).

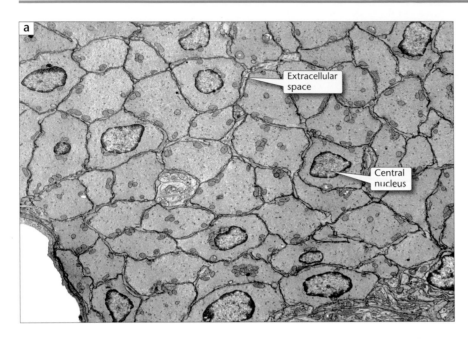

◀ **Fig 6.23a Ultrastructure of smooth muscle in the gut.** Typical arrangement of smooth muscle cells in this example from the external muscle wall of the gut. Nuclei are central within the cells and the cytoplasm is of moderate density representing myofilaments. Little extracellular space is noted. × 3,500.

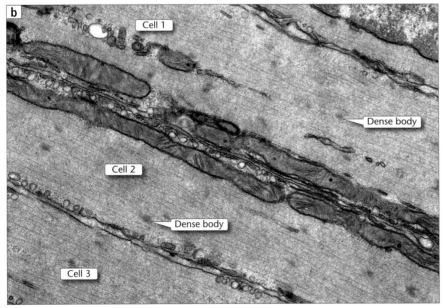

◀ **Fig 6.23b Smooth muscle cytoplasm in longitudinal section of several cells** shows many fine filaments of myosin and actin that are not organized into sarcomeres. Numerous small densities are found in the cytoplasm representing plaques, into which bundles of contractile filaments are attached. × 23,000.

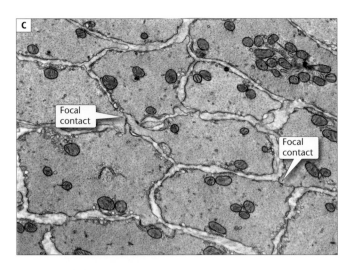

Fig 6.23c In cross section, smooth muscle cells are irregular in shape but make contact or close associations at focal points around the cell membrane. Extracellular regions contain collagen and reticular fibers. × 9,000.

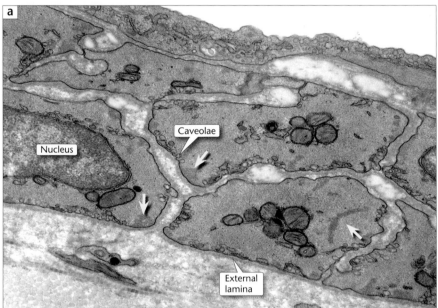

Fig 6.24a Contractile properties— vascular smooth muscle, showing wide extracellular spaces and an external lamina surrounding the cell membrane. Most of the collagen, reticular fibers, and elastin in the extracellular spaces are produced by the smooth muscle cells. Note the caveolae and the patches of dense material (**arrows**) associated with the cell membrane. These patches of dense material are described further in Figure 6.24b. × 19,000.

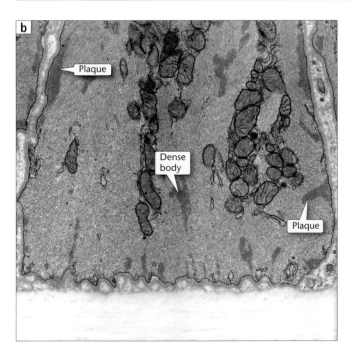

Fig 6.24b Part of a vascular smooth muscle cell, showing dense bodies and dense plaques within the cytoplasm. By providing anchorages for actin contractile filaments and attachment for filaments of the cytoskeleton, these dense patches resemble mini-sarcomeres in series, with networks of non-contractile structural filaments. Tension generated by the contractile filaments is transmitted throughout the interior and exterior of the cell, resulting in considerable shortening of the cell and, in turn, exerting force on any attached neighboring cells. × 15,000.

157

Calcium ion fluxes regulate actin–myosin interaction using calmodulin, a calcium-binding protein that stimulates myosin cross-bridges to interact with actin, thereby initiating the sliding-filament mechanism. Calcium entry and exit is a complex process controlled by channels and calcium-pumping mechanisms in the sarcolemma, augmented by the sarcoplasmic reticulum, which also releases calcium from membranous sacs associated with the sarcolemma. Caveolae are vesicular invaginations of the sarcolemma; these possibly regulate calcium entry into the cell by increasing its surface area (Fig 6.25).

Most smooth muscle is innervated by both sympathetic and parasympathetic components of the autonomic nervous system, whose axons pass close to or contact the cells. At these sites, norepinephrine (noradrenaline) and a variety of neuropeptides bind to sarcolemmal receptors, thereby effecting excitatory or inhibitory responses. Depending on local requirements, smooth muscle cells respond to other signals that do not necessarily involve an initial action potential stimulus; an example of this is the autorhythmicity, or spontaneous contractions, shown by visceral smooth muscle and other hollow tubes invested with smooth muscle. Hormones and agents released by endothelial cells and smooth muscle itself may stimulate or inhibit contractions, but an increase in intracellular calcium is required to initiate the contraction.

Modified smooth muscle cells

Myoepithelial cells are ectodermally derived stellate cells associated with the secretory cells of a variety of exocrine glands, such as sweat, salivary, and mammary glands. When contracted, they assist with the expulsion of secretory products into the glandular lumen and excretory passages. During lactation, myoepithelial cells in the mammary gland encourage milk secretion from the alveolar glands into the duct system. In the eye, myoepithelial cells in the iris contract to dilate the pupil. The walls of seminiferous tubules in some species contain myoid cells, which exert tension on the tubules, assisting with sperm and fluid movement toward the rete testis. At sites of wound healing, myofibroblasts produce collagenous matrix but are also contractile, serving to aid wound closure. Many capillaries and postcapillary venules have slender pericytes, which may contract in a similar way to smooth muscle.

DEVELOPMENT, GROWTH AND REGENERATION

In utero, skeletal muscles grow in length via multiple cell fusions, which are largely complete at birth and finalized by 1 year of age. The nuclei are postmitotic; hence increased bulk and length is achieved by the development of new sarcomeres and myofibrils but not by cell proliferation. Satellite cells, a separate mesenchymal cell line, may proliferate and contribute to muscle regeneration following injury or in various disease states, but their capacity is limited and significant tissue loss is replaced with connective or scar tissue.

During embryogenesis, cardiac myoblasts divide as they transform into myocytes and establish adhering junctions with their neighbors. Until recently, it was believed that in adults cardiac muscle cells could not proliferate or regenerate in response to damage to the myocardium. Injury or degeneration of cardiac muscle often leads to replacement with scar or fibrous tissue. Now it seems that there is a population of progenitor cells in the heart that serve to replace apoptotic cardiomyocytes at a low level. The presence of other types of progenitor cells originating from bone marrow mesenchymal cells remains controversial.

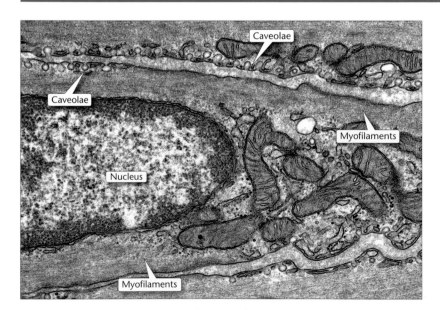

◀ **Fig 6.25 Cytoplasmic membranes.** Close apposition of plasma membranes of several smooth muscle cells, showing dense intercellular material, which possibly provides adhesion. Caveolae are numerous and resemble pinocytotic vesicles. They may increase the surface area of the membrane for the entry of calcium into the cytoplasm. Myofilaments are shown oriented in longitudinal section. × 27,000.

Smooth muscle cells develop and grow individually, and retain the capacity to proliferate. During pregnancy, the smooth muscle of the uterine myometrium shows cell hypertrophy and hyperplasia. Similar cell activities may occur in the smooth muscle of blood vessels and the gut, as well as in wound healing.

ABNORMALITIES AND CLINICAL NOTES
Skeletal muscle

Neuropathies, or disturbances of innervation, cause abnormal contraction and atrophy, and result in degeneration or replacement with connective tissue and fat.

Myopathies are primary disturbances of muscle cells. Myopathies may be of three types:
- Congenital, with decreased muscle tone, possibly related to altered autosomal genes
- Toxic, caused by alcohol or drugs
- Inflammatory, related to microbial infections or immune-related illness.

Myasthenia gravis

Myasthenia gravis is an autoimmune disease in which antibodies disrupt acetylcholine receptors in neuromuscular junctions. It chiefly affects women aged between 25 and 40 years. Weakness and muscle paralysis can be fatal if respiratory function is impaired.

Duchenne's muscular dystrophy

Duchenne's muscular dystrophy is a severe, inherited X-linked disorder affecting 1 in 3,500 male live births. There is muscle weakness, wasting, degeneration, and cell death, with fibrous tissue replacement. The disease is relentless, with death before or in the early 20s. The defective gene fails to produce dystrophin, an actin-binding protein associated with the sarcolemma. Dystrophin, together with syntrophin proteins (which are also reduced in this progressive myopathy), is thought to stabilize the muscle fiber membrane during contraction and relaxation. Dystrophin also occurs in the brain, and approximately one-third of patients with Duchenne's muscular dystrophy show mental retardation.

Fatigue

Muscle fatigue or weakness after repetitive contractions is accompanied by the build-up of excessive metabolic products (lactic acid, phosphate) and a declining response to calcium by the myofilaments. Fatigue (such as occurs in bicycle riding or marathon running) may also result from a calcium-induced inactivation of calcium release, thereby limiting vigorous exercise and counteracting possible muscle damage. When muscles are stretched during contraction (eccentric contraction such as walking down mountains), pain and weakness may persist for a day or more; this is called delayed onset muscle soreness. This is a result of sarcomere and myofilament disruption seen as sites of focal damage.

Chronic fatigue syndrome

Chronic fatigue syndrome is controversial. It affects physical and mental abilities, but muscle function appears normal, suggesting a nervous system disorder with an as yet unproven reaction to one or more viruses.

Tetanus

Tetanus (muscle spasm or rigidity), colloquially called lockjaw because of the spasms of the jaw muscles, occurs when inhibitory neurons are blocked by neurotoxins produced by *Clostridium tetani* infecting lacerations or puncture wounds. The toxins are many times stronger than most snake venoms and they enter the central nervous system through the peripheral nerves. The incidence of tetanus is greatly reduced following diptheria, pertussis, and tetanus (DTP) immunization during childhood.

Rigor mortis

After death, chemical changes occur in skeletal muscle, which cause them to harden and the body to stiffen. This stiffening commences in the face and spreads to the limbs and trunk. Excessive release of intracellular calcium activates muscle contraction, which is temporarily sustained since a supply of energy in the form of ATP (to reverse the contraction) is not available when metabolism ceases. Degeneration of the tissue slowly induces muscle relaxation.

Cardiac muscle
Cardiomyopathies

Cardiomyopathies are of several types, and often the cause or causes are unknown. Hypertrophic cardiomyopathy is a type of cardiomyopathy in which fibers enlarge in response to the excessive workload associated with deficient valves or high blood pressure. Dilated cardiomyopathy is more common; the heart expands in volume owing to muscle weakness. In restrictive cardiomyopathy, myocytes are non-compliant, resulting in decreased blood volume filling the heart during diastole.

Ischemia

In cases of ischemia (inadequate oxygen supply), contractile force is reduced and excessive intracellular calcium may arise, causing tissue damage. A cardinal symptom of ischemia is angina pectoris or chest pain. Severe restriction of blood flow and oxygen to cardiac muscle results in infarction or death of affected tissue with replacement by granulation and fibrous tissue. Angioblastic or bypass surgery can often re-establish blood supply, if performed prior to extensive tissue degeneration. However, myocardial infarction remains a common cause of death.

Heart failure

Chronic or congestive heart failure reduces pumping efficiency during systole and may result from diseased valves, cardiomyopathies, or inflammation.

Rheumatic fever

Rheumatic fever, a streptococcal infection, is an immunologic reaction against cardiac muscle antigens, resulting in focal inflammation, fibrosis, and tissue necrosis, including heart valvular deformities.

Smooth muscle

Disorders of vascular smooth muscle are common, especially in arteries, where proliferation of muscle cells and excessive production of extracellular matrix may result in intimal thickening and narrowing of the vessel lumen. Hypertension, endothelial disorders, and conditions contributing to atherosclerosis stimulate thickening of the vessel wall. Leiomyomas, or benign tumors of smooth muscle, may arise in the uterus as single or multiple tumors that form masses of estrogen-dependent smooth muscle, commonly known as fibroids. Leiomyomas may occur deep to the skin associated with arrector pili muscles; these present as small and often painful lumps.

Myofibroblasts have the histologic features of smooth muscle cells and fibroblasts; that is, they show contractile properties and synthesize various types of collagen. These properties enable myofibroblasts to contribute to the formation of granulation tissue in healing wounds. The collagen provides a measure of plasticity to the wound in the early phase of healing, and the contractile function, based upon actin filaments, enables granulation tissue contraction resulting in wound closure. Myofibroblasts disappear when the granulation tissue is reabsorbed following wound closure and are replaced by fibroblasts.

Nervous system

All nervous tissue consists of nerve cells (neurons), supporting cells (glial cells or neuroglia) and blood vessels, and in various arrangements is associated with connective tissue. Although estimates vary, there may be 100 billion neurons and many times this number of glial cells in the human nervous system. A basic understanding of the functional histology of the nervous system inevitably relies upon anatomy and physiology, but this chapter concentrates on material that is based upon histologic specimens normally available in slide class sets, or as demonstration slides, supplemented with material generated from neuroscience research.

To understand how the nervous system works, it is necessary to have a sound knowledge of the structure of neurons, axons, dendrites, and glia. Histology specimens help achieve this objective largely through the use of special stains; for example:

- Cell bodies are visualized with hematoxylin, or cresyl violet, which stains nucleic acids.
- Dendrites and axons are revealed with silver-based stains where these structures are stained black.
- Peripheral nerves are highlighted by Weigert stain or luxol fast blue, which stains lipid-rich myelin, and adding cresyl violet also emphasizes glial cells.

All of these components may further be displayed with the use of histochemistry, immunocytochemistry, and special fluorescence microscopy techniques.

ANATOMY OF THE NERVOUS SYSTEM

Anatomically, the nervous system is divided into the central nervous system (CNS), consisting of the brain and spinal cord, and the peripheral nervous system (PNS), which is defined as nerves that lie outside the CNS (Fig 7.1). Cranial nerves (12 pairs), spinal nerves (31 pairs), and the peripheral autonomic nervous system (ANS) belong to the PNS. Nerve tissue of the PNS is composed of sensory (afferent) and motor (efferent) nerves. These components are represented in the somatic nervous system, which supplies the musculature, skeleton, and skin, and in the visceral nervous system, which supplies the visceral organs, smooth and cardiac muscle, blood vessels, and numerous glands.

Afferent neurons convey impulses from a particular tissue or organ to the CNS (brain and/or spinal cord). Efferents of the somatic division conduct impulses from the CNS to control, for example, voluntary muscle action. Visceral efferents (i.e. motor fibers to the organs listed above) are not normally under conscious or voluntary control, and make up the autonomic nervous system (ANS). This system is anatomically and functionally separated into sympathetic and parasympathetic components, which in general show opposite effects upon the organs they innervate, but occasionally cooperative effects are noted. In a broad sense, the sympathetic system is associated with stressful or physical activity, whereas the parasympathetic system is active under normal or calm conditions. Nerves in the gastrointestinal tract are mostly intrinsic to it and are collectively referred to as the enteric nervous system (ENS). The ENS is a component of the peripheral autonomic nervous system, but because of its largely independent function it is sometimes considered to be a third division of the nervous system.

Cellular associations form defined tissues

Despite their obvious functional complexity, most of the components that form the CNS and PNS are highly organized into characteristic cellular associations, and careful examination of the histologic preparations listed here provides a firm foundation for understanding the cellular and tissue basis of the nervous system:

- Neuron and glial cell structure
- Peripheral nerves, myelinated and unmyelinated
- Ganglia, autonomic and sensory
- Gray matter and white matter
- Cerebral and cerebellar cortex, basal nuclei
- Spinal cord.

NEURONS

Neurons are the specialized anatomic and functional units of the nervous system that are able to receive information (signals from external or internal environments), process and integrate these signals, and conduct nerve impulses to designated target tissues. Thus, these cells are excitable (responsive to change), conductive (transmit nerve impulses), and secretory (communicate with other cells, using chemical messengers). A typical neuron has

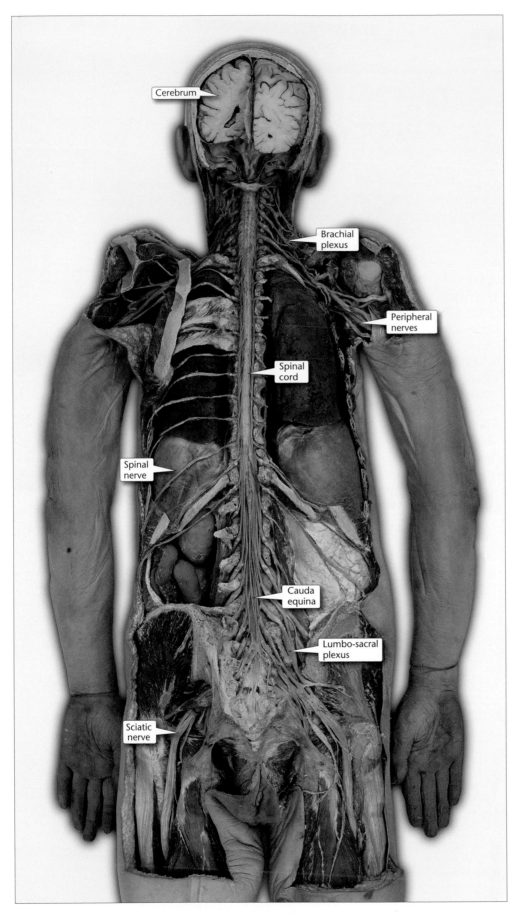

▲ **Fig 7.1 Human nervous system.** Overview of the nervous system showing the central nervous system of brain and spinal cord, the latter terminating between vertebral bodies L1 and L2. Peripheral nerves, such as the paired spinal nerves, give rise to the brachial and lumbosacral nerve plexuses.

a conspicuous nucleus surrounded by cytoplasm (the perikaryon), collectively referred to as the cell body or soma. Extending from the cell body are many branching processes called dendrites (tree-like morphology) and one larger, longer process termed the axon (Fig 7.2a–c).

Three main types

Neurons may be classified according to the morphology of the axon and dendrites or, more commonly, according to the number of cell processes extending from the cell body (Fig 7.3):

- *Multipolar* neurons, common in the CNS and ANS, have one axon and dozens of dendrites.
- *Bipolar* neurons, found in the olfactory epithelium and retina, have only two processes—one axon and one dendrite.
- *Pseudounipolar* neurons (also termed unipolar), found in the dorsal root ganglia (cluster of cell bodies) in the PNS, have a single short process that functions as an axon and branches as a T-shape, of which one process leads to the spinal cord and the other extends to a peripheral tissue.

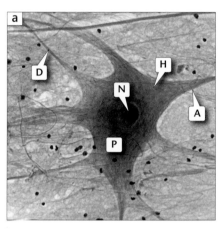

▲ **Fig 7.2a Typical neuron structure.** A motor neuron, grown in culture and spread as a whole-mount display. Shown are a central nucleus (**N**), cytoplasm or perikaryon (**P**) containing microtubules and neurofilaments, dendrites (**D**), often branching, and a slender axon (**A**) arising from an axon hillock (**H**). Surrounding neuropil contains glial cell nuclei embedded in a meshwork of fine dendritic processes. Via dendrites, electric impulses reach the cell body and are transmitted along the axon as action potentials, which arise in the axon hillock. Hematoxylin & eosin (H&E), spread preparation, × 490.

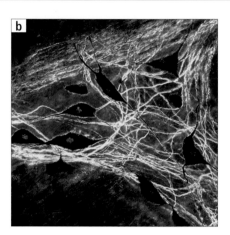

▲ **Fig 7.2b Neuron cluster.** Gold-impregnated whole mount of a ganglion (cluster) of neurons of the myenteric or Auerbach's plexus in the smooth muscle wall of the gut. Neuron cell bodies show dendrites and axonal processes, which form electrophysiologic circuits (note the Y-shaped pathways of nerve processes) that are important for intrinsic peristalsis of the musculature. The activity of these neurons is modified by extrinsic sympathetic and parasympathetic innervation. Gold chloride stain, whole mount, × 250.

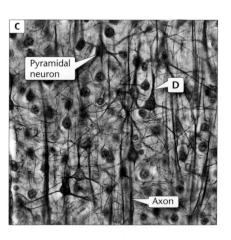

◀ **Fig 7.2c Pyramidal neurons.** Middle layer (layer III) of cerebral cortex showing pyramidal neurons that have single axons that exit the cortex and travel to white matter and numerous destinations (e.g. cortical fields in the opposite cortex), and with a dominant apical dendrite (**D**) that projects superficially. Other nuclei represent stellate neurons and astrocytes. Luxol fast blue/cresyl violet, paraffin, × 300.

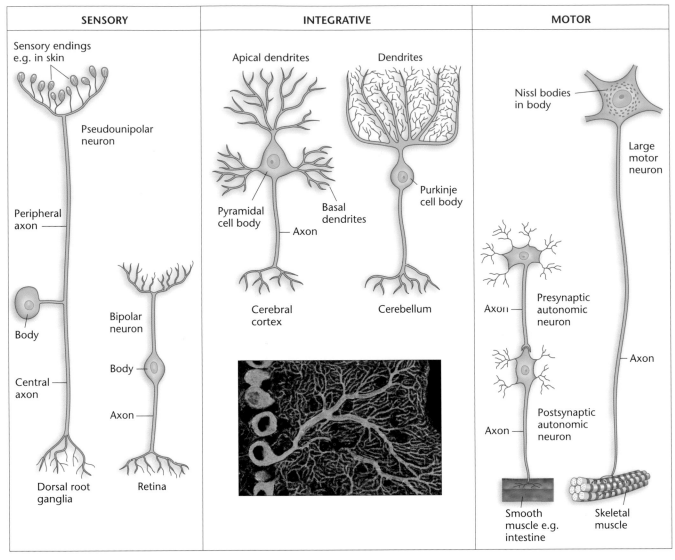

SENSORY	INTEGRATIVE	MOTOR

SENSORY

Sensory endings e.g. in skin

Pseudounipolar neuron

Peripheral axon

Body

Central axon

Bipolar neuron

Body

Axon

Dorsal root ganglia

Retina

INTEGRATIVE

Apical dendrites

Dendrites

Pyramidal cell body

Basal dendrites

Axon

Purkinje cell body

Cerebral cortex

Cerebellum

MOTOR

Nissl bodies in body

Large motor neuron

Axon

Presynaptic autonomic neuron

Axon

Axon

Postsynaptic autonomic neuron

Smooth muscle e.g. intestine

Skeletal muscle

▲ **Fig 7.3 Types of neurons.** Neurons are classified according to the number and morphology of their processes. Multipolar neurons have a single axon and two or more dendrites. Bipolar neurons have a single axon and one dendrite. Unipolar neurons (also called pseudounipolar) have an axon that divides near the cell body—one process passes centrally and the other originates peripherally. **Inset:** A multipolar Purkinje cell from the cerebellum. (Courtesy T Deerinck and M Ellisman, University of California, San Diego, USA; modified from Figure 3.3. in Standring S, ed. Gray's anatomy. 40th edn. Edinburgh: Elsevier, 2008.)

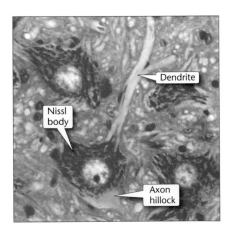

Dendrite

Nissl body

Axon hillock

◄ **Fig 7.4 Nissl substance.** Nissl substance or bodies are deeply stained structures in the perikaryon of the nerve cell body. The intensely basophilic appearance with dyes such as cresyl violet, methylene blue, or toluidine blue is due to many rhomboidal blocks of rough endoplasmic reticulum and associated polysomes. Nissl bodies also occur in dendrites but are absent from the axon. In large neurons, the origin of the axon may be identified because the axon hillock has no Nissl substance. Toluidine blue, araldite, × 470.

The cell body, axons, and dendrites

The cytoplasm of the cell body contains characteristic basophilic clumps of rough endoplasmic reticulum and polyribosomes called Nissl bodies (Fig 7.4) for synthesis of the proteins necessary for neuron function. The many thread- or antenna-like dendritic processes arising from the cell body usually branch profusely and intertwine with dendrites from adjacent neurons (Fig 7.5a & b). Dendrites conduct electric signals, transmitted through synapses with other nerve cell processes, toward the cell body. The neuron has a single axon, sometimes very long, up to a meter in

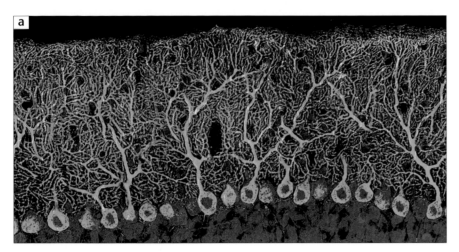

▲ **Fig 7.5a Dendrites.** Molecular layer of the cerebellar cortex. The main stems of the Purkinje cells send their dendritic trees to finely arborize within the outer layer of the cerebellar cortex. The dendrites establish many thousands of contacts (synapses) with other neurons in the molecular layer. Purkinje cells are colored green, nerve cell nuclei blue-purple, and glial cell processes red. Two-photon fluorescence microscopy, × 300. (Courtesy T Deerinck and M Ellisman, University of California, San Diego, USA.)

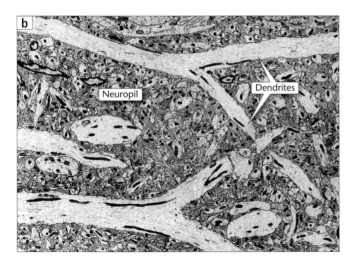

▲ **Fig 7.5b Ultrastructure of branching dendrites** of pyramidal neurons in the cerebral cortex. Microtubules and mitochondria are noted in the dendrites. The tissue between the dendrites is the neuropil, which consists of processes of many dendrites from other neurons. × 1,700. (From Peters A, et al. The fine structure of the nervous system. 3rd edn. New York: Oxford University Press, 1991.)

length, consisting of nerves arising from the spinal cord and terminating in the foot. Axons are the cell processes that conduct nerve impulses away from the cell body to reach their target (e.g. another neuron, a muscle cell, or gland) via synapses. Axons may be referred to as nerve fibers (Fig 7.6a & b).

Motor neurons carry impulses that stimulate their target cell, tissue, or organ. Sensory neurons receive stimuli from sensory receptors distributed throughout the tissues. Interneurons or association neurons interconnect motor and sensory neurons in the CNS.

Since axons lack protein synthesis machinery, all proteins and organelles required for the axon and synaptic terminals must be transported along the axon, that is away from the cell body following their synthesis in the cell body (referred to as anterograde axonal transport). Growth factors and some chemicals are transported from the synapses toward the cell body (this is called retrograde axonal transport). Microtubules serve as a rail system on which kinesin, a special motor protein, directs anterograde flow, and dynein conducts retrograde transport of organelles in the opposite direction.

NEUROGLIA

Glial cells are specialized, non-neuronal supporting cells within the CNS that are found in close association with neurons and blood vessels; in the past, they were considered to be substitutes for connective tissue with merely auxiliary functions.

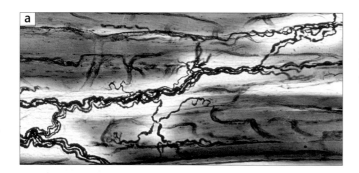

◀ **Fig 7.6a Axons.** Not readily visible in routine paraffin sections, individual axons, also called nerve fibers, may be demonstrated with heavy metal stains that show them as black structures. This tissue is skeletal muscle with numerous blood vessels. Silver stain, whole mount, × 90.

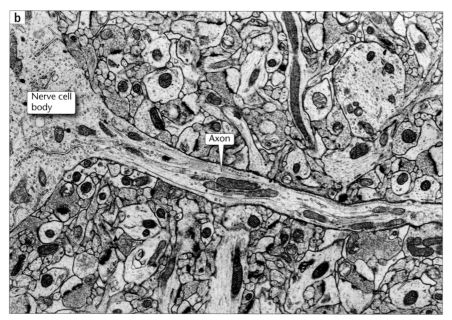

▲ **Fig 7.6b Ultrastructure of the axon hillock** emerging from the perikaryon of the nerve cell body. Mitochondria and microtubules are noted in the axon. Microtubules provide structural support and fast axonal transport of organelles and macromolecules using molecular motors called microtubule-associated proteins. × 10,000. (From Peters A, et al. The fine structure of the nervous system. 3rd edn. New York: Oxford University Press, 1991.)

Glial cells in the CNS arise from the neural tube. In the developing brain, neuroepithelial cells form special radial glial cells that act as scaffolds along which differentiating neurons navigate their way to their final destinations. Thus there is an intimate relationship between glial cells and neurons that persists for life. Although glial cells are at least 10 times more abundant than neurons, they do not convey electric excitation, but they are involved with CNS homeostasis and interactions with neurons, respond to lesions (leading to scar formation), and may proliferate to form certain brain tumors.

Glial cells also are abundant in the PNS and are mainly represented by the Schwann cells (see below). Schwann cells (and neurons) of the PNS develop from the neural crest.

Astrocytes

Astrocytes are stellate cells, often 50 μm or greater in diameter, and are of two varieties: the fibrous type is abundant in white matter and the protoplasmic type is found mainly in gray matter (Fig 7.7). Astrocytes send their processes to surround or contact surfaces of neurons not contacted by synapses, and to surround or contact about 99% of the brain capillary surface area (Fig 7.8). Their functions, which are far from well understood, include the following:

- Control of signal propagation and synapse formation between neurons
- Maintenance of ionic and transmitter metabolism
- Induction of vascular endothelial cells to form a seal or selective filter, called the blood–brain barrier, and therefore may play a role in stroke and ischemia
- A role in brain repair following injury and in the progress of neurodegenerative disease.

Human astrocytes release transmitters that regulate the activities of both neurons and adjacent astrocytes. These "gliotransmitters'"(glutamate, ATP, serine) may have widespread effects, because the largest astrocytes have processes that are up to 1 mm in length. Conventional Golgi-stained or glial fibrillary acidic protein (GFAP) immunolabeling of astrocytes actually reveals only about 15% of the total star-like volume of these cells. Most of the astrocytic processes are GFAP-negative, but new confocal

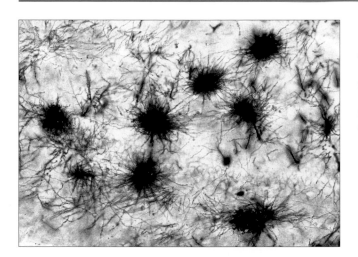

◀ **Fig 7.7 Protoplasmic astrocytes.** Known in general as neuroglia or glial cells, astrocytes, oligodendrocytes, and microglia are the three main types of neuroglia in the central nervous system. In this silver-based Golgi stain, mainly protoplasmic astrocytes are seen. Radially oriented processes of astrocytes make contact with neurons, surround their synapses, and make intimate contact with blood vessels and other astrocytes, but glial cells do not produce electric impulses. Golgi stain, paraffin, × 225.

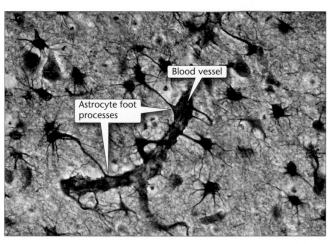

Blood vessel

Astrocyte foot processes

◀ **Fig 7.8 Fibrous astrocytes.** Rather than being simply space fillers or supporting cells, glial cells are known to mop up or inactivate neurotransmitters (glutamate, norepinephrine) to regulate nerve impulses, and help create a tight seal in blood vessels to form the blood–brain barrier that restricts entry of substances into the brain. Fibrous astrocytes are less complex than protoplasmic astrocytes, with fewer, less branched processes. Astrocytes maintain neuron survival by secreting neurotrophic factors, and guide migrating neurons during brain development. Bodian stain, paraffin, × 200.

microscopy techniques show that the astrocytes have an extraordinarily dense arborizing network of fine processes (Fig 7.9a & b).

Oligodendrocytes

Oligodendrocytes have branching processes that extend radially to wrap around several dozen or more axons in the CNS (mostly in white matter) to form segments of myelin sheaths (Fig 7.10). Axons are myelinated by consecutive oligodendrocytes, which exist in enormous numbers far exceeding those of astrocytes. Injury to oligodendrocytes may result in demyelination of axons in diseases such as multiple sclerosis and leukodystrophies.

Microglia

Microglia, the smallest of the glial cells, with rod-shaped nuclei, are specialized CNS phagocytes that remove cellular debris and damaged cells. Similar to macrophages, the microglia belong to the mononuclear phagocyte system. Microglia are considered to be immune effector cells in inflammatory-type responses, where they can secrete cytokines that inhibit neuron functions.

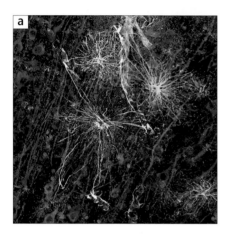

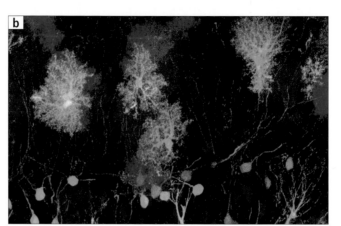

▲ **Fig 7.9a Astrocyte domains.** Protoplasmic astrocytes in human parietal cortex labeled with glial fibrillary acidic protein (GFAP) reveal some details of their processes. The glial cell nucleus is about 10μm in diameter, but the 40 or so processes extend for 100–200 μm in all directions. GFAP-positive processes reflect only 15% of the total volume of the cell, the remaining processes not being labeled. × 500. (Courtesy N A Oberheim, Department of Neurosurgery, University of Rochester Medical Center, USA; from Nature Neuroscience 2007; 11, cover image.)

▲ **Fig 7.9b Hippocampus astrocytes and neurons** in "brainbow" transgenic mouse, in which nerve cells randomly express fluorescent proteins of different colors. Astrocytes show extraordinarily dense packing of cell processes in contrast to fewer such processes seen in the neurons. The labeling of individual glial cells with this technique reveals the astrocyte domain, which overlaps only about 5% with an adjacent astrocyte. Each astrocyte "territory" is most clearly defined in brain areas of high density, suggesting that this organization is important for regulation of synaptic transmission. × 300. (Confocal microscopy by J Livet; from Livet J, et al. Nature 2007; 450:56–62.)

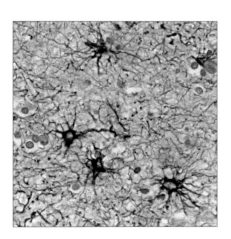

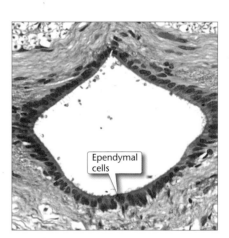

◀ **Fig 7.10 Oligodendrocytes.** Immunohistochemical demonstration of oligodendrocytes in white matter, showing the radial patterns of their cell processes. These glial cells myelinate axons in the central nervous system and, unlike Schwann cell myelination of peripheral nerves, a single oligodendrocyte may ensheath dozens of axons. Immunohistochemistry anti-tubulin, paraffin, × 400.

Ependymal cells

▲ **Fig 7.11 Ependyma.** The central canal of the spinal cord containing cerebrospinal fluid (CSF) is lined with ciliated, cuboidal, or columnar ependymal cells. Produced within the ventricles, CSF enters the central canal and subarachnoid space of the spinal cord. At puberty the central canal becomes obliterated, and the ependymal cells remain as clumps with rudimentary central spaces. H&E, paraffin, × 300.

Ependymal cells

The fourth type of glia in the CNS are ependymal cells (Fig 7.11). They line the ventricles of the brain and central canal of the spinal cord as cuboidal or columnar cells and, in certain locations, join with the pia mater (a delicate membrane that covers the brain and spinal cord) to form the choroid plexus, which secretes most of the cerebrospinal fluid (CSF). Tanycytes, or "stretch," cells are modified ependymal cells that send branches to form processes associated with subependymal capillaries.

Schwann cells and satellite cells

Schwann cells and satellite cells are special types of glial cells associated with the PNS. As they travel to their destinations, peripheral nerves require support, protection, and a suitable microenvironment—attributes provided by Schwann cells.

In myelinated nerves, individual Schwann cells wrap around the axon to form multiple, spiraling layers of Schwann cell membrane, called the myelin sheath. Schwann cells in series each envelop a small segment of one axon (Fig 7.12a–c). Small, oblique discontinuities

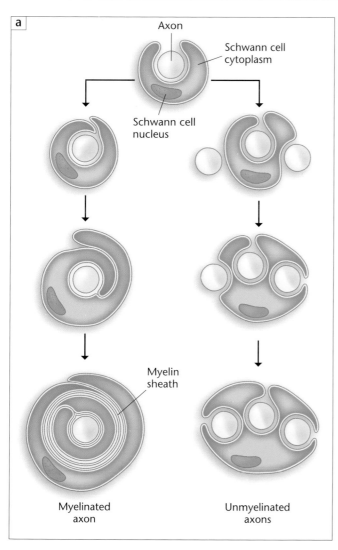

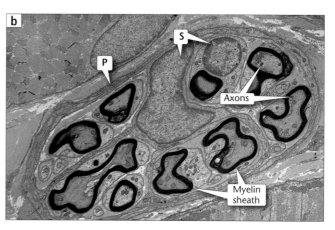

▲ **Fig 7.12b Myelinated axons.** Electron micrograph of myelinated axons invested with myelin sheaths. Schwann cell nuclei (**S**) are surrounded by the cell cytoplasm. The nerve fibers are enclosed by a thin covering of perineurium (**P**). × 4,000.

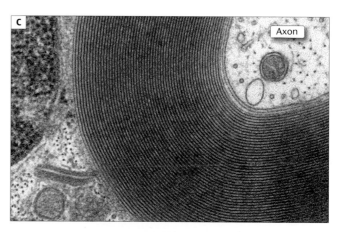

▲ **Fig 7.12c Ultrastructure of the Schwann cell myelin sheath**, showing many lamellae formed by the spiraled plasma membrane. The dense lines represent apposition of the inner leaflets of the plasma membrane as cytoplasm is extruded out during sheath formation. The less dense intervals between the dense lines represent the apposed outer membrane leaflets together with the obliterated intercellular space. × 45,000. (Courtesy K Tiekotter, University of Portland, USA.)

▲ **Fig 7.12a Schwann cell functions.** Derived from the neural crest, Schwann cells are a type of glial cell of the peripheral nervous system. If an axon is to be myelinated, it secretes neuregulin growth factors, which initiate and regulate the wrapping and growth of Schwann cell cytoplasm around the axon. The inner tongue of Schwann cell cytoplasm moves around the axon. The "g-ratio" is given by the diameter of the axon divided by the diameter of the axon and its myelin sheath. Most myelinated nerves in a given animal have a similar g-ratio, between 0.6 and 0.7. The thickness of the sheath varies with axon diameter such that bigger axons have thicker myelin, and smaller axons have thinner myelin. Unmyelinated axons are associated with Schwann cells, but no myelin sheaths are formed. Axons less than 1 μm in diameter are not myelinated.

of the myelin sheath that contain strands of Schwann cell cytoplasm are known as Schmidt-Lanterman clefts (Fig 7.13). These structures possibly provide areas of nutrient exchange between the axon, the Schwann cell, and extracellular fluid, and may facilitate flexion of the nerve fiber. Since the Schwann cells are arranged in succession, the length of the sheath may vary (in the range 0.2–1 mm) according to the growth of individual nerves in fetal and postnatal life.

The gap formed between these segments of myelin is called the node of Ranvier. Nodes occur where the axon is covered not by myelin, but by interdigitating extensions of Schwann cell cytoplasm and an external basal lamina. Nodes and myelin sheaths are physiologically important for the conduction of nerve impulses in myelinated nerves (Fig 7.14a & b, and see below).

Schwann cells also surround unmyelinated nerves, but they do not produce myelin. In these nerves or fibers, the axons are embedded in grooves or invaginations of the Schwann cell cytoplasm and the nucleus is usually located centrally (Fig 7.15), in contrast to the myelinated axons, where the Schwann cell nucleus, and most of its cytoplasm, is peripheral. Schwann cells originate from the neural crest, which forms precursor cells and then immature Schwann cells. Myelination proceeds only in Schwann cells that envelop large-diameter axons; those that ensheath small-diameter axons (1 μm or less) become non-myelinating cells.

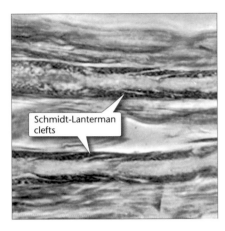

◀ Fig 7.13 Schmidt-Lanterman clefts. Focal disruptions of the myelin sheath lamellae are shown, forming oblique, linear clefts through the sheath. Clefts contain Schwann cell cytoplasm and may provide a route for continuity of cytoplasm from the outside of the myelin sheath to the inside, adjacent to the axon. Whole-mount nerve fibers, oblique incident light, × 300. (Courtesy K Tiekotter, University of Portland, USA.)

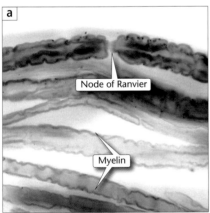

◀ Fig 7.14a Node of Ranvier. Preparation in which individual nerve fibers have been carefully separated by microdissection of a fresh nerve. The myelin that surrounds individual axons is clearly seen, as is the site called the node of Ranvier, where myelin is absent although the endoneurium is continuous. Nodes of Ranvier are spaced approximately 1 mm apart on each axon, and gaps in myelination ensure rapid transmission of electric impulses by a process termed saltatory conduction (action potentials "jump" from node to node). Each myelin segment, between two nodes, is provided by a single Schwann cell. The central nervous system counterparts of Schwann cells, which provide myelin, are oligodendrocytes. Unstained whole mount, × 300.

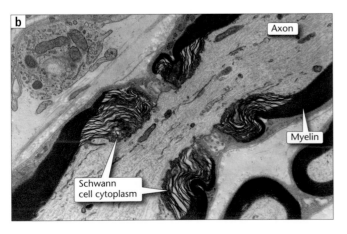

◀ Fig 7.14b Nodes of Ranvier are intervals between segments of myelin. At the node where myelin is absent, the axon is invested with processes of Schwann cell cytoplasm. Nodes function to propagate the action potentials along myelinated nerves by admitting Na⁺ ions through many localized membrane channels. Current density at nodes is very high, resulting in generation of action potentials that jump in a saltatory manner from one node to the next. × 6,700. (From Porter KR and Bonneville MA. Fine structure of cells and tissues. 5th edn. Lea and Febiger: Philadelphia, 1973.)

Satellite cells are specialized glial cells that surround the cell bodies found in ganglia. Ganglia are aggregations of neuron cell bodies that function like relay stations (Fig 7.16). The satellite cells probably play a role in metabolic exchanges between the neurons and surrounding nerve tissues.

Other glial cells of the PNS

Astrocyte-type cells known as olfactory ensheathing cells extend fine processes between groups of axons of the olfactory nerve. Axon terminals at skeletal neuromuscular junctions of skeletal muscle are covered by terminal glia (teloglia). Sensory nerve endings in the skin may be accompanied by glial cells that form the inner core of the Pacinian corpuscle. Ganglia of the enteric nervous system have glial cells, the enteric glia, that are similar to astrocytes.

> **Tip:** In the CNS the oligodendrocytes, derived from neuroepithelium, each myelinate several dozen or more nearby axons, but the many other unmyelinated axons are bare and not embedded in glial cells. In contrast, all myelinated and unmyelinated axons in the PNS are associated with Schwann cells (derived from the neural crest).

NERVE IMPULSES AND SYNAPSES
Nerve impulses

Depending upon its location and specialized function, a resting neuron may respond to a stimulus (e.g.

mechanical, chemical, electric, thermal, photons) by conducting an impulse or electric signal along the axon to its terminus. The biophysics of signal conduction encompasses a large body of knowledge and the general principles only are reviewed here in relation to neuron histology.

Resting potential

Neurons at rest expend energy to maintain an electric polarization across the plasma membrane, in which the internal surface is slightly more negative than the exterior. This is called the resting potential and results from:

- Unequal distribution of Na^+ and K^+ ions, in which at rest there are more K^+ ions and fewer Na^+ ions inside the cell than in the extracellular fluid
- Membrane sodium–potassium pumps, which export Na^+ and import K^+.

The net effect establishes a resting potential of about -70 mV.

Action potential

In response to a stimulus, extracellular Na^+ ions flow inward momentarily (about 1 millisecond), reversing the local membrane potential to $+30$ mV, which is followed by restoration of the resting potential by outflow of K^+ ions. An action potential is thus generated and the opening of Na^+ channels spreads to adjacent membrane regions along the axon, which thus propagates a new action potential slightly closer to the axon terminus.

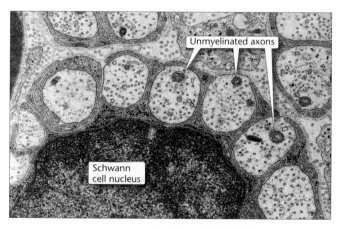

▲ **Fig 7.15 Schwann cells of unmyelinated nerves.** Six unmyelinated axons are shown embedded in Schwann cell cytoplasm. The axon at left is surrounded by a separate cytoplasmic process and is probably associated with another Schwann cell not seen in the section. × 23,000. (From Peters A et al. The fine structure of the nervous system. 3rd edn. New York: Oxford University Press, 1991.)

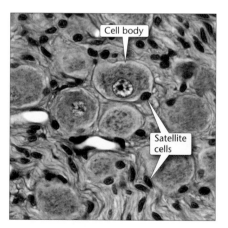

▲ **Fig 7.16 Satellite cells.** Nerve cell bodies in a dorsal (sensory) root ganglion of a spinal nerve. Each cell body is closely associated with one or more glial cells, termed satellite cells. These cells ensheath the nerve cells but do not myelinate them. H&E, acrylic resin, × 230.

Action potentials are analogous to oscillations generated along a skipping-rope, or the apparent "movement" of a Mexican wave through spectators at a football stadium. The action potential itself does not travel along the axon, but initiates new action potentials slightly ahead of it. A wave of electric excitation produced by a chain or series of action potentials is a nerve impulse. The magnitude of the depolarization associated with an action potential is not diminished as the impulse progresses along the axon and is comparable with the transmission of a flame along a burning fuse.

Speed of impulse conduction

The speed of impulse conduction varies according to the axon diameter and the presence or absence of a myelin sheath. In unmyelinated nerves, impulses travel as described above, but relatively slowly, around 0.5–2 m/s. Myelin sheaths greatly increase the velocity of nerve impulses by insulating the axon, which allows rapid intracellular diffusion of Na^+ ions from node to node, sufficient to trigger a new action potential at each node, a process which is called saltatory conduction (jumping from node to node). Larger, myelinated fibers, up to 20 μm in diameter, may conduct impulses faster than 100 m/s.

Synapses

When an impulse reaches a nerve ending, it must be conveyed to another nerve cell or to the tissue that it supplies (muscle, targeted blood vessel, glandular tissue); this is achieved by transmission of chemical substances known as neurotransmitters. Chemical synapses are specialized complementary regions between nerves or their processes, in which the end bulb of an axon, usually one of many endings derived from preterminal axon branchings, is parallel to and closely aligned (within 20 nm) with the postsynaptic membrane of the recipient cell. End bulbs contain synaptic vesicles filled with neurotransmitter and, in response to the action potential, vesicles discharge their contents into the synaptic cleft via exocytosis (Fig 7.17). Postsynaptic membranes bind the neurotransmitter substance and this triggers depolarization and excitation of the target cell.

Such chemical synapses are the most common way in which nerve impulses are conveyed from cell to cell; the effect can be either stimulatory where the postsynaptic neuron is electrically depolarized, or inhibitory where hyperpolarisation occurs.

Of the many chemical varieties of neurotransmitters, the main types are acetylcholine, biogenic amines (e.g. norepinephrine, dopamine), amino acids and derivatives (e.g. glutamate, gamma-aminobutyric acid), and neuropeptides (e.g. opioids).

Axon synapses may transmit to cell bodies, dendrites, or other axons; the common types are axodendritic and axosomatic, but various combinations between axons, soma, and dendrites are possible. Axon synapses are found in the CNS and in autonomic ganglia, including the enteric nervous system. Chemical signals across synapses travel in only one direction. The soma and, in particular, dendrites of the smallest neurons may have dozens or hundreds of synapses, but neurons in the CNS (e.g. the Purkinje cells) may have hundreds of thousands, visible as dendritic spines (Fig 7.18).

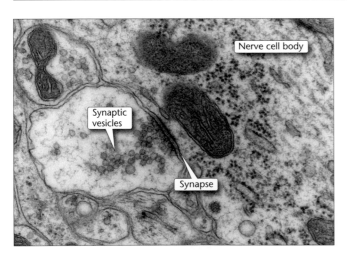

▲ **Fig 7.17 Synapse.** Ultrastructure of an axosomatic synapse of a Purkinje neuron. Note the synaptic vesicles within the axon and the associated membrane densities of the synaptic cleft. Neurotransmitters are packaged, stored, and released by synaptic vesicles. Upon stimulation of the synaptic terminal, neurotransmitter enters the synaptic cleft following exocytosis from vesicles. The neurotransmitter binds to postsynaptic membrane receptors and stimulates a response applicable to the target cell. × 30,000. (Courtesy K Tiekotter, University of Portland, USA.)

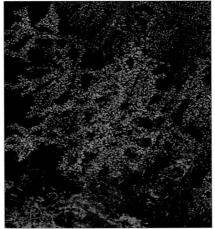

▲ **Fig 7.18 Dendritic spines.** A Purkinje cell of the cerebellum, showing thousands of short spines (green fluorescence) along the fine terminal branches of the dendrites (red fluorescence). Each spine is an outpocket, or small extension (1–2 μm), of the dendrite; the spines serve as synapses with dendrites of other neurons. A single Purkinje cell may have 100,000 dendritic spines. Confocal microscopy, × 650. (Courtesy F Capani, Institute for Cell Biology and Neuroscience, University of Buenos Aires, Argentina.)

Nerves of the enteric nervous system regulate the activity of the smooth muscle tissue in which they are embedded, but commonly do not make synaptic contacts with their target cells. In this case, the nerve fibers have small swellings, termed varicosities, that contain the neurotransmitters in many vesicles. Upon release, the neurotransmitter may diffuse for some distance, resulting in prolonged and widespread actions (Fig 7.19).

The neuromuscular junction

This is a special type of synapse, which may be considered as a peripheral synapse. A motor neuron that innervates muscle fibers forms branches that end as terminal swellings occupying recesses in the sarcolemma of the muscle fiber (Fig 7.20a–c). Such swellings have lost their myelin, but the Schwann cell cytoplasm persists and overarches along the upper aspect of the nerve terminal. The close apposition

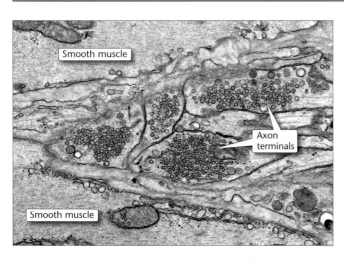

▲ **Fig 7.19 Axon varicosities**. Ultrastructure of axon terminals (boutons) of enteric nerves belonging to Auerbach's plexus in the external smooth muscle layer of the gastrointestinal tract. Varicosities have many vesicles containing neurotransmitters but lack specialized synaptic junctions typical of the nerve supply to skeletal muscle. Acetylcholine is a major neurotransmitter that regulates muscle contraction in the gut, but many other neurotransmitters are also involved, such as substance P, vasoactive intestinal peptide, other peptides and amines, and nitrous oxide. × 22,000.

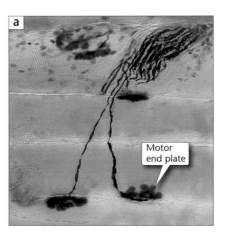

▲ **Fig 7.20a Motor nerve and terminal branches.** Histochemical preparation of a motor nerve and several of its terminal branches, which supply skeletal muscle fibers through the neuromuscular junction. Each junction, also known as a motor end plate, is stained blue owing to a positive reaction to acetylcholinesterase, an enzyme that degrades the neurotransmitter substance acetylcholine. The junctional regions are spread upon the muscle fiber with several individual extensions. Histochemistry for acetylcholinesterase, frozen section, × 450.

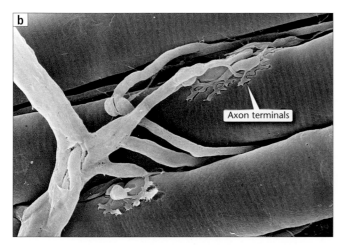

▲ **Fig 7.20b Motor nerve and neuromuscular junctions.** Scanning electron micrograph of a motor nerve and two neuromuscular junctions adherent to skeletal muscle fibers. Note the foot-like processes of the nerve terminals that locate within shallow depressions of the muscle sarcolemma. × 5,000. (From Desaki J and Uehara Y. J Neurocytology 1981; 10:101–10.)

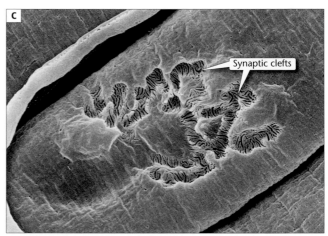

▲ **Fig 7.20c Motor nerve endings.** Scanning electron micrograph of a skeletal muscle fiber in which the motor nerve endings have been removed by acid digestion. The grooves and smaller clefts represent the interdigitation of nerve end processes of the junction. The clefts are narrow invaginations of the muscle sarcolemma, which serve to increase the surface area of sarcolemma exposed to neurotransmitter. × 12,000. (From Desaki J and Uehara Y. Dev Biol 1987; 119:390–401.)

between the axon and the muscle is called a motor end plate, and the 30–50 nm gap is the synapse across which the neurotransmitter (acetylcholine in the case of skeletal muscle) initiates depolarization of the sarcolemma. If an action potential is initiated in the sarcolemma, this is rapidly spread over the surface and deep within the muscle fiber, causing its contraction. A single motor nerve impulse results in a single muscle fiber action potential and therefore muscle contraction is regulated by the frequency of signals arriving from the motor neuron.

A motor unit is defined as all muscle fibers supplied by one motor neuron. For fine muscle control, small motor units (e.g. in eye movements) consist of three to six muscle fibers for each nerve fiber; for large skeletal muscles where strong contractions are required, each nerve fiber may supply many hundreds of muscle fibers.

PERIPHERAL NERVES AND GANGLIA
Peripheral nerves

In histologic sections stained with hematoxylin and eosin (H&E), peripheral nerves are often poorly stained and, to the untrained eye, may go unnoticed or be identified as connective tissue or even adipose tissue. The weak staining and hence minimal evidence of structural organization occurs because, regardless

of how many are aggregated together, individual axons are commonly very small in diameter (often 1–5 μm) and difficult to stain, and the myelin sheaths of myelinated nerves are virtually colorless with routine stains. As myelin is mostly lipid, the sheaths are dissolved during the tissue preparation process, which leaves empty spaces. Thus, a cross section through a whole nerve, large or small, gives the impression of tissue that lacks structural detail. A similar phenomenon occurs for nerves sectioned longitudinally, in which the parallel axons form multilayered, sinusoidal strands studded with nuclei.

Depending on the quality of specimen preservation and intensity of H&E staining, the characteristic features of nerves can be recognized, but the use of specific fixatives (such as osmium tetroxide) and various stains (such as Mallory, Masson, Van Gieson, or toluidine blue) greatly improves the structural detail, particularly for myelinated nerves (Fig 7.21a–e).

Ranging in diameter from a few micrometers to 15 mm (e.g. the sciatic nerve), nerves consist of multiple axons or nerve fibers bound together by connective tissue, and may be compared to an optic fiber cable that carries many individual filaments. Larger nerves are bound by a complete outer layer of dense connective tissue, called epineurium, deep to which is loose connective tissue that contains blood vessels and variable quantities of fat.

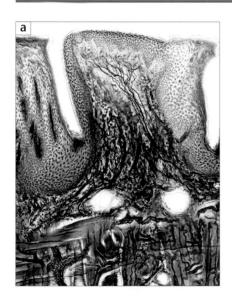

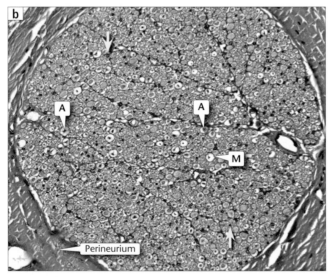

▲ Fig 7.21a Myelinated peripheral nerves. Fine nerves in paraffin sections may be traced with heavy metal staining techniques such as silver staining. Nerve fibers stain black with this method. This tissue is from the dorsum of the tongue showing nerve supply to a lingual papilla. Silver stain, paraffin, × 50.

▲ Fig 7.21b Myelinated peripheral nerve. A myelinated nerve in transverse section, with perineurium sending connective tissue septa into the nerve, transmits blood vessels and ramifies into a network of endoneurium. Many nerve fibers present as central dots, the axons (**A**) surrounded by an annulus of myelin (**M**), empty-looking because of the extraction of lipids during preparation. Small dense bodies (**arrows**) are Schwann cell nuclei; these cells wrap around the axons to form the myelin sheaths. Myelin insulates the axons in successive segments, which prevents loss of ions from the axoplasm to the extracellular tissue fluid, and, in the case of myelinated axons, action potentials are generated in the gaps or nodes between successive sheaths of myelin. H&E, paraffin, × 150.

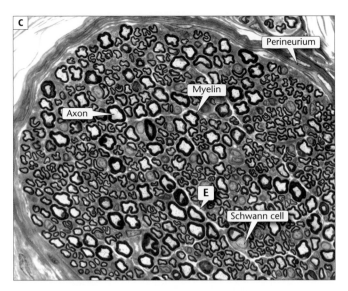

◀ **Fig 7.21c Myelinated axons.** Thin epon resin section of peripheral nerve contains myelinated axons of various diameters (myelin, axons, Schwann cells) supported by endoneurium (**E**). A histogram plot of axon diameter reveals a bimodal distribution, and larger fibers conduct impulses faster than smaller axons. An axon of 10 μm diameter conducts at 60 m/s to control muscle contraction, or conducts sensory information from tactile receptors in skin. In many nerves, small (0.5–1 μm), unmyelinated fibers predominate (not shown) and conduct at <3 m/s; they are involved with transmission of pain and they innervate blood vessels. Toluidine blue, epon section, × 300.

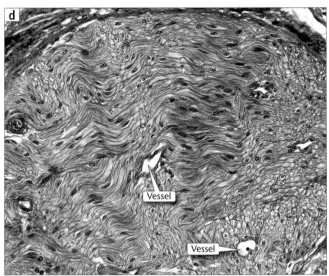

◀ **Fig 7.21d A bundle of nerve fibers** showing myelinated nerves in longitudinal, oblique, and transverse views. Many of the nuclei are of Schwann cells, the myelin sheaths staining weakly. Blood vessels are indicated. Masson's trichrome, paraffin, × 170.

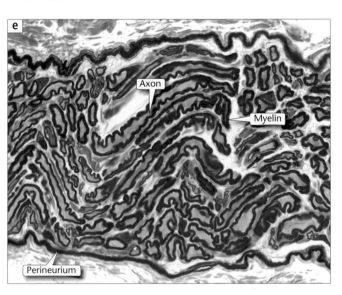

◀ **Fig 7.21e Motor and sensory peripheral nerve.** Thin epon resin section of a mixed motor and sensory peripheral nerve cut longitudinally, showing details of the complex arrangement of myelinated axons invested by the perineurium. In this plane of section, axons course both longitudinally and in transverse or oblique planes. The axons twist and spiral through the nerve to provide elasticity and extra length, which protects them from damage when, for example, a limb is extended, flexed, or laterally rotated. Myelin sheaths stain dark blue; the axons are stained pale blue-green. Empty-looking space between the axons is the connective tissue of the endoneurium, within which travel the capillaries. Toluidine blue, epon section, × 500.

In many nerves, axons are grouped together to form bundles, or fascicles, and each fascicle is invested by another connective tissue sheath called perineurium. Individual axons, together with their Schwann cells, are supported by thin, ramifying layers of endoneurium, through which capillaries supply the neural elements. For most nerves, the nerve fibers are a mixture of myelinated and unmyelinated types (Fig 7.22a & b), with the latter usually predominating.

Ganglia

Ganglia of the PNS are groups of cell bodies, associated with glial cells and often with a connective tissue capsule, that act as relay and integrative stations along sensory or motor nerve pathways. The sensory type is located in the dorsal root of each spinal nerve, and the motor type is found in the ANS.

Dorsal root ganglia (also known as spinal or sensory ganglia) contain many hundreds or thousands of pseudounipolar neurons, each surrounded by many satellite (glial) cells (Fig 7.23a & b). Each cell body, devoid of dendrites, has one process that resembles an axon that bifurcates within the ganglion, one branch extending peripherally to its site of origin

(i.e. a receptor in skin, muscle, etc), the other acting as an efferent branch and traveling to the gray matter in the spinal cord. The transmission of sensory information through a dorsal root ganglion does not involve synapses, and provides for the fastest signals transmitted within the nervous system.

Autonomic ganglia

Autonomic ganglia are associated with the sympathetic and parasympathetic divisions of the ANS. Sympathetic ganglia form the sympathetic chain (paravertebral), the prevertebral ganglia (associated with aorta), and cervical ganglia. Parasympathetic ganglia consist of the cranial and terminal ganglia; the former is associated with cranial nerves III, VII, and IX, and the latter occur near to or within the internal organs they supply and are associated with the vagus nerve or S2, S3, and S4 spinal segments.

In structure, autonomic ganglia are similar to sensory ganglia, except that the cell bodies are dispersed (Fig 7.24). There are fewer satellite cells because these neurons are multipolar, their radiating dendrites synapsing with motor signals that are transmitted by the preganglionic fibers that originate in the CNS.

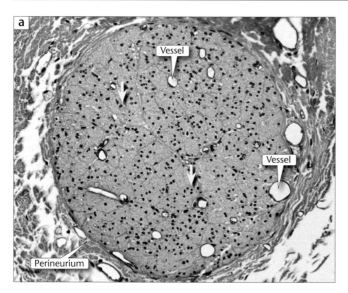

▲ **Fig 7.22a An unmyelinated nerve in transverse section**, showing perineurium extending inwardly to form a fine network of endoneurium. Numerous blood vessels are noted. The many small, scattered nuclei are of Schwann cells (**arrows**), but unlike myelinated nerves these cells invest the axons but do not form myelin sheaths. Thus, the material between these nuclei represents thousands of axons. Nerve impulses travel the length of each axon until they reach its terminal, usually a synapse. Impulses travel at 0.5–2 m/s, whereas in myelinated nerves the velocity may be over 100 m/s because of the rapid longitudinal diffusion of ions along the axon segments insulated by myelin sheaths, supplemented by successive action potentials at the non-myelinated segments (or nodes) between the sheaths. H&E, paraffin, × 150.

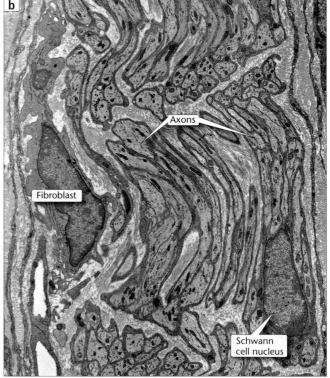

▲ **Fig 7.22b Ultrastructure of unmyelinated nerve fibers.** A Schwann cell nucleus is noted and its cytoplasm thinly invests the axons, between which is the supporting connective tissue of the endoneurium. × 4,000.

Enteric ganglia

The enteric nervous system (ENS) of the gut consists of many small ganglia of Auerbach's and Meissner's plexus (Fig 7.25). The ENS is often considered to be part of the parasympathetic system, but in functional terms the ENS, while operating independently of the ANS, is modified by both divisions of the ANS. Some investigators consider the ganglia of the ENS to be the third division of the ANS (see Ch 14 for additional information).

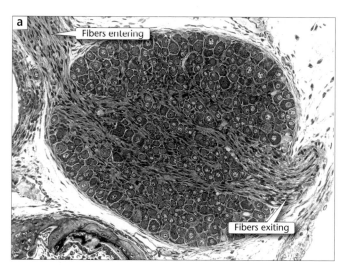

▲ **Fig 7.23a A dorsal root (sensory) ganglion of the afferent limb of a spinal nerve.** Spinal ganglia are swellings of the dorsal roots of spinal nerves. Ganglia vary greatly in size but they all show collections of nerve cell bodies, hundreds of which are seen here. Dorsal root ganglia are relay stations transmitting sensory signals from the periphery to the spinal cord. Entry and exit points for this afferent pathway are noted. Toluidine blue, araldite section, × 60.

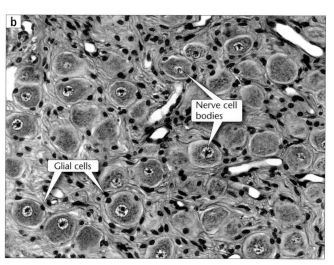

▲ **Fig 7.23b Detail of dorsal root ganglion**, showing large nerve cell bodies. These ganglia contain pseudounipolar neurons clustered together and surrounded by numerous glial cells called satellite cells. The single process of the neuron, its axon, is branched; one branch is the incoming pathway of the peripheral nerve, and the other joins the posterior root to reach the spinal cord. The nerve fibers, usually myelinated, run through the sensory ganglion, but do not synapse with the nerve cell bodies. H&E, paraffin, × 180.

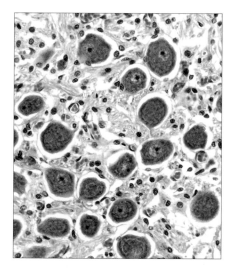

▲ **Fig 7.24 Autonomic (parasympathetic) ganglion in a salivary gland**, showing a cluster of nerve cell bodies associated with occasional neuroglial cells, called satellite cells. Nerve fibers, both afferent and efferent, synapse with the multipolar neurons, some fibers being sympathetic nerves from the cervical ganglion. Parasympathetic ganglia are located usually close to or within the organs that they innervate. The limited number of satellite cells reflects the presence of many dendrites emerging from the multipolar neurons. Ganglia of the sympathetic chain and prevertebral ganglia show similar histology, but the cell bodies are more dispersed. H&E, paraffin, × 270.

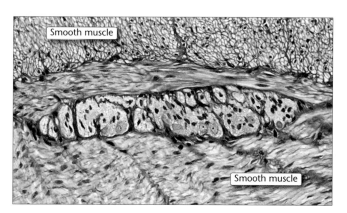

▲ **Fig 7.25 A ganglion of myenteric (Auerbach's) plexus in the muscle wall of the gut**, showing multipolar neurons, which form synapses with nerve fibers distributed into the plexus. Neuroglial cells, called satellite cells, associate with the nerve cell bodies. Although these ganglia primarily function as a parasympathetic plexus (stimulating muscle activity), sympathetic fibers from the sympathetic trunk also contribute to the plexus, and inhibit gut motility. The myenteric plexus regulates intrinsic gut movements and is in turn influenced by extrinsic inputs from the autonomic nervous system. Hematoxylin/PAS, paraffin, × 200.

CENTRAL NERVOUS SYSTEM

The CNS, which consists of the brain and spinal cord, performs the main functions of information correlation and integration. Most of the CNS is made up of two tissues—gray matter and white matter; in histologic sections, these are best studied using specially stained preparations in addition to conventional H&E specimens.

Brain

The brain consists of the cerebrum, cerebellum, and brainstem, and each part is made up of gray and white matter (Fig 7.26a & b). Gray matter is composed of neuron cell bodies, their dendrites and axons, neuroglial cells, and blood vessels, and is concerned with neural integration via enormous numbers of synapses (Fig 7.27a & b).

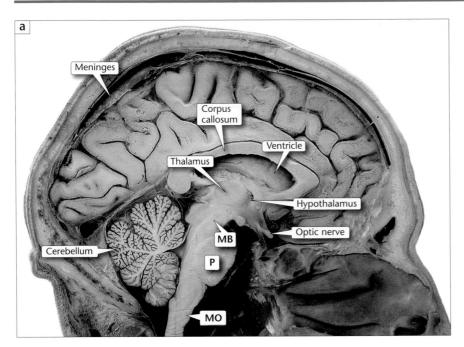

◄ **Fig 7.26a Architecture of the brain.** Sagittal section of brain illustrating meninges, cerebral hemisphere with folds of gray matter (gyri) and furrows (sulci), corpus callosum, lateral ventricle, thalamus and hypothalamus, optic nerve and infundibular stalk (cut), midbrain (**MB**), pons (**P**), and medulla oblongata (**MO**), and the cerebellum. At birth the brain weighs about 400 g, and grows to an average of 1,350 g in adults. The buoyant effect of cerebrospinal fluid in the meninges reduces the weight in situ to about 50 g.

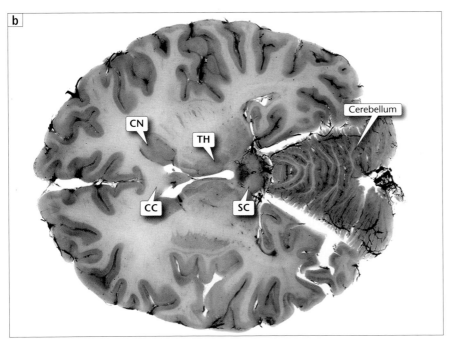

◄ **Fig 7.26b Gray matter distribution.** Angled horizontal section showing the distribution of gray matter (brown-yellow) in the cerebral cortex, in the central regions surrounding the third ventricle and in the cerebellum. Gray matter contains many billions of neurons and glial cells, densely packed in the cortical convolutions to form sulci (furrows) and gyri (folds), thereby increasing surface area. The cerebellar cortex of folia (ridges) contains cores of white matter (also found deep to the cerebral cortex) that consist mainly of myelinated fibers. Some functions of the indicated regions: the thalamus (**TH**) relays and processes most sensory input to the sensory cortex and influences the motor cortex; caudate nucleus (**CN**) is a basal ganglion that influences motor tracts to the cortex; the corpus callosum (**CC**) bridges between hemispheres, sharing information; the superior colliculus (**SC**) is for visual reflexes, tracking moving objects; the cerebellum coordinates skeletal muscle activity but does not initiate motor movements. (From a specimen prepared by S Robbins, Anatomy Department, University of Melbourne, Australia.)

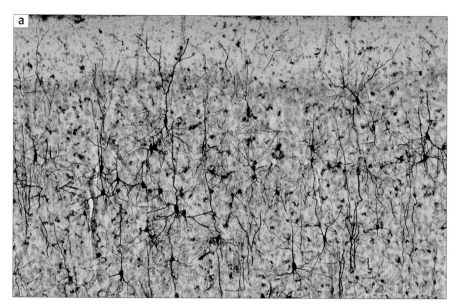

▲ **Fig 7.27a Gray matter.** Gray matter of the cerebral cortex is very richly populated with a variety of neurons and a larger population of glial cells. This specimen was stained with silver salts that for unknown reasons selectively stain black a small proportion (a few percent) of neurons and glia. Silver stain, paraffin, × 250.

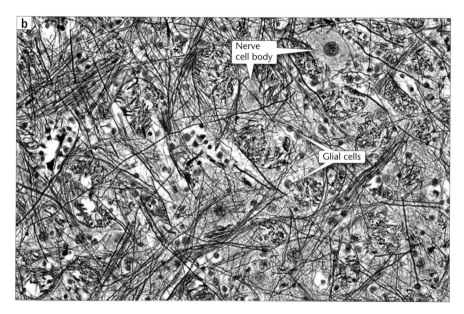

▲ **Fig 7.27b Neural circuitry.** Neurons and glial cells and their processes are shown in the cerebral cortex gray matter, illustrating the enormous complexity of neural circuitry. Most of the stained processes are branching dendrites that make synaptic connections between dendrites (dendodendritic), axons (axodendritic), and neuron cell bodies (dendrosomatic). Bodian stain, paraffin, × 400.

White matter is composed mainly of myelinated axons and neuroglial cells (Fig 7.28). It provides routes or nerve tracts that connect one part of the brain to another (e.g. superficial to deep, anterior to posterior), and also connects the brainstem to the spinal cord.

Neurons, glia, and capillaries are packed very tightly together. The tissue between the cell bodies is called the neuropil and consists of dendrites, axons, and glial processes (Fig 7.29). On average the width of the gaps between these processes is 20 nm. The space thus created is occupied by extracellular fluid, which comprises up to 20% of brain volume owing to the highly folded surface membranes of neurons and glial cells. Diffusion of nutrients, waste products of metabolism, and neurotransmitters occurs within the extracellular fluid. Accumulation of water in the brain, which includes swelling of the tissue, is termed cerebral edema. The brain (and the spinal cord) is covered by the meninges, which consist of three membranes—the tough dura mater, the delicate arachnoid mater, and the innermost pia mater. The pia, associated with a basement membrane, follows closely the contours of the CNS. Marginal glial cells of the brain extend foot-processes that adhere to the basement membrane, forming the glia limitans, which serves as structural support for the surface of the CNS.

Cerebrum

Over 80% of the volume of the brain is cerebrum. The two cerebral hemispheres each consist of the outer, folded cortex of gray matter (2–5 mm in thickness and up to 2 m² in surface area) covering the inner white matter. The primary sensory cortex is somewhat thinner compared with the motor cortex. Inside the white matter on the floor and medial walls of the hemisphere are additional collections of gray matter, called basal ganglia (or basal nuclei) and thalamic nuclei (Fig 7.30).

Histologically, the cerebral cortex is most easily studied because of its astounding concentration of neurons, which form six layers parallel to the cortical surface (Fig 7.31a & b). The ordered patterns of

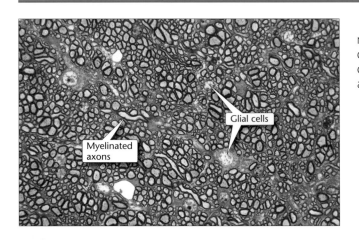

◀ **Fig 7.28 White matter.** Deep to the cerebral cortex the white matter is mostly myelinated axons, hence its color, which provide connectivity throughout the brain. Nucleated cells represent glial cells, some of which are the oligodendrocytes that myelinate the axons. Toluidine blue, araldite, × 200.

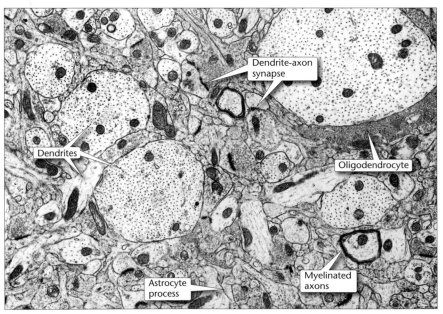

◀ **Fig 7.29 Neuropil of the cerebral cortex.** Ultrastructural view of the cerebral cortex, showing cross sections through five dendrites of pyramidal neurons. Note their plentiful supply of microtubules. Several dendritic spines are seen, some forming synapses with axons. Myelinated nerves are indicated, together with astrocyte processes and part of an oligodendrocyte. × 9,000. (From Peters A, et al. The fine structure of the nervous system. 3rd edn. New York: Oxford University Press, 1991.)

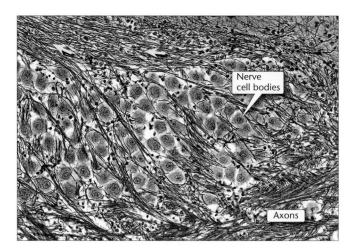

Nerve cell bodies

Axons

◀ **Fig 7.30 Thalamic nucleus.** Lateral geniculate nucleus (visual system) of the thalamus receiving optic tract fibers or axons. This nucleus processes visual information and transmits (**arrows**) to the visual cortex. Each nucleus receives axons from the retina of both eyes after passing through the optic nerves and chiasm. Connections from the retina to the visual cortex are highly ordered, with matching areas of retina mapped onto the cortex and a large cortical area devoted to processing information from the fovea. H&E/silver stain, paraffin, × 280.

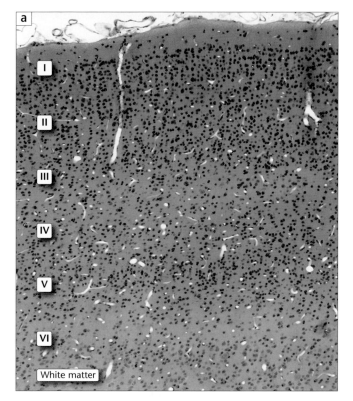

a

I

II

III

IV

V

VI

White matter

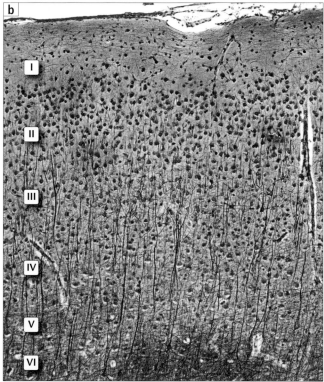

b

I

II

III

IV

V

VI

▲ **Fig 7.31a Cerebral cortex.** Vertical section of the somatosensory cortex, a region of the parietal lobe that occupies most of the postcentral gyrus. It is concerned with initial processing of tactile and proprioceptive (sense of position) information. Stimulation of this gyrus in conscious humans produces tingling and/or numbness sensations in contralateral parts of the body, which results in the familiar "map" on the cortex in which the body from tongue to toe is spread out linearly, forming the so-called homunculus (little person) often depicted in neuroanatomy texts. These regional specializations in part explain why the histology of the six horizontal layers (**I–VI**) vary in different regions of the cerebral cortex. Each layer has characteristic neurons with particular functions and unique connections. Signals enter first in layer **IV** (e.g. from the thalamus), and spread apically and basally. The six layers of the neocortex, preserved in most vertebrates, increase in surface area by folding as species evolve higher intelligence. The white matter contains myelinated axons that enter or leave the cortex. H&E, paraffin, × 60.

▲ **Fig 7.31b Somatosensory cortex.** Silver stain of somatosensory cortex shows some of the complexity of the neuronal dendrites and connections within and between cortical layers. The thick dendrites of pyramidal cells in layer **V** project toward layer **I**, where they ultimately bifurcate. Thousands of synapses terminate along these dendrites and play important roles in the integration of information. The laminar organization of the cortex reflects the layering of cells, dendrites, and connections. The vertical organization represents columns of cell bodies (perhaps 10,000 in each), the function of which is associated with particular sensations such as muscle stretch receptors, tendon or hair receptors, etc. These divisions of function are well separated in layer **IV**, but become integrated at other levels within the columns. Some of these incoming signals spread to the motor cortex located in the adjacent precentral gyrus. Layers: **I**, molecular; **II**, external granular; **III**, pyramidal; **IV**, internal granular; **V**, large pyramidal; **VI**, multiform. Silver stain, paraffin, × 60.

lamina such as those found in the hippocampus may be demonstrated with confocal fluorescence techniques (Fig 7.32). Regions of white matter have no corresponding morphological features.

Functionally, the cortical neurons and their connections are organized vertically or in columns (about 100–200 µm in width) with respect to the surface. In relation to the laminar organization of the cortex, the four outermost layers mainly receive afferent fibers from other regions of the cerebral cortex and brainstem, and the fifth and sixth layers provide efferent fibers that pass to the white matter. Identification of the types of neurons is essentially based on shape and size:

- Pyramidal cells—from 10 µm to 100 µm for the Betz cell variety in the motor cortex
- Stellate cells—diverse morphology, but typically small and multipolar
- Martinotti cells—with spinous soma and long, ascending axons
- Fusiform cells—in deep layer, spindle-shaped with axon entering white matter.

As a broad generalization, stellate cells are the interneurons of the cerebral cortex, and the pyramidal cells, which make up perhaps 70% of cortical cells, are the main output neurons.

The human brain, and particularly the cerebrum, is relatively and absolutely the largest among those of all primates. Higher neural function is associated not so much with cortical thickness or even absolute brain size (e.g. elephant, blue whale), but rather with communication between neurons via synaptic density. Special stains are required to reveal a tiny fraction of this connectivity, and in conventional histology preparations the silver metal impregnation methods usually work well.

A growing body of evidence suggests that certain regions of the cerebrum are the source of stem cells capable of supplying new neurons and glial cells. Neural precursor cells in so-called germinal niches in the subventricular zone of the lateral ventricle produce new neurons for the olfactory mucosa. The dentate gyrus of the hippocampus may also be a source of new neurons. Although much remains to be discovered, germinal niches could be a source of neurons and/ or glial cells following inflammatory or degenerative changes to brain tissue.

The thalamic nuclei are located adjacent (lateral) to the ventricles in the diencephalon. This collection of nuclei selects and integrates all information for the cortex of the cerebrum. The thalamus is involved in maintaining consciousness, and it directs information about movement from the basal ganglia and cerebellum to the cortex.

Basal ganglia, located deep within the white matter, are defined masses of gray matter that can be seen in dissected or sectioned specimens of the brain. These clusters of nuclei are heavily involved with coordinating muscle action, and appear to inhibit muscular tone, since disorders of the basal ganglia (as in Parkinson's disease) lead to tremor and rigidity of muscles when at rest.

Cerebellum

The cerebellum also consists of two hemispheres, deeply folded or corrugated into fissures and lobes. These are composed of an outer covering of gray matter (the cortex) and inner, branched cores of white matter (Fig 7.33a–c). Embedded deep in the white matter are the deep nuclei. Each hemisphere is connected to the brain stem by three cerebellar peduncles. All efferent and afferent pathways of the

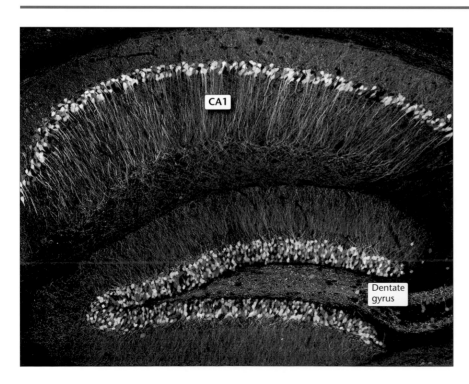

◀ **Fig 7.32 Neuron labeling.** The hippocampus (seahorse-shaped) from a "brainbow" transgenic mouse. The multicolor "brainbow" labeling reveals neurons of the cornu ammonis area (**CA1**) and dentate gyrus. This technique may be useful in studies of individual components of neural circuits. The hippocampus is involved with short-term memory and recalling spatial relationships. In primates and humans it is also a source of new neurons. × 40. (Confocal microscopy by TA Weismann; from Livet J, et al. Nature 2007; 450:56–62.)

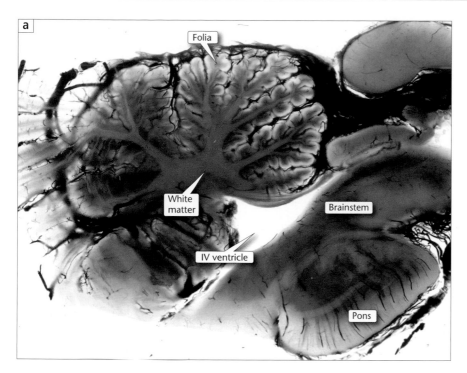

▲ **Fig 7.33a Cerebellum.** Cerebellum with its folia and central white matter, together with the brainstem, pons, and fourth ventricle are shown. Blood vessels stained black illustrate the extensive vascular supply required for the brain's high demand for energy, blood flow often being matched with neural activity and mapped using positron emission tomography (PET scanning). The lobulations of the cerebellar cortex and their folia together make up a surface area of about 1.5 m² (75% of cerebral cortex area), and this gray matter contains many more neurons than the entire cerebral cortex. (From a specimen prepared by S Robbins, Anatomy Department, University of Melbourne, Australia.)

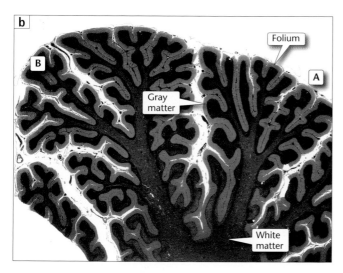

▲ **Fig 7.33b Cerebellum.** Hematoxylin and eosin stain of human cerebellum, showing folia and the central core of white matter covered by the cerebellar cortex of gray matter, with the granular layer and molecular layer visible. All folia have the same histologic structure within the three major lobes of the cerebellum, but functionally the cortex operates to coordinate muscle synergy along its entire longitudinal axis, indicated in the sagittal plane running from anterior (**A**) to posterior (**B**). Different axes regulate particular motor movements, such as of hands–fingers, feet–toes, or the trunk, for example. The most posterior lobe is concerned with equilibrium. H&E, paraffin, × 5.

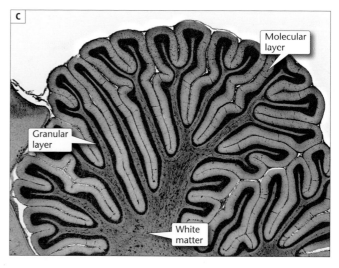

▲ **Fig 7.33c Surface area of cerebellar cortex.** This specimen of a monkey cerebellum shows the extensive surface area of the cortex, consisting of molecular and granular layers. If laid out flat, the surface area of the cerebellar cortex is about 75% of the surface area of the cerebral cortex, but the cerebellum is only 10% of the mass of the cerebrum. The inner white matter leads to four deeply placed gray cerebellar nuclei, which make up the output structures of the cerebellum. Modified Bielschowsky/neutral red, paraffin, × 8.

cerebellum run through them. In sagittal section, the whole mass resembles a cauliflower, since the white matter and covering gray matter branch out from a common stem. Although the cerebellum is concerned with numerous different but related activities (such as posture, equilibrium, and coordination of movement), its histology is remarkably homogeneous and orderly. The cerebellar cortex of gray matter has a surface area of more than 1 m² and consists of three layers:

- Outer molecular layer (mainly synaptic)

- Middle Purkinje layer—narrow, consisting of single, large Purkinje cells (dendrites in the molecular layer and axon passing into the white matter)
- Inner granular layer (synapses with a proportion of the afferent fibers to the cortex).

Numerous types of neurons, glial cells, and fibers are found in the cerebellar cortex (Fig 7.34a–d) and all are involved with the complex process of coordination of muscular activity, learning of movements, and cognitive functions.

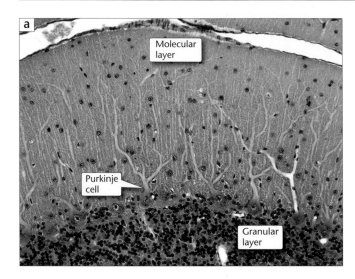

◀ **Fig 7.34a Cerebellar cortex.** A conventional histologic section stained with hematoxylin and eosin shows the three layers in more detail. Dendrites of Purkinje cells extend into the molecular layer, but only a tiny fraction of the dendritic tree is visible. Nuclei in the molecular layer are stellate and basket cell neurons, and the eosinophilic material between is the neuropil filled with dendrites and axons. The granular layer contains granule cells, and Golgi cells and afferent fibers from brainstem nuclei and the spinal cord. Axons from granule cells travel into the molecular layer to associate with the Purkinje cells. H&E, paraffin, × 150.

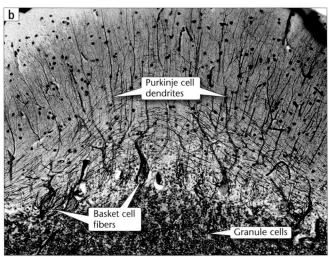

◀ **Fig 7.34b Cerebellar cortex—detail of the nerve fiber organization in the molecular layer.** Many parallel fibers arising from granule cells in the granular layer are noted. Passing perpendicular to the planar or fan-like dendritic tree of the Purkinje cells, parallel fibers make excitatory synapses with the Purkinje cells, and stellate and basket cells, and may extend for several millimeters along a folium. Basket cells of the molecular layer are inhibitory interneurons, with processes that synapse with the Purkinje cell body. Silver stain, paraffin, × 200.

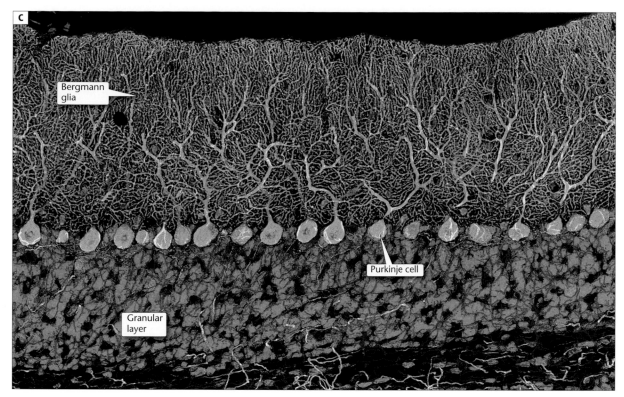

▲ **Fig 7.34c Cerebellar cortex—Purkinje cell dendrites.** Confocal fluorescence image of cerebellar cortex revealing the density and complexity of the Purkinje cell dendrites. These cells are the sole output neurons of the cerebellar cortex and are central to cerebellar cortical information processing. Indirect afferent fibers to Purkinje cells include the mossy fibers from the spinal cord and brainstem nuclei that terminate in the granular layer, thereby exciting granule cells, which in turn send ascending axons to Purkinje cells. Another major cerebellar afferent comprises the climbing fibers, arising from the inferior olivary sub-nuclei in the brain stem. Climbing fibers make direct synaptic contact with Purkinje cells, and each Purkinje cell receives input from just one climbing fiber. Climbing fibers convey signals about motor errors, adaptation, and motor learning. Bergmann glial cells wrap around synapses of Purkinje cells and modulate signaling across the synaptic clefts. The radial arrangement of Bergmann glia (and the retinal Muller glia) is unusual, but reflects their origin in the embryonic radial glia. It is possible that such glia are progenitor cells of neurons. Velate astrocytes cover the so-called glomeruli, a tangle of processes of interneurons, granule, and Golgi cells of the granular layer to which mossy fibers make many synapses. Two-photon fluorescence microscopy, × 300. (Courtesy T Deerinck and M Ellisman, University of California, San Diego, USA.)

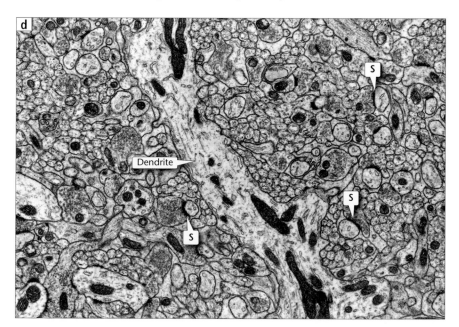

◀ **Fig 7.34d Ultrastructure of the neuropil of the molecular layer of the rat cerebellar cortex.** A dendritic process of a Purkinje cell passes through extraordinarily abundant numbers of parallel fibers (axons) originating from granule cells. Most of these are seen in cross section, reflecting their orientation, which is parallel to the surface of the cortex. Several synaptic contacts between granule cell fibers and Purkinje cell dendritic spines are noted (**S**). × 11,000. (Courtesy E Pannese, Instituto di Istologia, Embriologia, Neurocitologia, University of Milan, Italy.)

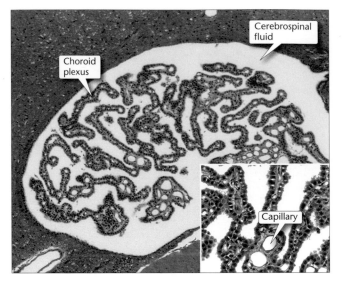

◀ **Fig 7.35 Cerebrospinal fluid.** The central nervous system is bathed in cerebrospinal fluid (CSF), a clear colorless fluid that is mostly water with small amounts of protein, numerous ions, and organic substances. The CSF is produced by the choroid plexus, elaborate folds of cuboidal epithelium derived from the pia mater of the brain and ependymal cells (glia) that line the ventricles, into which the villous-like choroid projects. Richly vascularized with fenestrated capillaries (see inset), blood perfuses through the choroid plexus to form the CSF, which circulates from the ventricles into the subarachnoid space (part of the meninges that surrounds the brain deep to the skull), where much is reabsorbed into venous blood of dural venous sinuses. Also, CSF circulates within the subarachnoid space of the spinal cord and cauda equina and in the central canal. In addition to providing buoyancy for the brain, CSF removes waste metabolites and maintains a stable physiologic environment for the CNS. H&E, paraffin, × 100. *Inset*, × 170.

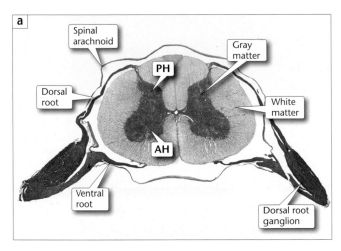

◀ **Fig 7.36a Spinal cord.** Transverse section through the spinal cord and dorsal root ganglia. The ganglion contains pseudounipolar sensory neurons (no synapses with associated nerves), which convey tactile, proprioceptive, temperature, and pain sensation to the spinal cord and brainstem via the dorsal root. The ventral root contains mainly axons of spinal motor neurons, which terminate in muscles. White matter contains myelinated nerve tracts and the gray matter, with a characteristic butterfly shape, contains the nerve cell bodies. **AH**, anterior horn; **PH**, posterior horn. Toluidine blue, paraffin, × 6.

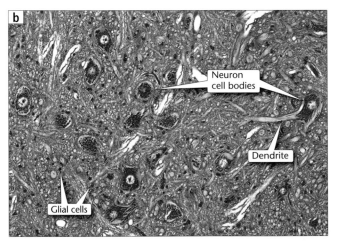

▲ **Fig 7.36b Gray matter of the spinal cord**, showing tight packing of the neurons, their dendrites, and the glial cells and their dendritic processes, which with the addition of blood vessels is called the neuropil. The deep staining of the cytoplasm around the nuclei of the neurons corresponds to rough endoplasmic reticulum and ribosomes, together comprising the Nissl body. Proteins, neurotransmitters, and components of organelles synthesized here are transported along the axons (axoplasmic flow) to their site of functioning. Toluidine blue, paraffin, × 170.

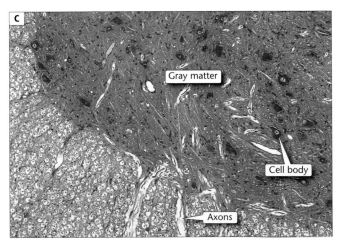

▲ **Fig 7.36c White matter of the spinal cord.** The transition from gray matter to white matter is abrupt; the latter is characterized by tracts or columns of axons surrounded by myelin sheaths— hence the white color. In white matter, myelin is formed by very fine cytoplasmic extensions of oligodendrocytes (glial cells), which wrap around the axons of up to 50 fibers. The lipoprotein plasma membranes collectively form the myelin sheath. Myelinated axons that originate from the cell bodies of neurons traverse the white matter on their path to a root of a spinal nerve. Toluidine blue, paraffin, × 110.

Cerebrospinal fluid

Found in the ventricles of the brain, and in the space that surrounds the brain and spinal cord, CSF is produced mainly by the choroid plexus—tufts of vascularized, epithelial-type cells called the ependymal cells that project from the wall into the lumen of each ventricle (Fig 7.35). Blood is selectively filtered through the choroid plexus and results in a total daily production of about 500 mL of CSF; this is constantly circulating and reabsorbed by arachnoid tissue within the meningeal coverings of the brain.

Spinal cord

At most vertebral levels, cross sections through the spinal cord show the distinctive, central, butterfly-shaped mass of gray matter, surrounded by the ascending and descending tracts of myelinated nerves, and the glial cells of the white matter (Fig 7.36a–c). The separation of gray and white matter is readily seen in the spinal cord, but this division is not absolute in the CNS, because signals traveling along descending nerve tracts pass through some gray matter before exiting the spinal cord.

Sensory fibers have cell bodies in the dorsal root ganglia (see Fig 7.23) and enter the cord via posterior (dorsal) roots to synapse with processes in the gray matter. Motor neurons of the gray matter send axons to the spinal nerves via anterior (ventral) roots. Long ascending and long descending tracts in the white matter carry sensory and motor impulses between brainstem and the cord, respectively.

DISORDERS AND CLINICAL COMMENTS

Alzheimer's disease

Alzheimer's disease (AD) is the most common cause of senile dementia, and affects an estimated one in ten people over 65 years of age, increasing to nearly one in two of those over 80 years of age. It is associated with the following pathologic features in the brain:

- Senile plaques of β-amyloid (starch-like fibrils) accumulating between neurons, surrounded by degenerative dendrites and glial cells
- Neurofibrils tangled within neurons
- Significant loss of neurons in the cerebral cortex and hippocampus.

The symptoms of AD include loss of memory, impaired reasoning, personality changes, and ultimately death through failure of physical function.

Currently, AD cannot be effectively treated with drugs. Deposition of amyloid may be the initiator of a cascade of biochemical reactions responsible for the neuropathology; in cases of early-onset AD, a hereditary component involves mutations in several genes that code for membrane proteins, which are expressed in high levels in the brain. Mutant forms of these genes seem to induce apoptosis. Whether amyloid deposition and cell death by apoptosis are independent or sequential steps in the production of brain lesions in AD remains to be determined.

Multiple sclerosis

Of the several demyelinating diseases that affect the CNS, multiple sclerosis (MS) is the most prevalent in North America, northern Europe, and Australasia. In MS, myelin sheaths of axons in the white matter of the brain and spinal cord are destroyed and replaced with fibrous tissue or glial tissue that forms sclerotic plaques. Conduction of nerve impulses is reduced in velocity or blocked, which leads to physical disabilities that are variable in extent and frequency of presentation, and often involve limb weakness, swallowing and speech difficulties, and disturbances of vision. Neurologic deficits may accumulate in chronic sufferers, who become severely disabled. Although a minority of cases of MS are familial, the etiology of MS is unknown and no cure is known.

Motor neuron disease

Motor neuron disease is a degenerative disease in which the motor neurons in the anterior horns of the spinal cord progressively degenerate, particularly at the cervical and lumbosacral level. This results in wasting and weakness of limb muscles, but many more muscle groups show atrophy as the disease advances. In histologic sections of the spinal cord, a loss of axons is evident in the crossed and uncrossed corticospinal tracts, which gives rise to the alternative name for the disease—amyotrophic lateral sclerosis. The cause(s) remain unknown and the condition is eventually fatal, usually from respiratory failure following the loss of respiratory motor neurons.

Parkinson's disease

Progressive loss of motor function, rigidity, and involuntary continuous tremor are among the symptoms associated with Parkinson's disease, the cause of which is unknown. The pathologic features are seen in the substantia nigra (found in the basal ganglia or nuclei), where significant destruction of dopamine-secreting neurons occurs, but the mechanisms that lead to abnormal motor effects are not understood. At present there is no cure, but amelioration of symptoms may be achieved with l-dopa and dopamine agonists (dopamine is ineffective since it cannot cross the blood–brain barrier).

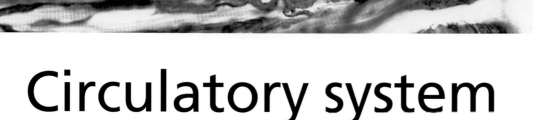

Circulatory system

From a functional perspective, the circulatory system is responsible for maintenance of homeostasis, using two systems:

- The *cardiovascular system*, which consists of the heart, arteries, capillaries, and veins collectively forming a closed system of tubes. The two subdivisions are the pulmonary circulation of the lungs and the systemic circulation for the body, both of which rely upon the heart as the pump for blood distribution.
- The *lymph vascular system*, comprising vessels acting as a drainage apparatus for the extracellular fluid originating from the capillaries. This fluid, called lymph, moves from the periphery and drains into certain veins in the base of the neck.

CARDIOVASCULAR SYSTEM

The heart and blood vascular network is the dominant anatomic component, but both systems have basic histologic similarities, subject to regional variations serving specialized functions. Circulation of blood through arteries, capillaries, and veins with the heart as the pump now seems self-evident, but for 1,400 years (since Galen) venous and arterial blood vessels were thought to comprise separate ebb and flow systems linked by invisible pores between the right and left ventricle. In 1628, the English physician William Harvey concluded—without the benefit of microscopy—that the blood, in actuality, circulates in a closed system of vessels, both pulmonary and systemic, and returns to the heart by the venous route.

Although the blood vascular system is essential for gas exchange (lungs, placenta), temperature control (skin), hormone distribution, immune function, and general control of metabolic activity, the total volume of blood in the body for males is only 5–6 liters (Fig 8.1a & b)—less than half the volume of extracellular fluid within most of the organs and tissues.

The principal differences in the histologic organization of the two vascular systems are based upon the requirement that the cardiovascular system pumps and transports more than 5 liters of blood per minute, whereas the lymphatic system drains lymph fluid into the venous system at the very slow rate of about 100 mL/h. To accommodate major differences in pressure, resistance to flow, and vessel diameter, as well as the varying capacity for transvascular exchange, both circulatory systems show characteristic histologic features (Fig 8.2).

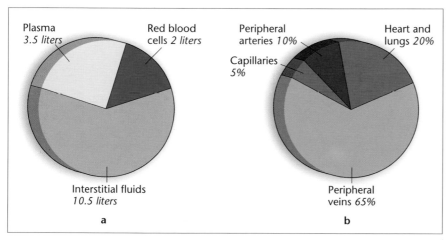

▲ **Fig 8.1 Blood and extracellular fluid volumes. a** The volume of blood varies with body mass: in females it is 4–5 liters, in males 5–6 liters. In an average adult, total extracellular fluid volume is about 14 liters. The extracellular fluid consists of blood plasma and interstitial fluids (extracellular fluids, lymph, cerebrospinal fluid, sweat, secretions of the gut and peritoneum, and other fluids). **b** The peripheral or systemic circulation (i.e. excluding the heart and lungs) contains about 80% of total blood volume. The venous system accounts for most of the peripheral blood volume. The capillaries, although associated with only 5% of blood volume, present by far the largest surface area for substance exchange, estimated to be about 600 m².

Heart

The heart can be considered as a tube that undergoes complex modification during its development to become divided into two longitudinal compartments folded back on themselves such that the inflow and outflow vessels are located next to one another. The chambers of the heart share several features commonly seen in various other blood vessels, including a three-layered wall, valves, and a nerve supply (Fig 8.3). As an organ responsible for propelling blood through the circulatory system, the heart resembles a demand pump, since its pumping mechanism is not fixed in terms of outflow but responds to variations in circulatory flow in periods of rest or exercise. In an average lifetime the heart pumps up to 250 million liters of blood, equivalent to the displacement tonnage of three cruise liners the size of the *Queen Mary*.

Walls of the heart

The histology of the heart walls is shown in Figure 8.4a & b.

The external layer is the epicardium, which consists of squamous-type mesothelium and basal lamina, together with connective tissue containing the blood vessels that supply the heart and nerves that innervate it. The middle and thickest layer of the heart wall is the myocardium, made up of bundles and layers of cardiac muscle, as described in Chapter 6. The endocardium lines the inner surfaces of the heart; it comprises an endothelial layer that is continuous with the lining of the major veins and arteries entering and leaving the heart. Deep to the basal lamina of the endothelium is a thin layer of collagen fibers followed by a wider zone of denser connective tissue with elastic fibers and some smooth muscle. Where the endocardium meets the myocardium, a subendocardial

Component	Inner lining	Wall	Nerves	Valves	Function
Heart	Endothelium	Cardiac muscle	Intrinsic, autonomic	Yes	Pump
Artery	Endothelium	Smooth muscle, elastin	Autonomic	No	Blood flow (high pressure)
Arteriole	Endothelium	Smooth muscle	Autonomic	No	Resistance, blood pressure control
Capillary	Endothelium	Endothelium, pericytes	No	No	Substance exchange
Venule	Endothelium	Pericytes or smooth muscle	Autonomic	No	Substance exchange, reservoir
Vein	Endothelium	Smooth muscle, fibrous tissue	Autonomic	Yes	Blood flow (low pressure)
Lymphatic capillary	Endothelium	Endothelium	No	No	Collection of extracellular fluid
Lymphatic vessel	Endothelium	Smooth muscle	No	Yes	Lymph flow

▲ **Fig 8.2** Characteristic features of the cardiovascular and lymph vascular systems.

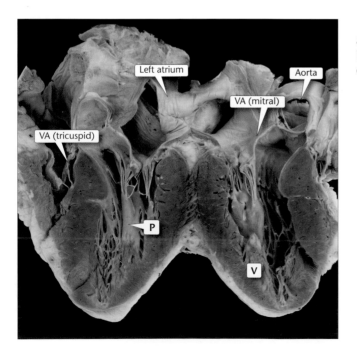

◀ **Fig 8.3 Anatomy of the heart.** The walls of the ventricles (**V**) are composed mainly of cardiac muscle, which within the chambers is formed into a variety of extensions, including papillary muscles (**P**) connecting to valves (**VA**).

layer is described, consisting of loose connective tissue. In the ventricular walls the subendocardium contains small blood vessels and nerves, and the branches of the impulse-conducting system of the heart.

Conducting system

The distal cells of the conducting system are modified cardiac muscle cells referred to as Purkinje fibers (Fig 8.5a). Intrinsic waves of excitation (depolarization), which are independent of autonomic innervation but may be modified by it, originate in the sinoatrial node (the heart pacemaker), which transmits electrical impulses to the atrioventricular node and then to the atrioventricular bundle of His. The nodes and bundle are comprised of small myocytes, whereas the terminal branches of Purkinje fibers are made up of myocytes that are larger than normal (Fig 8.5b).

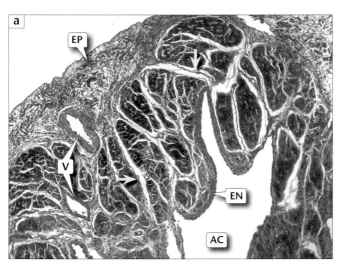

▲ **Fig 8.4a Heart walls.** Section through the wall of the atrium, showing the thin, inner lining of endocardium (**EN**) facing the atrial chamber (**AC**), with thin collagenous septa (**arrows**) extending between the cardiac muscle to merge with the outer wall, or epicardium (**EP**). The endocardium contains collagen, elastic fibers, and occasional smooth muscle cells, whereas the epicardium contains loose connective tissue, elastic fibers, some adipose tissue, and branches of coronary vessels (**V**). Both layers are bordered by a simple squamous epithelium. Azan, paraffin, × 30.

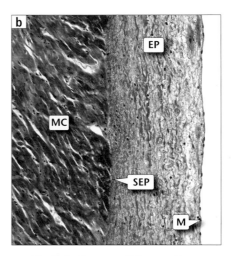

▲ **Fig 8.4b Heart wall layers.** The epicardium (**EP**) is shown external to the myocardium (**MC**). These are attached to each other in the subepicardial region (**SEP**) via septa of collagen bundles. The mesothelium (**M**) on the external surface is moist and slippery, allowing the heart to move with minimal friction within the pericardial sac. Azan, paraffin, × 150.

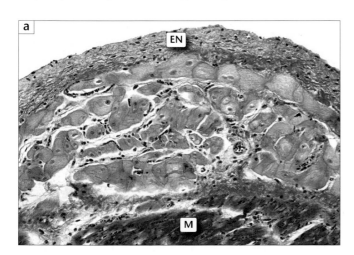

▲ **Fig 8.5a Purkinje fibers.** The tract of Purkinje fibers (modified myocytes), between the endocardium (**EN**) and myocardium (**M**), transmits and distributes action potentials to the ventricles from the atrioventricular node. The action potentials are originally generated by the cardiac pacemaker cells of the sinoatrial node. Azan, paraffin, × 180.

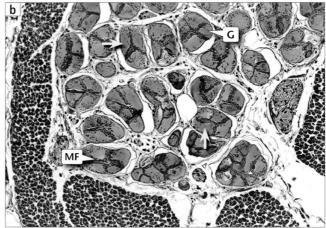

▲ **Fig 8.5b Purkinje myocytes** are large cells with abundant glycogen (**G**), sparse myofilaments (**MF**), and extensive gap junctional sites (**arrows**). These cells conduct action potentials rapidly (3–4 m/s, compared to 0.5 m/s for cardiac muscle) to all regions of both ventricles, causing ventricular depolarization and then contraction. Hematoxylin and eosin (H&E), paraffin, × 180.

Fibrous "skeleton" of the heart

The "skeleton" of the heart comprises thick, fibrous connective tissue bands around the heart valves, supporting them, providing for the attachment of cardiac muscle fibers, and preventing the spread of electrical impulses (except via the conducting system) from the atria to the ventricles. Each valve is a plate, or flap, of fibroelastic connective tissue extending from the fibrous skeleton and covered by endocardium (Fig 8.6).

> **Tip:** Heart muscle is identified by (i) central nuclei in the cardiomyocytes, (ii) intercalated discs (junctions) between successive cells, (iii) branching of the cells, and (iv) striated cytoplasm, best seen if the condenser diaphragm of the microscope is closed to about one-third of its maximum aperture.

Blood vessels

The histology of the arterial, capillary, and venous systems reflects their specialized duties and conforms to physiologic principles of hemodynamics that relate blood flow to pressure. Blood–tissue exchange depends on diffusion (Fick's law), and capillary filtration depends on a balance between hydrostatic and osmotic forces (the Starling hypothesis).

A good example of how these variables are regulated is the observation that following a minor cut to a finger blood flow is very slow, in contrast to that seen in severance of a major artery where blood loss may be copious. The marked difference in the velocity of blood flow is in large measure due to changes in pressure and vessel diameter, although the length and shape of the vessels, and blood viscosity are also important factors.

The relationship between pressure and flow in a vessel is given by Poiseuille's law:

$$\text{flow} = \frac{k\Delta P r^4}{\eta l}$$

where ΔP is the pressure gradient, r is the vessel radius, l is the vessel length, η is the fluid viscosity, and k is a constant.

For constant pressure, a small change in vessel radius produces a large change in the blood flow. For example, if the radius is decreased from 2 mm to 1 mm (and all other values remain constant), there is approximately a 16-fold decrease in blood flow.

It is important to recognize that the functional properties of blood vessels are greatly influenced by their diameter (and hence by their radius), and that this is governed by the histology of their walls. The principles of hemodynamics and the functions and control mechanisms relating to the cardiac, systemic, and microcirculatory systems encompass a large body of knowledge and are discussed in texts of medical physiology. Physical characteristics of blood vessels are presented in Figure 8.7.

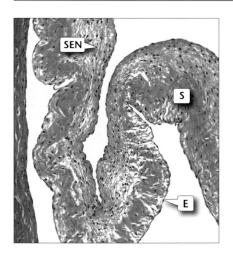

◀ **Fig 8.6 Heart valves.** A heart valve is a flap-like extension of endocardium covered by endothelium (**E**) and containing a subendocardial layer (**SEN**) of collagen and elastin, and a valve skeleton (**S**) of dense connective tissue in continuity with the fibrous, ring-like skeleton of the heart (between atria and ventricles). Valves contain no blood vessels. H&E, paraffin, × 30.

Blood vessel	Diameter	Wall thickness
Aorta	2.5 cm	2 mm
Elastic arteries	1 cm	1 mm
Muscular arteries	0.5–10 mm	0.5 mm
Arterioles	30–200 μm	10–20 μm
Capillaries	<10 μm	<1 μm
Postcapillary venules	10–30 μm	1–2 μm
Venules	>50 μm	2–5 μm
Veins	1–10 mm	0.5 mm
Vena cava	3 cm	1.5 mm

▲ **Fig 8.7** Structural differences between blood vessels of various types.

Arteries

Arterial vessels have thick walls and variable quantities of elastic fibers. Their walls have three layers:

- Inner tunica intima, which includes the endothelial lining
- Intermediate tunica media with smooth muscle
- Outer tunica adventitia of connective tissues.

In arteries of medium size, a distinct strip of elastic material, the internal elastic lamina, lies between the tunica intima and media, and a similar external elastic lamina is found between the tunica media and adventitia.

In elastic arteries such as the aorta, the tunica media is very thick, showing between 30 and 50 fenestrated layers of elastin with smooth muscle cells, collagen, and extracellular matrix between each elastin layer (Fig 8.8a–c). Smaller elastic arteries are recognized by their variable quantity of elastic lamellae in the tunica

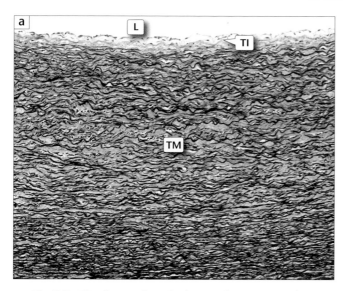

▲ **Fig 8.8a Elastic arteries.** The largest elastic artery is the aorta, which can be readily identified by its thick wall. At low power, this shows dozens of sheets, or lamellae, of elastic fibers, which stain black with appropriate staining methods. The thin, non-elastic region next to the lumen (**L**) is the tunica intima (**TI**); the lamellae are in the broad tunica media (**TM**). Elastic fibers recoil after the vessel is stretched when blood is pumped from the heart. Verhoeff's/Masson trichrome, paraffin, × 50.

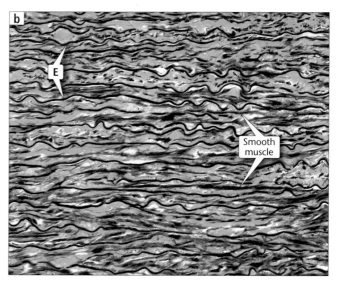

▲ **Fig 8.8b Tunica media of the aorta**, showing many lamellae of elastin (**E**), stained black. In between are layers of collagen and extracellular matrix, stained green, and smooth muscle cells, stained red. The smooth muscle cells produce the elastin, collagen, and matrix. Blood ejected into the aorta during systole increases the volume of a segment of the aorta by stretching its wall. In diastole, this stored potential energy is converted to kinetic energy when the elastic lamellae recoil, maintaining and at the same time dampening pulsatile arterial flow. Verhoeff's/Masson trichrome, paraffin, × 200.

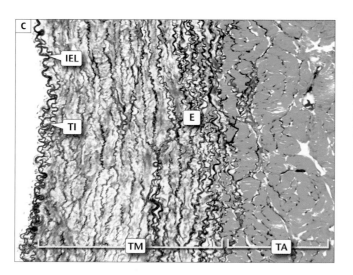

◀ **Fig 8.8c The subclavian artery** is an elastic artery with sheets of elastic lamellae (**E**) in the tunica media (**TM**) that are often discontinuous. The tunica intima (**TI**) adjacent to vessel lumen shows an internal elastic lamina (**IEL**). Unlike muscular arteries, there is no distinct external elastic lamina marking the region called the tunica adventitia (**TA**), a layer of connective tissue with neurovascular supply and some elastin. Van Gieson's and Augustin's trichrome, paraffin, × 100.

media, which may be of similar or greater thickness than the surrounding tunica adventitia (Fig 8.9a & b).

Muscular or medium-sized arteries (with diameters of more than 0.5 mm) have between 10 and 40 layers of smooth muscle cells, arranged spirally within the tunica media with small amounts of elastin (Fig 8.10a–d). The internal and external elastic laminae are usually prominent, and the tunica adventitia is relatively thick. The smooth muscle cells of the tunica media are enveloped by a basal lamina, which they secrete (Fig 8.11).

Arterioles (with diameters of 30–200 μm) show only one or two layers of smooth muscle cells in the tunica media. The elastic laminae may be absent and the tunica adventitia is thin (Fig 8.12a & b). The smaller arterioles act as sphincters and exercise fine control of blood flow in a manner analogous to turning a tap connected to a garden hose. These vessels are surrounded by discontinuous smooth muscle cells and, together with larger arterioles, contribute significantly to vascular resistance according to the state of relaxation or contraction of their smooth muscle (Fig 8.13a & b). Because of this resistance to flow, large falls in pressure occur such that, under normal conditions, the blood pressure in the arterioles is only 30% of that in the aorta.

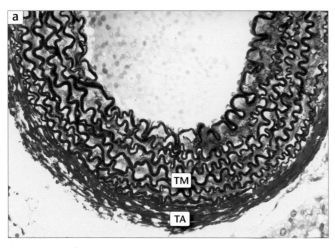

▲ **Fig 8.9a Small elastic artery.** Elastic artery stained with Gomori trichrome showing numerous folded elastic lamellae in the tunica media (**TM**) and collagenous material in the tunica adventitia (**TA**). Examples of these elastic arteries are the renal, common iliac, brachiocephalic, and pulmonary arteries. Gomori trichrome, paraffin, × 120.

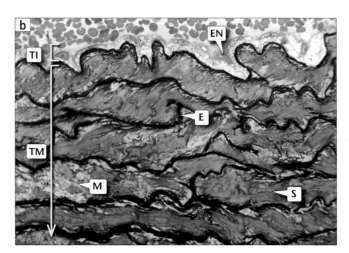

▲ **Fig 8.9b The inner wall of an elastic artery**, showing the tunica intima (**TI**), which consists of endothelial cells (**EN**) facing the lumen and resting on a thin subendothelial layer of collagen. The tunica media (**TM**), only part of which is shown, contains branching elastic lamellae (**E**) and extracellular matrix (**M**), both of which are synthesized by the layers of smooth muscle cells (**S**). Nutrients for the inner half of the tunica media (in large elastic arteries) diffuse from the blood plasma; the outer half is supplied by capillaries of the vasa vasorum (the vessels of the blood vessels). Toluidine blue, araldite, × 400.

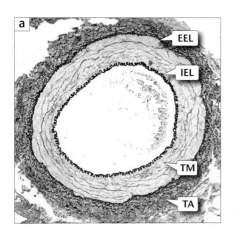

◀ **Fig 8.10a A medium-sized muscular artery**, stained for elastin and showing the internal elastic lamina (**IEL**) and external elastic lamina (**EEL**). The tunica media (**TM**) contains little elastin, but the tunica adventitia (**TA**) contains rather more in the form of discontinuous profiles. Muscular arteries chiefly maintain blood flow to organs, their smooth muscle cells in the media providing limited dilatory or constrictive effects on vessel diameter. Van Gieson's, paraffin, × 50.

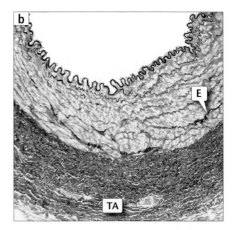

▲ **Fig 8.10b Higher magnification of a muscular artery**, with interrupted elastic lamellae (**E**) in the tunica media. The thick tunica adventitia (**TA**) of connective tissue counteracts wall stress when the vessel is relaxed. When the vessel is constricted, wall stress is reduced (if the blood pressure is unchanged) and carried by the smooth muscle contraction within the tunica media. Verhoeff's, paraffin, × 50.

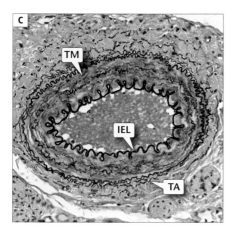

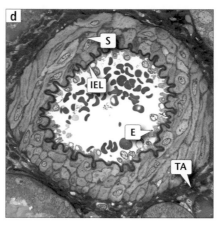

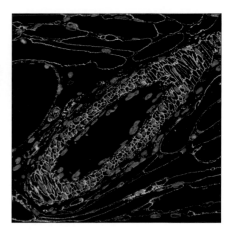

▲ **Fig 8.10c Muscular arteries become arterioles** when the tunica media (**TM**) is reduced in thickness to one layer or several layers of smooth muscle cells. An internal elastic lamina (**IEL**) remains and the tunica adventitia (**TA**) begins to reduce in thickness. Gomori trichrome, paraffin, × 100.

▲ **Fig 8.10d Arterial vessel in transition.** Thin epoxy resin section of an arterial vessel in transition between a muscular artery and an arteriole, showing several layers of smooth muscle cells (**S**) of the tunica media and a thin tunica adventitia (**TA**). Note undulating internal elastic lamella (**IEL**) and protruding endothelial cells (**E**), indicating vasoconstriction of the vessel. Toluidine blue, araldite, × 290.

▲ **Fig 8.11 Tunica media.** A muscular artery showing immunofluorescence labeling of laminin (yellow) surrounding the smooth muscle cells with their nuclei stained blue. Laminin is an extracellular protein of basal lamina; it provides adhesion and resists tensile forces experienced by the vascular wall. The laminin seen peripherally is bordering skeletal muscle fibers. × 250. (Courtesy J Zbaeren, Inselspital, Bern, Switzerland.)

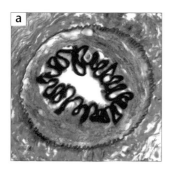

◀ **Fig 8.12a Constricted ateriole.** Gomori trichrome staining of a constricted arteriole with a highly folded internal elastic lamella and a thin external elastic lamina. Between these layers is the tunica media. Arterioles control blood flow by dilatation or constriction, and contribute to peripheral resistance and significant changes in blood pressure. Gomori trichrome, paraffin, × 300.

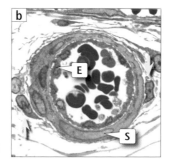

◀ **Fig 8.12b A small arteriole** (30 μm diameter), showing a single smooth muscle layer (**S**) surrounding the tunica intima, with endothelial cells (**E**) facing the lumen. Pericytes (**arrows**) surround the vessel wall and contract or relax in response to changes in blood pressure, local metabolites (including oxygen and carbon dioxide), factors from the endothelium, sympathetic nerve activity, and various vasoactive hormones. Toluidine blue, araldite, × 550.

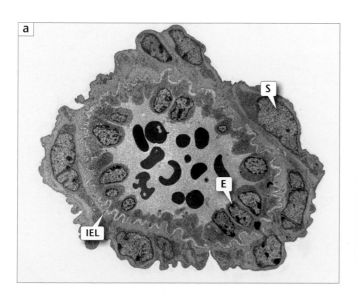

▲ **Fig 8.13a Ultrastructure of an arteriole.** A contracted arteriole showing the folded internal elastic lamina (**IEL**) and associated compressed endothelial cells (**E**). The tunica media is a single layer of smooth muscle cells (**S**). × 2,800.

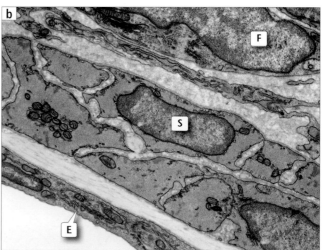

▲ **Fig 8.13b Ultrastructure of an arteriole.** Part of the tunica media of an arteriole showing a double layer of smooth muscle cells (**S**), the endothelium (**E**) and fibroblasts (**F**) of the tunica adventitia. Vascular smooth muscle contracts in response to releasable intracellular stores of Ca^{++} but also requires these ions to be imported. Coordinated contraction is mediated via the gap junctions linking the tip processes between the cells. × 9,500.

The crucial role of the arterial system is to distribute blood to various capillary networks and to act as a hydraulic filter (i.e. resistance and compliance properties, which are especially important in the small arteries and arterioles). These properties change intermittent high-pressure flow into steady, low-pressure flow in the capillaries and veins. Several mechanisms constrict (close) or dilate (open) most vessels with a smooth muscle component:

- Changes in blood pressure may stretch smooth muscle, causing its contraction and thereby vessel constriction (myogenic hypothesis).
- Endothelial cells release nitric oxide (e.g. in response to stimulation by histamine or acetylcholine), which dilates blood vessels; this release of nitric oxide is involved in the process of penile erection and also may be involved in increasing cerebral blood flow in regions of the brain concerned with memory.
- In the cerebral and coronary vessels, blood flow is autoregulated in response to pressure changes; this is thought to be a combination of local metabolic and myogenic control.
- Constriction of most vessels is primarily regulated by sympathetic innervation via the release of norepinephrine (noradrenaline).

Capillaries

The terminal arterioles (the smallest arterioles, with a diameter of approximately 30 µm) reduce in size to give rise to the capillaries, which usually have a diameter in the range 4–8 µm (Fig 8.14).

A network of capillaries can be formed in two ways (Fig 8.15):

- By direct branching from an arteriole, which is marked by a terminal precapillary sphincter of smooth muscle
- By branching from a metarteriole that has a discontinuous coating of smooth muscle in its wall, regulating blood flow through its derivative capillaries.

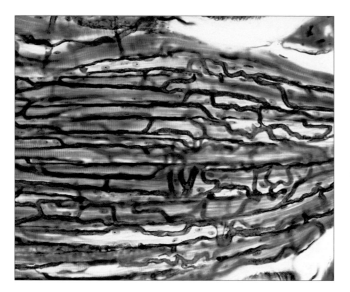

◀ **Fig 8.14 Capillaries**. Teased preparation of striated muscle showing a capillary network of thin, endothelium-lined tubes, which branch and anastomose to provide a large surface area for exchange of substances—water, gases, and solutes. Capillary blood flow is relatively slow, blood pressure is low and substance exchange occurs via diffusion, osmosis, or transcytosis (transfer of vesicles between luminal and peripheral surfaces of endothelial cells). The capillaries here are the continuous type (non-fenestrated). Other types are fenestrated capillaries (endocrine glands, kidney, gut), discontinuous capillaries (liver, spleen, bone marrow), and tight-junctional capillaries (central nervous system and retina). Silver stain, whole mount, × 150.

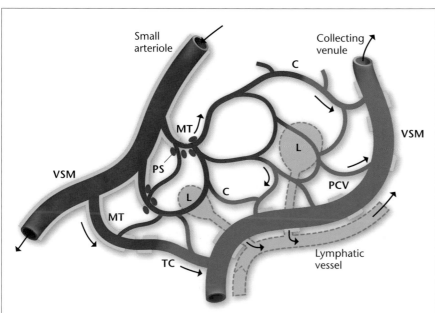

◀ **Fig 8.15 General scheme of the microvasculature.** Oxygenated blood from terminal arterioles with vascular smooth muscle in their walls (**VSM**) branch to form capillaries (**C**) or metarterioles (**MT**), which in turn contribute to the capillary beds. The commencement of a capillary is usually associated with a precapillary sphincter (**PS**) of smooth muscle. Capillary blood enters postcapillary venules (**PCV**); these drain into collecting venules, which have a few vascular smooth muscle cells in their walls. These vessels lead to muscular venules, then to small veins. Some metarterioles form thoroughfare channels (**TC**) that connect directly to venules, bypassing capillaries. Blind, dilated ends of lymphatic capillaries (**L**) are shown, draining into a larger lymphatic vessel, at times containing valves.

Capillaries are endothelial tubes encircled by a basement membrane (Fig 8.16). They are often associated with pericytes, which are contractile-type cells located at intervals along the outer circumference of the capillary wall. Pericytes are mesenchymal (connective tissue) cells capable of differentiating into smooth muscle cells or fibroblasts during angiogenesis, tumor growth, and wound healing.

Capillaries are well adapted for the exchange of diffusible substances between blood and the surrounding environment because of slow blood flow (see below), their large surface area, and their very thin walls. Individual capillaries may show spiral, curved, or right-angled shapes with accompanying high resistance to blood flow, but their enormous volume density in tissues reduces their collective resistance. Since the total cross-sectional area of all capillaries is very much greater than that of the aorta yet the total blood flow is the same, the velocity of flow in capillaries is much reduced. This assists with capillary–tissue exchange, for which the capillaries show three different histologic types (Fig 8.17):

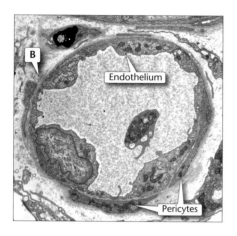

◀ **Fig 8.16 Capillary morphology.** Ultrastructure of a capillary (continuous type) showing the endothelial cell lining surrounded by an extracellular matrix or basal lamina (**B**) and the cytoplasmic processes of pericytes. Capillaries are invisible to the naked eye and often reach 0.5–1 mm in length. Transendothelial transport in both directions occurs chiefly by diffusion and also by filtration and via vesicles exhibiting pinocytosis. Most gases, wastes, and substrates are exchanged across capillary walls by diffusion. Pericytes are mesenchymal cells with the ability to differentiate into fibroblasts or myoid cells. × 4,800.

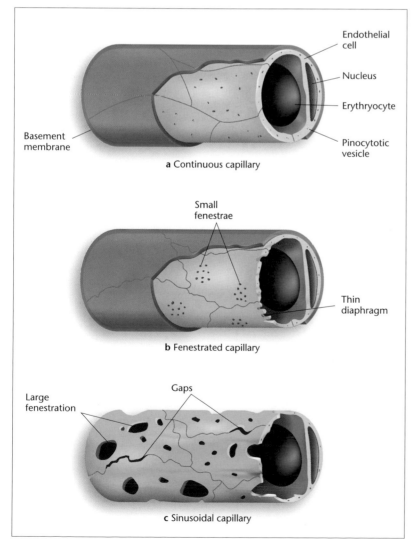

a Continuous capillary

b Fenestrated capillary

c Sinusoidal capillary

◀ **Fig 8.17 Types of capillaries. a** The *continuous* capillary is a common variant and is found in muscle, connective tissues, lung, skin, and nerve tissue. Endothelial cells form a continuous ring of one or more cells linked by tight junctions. Transcapillary diffusion of many substances is faster than the slower pinocytotic vesicle transfer of macromolecules. **b** In *fenestrated* capillaries found in the gut mucosa, most endocrine glands and the kidneys, fluid filtration is rapid via small 50 nm pores, which are usually bridged by a thin spoke-like diaphragm. **c** *Sinusoidal* or discontinuous capillaries occur in bone marrow, spleen, and liver. Large gaps and fenestrae are permeable to large-molecular-weight compounds and, in some cases, blood-borne cells such as red and white blood cells. These capillaries lack a basal lamina (basement membrane).

- Continuous capillaries are the most common type; they exhibit a continuous endothelial layer where endothelial cells are joined together by tight or occluding junctions (Fig 8.18).
- Fenestrated capillaries are seen in parts of the gut, and in endocrine glands and the renal glomerulus, and show interruptions across the attenuated parts of the endothelium, which are bridged by a thin diaphragm (Fig 8.19).
- Sinusoidal capillaries are of larger diameter; they are seen in the liver, the spleen, and bone marrow (Fig 8.20). Gaps or discontinuities appear in their walls allowing transport of whole cells between blood and tissue.

The permeability of the capillary wall is selective with respect to the size and organic properties of potentially permeant molecules. Gases and many small molecules readily diffuse across the endothelium of continuous or fenestrated capillaries, but larger molecules and water-soluble substances are selectively transported either via segments of the tight junctions through the fenestrations, or by way of vesicle transcytosis through the endothelium. Capillaries in the brain, estimated to be 600 km in total length, serve the important function of maintenance of the blood–brain barrier. The barrier consists of tight junctions between capillary endothelial cells and restricts entry into the brain and spinal cord of many molecules with a large molecular weight as well as highly charged ions. The selectively impermeable blood–brain barrier prevents transfer of many blood-borne harmful substances, but nictotine, ethanol, heroin, and caffeine easily cross the barrier.

Veins

The venous system should not be considered simply as a series of vessels returning blood to the heart. In addition to this function, parts of the venous system are involved with fluid and nutrient exchange and the transfer of leukocytes, serve as reservoirs for blood, and are the main blood vessels involved in inflammatory responses—they are far more distensible than arterial vessels of the same caliber.

Once blood leaves a capillary network it enters the first and smallest-diameter vessels of the venous vascular system, the postcapillary venules, which are

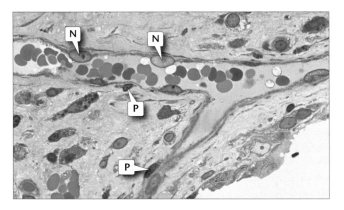

▲ **Fig 8.18 Continuous capillary**. Thin epoxy resin section, showing a branched capillary within a region of loose connective tissue. The wall is a thin endothelial tube whose nuclei (**N**) bulge into the lumen, where erythrocytes are noted. Slender strips of reticular fibers are associated with the endothelium, but there is no media or adventitia. Round or fusiform pericytes (**P**) are present; these are known to be myoid-like in function and capable of contributing to angiogenesis. Toluidine blue, araldite, × 510.

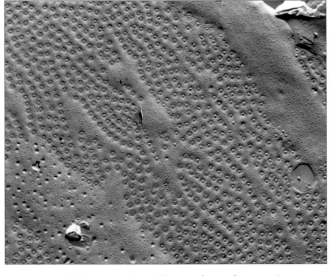

▲ **Fig 8.19 Fenestrated capillary**. A freeze-fracture electron micrograph of the endothelial surface of a fenestrated capillary in the kidney. Non-fenestrated areas separate many small pores. The pores are of uniform size and spacing. × 15,000. (Courtesy L Orci, University of Geneva, Switzerland; from Orci L & Perrelet A. Freeze-etch histology. Heidelberg: Springer-Verlag, 1975.)

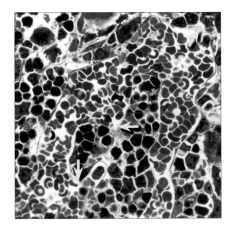

◀ **Fig 8.20 Sinusoidal capillary**. The example shown is in bone marrow, where the blood-filled capillary is wide and of variable shape, and gaps in the endothelium are noted (**arrows**). Gaps allow the emigration of all types of formed elements from the marrow to the capillaries. Toluidine blue, araldite, × 430.

10–30 μm in diameter. They contain pericytes but have no intimal layers and, since their pressure is lower than that of either capillaries or the surrounding tissue, fluids tend to enter these venules (Fig 8.21a & b). Conversely, leukocytes normally migrate into the tissues from these small venules (e.g. in the gut), and postcapillary venules leak fluids, proteins, and cells during the course of an inflammatory response. The transfer of leukocytes from the vessel to the surrounding tissues can be recognized histologically.

The cells adhere to the endothelium (margination) and then cross the vessel wall using ameboid-type movement (diapedesis).

Larger venules, with diameters of more than 50 μm, begin to show some smooth muscle fibers, and progressively larger-diameter vessels form veins (Fig 8.22a & b).

Veins show considerable variation in structure depending upon the venous pressure. It is customary to describe small-to-medium and

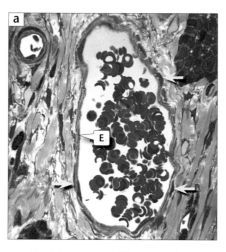

▲ **Fig 8.21a Postcapillary venules.** Venules are formed from one or more postcapillary venules emerging from capillary beds. They have very thin walls, and their endothelium (**E**) is associated with pericytes (**arrows**), or thin smooth muscle cells, which are often incomplete, not forming a distinct media. Postcapillary venules are important sites for blood–interstitial substance exchange. Toluidine blue, araldite, × 400.

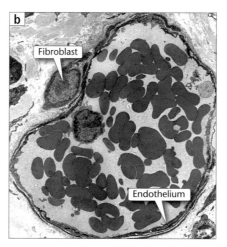

▲ **Fig 8.21b Ultrastructure of a venule** showing the attenuated wall consisting of endothelium and one or two layers of pericytes. Occasional fibroblasts are the source of collagen fibers that occupy much of the extracellular tissue space. × 1,500.

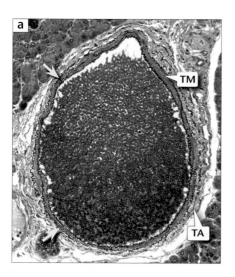

◀ **Fig 8.22a A medium-sized vein** filled with blood that has prevented its collapse. Note the thin tunica media (**TM**), the somewhat thicker tunica adventitia (**TA**), and the fenestrated elastic lamellae (**arrows**). This vein is probably maximally stretched, accommodating a large volume of blood—veins have high capacitance. Sympathetic nerve supply to the tunica media causes smooth muscle contraction and reduces the blood-carrying capacity of the venule, allowing redistribution of blood elsewhere. Gomori trichrome, paraffin, × 70.

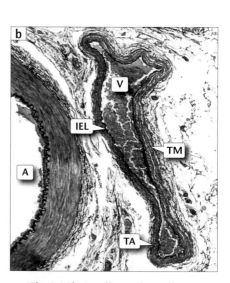

▲ **Fig 8.22b A collapsed small vein** (**V**) is shown next to the wall of a muscular artery (**A**). Staining for elastin reveals a thin internal elastic lamina (**IEL**). Several layers of smooth muscle make up the tunica media (**TM**), which is surrounded by connective tissue of the tunica adventitia (**TA**). Van Gieson's, paraffin, × 130.

large veins. As a general rule, veins have a larger diameter than any accompanying artery, with a thinner wall that has more connective tissue and fewer elastic and muscle fibers.

Small- and medium-sized veins have a well developed adventitia (Fig 8.23). The tunica intima lacks a continuous internal elastic lamina and the tunica media is thin, consisting of two or three separated layers of smooth muscle.

Large veins include the portal vein, the pulmonary veins, the venae cavae, and several others associated with the viscera. Large veins have diameters greater than 10 mm. These vessels have a thicker intima and a poorly developed media, but tunica adventitia is very thick and contains collagen, elastic fibers, and a variable amount of smooth muscle (Fig 8.24).

The vessel wall structure renders veins very flexible and capable of accommodating large volumes of blood. Consequently, veins contain most of the total blood volume in the body. Sympathetic innervation causes veins to constrict, which contributes to increased venous return and hence to cardiac output, thereby ensuring that enhanced arterial perfusion of vital organs is matched by drainage into the venous segment of the circulatory system.

Valves

Valves assist venous function. They are found in most medium-sized veins but are generally absent from very small and very large venous structures. Valves are inward extensions of the tunica intima with elastic fibers. They form semilunar pockets by occurring in pairs (Fig 8.25). In addition to preventing backflow (important in directing blood flow against gravity), valves also serve to inhibit excessive back-pressure in more distal veins and act as a type of partition pump, momentarily isolating segments of blood in the vein during its normal one-way passage toward

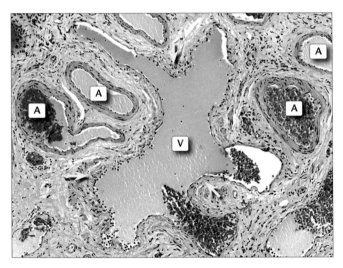

▲ **Fig 8.23 Larger veins**. A medium-sized vein (**V**) showing an irregular outline, indicating confluence of other venous branches into the main vessel, and variations in the distension of its wall. This variation occurs in response to blood pressure and sympathetic innervation of the sparsely supplied smooth muscle cells (**arrows**). Note the uniform thickness of the tunica media in adjacent arterioles (**A**). H&E, acrylic resin, × 100.

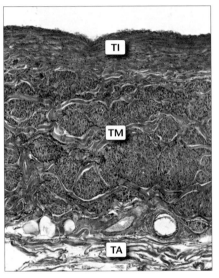

▲ **Fig 8.24 Vena cava**. The tunica intima (**TI**) and tunica media (**TM**) of the inner wall of the vena cava. The tunica media contains smooth muscle and collagen. Vessels in the tunica adventitia (**TA**) constitute the vasa vasorum, supplying the vessel wall with nutrients and oxygen not available from venous blood in the lumen. The tunica adventitia may also contain smooth muscle and collagen, but this varies along the length of the vena cava. H&E, acrylic resin, × 120.

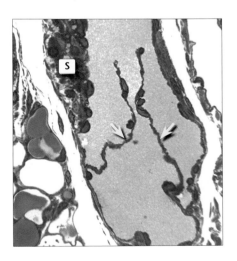

◀ **Fig 8.25 Valves**. As venules become larger, their wall gains smooth muscle cells (**S**), seen here in cross section. A valve is noted (**arrows**); it consists of thin intimal extensions, which are relatively inelastic. When pressed together by restriction of more proximal blood flow, these intimal extensions prevent retrograde transport. Toluidine blue, araldite, × 550.

the heart. In many veins unidirectional flow of blood is a consequence of the vessels being compressed by surrounding tissues (e.g. within muscle, between muscle or organs and fascia, or within certain organs that contain some muscle, such as the spleen).

Blood supply of blood vessel walls

The vasa vasorum (the blood vessels of the larger blood vessels) is a system of microvessels, usually capillaries from adjacent small arteries. They supply nutrients, especially oxygen, to the walls of medium and larger arteries and veins. The vasa vasorum are much more extensive in the veins than in the arteries because of the poor oxygen content of venous blood. In arteries, the vasa vasorum do not penetrate much beyond the tunica adventitia, whereas in veins these vessels may approach the tunica intima.

Anastomoses

Vascular anastomoses are pathways linking arteries with veins or arterioles with venules, thus bypassing a capillary network and hence providing an alternate channel of blood supply. Arteriovenous anastomoses occur mainly in the skin of the digits, nose, and lips. Here they regulate heat loss by directing arterial blood into the venous plexus beneath the skin. A similar direct connection between arterial and venous vessels is seen in the thoroughfare channels, modified lengths of metarterioles in which the smooth muscle component of the walls is diminished or absent (see Fig 8.15).

Innervation of blood vessels

Vasoconstrictor nerves acting on blood vessels belong to the sympathetic system. They act mostly on small arterial vessels, arterioles, and veins, with the last being more responsive. Sympathetic vasoconstrictor nerves have less influence on larger vessels. At their target vessels, such as terminal arterioles, the nerves show varicosities with dense core vesicles that release norepinephrine (noradrenaline), which decreases blood flow by constricting the vessel. Subsequently, capillary blood flow declines or may be arrested. Blood vessels of skeletal muscle present a special case. During exercise, sympathetic innervation of arterioles causes them to dilate and increase blood flow to the tissue. Parasympathetic vasodilator nerves are cholinergic and decrease vascular resistance. The cranial outflow innervates cerebral and coronary arteries, salivary glands, the pancreas, and much of the gut. Sacral outflow supplies the genital tissues, bladder, and large bowel. Parasympathetic nerves do not supply the skin and skeletal muscle.

Endothelial cells

Strategically positioned between the blood compartment and the vascular wall, endothelial cells are exposed not only to the biochemical milieu in both of these compartments but also to changes in physical factors such as pressure, stretch, and tissue damage. In addition to their obvious barrier and nutrient exchange roles, endothelial cells perform a wide range of important synthetic and secretory functions that provide a balance between stimulation or inhibition of vascular tone, inflammatory reactions, angiogenesis, blood clotting, and thrombus formation.

The diversity of endothelial cell function is, in part, related to the histologic organization of the tunica intima, where endothelial cells and their basement membranes act as a superficial component or barrier. The subendothelial layer forms a secondary barrier (Fig 8.26). Tight junctions are especially prominent in the brain between apposed endothelial cells of the capillaries, forming the blood–brain barrier. The capillary endothelium acts like a superfine filter, restricting entry of many substances including certain ions and lipophilic molecules larger than 4 nm.

Endothelium is an important regulator of vascular homeostasis, maintaining a balance between vasodilation and vasoconstriction, and is also involved with blood coagulation. Endothelial cells secrete the potent vasorelaxant nitric oxide and vasoconstrictive agents (endothelin proteins) that counteract the effects of nitric oxide. The adluminal surface of glycocalyx (glycoproteins and glycosaminoglycans) and its secreted prostacyclin are antithrombotic (i.e. they prevent the adherence of platelets). The subendothelial layer, normally shielded by the endothelium, contains glycoproteins such as fibronectin and von Willebrand factor (vWF), synthesized by endothelial cells. Endothelial cells contain small organelles about 0.1–0.2 μm in size, called Wiebel-Palade bodies, that store vWF and secrete it into blood, where it stabilizes clotting factor VIII, an essential part of the clotting cascade reaction.

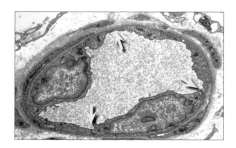

◀ **Fig 8.26 Endothelium.** Ultrastructure of endothelial cells of a capillary. These squamous epithelial cells are very thin, often less than 0.5 μm, except for their nuclear regions. Adjacent endothelial cells form narrow intercellular clefts and tight junctions (**arrows**) where they meet. The cytoplasm is often richly supplied with vesicles for macromolecular transport. Endothelium may proliferate in response to the secretion of vascular endothelial growth factor (VEGF), for example, by cancer cells, thereby promoting tumor growth. The surface of endothelium is the entry point for migration of leukocytes into tissues; this involves cell collision, rolling, and adherence, followed by diapedesis of the leukocyte. Extravasation occurs normally and is greatly enhanced in inflammatory reactions. × 4,000.

These compounds and others are prothrombotic and induce platelet plug formation if the vessel is injured. While endothelial cells synthesize anticoagulant and procoagulant factors, under normal physiologic conditions anticoagulant factors predominate.

Endothelial cells present the first barrier to leukocyte infiltration into tissues. Attraction, adherence, and migration of leukocytes through the tunica intima is a key feature of inflammatory reactions, mediated partly by activated endothelial cells. Leukocytes cross the endothelium by the transcellular pathway through endothelial cytoplasm, or via the paracellular route in which the leukocytes squeeze through apposed endothelial plasma membranes. The latter activity, referred to as diapedesis, requires the opening and closing of endothelial tight and adherens junctions. Formation and repair of the vascular wall, and the growth of tumors require rapid proliferation of endothelial cells. Because the normal endothelium has limited regenerative capacity, vascular repair relies upon endothelial progenitor cells, which are derived from bone marrow stem cells or from resident progenitor cells within organs and the systemic vasculature. Endothelial progenitor cells circulate in blood after vascular injury or during tumor growth.

While vasculogenesis refers to the growth of endothelial tubes, angiogenesis is the process of vascular growth by vessel sprouting and stabilization by associated smooth muscle. These processes are stimulated by various endothelial-derived cytokines and other growth factors, secreted by macrophages and tumor cells that specifically stimulate endothelial cell proliferation.

LYMPH VASCULAR SYSTEM

The fluid in the interstitial or extracellular spaces is mainly derived from capillaries and small venules (Fig 8.27). It contains electrolytes, lipids, proteins, and cells. Most of this fluid is returned to the venous vessels and the remaining fraction is continuously drained by the lymphatic system. Lymph is the term applied to interstitial fluid in a recognizable lymph vessel, the smallest of which resembles a capillary and the largest of which is similar to a vein.

One of the functions of the lymphatic system is to control the hydrostatic and osmotic pressure within the interstitium; other functions are to gather lymphocytes from the tissues and to supply antibodies via the lymph nodes that eventually enter the venous system.

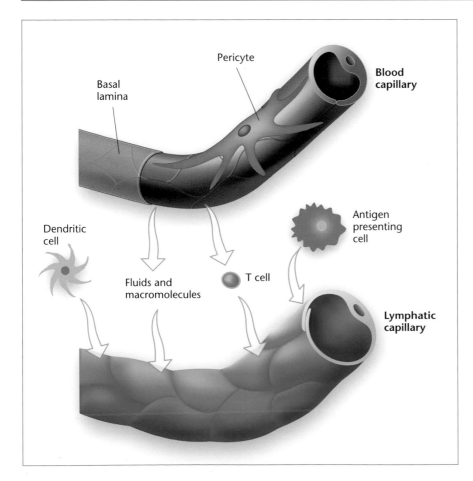

◀ **Fig 8.27 Structure and function of lymphatic capillaries.** The fluid and cells arising from capillaries enter the interstitial or extracellular spaces. Lymphatic capillaries are simple squamous endothelial tubes with very thin walls. They are able to receive each of these components and serve to drain the interstitium. Lymph vessels carry lymph to lymph nodes for presentation to cells of the immune system.

Lymph capillaries are lined by a thin endothelium and range in cross section from collapsed slit-like spaces to recognizable capillary-type vessels. They are usually wider than blood capillaries, but lack pericytes (Fig 8.28). Interstitial fluid enters the blind-ending lymph capillaries in two ways:

- By passive diffusion through minute gaps between adjacent endothelial cells
- By being drawn into the capillary lumen across the transient negative pressure gradient created whenever the vessel is relaxed.

With increasing diameter, the walls of lymph vessels become thicker and contain collagen, elastin, and variable quantities of smooth muscle. Transport of lymph is ensured by compression of the vessels and by the presence of valves in the smaller vessels. In larger-caliber lymph vessels entering lymph nodes and in the main lymphatic trunks, the smooth muscle in the vessel walls constricts the vessels via both intrinsic mechanisms and extrinsic mechanisms (i.e. via the sympathetic nervous system). Lymph nodes filter the collected lymph; their functions as lymphoid tissues are discussed in Chapter 11.

Lymphatics are absent from bone, the brain, the thymus, and the eyes. Tissues in which lymphatics can be seen reliably include the portal triads of the liver, the core of the gut villi, and the intertubular tissue of the testis (Fig 8.29). For further details see the corresponding chapters.

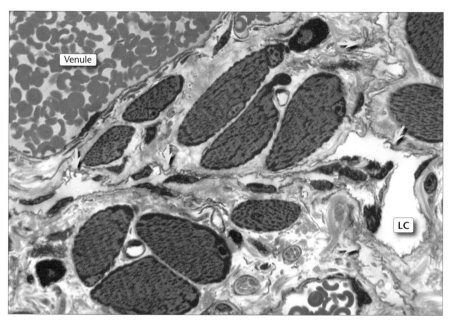

▲ **Fig 8.28 Lymphatic capillary.** Initial lymphatics are lymphatic capillaries (**LC**) with blind endings, in which the endothelial cells overlap and interdigitate (**arrows**) with the surrounding extracellular space. Gaps between the endothelial cells allow transfer of fluid, macromolecules, bacteria and particles from the interstitial fluid into the lymphatic capillary. This leakiness occurs when intralymphatic pressure is low, but the endothelial cells are not sucked into the lymphatics because they are anchored by fibrils to collagen in the interstitial space. Overlapping endothelial cells seal the lymphatic wall when primary lymph pressure is higher than extralymphatic tissue pressure. Lymph also contains lymphocytes, which are circulated between lymphoid tissues and stored in lymph nodes. The circulation time of lymph is 2–3 days, whereas blood recirculates in about 1 minute. Lymph flow is generated by interstitial hydrostatic pressure, vascular pulsations, tissue movements, valves in conducting lymphatics and smooth muscle in the walls of large lymphatic vessels (the lymphatic and thoracic ducts). Toluidine blue, araldite, × 550.

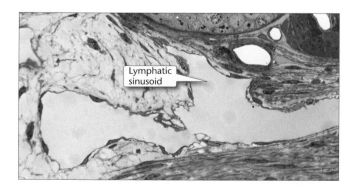

◄ **Fig 8.29 Lymphatic sinusoid.** In certain tissues, such as the testicular intertubular space seen here, the lymphatic vessels may attain considerable size, resembling sinusoids. In some rodent species the sinusoids are discontinuous and in communication with the interstitial connective tissue. The function of the lymphatic sinusoids is to regulate the fluid and protein content within the interstitium. Toluidine blue, araldite, × 400.

Comparing arteries and veins

Arteries and veins often occur together in the tissues, so it is necessary to be able to distinguish between them. They cannot be classified reliably on the basis of their diameter, shape, or position. The relative thickness of their walls compared with their overall size is only a rough guide to their classification. In general, arteries are recognized by the presence of the cellular nature of the tunica media, which consists of smooth muscle cells that are more abundant in numbers and concentric layers than in veins. By contrast, veins have thinner walls in association with a wider lumen. Examples of these differences are seen in Figure 8.30a–c.

> **Tip:** All blood and lymphatic vessels can be identified quickly because they always show an internal lining of endothelium—squamous endothelium. Other types of hollow tubes, such as the ducts of many glands, show a cuboidal or columnar epithelial lining regardless of how the duct has been cut in the tissue section.

DISORDERS AND CLINICAL FEATURES

Heart and arterial vasculature

Many conditions affect the heart and its vasculature.

Cardiac failure occurs when the heart cannot fulfill its function of supplying all the tissues of the

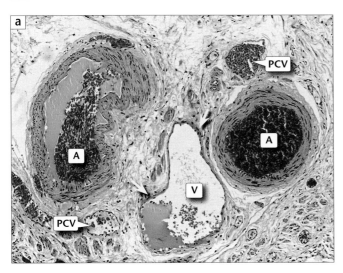

▲ **Fig 8.30a Arteries and veins.** In contrast to small muscular arteries (**A**), muscular venules (**V**) have scant smooth muscle forming a rudimentary media (**arrows**), which often blends with a thin adventitia when viewed at low magnification. Postcapillary venules (**PCV**) are shown for size comparison. H&E, acrylic resin, × 70.

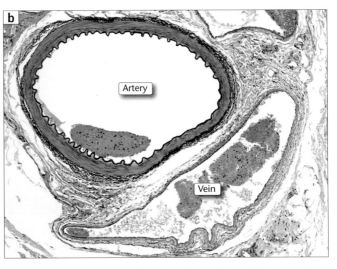

▲ **Fig 8.30b Arteries and veins.** Although of similar size to the muscular venule, the muscular artery has a thicker wall compared with the vein, and the artery shows a convoluted internal elastic lamina and external elastic lamina, both stained black for elastin. The vein has a thin wall of connective tissue and, while not visible at this magnification, has few smooth muscle cells. Van Gieson's, paraffin, × 80.

◀ **Fig 8.30c Arteries and veins.** The small muscular artery shows a folded internal elastic lamina and elastin in the tunica media and distinctly in the adventitia. In contrast, the larger vein has elastic lamina in a tunica that is thin in comparison with the diameter of the vessel. Note also numerous venules with very thin walls that do not contain elastic fibers in their walls. Gomori trichrome, paraffin, × 65.

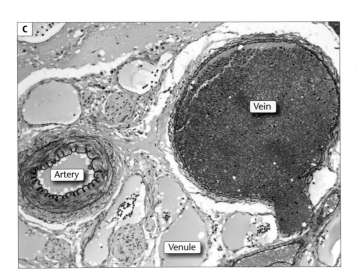

body with an adequate flow of oxygenated blood. Congestive heart failure occurs when blood flow from one or both ventricles is inadequate, leading to excessive venous dilatation and edema in the pulmonary or systemic circulation.

Damage to the valves can result from inflammation (often caused by rheumatic fever in childhood, a bacterial pharyngeal infection). The inflammation distorts their shape with scar tissue, and their impeded function causes regurgitation and volume overload, which contributes to heart failure. Cardiac failure can also occur if valves become stenotic (narrow), as this causes a pressure overload.

Cardiac failure often results from long-term essential hypertension, where a high peripheral resistance imposes a pressure overload on the heart.

In general, arterial disorders are broadly referred to as arteriosclerosis (hardening of the arteries), a term used to describe the progressive thickening of the intima that occurs from middle age onward. In arteriosclerosis, the walls of small arteries and arterioles become thicker with additional collagen. There is a resultant loss of elasticity, which leads to elevated blood pressure, and, in turn, to secondary hypertension (as distinct from primary or essential hypertension, in which the increased vascular resistance of organs and tissues cannot be linked to any single cause). With elevated blood pressure, blood vessels may hemorrhage.

Atherosclerosis (atheromata) is the most common pathologic variant of arteriosclerosis. It is a gradual narrowing of the arterial lumen by a build-up of an atheroma (fibrous–fatty tissue) on the inside of the vessel. It often affects the abdominal aorta and the coronary, popliteal, cerebral, and carotid arteries.

Atherosclerosis is by far the major cause of morbidity and death in industrialized societies. A thrombus (blood clot) may block an artery (thrombosis), or an embolus (mobile clot) may be transported to other sets of vessels (e.g. vessels in the brain, causing a stroke). Myocardial infarction (heart attack) results from an atheromatous plaque (or thrombus or embolus) occluding a major coronary artery (which can also cause vessel rupture or hemorrhage). This occlusion leads to myocardial ischemia (inadequate supply of blood to the heart muscle), which causes a reduced contractile response. Ultimately, myocardial tissue necrosis (an infarct) will occur if blood flow is not restored to adequate levels.

In some cases of arterial disease, a ballooning out of a weakened arterial wall (aneurysm) occurs. The aorta is often affected, the rupture of which may cause massive and even fatal hemorrhage.

Veins

Varicosities and thromboses are the most common clinical disorders of veins. Varicose veins usually occur in superficial vessels of the leg. They can be seen as dilatations and contortions. They are caused by a loss of valve function between deep and superficial veins. This disorder may be temporary (as in pregnancy, where venous pressure in the legs is increased); in chronic cases it may be hereditary.

Portal hypertension, which is commonly associated with cirrhosis of the liver, can cause varicosities in the esophageal and hemorrhoidal veins. Thrombi, together with venous inflammation (phlebitis), may also occur in the legs, causing swelling and discomfort. If an embolus develops it may result in a pulmonary embolism, which can be fatal. Pregnancy and constipation may cause enlargements of the anal venous plexus, forming hemorrhoids.

Lymphatic vessels

Obstruction of lymphatic vessels causes edema, an excessive accumulation of interstitial fluid, and may follow regional inflammation, infection by parasites, or surgical removal of lymph nodes. Lymphangitis, or "blood poisoning," may occur in response to an infected wound, particularly if the infection is caused by bacteria. The inflammation of the lymph vessels presents as painful red streaks in the subcutaneous tissue.

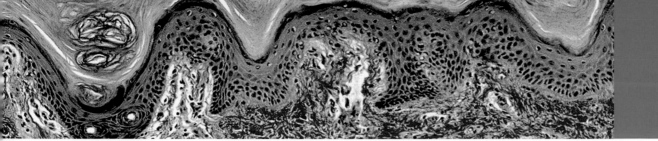

Skin

Skin is the largest of all human organs, with a surface area of about 2 m² in adults and a thickness that varies from 0.5 mm to 4 mm. The skin contains the following major components:

- The epidermis, a superficial layer of stratified squamous keratinized epithelium
- The dermis, an underlying layer of fibroelastic connective tissue, which is often quite thick and contains blood vessels, nerves, a variety of glands and, in most areas, hair follicles.

Deep to the dermis is the hypodermis, a layer of subcutaneous adipose connective tissue contributing to the superficial fascia (Fig 9.1). Depending on location, the hypodermis blends with deep fascia or periosteum of bone.

The upper two layers have been likened to a double-layered cake with icing: the "layers" contain living tissues and the "icing" is formed of insoluble scales of keratin protein.

Because the skin is exposed to the environment, it must be capable of responding to changes in the outside world as well as from within the body, all the while maintaining a physiologic balance between these two environments. Its major functions include protection, sensory awareness, thermoregulation, production of the precursor of vitamin D, various properties of secretion and permeability, immunologic defense, and wound healing. The skin also develops hair and nails, which serve a specialized protective function.

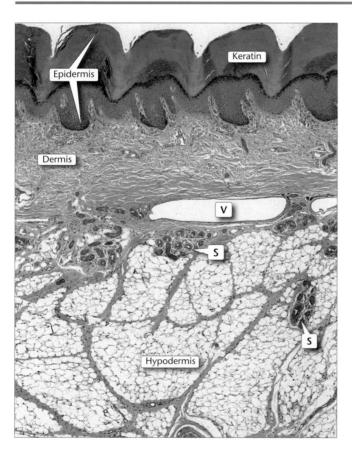

◀ **Fig 9.1 Architecture of skin.** The epidermis in this specimen is a highly cellular epithelial layer. It is sharply demarcated from the deeper dermis, which contains strands of dense connective tissue. The surface of the epidermis shows a thick, non-cellular keratin layer. Undulations of the dermis form dermal ridges with upward extensions—dermal papillae. The ridge and groove arrangement resists the wear and tear forces applied to the epidermis. The hypodermis comprises adipose tissue surrounded by connective tissue. A blood vessel (**V**) and sweat glands (**S**) are shown. Hematoxylin and eosin (H&E), paraffin, × 20.

Histologically, skin is classified as either thick or thin (Fig 9.2a & b). Thick skin is always seen on the palms of the hand and the soles of the feet; it lacks hair. Thin skin exists in most other locations and usually contains hair—thin skin without hair occurs in parts of the genital region, in the lateral and terminal regions of fingers and toes, and in the lips.

EPIDERMIS

The most superficial layer of skin is a keratinized stratified squamous epithelium of variable depth (Fig 9.3a). It is avascular, but is supplied by very fine nerve endings that penetrate through most of the epithelial cell layers. The true epithelial (ectodermal) skin cells are referred to as keratinocytes and are accompanied by various other cell types involved with skin pigmentation, sensory perception, and immune functions.

Basal layer—stratum germinativum

The epidermis exhibits up to five main layers, and it is attached to the underlying dermis. Blood vessels do not enter the epidermis. The deepest or basal epidermal layer is the germinal or proliferative cell

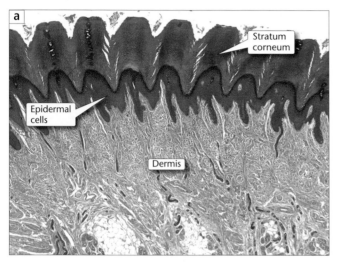

▲ **Fig 9.2a Thick skin.** Thick skin from the palm of the hand is characterized by a substantial superficial cornified layer of keratin, which usually desquamates or exfoliates into strands or flakes. This layer of keratin is the stratum corneum and serves as a protective, waterproof barrier. Deep to the epidermis, the dermal tissue displays bundles of collagen and contains nerves and vascular elements, the latter providing a source of nutrients to the epidermis, which itself is avascular. H&E, paraffin, × 20.

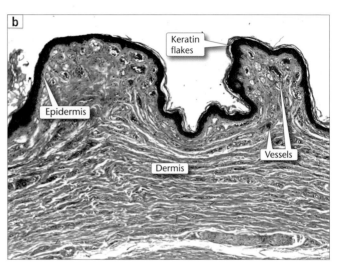

▲ **Fig 9.2b Thin skin.** Specimen of thin skin from the abdominal region, showing an irregular, folded epidermis covered by a thin, compact stratum corneum, its superficial layers showing desquamation of keratin flakes. The dermis comprises collagen bundles and blood vessels, particularly in the upper dermis. H&E, paraffin, × 40.

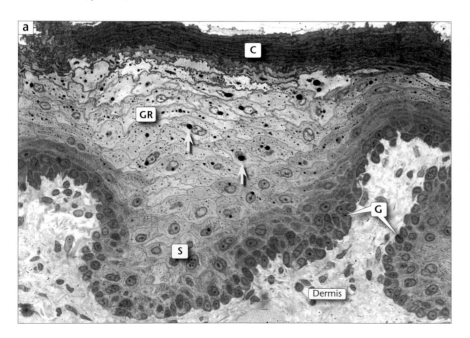

◀ **Fig 9.3a Cells of the epidermis.** Thin epoxy resin section of thin skin, showing cells of the stratum germinativum (**G**), stratum spinosum (**S**), stratum granulosum (**GR**), and stratum corneum (**C**) with non-viable layers of keratin. Note the keratohyalin granules (**arrows**), which contain profilaggrin, a protein that associates with cytoplasmic keratin filaments. In the dermis, connective tissue comprises loosely arranged collagen. Toluidine blue, araldite, × 500.

layer—the stratum germinativum (Fig 9.3b). This comprises a single row of cells resting on a basal lamina, which is strongly adherent to the underlying dermis. These are stem cells, and divide by mitosis to produce most of the cells of the epidermis, which are destined to mature into the uppermost layer of keratin. Hence all epidermal cells of this type are referred to as keratinocytes. Above the germinal layer, the keratinocytes are postmitotic.

It is within the cells of the germinal layer that small amounts of cytoplasmic intermediate filaments of the keratin type are found. These are tonofilaments, which go on to form a component of the keratin and, in the basal layer, are connected to surface desmosomes between adjacent cells.

Second layer—stratum spinosum

As upward displacement occurs, the second layer of keratinocytes—the stratum spinosum—is formed (Fig 9.3c). This layer is about five cells thick and is so named because the cells appear to have spines or prickles projecting from their surface. These are desmosomes on fine spike-type cytoplasmic processes;

they interdigitate and attach to neighboring cells.

Keratin filaments are abundant and provide an internal supporting framework within these cells via their insertion into the desmosomes. Occasional lamellar granules are seen in the spinous cells, representing initial development of lipid-rich substances, which continues in the more superficial cells.

Third layer—stratum granulosum

Transformation of the spinous cells into the cells of the third layer—the stratum granulosum (Fig 9.3d)—is characterized by accumulation of numerous dense bundles of keratin, which become associated with a protein called profilaggrin that induces the formation of keratohyalin granules. These contain filaggrin proteins that are anchored to desmosomes. At the same time, the nucleus and organelles break down and their ultimate destruction results in cells filled only with keratin. The cells of the granular layer have the distinction of being programmed to destroy their nuclei and organelles, yet at the same time to synthesize keratin and lamellar bodies.

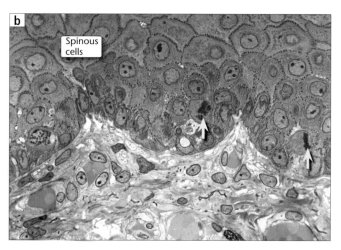

▲ **Fig 9.3b Basal germinal layer.** Cells of the basal germinal layer proliferate by mitosis (**arrows**) to provide a constant supply of keratinocytes which undergo differentiation and upward displacement. The spinous (or prickle) cells show serrated edges because of interdigitated desmosomes. Toluidine blue, araldite, × 650.

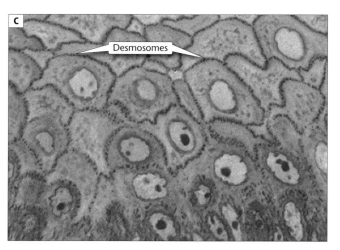

▲ **Fig 9.3c Stratum spinosum.** Keratinocytes of the stratum spinosum show serrated surface profiles that give spinous or prickle-type morphology. These are formed by the desmosomes in between the cells. Keratin filaments are abundant in spinous cells and, via attachment to the desmosomes, they provide a relatively rigid cytoskeletal framework that is resistant to mechanical deformation. Toluidine blue, araldite, × 1,200.

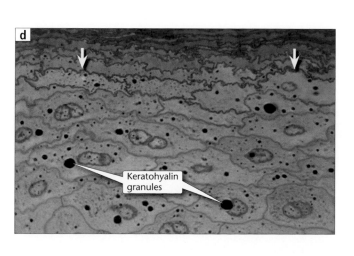

◀ **Fig 9.3d Stratum granulosum.** Cells of the stratum granulosum contain variable quantities of granules representing keratohyalin together with many smaller lamellar granules, about 0.5 μm in diameter. These lamellar granules contain several types of proteins and are visible as particulate matter in the cytoplasm. These granules will fuse with the plasma membrane and form an impermeable barrier that restricts water loss from the epidermis. Note the greater density and thickness of the plasma membranes (**arrows**). Toluidine blue, araldite, × 1,200.

The contents of the lamellar granules in the granular cells are discharged into the extracellular space and provide a lipid layer between the succeeding cell layers. This is effective in establishing a permeability barrier for the skin.

Fourth layer—stratum lucidum

In thick skin, a narrow fourth layer, the stratum lucidum (Fig 9.3e), is sometimes observed above the granular layer. It consists of flattened, dead cells with abundant keratin proteins, and it presents as a thin undulating line of poor staining intensity.

Fifth layer—stratum corneum

The fifth and most superficial layer is the stratum corneum (Fig 9.3f), which consists of dead, anucleate squamous cells containing keratin. It is especially thick (more than 1 mm) on the soles of the feet and quite thin (about 0.1 mm) over much of the body surface. Thus, the number of individual cell layers making up the fifth layer can range from about 10 to a few hundred. The association of disulfide-bonded keratin and matrix of proteins including filaggrin form thick cell membranes with protective properties and impermeability to fluids.

These plates of keratin, which are also referred to as the horny layer of cornified cells, are constantly shed from the surface and replaced by new cells arising from the deeper layers. Normally the transit time from a stem cell to desquamation is about 1 month.

Cells resident in the epidermis

The color of skin in healthy people is determined by the following:

- Oxygen content of underlying blood vessels
- Presence of carotene (yellowish pigment) from the diet
- Pigmentation of the epidermis derived from the melanocytes.

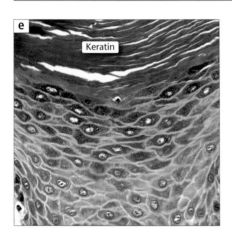

◀ **Fig 9.3e Upper stratum granulosum.** In the upper region of the stratum granulosum, the cell nuclei disintegrate (probably by a type of programmed cellular degeneration), but the keratohyalins and lamellar granules persist, and the cells become increasingly flattened or squamous. In consequence of the keratinocytes losing their nuclei and organelles, the cells are reduced to shells containing keratin–filaggrin protein complexes. H&E, paraffin, × 500.

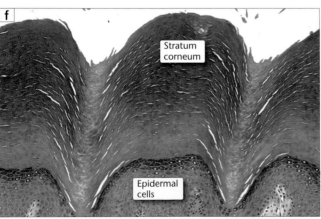

◀ **Fig 9.3f Stratum corneum.** Layers of stratum corneum are shown, consisting of flattened, irregular scales filled with keratin and bordered by a rigid, resistant, cornified plasma membrane, which protects the deeper cellular layers from abrasion, dehydration, and the entry of many solvents. The precise means of degradation of all the organelles and inclusions and the nucleus is not known. Exfoliation of the plaques of keratin involves enzymatic breakdown of the adhesive properties, including the desmosomes, between the cornified cells. The continual loss of cells is compensated for by proliferation and upward migration of keratinocytes from the deeper strata. H&E, paraffin, × 80.

Melanocytes

Melanocytes, which originate in the neural crest but are capable of division in adult life, are dendritic in structure and reside at the level of the basal layer of the epidermis (Fig 9.4a & b). Melanocytes synthesize melanin pigment from precursors such as tyrosine and dihydroxyphenylalanine (dopa), and transfer the pigment to surrounding keratinocytes within granules called melanosomes. Melanin exists in two forms: red–yellow melanin or pheomelanin, and eumelanin, which is brown–black.

Melanin absorbs and scatters the ultraviolet radiation that is present in sunlight and thereby protects cells from the possible mutagenic effects of ultraviolet light. The ratio of melanocytes to basal epithelial cells varies between about 1:5 and 1:10, depending on which region of the body is examined. However, differences in skin color are related to the amount of melanin produced, since the number of melanocytes is similar in light and dark skin but dark-pigmented skin may have 40 times as much melanin as light skin. Melanin production is increased in response to prolonged solar radiation, causing a suntan, whereas lack of melanin in albino conditions is associated with greater risk of epidermal damage and skin cancer.

Langerhans cells

The immunologic defense of the skin is in part attributed to Langerhans cells, which are found among the cells of the stratum spinosum (Fig 9.5). These dendritic-type cells represent about 5% of epidermal cells and migrate into the epidermis from the bloodstream; they function as antigen-presenting cells and may stimulate T cell responses in various allergic and inflammatory conditions.

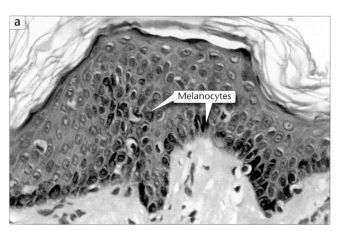

▲ **Fig 9.4a Pigmented skin.** In pigmented skin, melanosomes containing either red–yellow or brown–black melanin are transferred to surrounding keratinocytes (by means of a type of phagocytosis) and often form a pigmented layer deep in the epidermis and in more superficial cells. In darker skin, the melanin is even more widespread. Melanin provides protection from the potentially harmful effects of ultraviolet radiation, which stimulates melanin production. Synthesis of melanin is also under endocrine control; for example, in pregnancy increased pigmentation of facial skin may occur. H&E, paraffin, × 400.

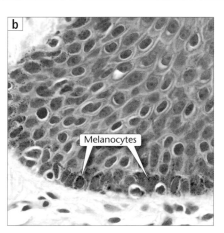

▲ **Fig 9.4b Melanocytes.** Melanocytes reside in the basal aspect of the epidermis and show a pale cytoplasm. In specimens of fair skin, the production of melanin pigment in cytoplasmic melanosome granules is minimal but in this specimen melanin granules within the basal keratinocytes are easily seen. H&E, paraffin, × 500.

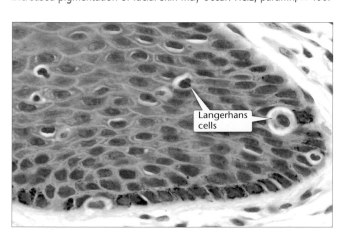

◀ **Fig 9.5 Langerhans cells.** These cells are pale-staining in routine histologic sections and, unlike melanocytes, are located not on the basal lamina but deeper within the stratum spinosum. Langerhans cells are antigen-presenting cells and are involved with inflammatory reactions. After capturing antigen they migrate to lymph nodes, where they become dendritic cells. H&E, paraffin, × 600.

Merkel cells

A third cell type, the Merkel cell, is a specialized sensory transducer positioned among the cells of the basal epidermal layer. Although uncommon in most areas of the skin, Merkel cells are often present in the skin of the digits and the lips, and around hair follicles. Merkel cells are in communication with afferent nerve endings and are thought to modify the stimulus received by the sensory neurons.

> **Tip:** The color of skin is not determined by the abundance or lack of melanocytes. The number of melanocytes is about the same in all humans. It is the amount and distribution of the melanin granules in the epidermis that gives differences in skin color.

DERMIS

The dermis lies beneath the epidermis and contains abundant collagen and lesser amounts of elastic and reticular fibers, together with extracellular matrix and the cell types commonly found in dense irregular connective tissue (Fig 9.6a & b).

In areas subject to constant wear and tear, such as thick skin, the dermis interdigitates with the epidermis to form an uneven border of dermal papillae that are not unlike a sawtooth arrangement. Together with hemidesmosomes positioned between the basal keratinocytes and the basal lamina facing the dermis, the interface between dermis and epidermis is a site of strong attachment.

The more superficial part of the dermis is called the papillary region and consists of loose connective tissue with nerves and numerous blood vessels supplying nutrients to the epidermis.

Depending on the type of skin, the deeper and more extensive reticular part consists of many more collagen bundles with a meshwork or reticulum of coarse elastic fibers. The dermis is well suited to withstand mechanical stresses, being flexible and elastic, and it provides support for neurovascular components, all the glands of the skin, and hair follicles.

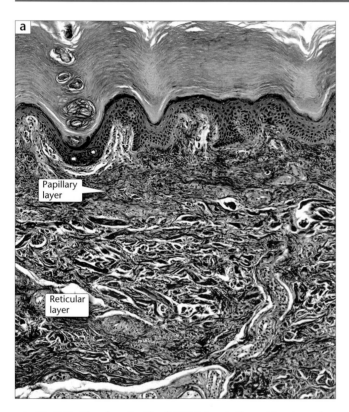

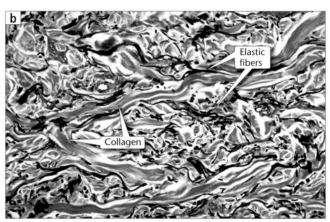

▲ **Fig 9.6b In the reticular layer of the dermis,** note the very thick irregular bundles of collagen, between which are elastic fibers. These proteins respectively provide resistance against deformation with wear and tear, and elasticity when skin is stretched. Van Gieson's, paraffin, × 500.

▲ **Fig 9.6a The dermis.** The dermis supports the epidermis, and its content of collagen, extracellular matrix, and variable quantities of elastic fibers give skin its remarkable mechanical properties. The upper papillary region can be recognized by its finer collagen fibers. Deeper in the dermis is the reticular layer, identified by its greater depth and coarser collagen bundles. Collagen confers strength and the elastin gives skin its flexibility. Van Gieson's, paraffin, × 90.

Several important functions of the skin are attributable to structural components intrinsic to the dermis. The arrangement of blood vessels in the dermis into vascular plexuses provides capillary networks directed toward, but not penetrating, the epidermis, and other vessels occur around the various glands and the hair follicles in the deep dermis. Blood within the dermis can bypass many of the capillaries by entering numerous arteriovenous anastomoses (shunts). Thus, when blood is flowing in the uppermost capillary plexuses, it may be cooled by the evaporation of sweat upon the surface of the skin. Conversely, when the air temperature is low, blood can bypass the capillaries, so it is not cooled, thus helping to retain body heat.

Tissues in the dermis can also participate in immunologic defense by maintaining inflammatory responses.

In addition, the dermis shows remarkable regenerative capacity in the healing of wounds and in cases of skin grafting.

Sweat glands

Sweat glands are of two types:
- Eccrine glands, which expel sweat onto the surface of the skin
- Apocrine glands, which deliver a milky secretion directly into certain hair follicles.

Both types are resident in the dermis but are derivatives of the epidermis, forming ducts that terminate inferiorly as coiled structures in the reticular portion of the dermis or the hypodermis (Fig 9.7).

Eccrine glands

The eccrine glands resemble a tube (the duct) ending in a coiled portion (the secretory unit), the latter forming circular or elliptical profiles in sections, with cuboidal secretory cells surrounding a small central lumen (Fig 9.8). Modified smooth muscle cells (myoepithelial cells) form a margin around the secretory units and, on contraction in response to cholinergic and sympathetic stimulation, assist with expulsion of the sweat. As they pass to the epidermis,

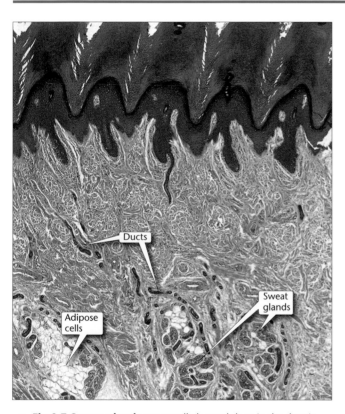

▲ **Fig 9.7 Sweat glands** are usually located deep in the dermis, but their connection with and origin from the epidermis are marked by their slender ducts, which pass through the dermis and penetrate the epidermis to reach the skin surface. Sweat glands often occur in small clusters and are associated with adipose tissue. H&E, paraffin, × 80.

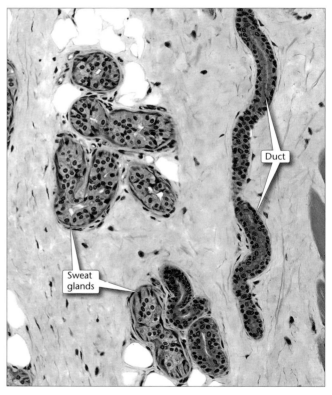

▲ **Fig 9.8 Eccrine glands.** The secretory coil of the eccrine sweat gland occurs as an ovoid hollow tube with one or more layers of cuboidal or low-columnar cells. The primary secretion is isotonic sodium chloride solution, but the salt is reabsorbed in the duct, resulting in a watery solution that evaporates at the surface of the skin to prevent overheating. Sweating is controlled mainly by sympathetic cholinergic fibers. The sweat ducts are straighter, narrower, and more densely stained than the secretory coils. Ducts reduce the concentration of sodium chloride by active absorption; the final sweat thus has little salt content. Thermoregulation, by evaporative cooling, is essential for homeothermy and in physical exercise; it is altered in climate variations. H&E, paraffin, × 200.

213

the ducts are lined by a double layer of cuboidal cells; these are replaced by keratinocytes as the duct passes upwards through the epidermis.

Eccrine sweat glands occur all over the body and are especially abundant on the forehead, axillae, palms and soles. Their initial secretion is water, and sodium and potassium ions, but at the surface the sweat is 99% water, the ions having been absorbed by the epithelial lining of the ducts. Sweat is colorless, has no odor, and as it evaporates it dissipates heat from the skin. Water loss via diffusion through the skin may amount to several hundred milliliters per day. Normally about 100 mL per day is lost via the sweat glands, but with strenuous exercise in a hot climate, this may increase to 1–2 L per day.

Apocrine glands

Apocrine glands have a larger secretory coil than eccrine glands. The secretory coil is lined by a cuboidal or columnar epithelium associated with myoepithelial cells, and it usually empties via a duct connected to a hair follicle (Fig 9.9). These glands are numerous in the scalp, neck, groin, and axillae.

Apocrine gland secretion is a milky, odorless fluid, which is broken down by surface bacteria into various substances with distinctive odors. Formerly, the secretion of this fluid was thought to involve blebbing or fragmentation of part of the secretory cells (a mechanism of secretion known as "apocrine" secretion), but in fact the secretory mechanism has been found to be exocrine (merocrine) in nature. In the axillae, apo-eccrine glands may occur, emptying via ducts directly onto the surface of the skin. These glands develop around puberty and are possibly derived from eccrine sweat glands.

Sebaceous glands

Sebaceous glands are also derived from the epidermis. They are flask-shaped and packed solidly with cells that often have a foamy appearance in sections (Fig 9.10a–d). Sebaceous glands commonly empty into the upper regions of hair follicles. They may also be seen in certain non-hairy sites such as the nipples and eyelids. They are most numerous on the face and upper thorax; they are absent from the palms of the hands and soles of the feet. Becoming active at puberty, the secretory product contains whole cells released as disintegrated matter from the glands by the so-called holocrine process. These exfoliated cells form an oily or greasy product called sebum, which serves as a softening and waterproofing agent for the skin.

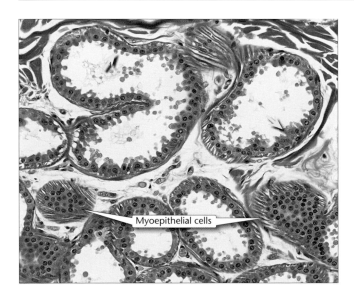

Myoepithelial cells

◀ **Fig 9.9 Apocrine glands.** These glands have large lumens, and are otherwise similar to eccrine sweat glands, except that they usually empty into hair follicles. They occur in the axillae, the areolae of the nipples, and the genital and perineal regions. Cytoplasmic blebbing (**arrows**) is not indicative of true apocrine secretion; these glands secrete via a merocrine process. Apocrine sweat is a milky non-odorous secretion that is (sometimes) converted to an unpleasant odor by bacteria on the skin surface. Note myoepithelial cells that, via adrenergic innervation, contract to facilitate secretions. H&E, paraffin, × 220.

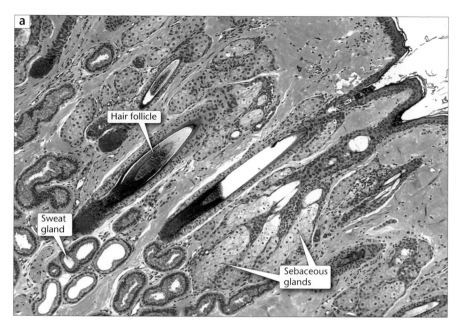

◀ **Fig 9.10a Sebaceous glands.** These are often, but not exclusively, associated with hair follicles, the external sheath of which is continuous with the gland. They are characterized by being filled with cells, unlike sweat glands, which are hollow structures. Areas of skin with sebaceous glands not found with hair include parts of the face, the nipples, and trunk. H&E, paraffin, × 100.

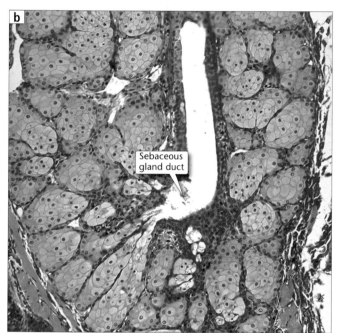

◀ **Fig 9.10b Sebaceous glands.** Sebaceous glands are lobulated and filled with cells that secrete sebum (a greasy liquid), often into the canal of a hair follicle with which they are often associated. This provides the hair shaft and skin surface with a coating of sebum, acting as a lubricant and as a protective layer. As is the case with hair follicles, sebaceous glands are of epidermal origin and, together with arrector pili muscles and apocrine glands, they constitute the pilar unit. The sole of the foot and the palm of the hand are the only areas of skin that do not contain sebaceous glands. H&E, paraffin, × 170.

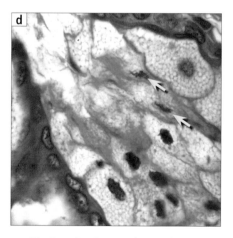

▲ **Fig 9.10d Sebum.** Sebum is the end-product of disintegration of sebaceous cells, which exit the gland by means of a holocrine secretory process (i.e. the whole cell is the secretory product). Note the shrinkage and destruction of the nuclei (**arrows**) and the rupture of the cell membranes with discharge of the sebum into the excretory passage. H&E, paraffin, × 550.

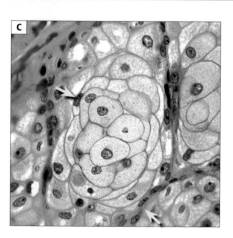

◀ **Fig 9.10c Sebaceous cells.** These are filled with lipid-rich droplets, giving a multivacuolated appearance with a central nucleus. Cells at the periphery (**arrows**) are the germinative cells, which are stimulated during puberty to proliferate by the elevated levels of sex steroid hormones. Excessive sebum production may cause skin spots on the face or acne (duct disruption). Masson's trichrome, paraffin, × 300.

215

Hair follicles

Hair follicles are specialized downgrowths of the epidermis extending deep into the dermis (Fig 9.11a–c). Growth of the hair shaft originates from the bulb region located about midway or deeper along the shaft. Stem cells in the bulb supply proliferative cells to the hair root, seen as a terminal bulb of proliferating cells (the matrix). These proliferating cells in the matrix are similar to the germinal cells of the epidermis.

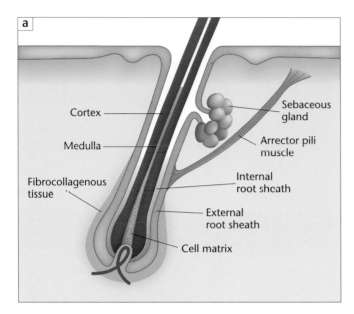

a

Cortex

Medulla

Fibrocollagenous
tissue

Sebaceous
gland

Arrector pili
muscle

Internal
root sheath

External
root sheath

Cell matrix

◀ **Fig 9.11a Diagram of the main parts of a hair follicle**, showing external and internal root sheaths, supported by the dermal connective tissues. The root sheath region near the sebaceous gland is known as the follicle bulb and is the source of stem cells that may supply cells to the local epidermis, the sebaceous glands, and the matrix zone of the growing hair follicle. In response to cold, fear, or anger, sympathetic innervation to the smooth muscle of the arrector pili elevates the hair to an upright position, a phenomenon well demonstrated in feline species.

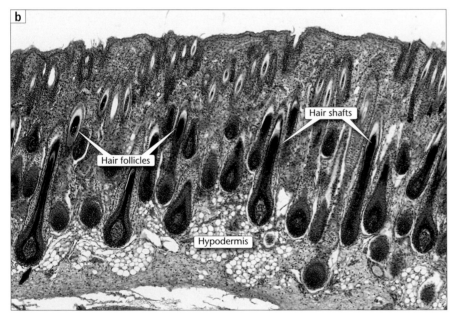

b

Hair shafts

Hair follicles

Hypodermis

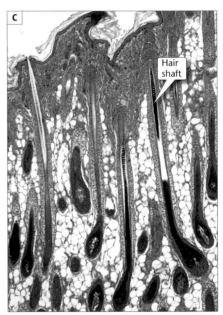

c

Hair
shaft

▲ **Fig 9.11b Scalp skin.** The scalp shows hairy skin with numerous long hair follicles and hair shafts. Follicles are epidermal invaginations into the dermis and hypodermis. The hypodermis is equivalent to the fibrous fatty tissue of the superficial fascia. Septae of connective tissue from the deep fascia connect with the dermis. H&E, paraffin, × 30.

▲ **Fig 9.11c Scalp skin.** Hairy skin from the scalp, showing the deep penetration of follicles into the hypodermis, recognized by the extensive adipose tissue. Heavy pigmentation of the hair shafts is attributed to melanin. Note that the epidermis is thin, a feature always associated with hair follicles. H&E, paraffin, × 40.

Melanocytes populate the matrix and provide pigments to the matrix cells, which, with upward displacement, are transformed into hard keratin to form the outer cortex and cuticle layers of the hair.

Hair follicles are multilayered cylinders of cells, the histology of which is understood from longitudinal and cross sections (Fig 9.12a–d).

The central medulla of the hair contains soft keratin. Immediately surrounding most of the length of the hair shaft is a sleeve of soft keratin—the internal root sheath, which is also derived from the deeper matrix.

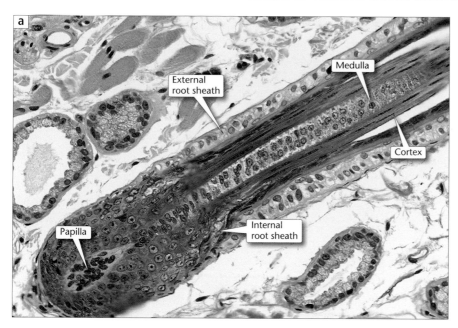

▲ **Fig 9.12a Hair follicle**, showing the hair shaft with a prominent medulla of vacuolated cells with soft keratin, and a deeply staining cortex with hard keratin. An internal root sheath and external root sheath are shown; the latter is a downward extension of the epidermis. In the bulbous portion there is a connective tissue papilla surrounded by matrix cells, which proliferate and mature into the hair cortex and medulla. H&E, paraffin, × 200.

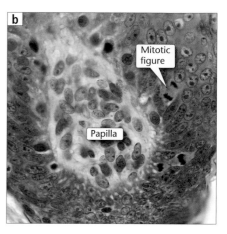

▲ **Fig 9.12b Bulb of hair follicle**, showing central connective tissue papilla providing nutrients from its capillaries. Mitotic figures in the cell matrix contribute new cells, which are destined for the hair shaft and inner root sheath. The matrix contains melanocytes, their melanosomes transferring melanin to the hair cortex. Blond hair contains incompletely melanized pigment; red hair contains yellow-red melanin; and in gray hair, the melanocytes have a reduced ability to synthesize pigment. H&E, paraffin, × 400.

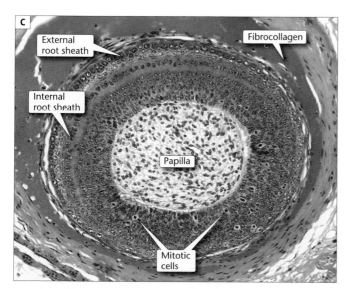

▲ **Fig 9.12c Cross section of a hair follicle through the level of the bulb**, showing outer fibrocollagenous dermis, external root sheath and internal root sheath, cell matrix with mitotic keratinocytes, and the central connective tissue papilla. H&E, acrylic resin, × 200.

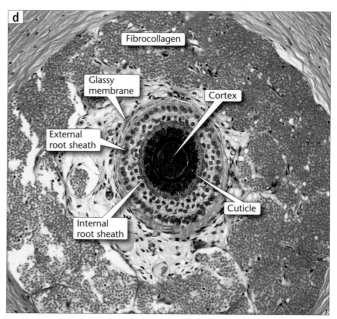

▲ **Fig 9.12d Cross section of hair at mid-shaft level**, showing fibrocollagenous tissue, the glassy membrane, a thick basal lamina surrounding the external root sheath, the granular inner root sheath, and the cuticle and cortex of the hair shaft. H&E, acrylic resin, × 200.

The external root sheath is formed by the cellular walls of the hair follicle and is similar to a deep, narrow pit extending down from the surface epidermis. A thick basement membrane—the glassy membrane—separates the external sheath from the dermis.

In many instances, hair follicles are associated with a thin bundle of smooth muscle—the arrector pili muscle, which extends obliquely from the follicle to the papillary dermis. Upon contraction, the hair is straightened, forming "goose bumps" in cold temperatures and making the hairs "stand on end" via sympathetic discharge in response to fright or panic. In animals with fur, the elevation of the hairs helps to trap air, which reduces heat loss in cold weather.

Tip: Hair follicles are normally found only in (most) body regions of thin skin. Remember that the scalp is thin skin. Hair follicles are usually accompanied by sebaceous glands.

Nails

Nails are plates of hard keratin equivalent to the stratum corneum (Fig 9.13a & b). Beneath the nail is the nail bed, consisting of the deeper layers of the epidermis. Deep to the ridge of soft skin (cuticle) at the proximal end of the nail is the nail matrix, containing the proliferative cells that form the growing nail. The white crescent-shaped lunula is the distal portion of the matrix; its color is determined partly by light scattering and partly by the thickness of the epithelial cells of the matrix. Normally nails grow 2–4 mm per month. A fingernail grows out completely in about 6–12 months, whereas toenails do the same in 12–18 months.

Cutaneous innervation

Sensory receptors in the skin are of two general types:
- Free or bare nerve endings
- Encapsulated nerve endings.

Free nerve endings

Small, bare nerve endings that are sensitive to pain are found in the epidermis and the dermis (Fig 9.14). They are also associated with hair follicles, where they act as mechanoreceptors. Sweat glands and vascular elements are associated with both sensory and autonomic nerve fibers.

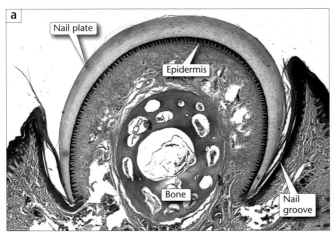

▲ **Fig 9.13a Cross section of nail plate.** Cross section through the distal end of a finger showing the hard keratin of the nail plate, deep to which is the serrated profile of the epidermis and the dermis of the nail bed. The epidermal stratum corneum moves distally with the growing nail. Between the nail and lateral skin fold is the nail groove. Cancellous bone of distal phalanx is indicated. H&E, paraffin, × 20.

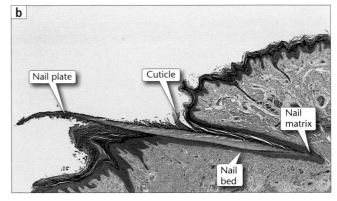

▲ **Fig 9.13b Longitudinal section of nail plate**, showing named parts. The matrix generates the nail plate, the eponychium is the cuticle, and the nail bed epidermis lacks the stratum granulosum, which is present in the other regions of skin. Masson's trichrome, paraffin, × 20.

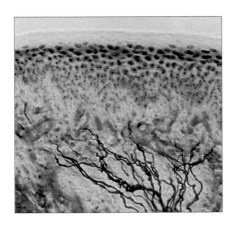

◀ **Fig 9.14 Free nerve endings.** The skin is supplied with free nerve endings that contribute to sensory perception, as evidenced by the patterns of the dermatomes (cutaneous branches of a spinal nerve). The fibers are often non-myelinated and branch profusely, and may respond to temperature and mechanical forces. Silver stain, paraffin, × 300.

Thermoreceptors are of two classes, warm and cold. They are supplied by afferent fibers that are related to spot-like receptive fields, called warm or cold spots. The receptor terminals are unencapsulated (i.e. they are free nerve endings) and are located in the epidermis 0.1–0.5 mm below the surface of the skin.

Encapsulated nerve endings

Encapsulated nerve endings include a variety of types that are mostly found in the dermis.

Meissner's corpuscles are bulbous nerve endings located in the papillary dermis just beneath the epidermis (Fig 9.15). Schwann cell processes surround the sensory nerve fiber and are arranged in stacks parallel to the skin surface. These receptors are sensitive to touch.

Pacinian corpuscles are about 1 mm in length and their internal structure resembles that of a sliced onion, with many concentric lamellae surrounding a central terminal axon (Fig 9.16a & b). Located deep in the dermis or in subcutaneous tissue, they tend to be more frequently seen in the fingers, but may occur throughout the dermis and in numerous organs and supporting tissues. These corpuscles are sensitive to pressure and vibration.

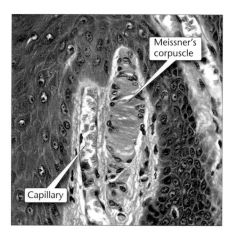

◀ **Fig 9.15 Meissner's corpuscle.** Meissner's corpuscles are encapsulated nerves that occur in the dermis, just beneath the epidermis. They are abundant in the tactile areas of the fingers and toes, and in the glabrous skin. An afferent nerve fiber may be linked to 14–25 corpuscles, forming flat discoidal sensory nerve endings with Schwann cells. The receptive fields of Meissner's corpuscles range from 2 mm to 8 mm in diameter. A capillary is also seen in this section. H&E, paraffin, × 250.

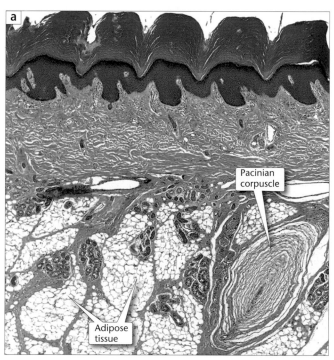

▲ **Fig 9.16a Pacinian corpuscles.** Located deep beneath the epidermis–dermis, Pacinian corpuscles are easily identified by their concentric layers of very thin cell processes surrounding a central axon. This specimen was selected from the palmar skin of the hand. These receptors are rapidly adapting, in that they discharge their signal at the onset of a stimulus, in this case high-frequency vibrations. H&E, paraffin, × 80.

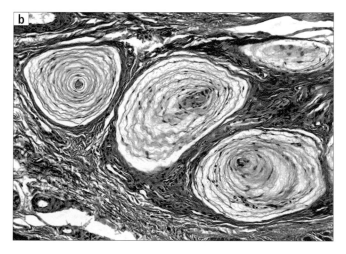

▲ **Fig 9.16b Pacinian corpuscles.** These encapsulated sensory nerve endings are about 1 mm in length. They are sensitive to deep pressure and vibration, and they occur in the subcutaneous tissue, particularly in the palms and soles, near joints and tendons, and in parts of the genital region. The core is an afferent axon, which disperses its processes into concentric lamellae that are associated with flat, adherent cells, giving the appearance of a sliced onion. H&E, paraffin, × 120.

Ruffini corpuscles, also found in the dermis, are encapsulated mechanoreceptors similar in structure to Golgi tendon organs (they are spindle-shaped), and their nerve fibers are associated with collagen fibrils.

Krause end-bulbs, located in the superficial parts of the dermis, show an arborizing pattern of sensory nerve fibers within a capsule; they are also thought to be mechanoreceptors.

SKIN DISORDERS
Eczema

Inflammation of the skin is commonly due to eczema or dermatitis; the two terms are medically synonymous. Eczema can run in families.

In infants it may occur in the skin creases of the knee and elbow, the trunk, and the face. Occasionally it occurs in conjunction with hay fever and asthma, and thus it may be symptomatic of an allergic reaction. In adults, it can occur in response to a range of chemicals, to jewellery, or to certain foods.

Cortisone applied directly to the affected skin can be very effective in reducing the inflammation.

Psoriasis

Psoriasis of the skin is associated with accelerated proliferation of keratinocytes producing pink-red inflammatory areas with flakes or plaques. Various treatments are effective in relieving symptoms, but the cause of this disorder remains unknown. The effectiveness of immunosuppressive agents in alleviating this disorder supports the notion that T cells may be involved.

Acne

Acne is associated with overactivity of the sebaceous glands, causing the sebum that is produced to block the excretory duct. The acne "spots," clinically known as comedones, that are seen on the skin may be black because of the presence of melanin (not dirt), or they may be white because of accumulated sebum. If the duct is ruptured, local inflammation occurs, because the skin bacteria convert the sebum into tissue-destructive agents, thereby causing increased inflammation and pus. Acne may be associated with increased production of sex hormones at puberty or with individual differences in skin sensitivity to the bacteria that promote inflammation. Antibiotic preparations can reduce the bacteria. "Spots" and acne usually disappear with age.

Abnormalities of pigmentation

Pigmentation of the skin may be increased or reduced in a number of conditions. In suntanning, more melanin than usual is produced in order to protect the skin from ultraviolet radiation. The ultraviolet-B (UVB) wavelength (290–320 nm) is the most dangerous with regard to the development of sunburn, dry and wrinkled skin, and skin cancer. Topical application of a sunscreen in conjunction with protective clothing and a hat is recommended for Caucasians before exposure to the sun.

Basal cell carcinoma, or solar keratosis, is a slow-growing cancer of the epidermis caused by cumulative sun exposure. It is non-malignant, and it may be removed surgically and repaired with skin grafting.

Malignant melanoma is a tumor of the melanocytes and, if untreated, is very often fatal. Melanomas are frequently associated with a history of sunburn or excessive sun exposure, but they may occur spontaneously (e.g. on the sole of the foot), possibly originating from a pigmented mole or nevus.

Yellowing of the skin is associated with jaundice and represents accumulation of bilirubin in the blood and tissues of the dermis. Neonates who are jaundiced may be treated by exposure to blue light, which is absorbed by the water-insoluble bilirubin, causing it to fade and become water-soluble. In this form, the bilirubin is removed from the dermis and blood, and excreted in the urine.

Owing to genetic mutation, people with albinism have an enzyme deficiency, which means that they fail to produce melanin. This affects the color of the skin, hair, and eyes. The skin is pale, the hair is silvery white, and the iris is pink.

Skin cancer

Cancer of the skin in Western countries is the most common cancer. About 80% of non-melanoma skin cancers are basal cell carcinomas and 20% are squamous cell carcinomas (SCCs), the latter being a common cancer in Caucasians. SCC is associated with a serious risk of metastasis. Exposure to UVB is a main causative factor and ultraviolet-A (UVA, 320–400 nm) adds to the risk. Mutations in DNA involving the p53 gene suppress cell apoptosis, leading to cell proliferation seen as keratoses, which are abnormal scale-like lesions. If untreated these may form tumors with invasive properties.

Vitamin D deficiency

With appropriate exposure to sunlight, the skin provides the body with vitamin D_3, which is later converted in the liver and, finally, in the kidneys, to the active form of vitamin D. Vitamin D is in fact a hormone, not a vitamin, and is essential for normal mineralization of bone and maintenance of calcium homeostasis. Chronic lack of exposure of the skin to solar radiation may result in rickets if dietary intake of vitamin D-rich foods (fish-liver oils, egg yolks) is inadequate. Commercial milk supplies are commonly fortified with vitamin D, and this essentially eliminates the development of rickets.

Wounds

Healing of the skin is required in response to a wound or to burning. Superficial cuts or abrasions repair relatively quickly, depending on their severity and skin age. These wounds may show blood clots followed by scab formation, the latter being a mixture of clotting proteins and fibroblasts. Pus forms if bacterial infection occurs; the pus contains dead white blood cells and bacteria. The epidermis regenerates beneath the scab.

Scar tissue forms in response to more severe wounds and contains more collagen than its surroundings. Overproduction of the connective tissue in a scar forms a keloid—a firm, raised area of the skin. Recent studies on experimentally induced wounds in mice have shown that re-epithelialized skin in healed wounds generates new hair follicles in the center of the wound.

This suggests that healing with repair (scar tissue) is a different process from healing with regeneration.

Burns

Burns are classified as superficial (previously known as first degree), partial thickness (previously second degree) and full thickness (previously third degree), reflecting their severity. Sunburn is a superficial burn and does not require special treatment. Partial-thickness burns involve partial destruction of the epidermis and the dermis; they result in blistering and, in some cases, the healing process forms scar tissue. In full-thickness burns, the subcutaneous tissues are destroyed as well, and fluid loss, infection, and loss of cutaneous sensation are serious complications. Skin transplantation is usually required.

Skeletal tissues

The skeleton is a remarkable example of specialized connective tissues brought together to form a living tissue with great strength, yet minimal weight. Bone is a masterpiece of biomechanical engineering that provides support, protection, locomotion (acting as levers through muscle action), a repository for hemopoietic tissues, and storage for calcium and phosphorus. Mature bone is a dynamic, living tissue that is constantly turning over—older bone is resorbed but is continuously replaced by deposition of new bone. The ability of bone to regenerate and repair following fracture is self-evident, and it is one of few tissues that can heal without scar formation. Bone is a source of pluripotent mesenchymal stem cells, which proliferate and differentiate into various cell lineages that include bone marrow, vessels, adipose tissue, cartilage, and cells specialized to make bone. In many joints, the bony articular surfaces are covered with articular hyaline cartilage, which acts as a shock absorber with almost frictionless surfaces for joint movement. Unlike bone, articular cartilage cannot regenerate itself if damaged or diseased, and this can lead to osteoarthrosis.

As an organ, bone consists of bone tissue (mineralized connective tissue), cartilage, vessels, an adherent covering of connective tissue, bone marrow, and fat. For medical and paramedical students, an understanding of skeletal structure and function is essential in clinical practice (e.g. for the diagnosis and management of fractures, the recognition of growth abnormalities, and a proper appreciation of pathologic changes and metabolic disorders that affect bone function).

In this chapter, skeletal biology is reviewed, considering first the histology of adult bone and then the mechanisms by which bone is developed. A common area of confusion in bone histology is bone's relationship to cartilage, because for most bones (except most of the skull, the facial bones, and the clavicle) a cartilaginous precursor is formed in the embryo. This cartilaginous precursor is replaced by bone as the embryo grows. An understanding of this process is facilitated by a closer examination of the fully formed tissue—the mature bone.

ADULT BONE
Basic structure

All adult bone tissue has a similar structure, consisting of cells and matrix with a neurovascular supply.

Bone formation always follows the same pattern—the synthesis of an initial, non-mineralized (non-calcified) organic matrix that is rich in collagen—osteoid (prebone or preosseous tissue)—which is then converted to mineralized or calcified bone. Bone deposition depends on the prior availability of a suitable base, which is either collagen-rich connective tissue or a cartilaginous matrix. Most bones are formed from the latter.

Macroscopically, two types of adult bone can be distinguished. Cortical bone (also known as compact or dense bone) is hard and commonly thick (e.g. the tubular shaft of long bones) and represents about 80% of skeletal weight. The inner cancellous bone (also known as spongy or trabecular bone) forms a honeycomb-type network enclosing cavities filled with bone marrow. It resembles a scaffold with a large surface area, and the orientation of trabeculae relate to the mechanical loads placed upon the bone. The principal components are shown in Figure 10.1a–c.

Components of bone

Bone is a natural composite material, comprising about 90% extracellular matrix and 10% water by weight (Fig 10.2).

The matrix is about 65% inorganic mineral, predominantly microcrystalline calcium phosphate in the form of hydroxyapatite $[Ca_{10}(PO_4)_6(OH)_2]$ with traces of sodium, magnesium, fluoride, and other ions.

The organic component of the matrix, about 25% of bone weight, is type I collagen, with non-collagenous proteins (glycosaminoglycans and other matrix proteins) that are uniquely found in bone and assist with mineralization.

Woven (immature) bone

Cortical and cancellous bone display a consistent structure that results from the transformation of osteoid matrix into an ordered pattern of mineralized bone. Immature bone of the fetus has collagen fibrils arranged in random patterns, in contrast to mature bone, which is characterized by regularly arranged sheets or layers/lamellae containing collagen fibrils. The former type of bone is classified as woven bone if collagen fibrils run in various directions or if they are parallel but not yet frequently or consistently layered (this is also occasionally termed bundle or parallel-fibered bone). This arrangement is referred

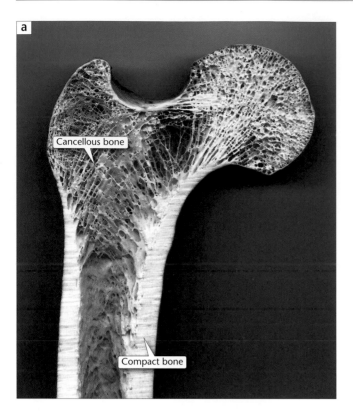

◀ **Fig 10.1a Architecture of bone.** Coronal section through adult dried femur, showing internal organization of plates and struts of cancellous bone with cavities between for bone marrow. Trabeculae of cancellous bone are aligned parallel to the forces applied to the bone. The head and greater trochanter have a thin shell of compact bone. From the inferior neck region and distally along the shaft (diaphysis), the cortex consists of a thick cylinder of compact bone.

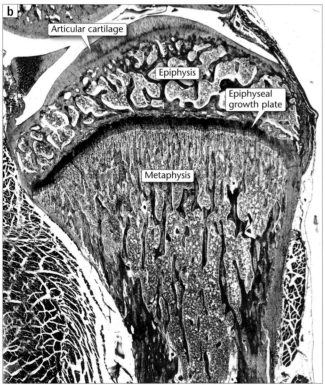

◀ **Fig 10.1b Architecture of bone.** Histologic section of rat tibia, showing epiphyseal growth plate separating epiphysis and metaphysis. Internally the cancellous bone forms networks of interconnected trabeculae, the gaps between which are filled in with bone marrow. Facing the joint space, the bone end is covered with hyaline articular cartilage. Masson's trichrome, paraffin, × 12.

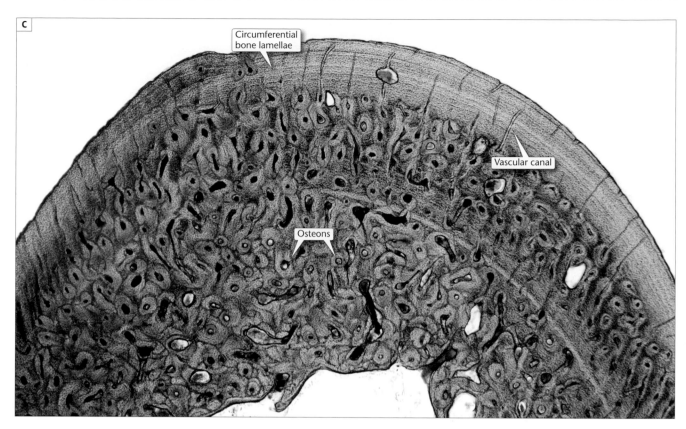

c

Circumferential bone lamellae

Vascular canal

Osteons

▲ **Fig 10.1c Architecture of bone.** Unstained slice of cortical bone about 200 μm thick, after formalin fixation and extraction and removal of fibro-fatty tissues. Osteons (cylinders of bone tissue) cut in various planes show a central vascular Haversian canal surrounded by concentric lamellae of bone. Entering via the circumferential layers of bone are numerous vascular canals that supply the whole tissue. × 30.

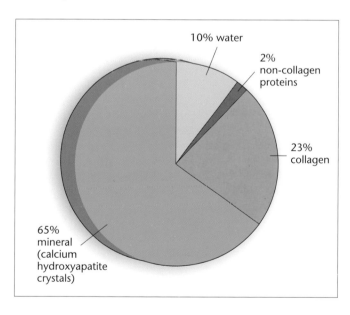

10% water

2% non-collagen proteins

23% collagen

65% mineral (calcium hydroxyapatite crystals)

◀ **Fig 10.2 Composition of bone.** Approximate proportions by weight of adult cortical bone. About 25% is organic, 10% is water, and 65% is mineral. The organic matrix is mostly collagen type I and the non-collagenous proteins are concerned with regulating mineralization or stabilizing the mineralized matrix, or with bone resorption.

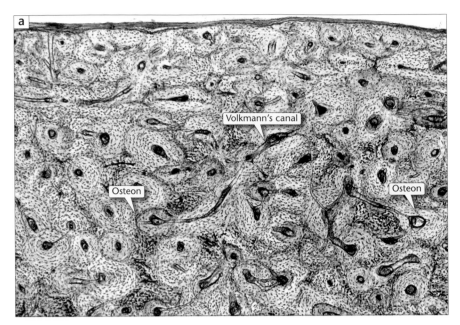

▲ **Fig 10.3a Adult compact bone.** Unstained ground section of compact bone with osteons (cylinders of bone tissue), the fundamental structural units of mature compact bone. Osteons show central vascular Haversian canals that communicate with other osteons via Volkmann's canals. The particulate nature of osteons represents their many osteocytes embedded in the bone matrix. × 50.

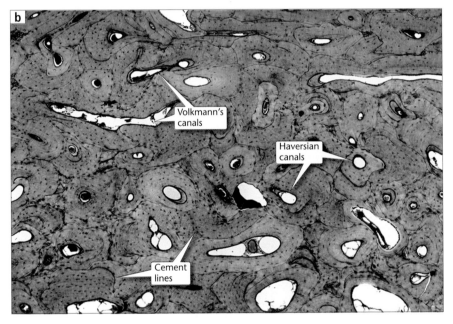

▲ **Fig 10.3b Adult compact bone.** Decalcified histologic section of compact bone, with the boundaries of osteons identified by thin, dense cement lines that are hypermineralized with less collagen than normal bone matrix. Empty spaces are vascular (Haversian) canals in the center of osteons and form linkages (Volkmann's canals) between osteons. Many dark spots in osteons represent the osteocytes. Hematoxylin and eosin (H&E), paraffin, × 60.

to as nonlamellar bone. Woven bone is formed in the growing skeleton, particularly in the fetus, and in adults during phases of rapid bone remodeling such as post-fracture repair. Immature bone is mineralized, but is eventually replaced with mature, lamellar bone.

Lamellar bone

As the name suggests, lamellar bone consists of orderly strata or layers of bone matrix and densely aggregated collagen fibers.

Compact bone

Compact bone is found in the shaft of long bones and at the surface of flat or irregular-shaped bones (Fig 10.3a & b). It consists of cylinders (oriented mainly parallel to the long axis) that have concentric layers, or lamellae, of mineralized bone matrix. These layers resemble the growth rings of a tree trunk (Fig 10.4a–e). Scattered rather uniformly throughout the lamellae are minute cavities occupied by bone cells called osteocytes. Their numerous thin processes extend into the surrounding bone matrix inside tiny canaliculi. (The physiologic significance of osteocyte

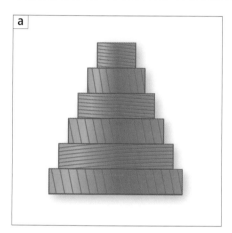

◀ **Fig 10.4a Collagen orientation.** Scheme of orientation of collagen in individual concentric bony lamellae that make up the osteon. Each lamella shows different directions of its collagen that in combination confer on bone greater resistance to stress applied from any direction. During osteon construction, the outermost lamella is formed first, with inner lamellae deposited within one another in succession.

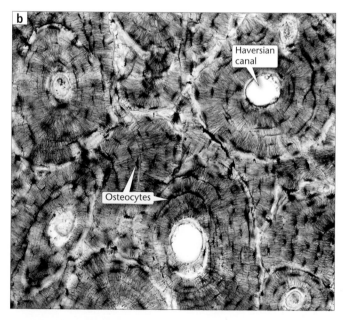

▲ **Fig 10.4b Osteons in compact bone.** Fixed, undecalcified, ground section of compact bone showing osteons with central Haversian canals. Arranged in concentric circles the flat nuclei of osteocytes trapped in small cavities or lacunae are noted. Many fine processes extend from osteocytes into the tissue. These are narrow spaces in the bone matrix called canaliculi and they contain cell processes arising from the osteocytes. × 165.

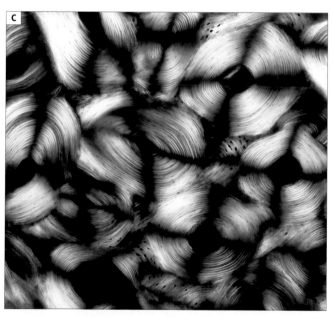

▲ **Fig 10.4c Structure of osteons.** Unstained, ground section viewed with plane-polarized light, which emphasizes the concentric lamellae of bone in each osteon. Cell nuclei are not visible in osteons but are seen in the interstitial bone lamellae between osteons. Alternating bright and black rings arise owing to orientation of mineralized collagen with respect to the polarized light waves. Bright rings have collagen that transmits light (i.e. oriented transversely to the axis of light direction). Black rings represent collagen oriented in a direction that absorbs light (i.e. aligned along the axis of light direction). Bone matrix collagen is thus organized in different directions, both within and between osteon lamellae. × 165.

morphology is discussed in the section below on bone cells.) Passing centrally through each of the bone cylinders, a neurovascular canal provides nutrient supply to the tissue. In compact bone each cylinder is termed an osteon or Haversian system (named after Havers, who first described them in 1691). Osteons are typically 200–250 µm in diameter, and often 3–5 mm in length, but they can be 10 mm or longer. Woven bone in neonates is progressively replaced during postnatal life, and in 2-year-olds the femoral cortex consists largely of osteons.

Osteons occur in large numbers, depending on bone thickness. In a cross section of the midshaft of the adult femur, the cortical bone may be 1 cm in width and display many thousands of osteon profiles (Fig 10.5).

Osteons may end blindly, often show multiple branching into four or five descendants, and tend to follow a gentle spiral around the long axis of a bone (Fig 10.6). This structural feature may contribute to the spiral or oblique course commonly taken by fractures of long bones. In adult bone several bony lamellae (like layers of plywood) may extend around the outer limits of the bone. These are known as the circumferential lamellae and may also be found lining the inner circumference of the bone shaft.

The branching patterns of osteons are evident from the continuity of the central vascular (Haversian) canals between osteons, the external bone surface, and the bone marrow cavity. The channels that link osteons are called Volkmann's canals and are the route by which blood vessels supply the osteons. Volkmann's canals are not usually surrounded by concentric bone lamellae, which distinguishes them from Haversian canals.

Osteons are not permanent, but are continuously being replaced by bone remodeling (i.e. a process of bone resorption and deposition of new bone). Between the osteons are angular pieces of lamellar bone, which are termed interstitial lamellae. These are persistent remnants of older osteons that have been partly obliterated during the lifelong internal reorganization of bone. In adult bone, loss is normally matched exactly by new bone deposition.

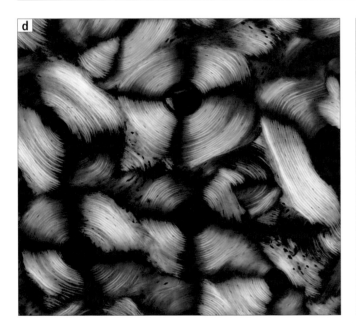

▲ **Fig 10.4d Collagen bundles in osteons.** Osteons viewed with polarized light using a 530 nm tint plate inserted between specimen and analyzer. The mineralized collagen bundles are yellow if parallel to the vibration direction of light, and blue when perpendicular to this direction. Orientation of collagen bundles in osteons is non-random and contributes to the strength and hardness of compact bone. × 200.

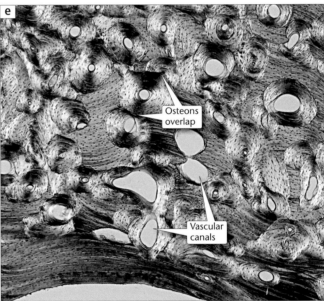

▲ **Fig 10.4e Osteons and lamellar bone.** When the specimen is viewed with partly crossed polarized light optics, the relationship of osteons to interstitial lamellar bone is revealed. Note how some osteons overlap others, illustrating that osteons are not highly organized in space but are arranged in somewhat random positions. The location and size of osteons is determined by their resorption (obliteration) and renewal (reconstruction), both normal processes in healthy bone. × 75.

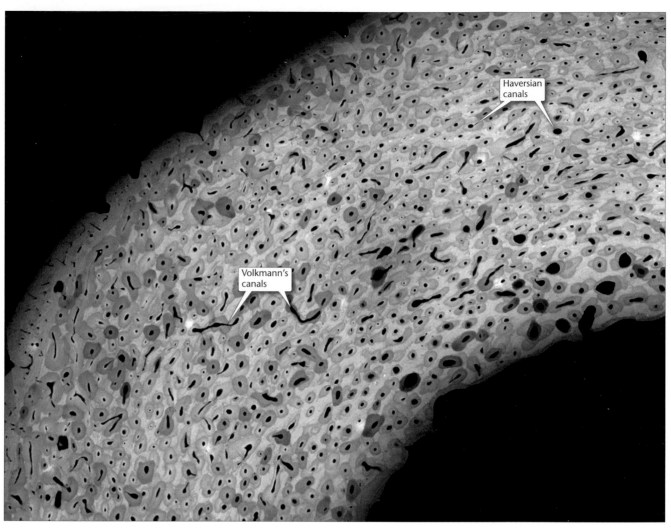

▲ **Fig 10.5 Osteon populations.** Microradiograph of adult human femoral midshaft fixed in 70% alcohol and ground to 100 μm in thickness. Areas of black in the tissue represent Haversian or Volkmann's canals of osteons, or tissue being remodeled by resorption. Osteons are densely packed and lie within surrounding interstitial lamellar bone. In the complete cross section there are tens of thousands of osteons, most of which are aligned parallel to the long axis of the bone. × 20. (Courtesy S Feik, D Thomas, J Clement, School of Dental Science, University of Melbourne, Australia.)

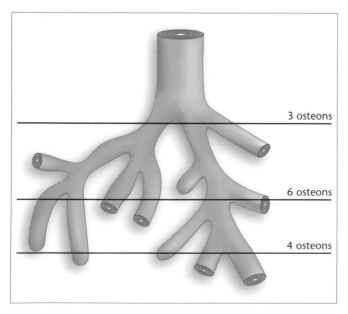

◀ **Fig 10.6 Branching of individual osteons.** Individual osteons may branch and intertwine, as tree roots do, so that in various sectional planes different numbers of osteons are observed. Some osteons end blindly; others may terminate as non-osteonal vascular channels. Depending on the species and the particular bone, groups of osteons may be longitudinally or spirally oriented with respect to the long axis of the bone. This arrangement explains why, in thick transverse sections of bone, osteons may appear circular or elliptical in cross section.

Cancellous bone

Cancellous bone, also known as spongy or trabecular bone, is lighter than compact bone, but is irregular in structure. It consists of bone matrix in the form of struts or plates called trabeculae, which are commonly 100–300 µm in thickness and spaced 300–1,500 µm apart (Fig 10.7a & b). The matrix of cancellous bone often shows a pattern of parallel lamellae, in contrast to the concentric arrangement in compact bone.

Cancellous bone is very porous; about 80% of its volume is made up of pores filled with bone marrow. The many beams and bridges characteristic of cancellous bone serve to minimize mass, but it retains considerable resistance against disruptive forces placed upon it (Fig 10.8a & b). Occasionally cancellous bone shows remnants of osteons remodeled into trabeculae that lack central canals. This is the result of bone remodeling that is probably controlled by matrix strain

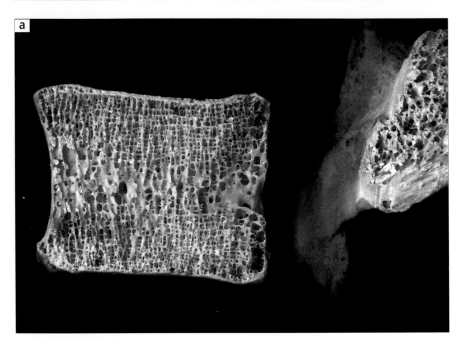

◀ **Fig 10.7a Cancellous bone.** Sagittal view of human lumbar vertebral body. In contrast to long bones the cortical compact bone with the medulla is mainly spongy-type bone resembling a honeycomb. The porous structure reduces bone weight but retains strength and is a repository for hemopoietic tissue. In situations of bone loss such as osteoporosis, the trabeculae of the cancellous bone become thin, reduced in number, and may result in "compression fracture."

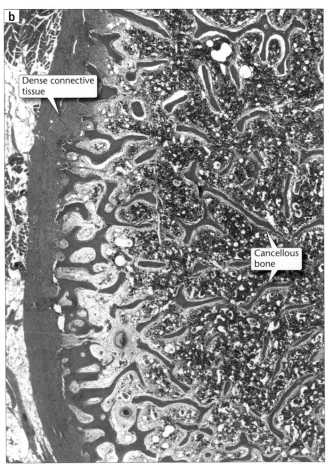

Dense connective tissue

Cancellous bone

◀ **Fig 10.7b Trabeculae in cancellous bone.** Histologic section of a growing rib showing many profiles of trabeculae typical of cancellous bone. Bone marrow occupies the intervening spaces. Although the bone in trabeculae is lamellar, there are no osteons owing to the lack of blood vessels within the bone matrix. Accordingly, the supply of nutrients to cancellous bone places an upper limit on trabecular thickness. H&E, paraffin, × 30.

caused by mechanical loading; it produces irregular associations of lamellae. As a general rule, cancellous bone lacks true osteons because it is not penetrated by blood vessels.

Periosteum and endosteum

Periosteum is a layer of vascularized connective tissue covering the outer surfaces of bones, except for articular surfaces and the insertion sites of tendons and ligaments. The periosteum is the route by which blood vessels and nerves gain access to bone tissue and the bone marrow. It has a superficial fibrous component and an inner osteogenic layer adjacent to the bone. Depending on the size and type of individual bone, periosteum may be a delicate, loose connective tissue sheet or a dense, fibrous membrane (Fig 10.9a & b). Both may be stripped from the

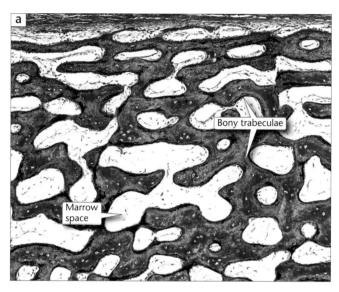

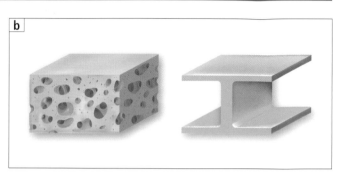

▲ **Fig 10.8b Strength of cancellous bone.** The structure of cancellous bone can be compared to that of a steel beam; while providing rigidity, the bone structure weighs less than an equivalent body constructed entirely as a solid mass.

▲ **Fig 10.8a Strength of cancellous bone.** In adult spongy bone, fully developed trabeculae are united to form a structure that is lighter in weight compared with dense compact bone, but which remains resistant to mechanical loading. The blue-stained core is fully mineralized bone with embedded osteocytes; red-stained surface segments are not fully ossified, representing sites of new bone deposition. Marrow spaces have been extracted during tissue preparation. H&E/alcian blue, paraffin, × 60.

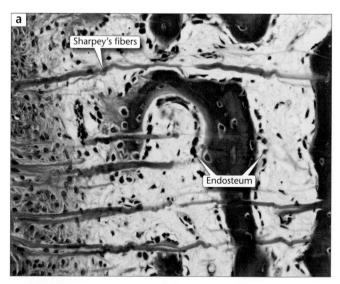

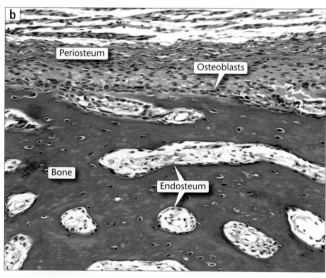

▲ **Fig 10.9a Periosteum and endosteum.** Attachment of periosteum to bone is reinforced by Sharpey's collagen fibers, which penetrate deeper bone much like nails driven through plywood. Rows of osteoprogenitor cells follow the contours of bone and constitute the endosteum. When required, endosteal cells are the source of osteoblasts, which produce new bone, which is added in layers to the surface of preexisting bone. H&E, paraffin, × 200.

▲ **Fig 10.9b Periosteum and endosteum.** An outer fibrous and inner cellular layer make up the periosteum, both layers containing blood vessels and nerves. At the interface with bone, rows of osteoblasts and osteoclasts are present. Osteoblasts add bone and osteoclasts resorb it, thereby contributing to the modeling process (shape) and remodeling process (internal architecture). Spaces within the bone tissue are lined with endosteum. H&E, paraffin, × 110.

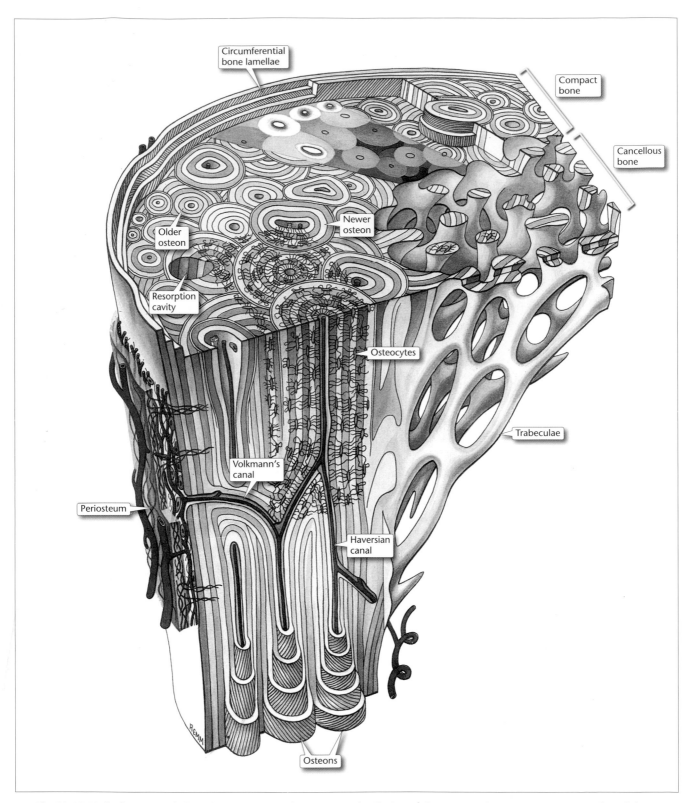

▲ **Fig 10.10 Main features of the microstructure of mature lamellar bone.** Areas of compact and trabecular (cancellous) bones are included. The central gray area in the transverse section simulates a microradiograph, the densities reflecting variations in mineralization. Note the general construction of the osteons; distribution of the osteocyte lacunae; Haversian canals and their contents; resorption cavity; and the different views of the structural basis of bone lamellation. (Reproduced with permission from Gray's anatomy: the anatomical basis of clinical practice, 39th edn. Susan Standring, editor-in-chief. Churchill-Livingstone, Edinburgh, 2005.)

bone surface, but the boundary with the bone is anchored to varying extent by bundles of collagen called Sharpey's fibers. These may extend for several millimeters into the bone tissue. Endosteum lines the internal surfaces of bone, including the Haversian canals, but is very much thinner and more cellular. Periosteum and endosteum are characterized by osteoprogenitor or bone-lining cells, which act as stem cells for the generation of bone-forming cells of the osteoblast lineage.

Generic morphology of adult bone

When all the above features are combined, an overall picture of the histology of adult bone can be represented schematically (Fig 10.10).

STRUCTURE AND FUNCTION OF BONE CELLS

Adult bone contains four types of cells, which are classified according to their location and function:

- Osteoprogenitor cells—precursor cells that self-replicate or differentiate into bone-forming cells
- Osteoblasts—bone-forming cells that deposit osteoid and control subsequent mineralization
- Osteocytes—modified osteoblasts that become surrounded by newly formed bone
- Osteoclasts—macrophage-type cells that resorb bone.

Each of these cell types is in various ways interactive and their functions are coordinated to fulfill the major role of maintenance of healthy bone tissue. In this dynamic organ, with a significant turnover of its tissues through bone formation and resorption, the functions of osteoblasts, osteocytes, and osteoclasts are coupled and regulated in space and time. Together these cells form a basic multicellular unit (BMU), which is a site for bone remodeling that occurs asynchronously throughout the skeleton. The role of the BMU in remodeling is reviewed later.

Osteoprogenitor cells

Osteoprogenitor cells are mesenchymal cells of bone and bone marrow that develop into osteoblasts if new bone is being formed. Where new bone is not required, these cells are quiescent and are called bone-lining cells; in these cases they are located in the layers covering the external bone surface, the periosteum (Fig 10.11) and in the internal surfaces facing the marrow cavities, the endosteum. They resemble fibroblasts and are called periosteal or endosteal cells. Bone-lining cells of the endosteum are accompanied by collagen fibers apposed to the bone surface. Osteoprogenitor cells are activated following fracture, during growth, or in various disorders of bone growth.

Osteoblasts

Osteoblasts are derived from osteoprogenitor cells and also line periosteal and endosteal surfaces, forming a single layer of cuboidal-type cells that produce unmineralized organic osteoid matrix. Osteoid is deposited or apposed to a suitable surface only when new bone is required during growth, in response to fracture, or in remodeling of adult bone (Fig 10.11, Fig 10.12a & b). Osteoid matrix consists of type I collagen and non-collagenous matrix proteins that include proteoglycans, glycoproteins, and bone-specific proteins.

Osteoblasts regulate the way in which osteoid becomes mineralized bone. Woven bone forms more

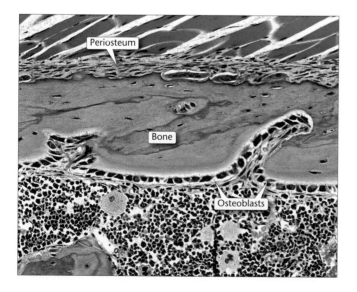

◀ **Fig 10.11 Osteoprogenitor or bone-lining cells.** These cells are of mesenchymal origin and differentiate into osteoblasts, which produce bone matrix. When quiescent they are small fibroblast-type cells found in the deep periosteum, where they may coexist with osteoclasts, the latter derived from bone marrow. The row of epitheloid-type cells following the endosteal bone surface are the activated osteoblasts, among which are slender osteoprogenitor cells. H&E, paraffin, × 190.

rapidly than lamellar bone, with osteoid becoming mineralized within several days; however, full mineralization in adults may take up to 100 days. Osteoblasts release matrix vesicles, which are 100 nm in diameter and rich in calcium-binding proteins (annexin, phosphatidyl serine) and phosphatases (alkaline phosphatase, pyrophosphatase) concentrated in or near the vesicle membrane. At this time matrix vesicles do not contain mineral. The release of polarized matrix vesicles toward recently formed osteoid matrix ensures the non-random commencement of mineralization. In phase I of mineral crystal formation, calcium and phosphate ions accumulate in vesicles, resulting in the precipitation of $CaPO_4$ non-crystalline mineral, which is then transformed into insoluble hydroxyapatite crystals. Phase II is initiated when matrix vesicles are ruptured by the crystals, thereby exposing them to the extracellular fluid, which is supersaturated with respect to apatite. This encourages further crystal nucleation to occur, and is additionally promoted by contact with osteoid collagen, which serves to nucleate and orient newly forming apatite crystals. As osteoid is mineralized into mature bone, the proportion of collagen as matrix is reduced (from 30% to about 20% dry weight) and other matrix proteins decline (from 10% to 1%), but mineral (in the form of calcium salts) increases from 10% to about 65%.

Lamellar bone formation takes around 10–15 days between osteoid production and mineralization, with full mineralization achieved after several months. Upon cessation of bone formation, osteoblasts transform into either osteocytes or bone-lining cells.

Osteocytes

Osteocytes are recognized when osteoblasts become entombed by mineralized matrix, where they may remain as terminally differentiated cells for years, sometimes decades. The spaces they occupy in the bone, called lacunae, are distributed in concentric patterns in the lamellae of cortical bone but randomly in lamellar cancellous bone.

Cytoplasmic processes extend from osteocytes inside thin tunnels, or canaliculi, that radiate from the lacunae into surrounding bone (Fig 10.13a–d). Canaliculi of adjacent osteocytes are continuous channels containing fluid in communication with the extracellular fluid space in the central canal.

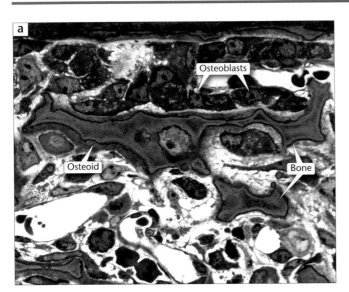

◀ **Fig 10.12a Osteoblasts.** Osteoblasts are closely apposed to preexisting bone and separated from it by a seam of osteoid (unmineralized matrix), which osteoblasts secrete. Note how osteoid is of uniform thickness and shows a different staining response compared with mineralized bone because of its initial low mineral content. The osteoid seam is progressively mineralized facing the bone, with new osteoid matrix added on the opposite aspect. Osteoblasts direct the mineralization of osteoid by accumulation and growth of $CaPO_4$. Toluidine blue, araldite, × 570.

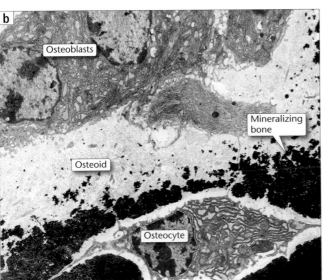

◀ **Fig 10.12b Ultrastructure of osteoblasts and the mineralization front.** Packed with rough ER, the osteoblasts are secreting osteoid, which partly surrounds one cell that is destined to become embedded in mineralizing osteoid. At that time it will be identified as an osteocyte, and may remain there for months or years. Mineralizing bone is very electron-dense, and many individual spots represent sites of mineral nucleation and crystallization that originate from matrix vesicles (not visible) secreted by the osteoblasts. × 4,700. (Courtesy Pavelka M and Roth J. Functional ultrastructure. Vienna: Springer-Verlag, 2005.)

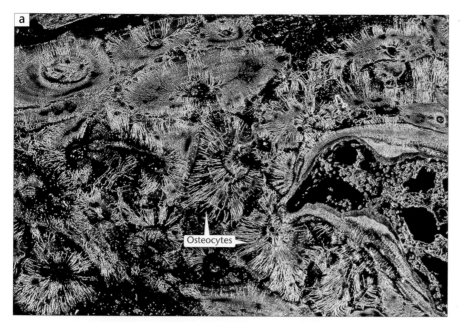

◀ Fig 10.13a Osteocytes. Silver-stained ground section of compact bone viewed with darkfield microscopy. This optical technique shows to advantage the enormous surface area presented by the thin, cytoplasmic extensions of osteocytes. One purpose of this arrangement is to provide an interface between the bone matrix through which they pass and the extracellular fluid that bathes the extensions. Because bone is a living tissue with a rich blood supply, the osteocytes provide the mechanism by which the levels of calcium and phosphate in blood and their storage in bone are kept in balance. A filtrate of blood reaches the osteocytes via the vascular Haversian canals. × 100.

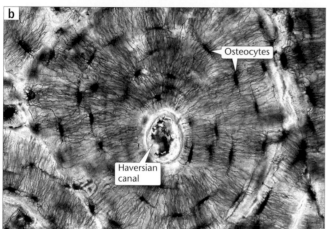

◀ Fig 10.13b Osteocytes. Unstained ground section of an osteon with a central Haversian canal surrounded by several rings of dense, flattened lacunae in which osteocytes are trapped. Fine canaliculi extend radially from the lacunae and interconnect with continuity to the Haversian canal. × 280.

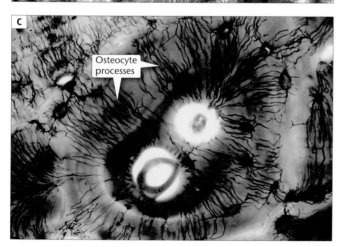

▲ Fig 10.13c Canaliculi. Histologic section of compact bone after the tissue was infiltrated with silver salt solution. Silver stains the lacunae and their canaliculi, many of which appear to be in contact with the central vascular spaces of the Haversian canals. Tissue fluid derived from blood may therefore access all regions of osteons through the canalicular system, which contains gap junction–linked cytoplasmic extensions of the osteocytes. Silver stain, paraffin, × 360.

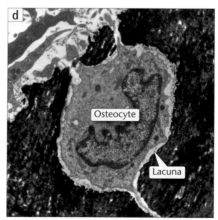

▲ Fig 10.13d Ultrastructure of the osteocyte, separated from the bone matrix by a narrow space called the lacuna. Thin cytoplasmic extensions within canalicular spaces are noted. At their termination these extensions are attached via gap junctions to corresponding extensions from nearby osteocytes. Canaliculi and their cell processes are the structures that maintain physiological links between the living osteocytes and serve to distribute nutrients to and from Haversian canals. × 8,000. (Courtesy A Pierce, Dental School, University of Adelaide, Australia.)

Nutrient supply of lamellar bone is derived from blood vessels in the canals or from periosteal and endosteal surfaces. Cytoplasmic processes of neighboring osteocytes make contact via gap junctions, allowing ionic exchange.

Osteocytes are considered to be mechanosensory cells that regulate the composition of bone matrix via ion–nutrient exchange, thereby ensuring maintenance of serum calcium and phosphate levels via the effects of parathyroid hormone and vitamin D analogs. The total surface area of the osteocyte–canalicular system available for calcium exchange is 300–500 m².

With aging and reduction in blood supply, osteocytes may die and be replaced with mineral (micropetrosis), making bone more brittle. Alternatively they may be destroyed as bone is remodeled via the resorption action of osteoclasts.

Osteoclasts

Osteoclasts are large (>40 μm in diameter) multinucleated phagocytic cells that break down calcified matrices. They originate from hemopoietic progenitor cells and are not related to bone-forming cells. In order for osteoclasts to resorb bone, a mechanism must exist that determines which bone surface will be targeted. This is one of the functions of the BMU, which is activated by mechanical forces, bone cell turnover, hormones (e.g. parathyroid hormone), cytokines, and local factors. In cases of microcracking or reduction in mechanical loading, the lining cells of endosteum are retracted with digestion of the endosteal collagen membrane by matrix metalloproteinases. Osteoclasts are recruited to these sites and attach to bone via actin-based adhesion structures called podosomes. The foot-like podosomes form a tight annular seal, analogous to certain molluscs such as rock-clinging limpets. The interface between the osteoclast and bone is the site of resorption, creating a recess known as Howship's lacuna (Fig 10.14a–d). Erosion of bone starts with its demineralization, which the osteoclast achieves by acidification within the lacuna. The osteoclast forms carbonic acid from CO_2 and water; the carbonic acid dissociates to bicarbonate and a proton. Protons are transported across the cell membrane into the lacuna, raising the pH to 4–5 in the extracellular space, where the bone apatite is degraded. After digestion of the mineral, the organic matrix is exposed and is degraded by lysosomes, particularly cathepsin K, and metalloproteinases secreted by the osteoclast. Having excavated a lacuna, the osteoclast may move to a new site or undergo apoptosis.

In cancellous bone, the cavities produced in trabeculae are replaced with new lamellae. In cortical bone, osteoclasts bore a tunnel, or resorption canal (about 200 μm in diameter), through the bone; in this canal capillaries and bone-forming cells are carried.

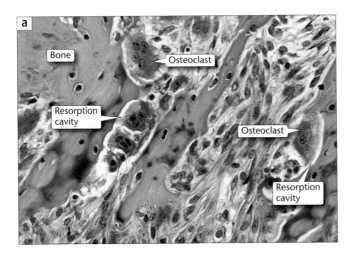

▲ **Fig 10.14a Osteoclasts.** As a type of phagocytic cell, the osteoclast is derived from the monocyte lineage in bone marrow and therefore is separate from the osteoprogenitor cell lineage. Osteoclasts are identified by their position close to a bone (or calcified cartilage) surface and by their multiple nuclei that arise by fusions of precursor cells when osteoclast activity is required. The gap between the osteoclast and bone is the Howship resorption cavity (Howship's lacuna), in which mineral and organic components of bone are degraded by the cell. Masson's trichrome, paraffin, × 350.

Tunnels are refilled with layers of lamellar bone, starting peripherally and advancing inward toward the capillaries, forming a new osteon (see section on remodeling below).

Osteoblast–osteoclast communication

Osteoclast and osteoblast activities are coordinated such that bone resorption is normally followed by new bone deposition—therefore bone mass remains stable. Osteoclastogenesis is dependent on two cytokines, both produced by osteoblasts: receptor activator of nuclear factor-κB ligand (RANKL) and monocyte-colony stimulation factor (M-CSF). M-CSF controls proliferation of osteoclast precursors and RANKL directly controls osteoclast differentiation by activating RANK on osteoclast precursors.

Parathyroid hormone and vitamin D derivatives stimulate bone resorption, whereas calcitonin inhibits osteoclast activity directly or via local interactive effects mediated through osteoblasts. Leptin (a protein hormone produced by adipose cells), acting on the hypothalamus, stimulates bone resorption via sympathetic nerves that activate the osteoblast–osteoclast RANKL/RANK pathway. Conversely, recent research has shown that leptin and sympathetic tone (basal nerve activity) regulate the molecular circadian

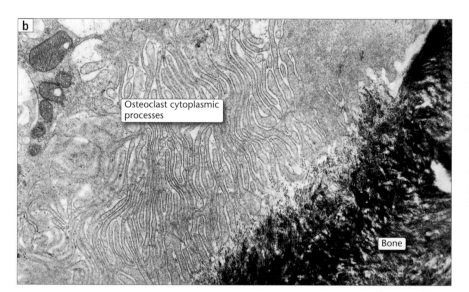

◀ **Fig 10.14b Ultrastructure of osteoclast cytoplasm within a resorption cavity**, showing the typical "ruffled" membrane across which the cell secretes acid to dissolve mineral, and a range of lysosomal enzymes for digestion of the organic components of bone. The clear zone has abundant actin filaments and is the limit of the resorption cavity, which is defined by the ring-like attachment of the osteoclast to the bone. × 15,000. (Courtesy Pavelka M and Roth J. Functional ultrastructure. Vienna: Springer-Verlag, 2005.)

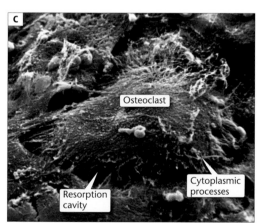

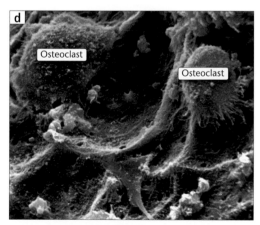

▲ **Fig 10.14c Osteoclast with membrane ruffling.** Scanning electron micrograph of an osteoclast, showing the peripheral fringe of membrane ruffling associated with the ventral surface, deep to which is the Howship resorption cavity on the bone surface. × 1,000. (Courtesy A Pierce, Dental School, University of Adelaide, Australia.)

▲ **Fig 10.14d Bone surface excavations by osteoclasts.** Scanning electron micrograph of excavations of bone surface made by osteoclasts, several of which are actively resorbing bone to form new concavities. × 1,000. (Courtesy A Pierce, Dental School, University of Adelaide, Australia; from Pierce AM, et al. Electron Microsc Rev 1991; 4:1–45.)

clock genes in osteoblasts to increase bone formation and mass. Estrogen exerts a bone-protective effect by inhibiting osteoblast RANKL production. It also stimulates osteoblasts to produce osteoprotegerin, a cytokine that masks RANKL and thus prevents osteoclast differentiation. Estrogen deficiency accompanying menopause is associated with net bone loss and increased risk of fracture.

> **Tip:** The processes of biomineralization, directed by osteoblasts, have some parallels with the simple recipe for growing crystals such as copper sulfate. To start the process, a seed crystal is introduced into a saturated solution and acts as a nucleating point for crystal growth. Similarly, rupture of tiny crystal needles from osteoblast-derived matrix vesicles act as the nucleators for early growth of hydroxyapatite crystals (up to 40 nm) in extracellular fluid.

DEVELOPMENT AND GROWTH OF BONE

Bone can normally be formed only by deposition on a suitable, preexisting, naturally occurring matrix (e.g. bone matrix or calcified cartilage) or solid surface (e.g. a prosthesis) that is in close proximity to a blood supply. These two criteria place limitations on the shape and size of developing bone; that is, newly formed bone is deposited in layers with a variety of shapes (flat, curved, undulating), and mineralization sites must be within 200 μm of a capillary to receive nutrients via diffusion. Most skull and facial bones and the clavicular bones form by intramembranous ossification in areas of mesenchyme. The axial and appendicular skeleton, especially the long bones, forms by endochondral ossification in areas of cartilage (Fig 10.15).

These descriptive terms do not imply that the ossification process in the skull or long bones differs, since the mechanisms of bone formation are the same regardless of the site of development. The morphology of bone is specified in the genetic blueprint; fetal limb buds grown in vitro are programmed to develop into the shapes of the respective adult bones. The terms intramembranous ossification and endochondral ossification refer to the environment in which bone formation occurs, not the process of ossification itself.

Occasionally intramembranous ossification is described as forming "membrane bones" and

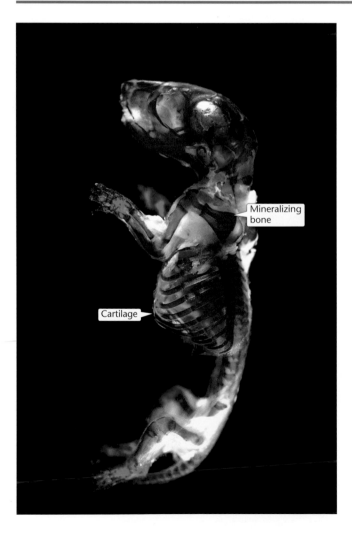

◄ **Fig 10.15 Bone development.** Rodent specimen demonstrating the locations of bone tissue (stained pink-red with alizarin dye) and cartilage tissue (stained blue with alcian blue dye). Many parts of the developing skeleton are part bone and part cartilage, illustrating a role for cartilage in bone formation, specifically in endochondral ossification. As bone deposition and ossification proceeds, much of the cartilage is slowly replaced with bone tissue. Where articulation between bone surfaces is required, cartilage is retained at articular surfaces. This is termed articular hyaline cartilage. Fibrocartilage and elastic cartilage are retained in specific anatomical locations. Alizarin/alcian blue, × 3.

endochondral ossification as forming "cartilage bones." These descriptions suggest that bone formation in these locations differs, when in fact it is the same. Ossification and calcification are sometimes used interchangeably, but the processes are not synonymous. Certain pathological changes of soft tissues may result in their calcification, although no bone is formed. Similarly, specialized cartilage cells in growing bone produce calcified, cartilagenous extracellular matrix that is mineralized but is distinct from bone. Ossification is the process by which cells of skeletal tissues secrete an organic matrix specific to bone and by which the matrix is subsequently calcified or mineralized by deposition of calcium salts.

The onset of ossification in the embryo and fetus

The initial appearance of ossification in the human occurs in the clavicle at about 6.5 weeks post conception. Although there is individual variation, the next bones to show early ossification are the mandible and maxilla. Toward the end of the embryonic period (first 8 weeks), the beginning of ossification is then noted in the humerus and radius, then in the femur, tibia, and ulna. Widespread ossification proceeds during the fetal period. At 9 weeks, ossification is detected in the developing vertebral bodies, and in the skull in the interparietal, supraoccipital, squamous temporal, zygomatic, and frontal bones. At birth most of the long bones show ossification at the center of the body or shaft, but most of the ends lack bone tissue and are still cartilaginous. In the developing embryo the ossification process commences from condensations of mesenchymal cells that are bipotential in the sense that they may differentiate into either osteoblasts or chondrocytes. Together these specialized cells can be said to arise from common progenitor cells that are sometimes called osteochondral progenitors. One of the factors that directs differentiation of the progenitor cells is the signaling molecule Wnt (a combination of *Drosophila* wingless gene Wg, and the vertebrate integrated gene Int; the genes are homologous). If Wnt signaling is high in the mesenchymal condensate, osteoblasts are formed; if Wnt signaling is low, chondrocytes differentiate.

Intramembranous ossification

Commencing at about 7 weeks of gestation at sites where the cranial vault or facial bones will appear, a primary center of ossification will form within a "slab" of mesenchyme tissue. Here, the cells differentiate into osteoblasts capable of making woven bone matrix (osteoid), which in subsequent weeks is mineralized into bone (Fig 10.16a & b). As osteoblasts are

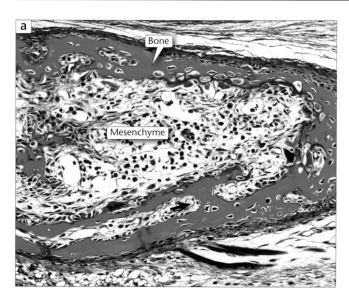

▲ **Fig 10.16a Intramembranous ossification.** Section of a growing flat bone in the fetal skull, showing the outer cortex of newly formed woven bone, which contains osteocytes with osteoblastic cells lining the bony surfaces. A core of mesenchymal tissue, supplied with capillaries and hemopoietic tissues, is noted. New spicules of bone are seen (small masses of tissue), together with a strut-like connection (**arrow**), which defines newly forming trabeculae. Masson's trichrome, paraffin, × 120.

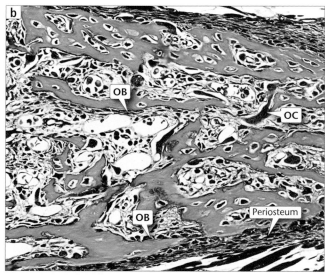

▲ **Fig 10.16b Bone from the fetal skull**, illustrating how bony spicules become interconnected to form trabecular bone, which defines the cavities for bone marrow and other areas containing blood vessels and mesenchymal tissue. Bone-lining cells, or osteoblasts (**OB**), are indicated, together with larger cells representing osteoclasts (**OC**). The osteoclasts resorb bone to allow for remodeling of the trabeculae as the bone grows in size during development. Note the thick periosteum, which contains osteogenic cells for bone deposition on the subperiosteal bone layer. Masson's trichrome, paraffin, × 170.

surrounded by the mineralized matrix, they transform into osteocytes linked by canaliculi. The small masses of bone, now needle-like, are called spicules; these unite to form interconnected trabeculae, resulting in complex radial networks of strut-like components, between which is hemopoietic tissue. At this time the many trabeculae characteristically seen in the flat bones of the fetal skull are referred to as the primary spongiosa (Fig 10.17). This new woven bone is later remodeled into lamellar bone, where concentric layers of bone matrix are deposited (i.e. growth by apposition) by osteogenic cells on the surface of trabeculae.

With maturation and enlargement, removal and resorption of some bone is accomplished by osteoclasts, and new bone, forming osteons, is added where growth is required. In the cortex of these bones the gradual change from woven to lamellar bone continues during postnatal development, and in adults definitive Haversian systems are formed by internal remodeling (Fig 10.18). Thus organized osteons of

adult bone are formed from the poorly organized early woven bone (which involves gene activity and mechanical loading). This is referred to as secondary bone formation.

Endochondral ossification

Bones of the fetal axial skeleton and developing limbs need to grow in length and diameter. In order to achieve this, cartilage is formed as an intermediary tissue between the initial appearance of mesenchyme and the formation of bone. Bone is rigid and, because it cannot expand from within, it grows in bulk by apposition of layers of new bone on its surface. This type of growth is too slow to cope with the relatively rapid growth of ribs, long bones, and vertebrae during fetal development and childhood. Cartilage, however, can grow substantially by adding new cells internally and by producing extracellular matrix to increase its bulk.

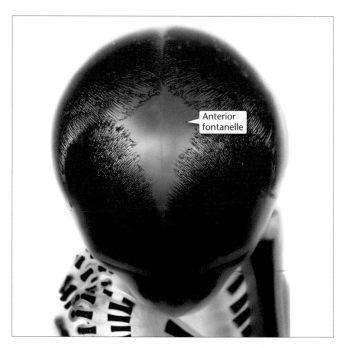

◀ **Fig 10.17 Primary spongiosa in fetal skull.** At about 16 weeks the flat bones of the skull (stained with alizarin dye to show ossification) show fine needle-like bone growths, known as the primary spongiosa. This is a network of woven or immature bone in the form of trabeculae. It is the foundation for the later development of lamellar-type bone that will be termed cancellous or spongy bone. The anterior fontanelle is composed of fibrous connective tissue into which the surrounding curved bones grow until 18 months–2 years of age, when it is closed and the bones interlock at sutures.

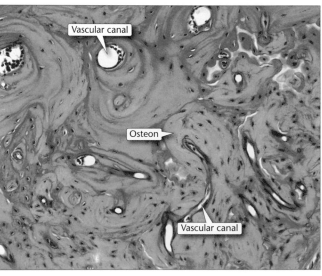

◀ **Fig 10.18 Postnatal skull.** With continued growth of skull bone in postnatal life, the previously cancellous bone in the fetus is converted into plates with compact lamellar bone in the cortex. Spaces in the earlier cancellous bone are progressively filled in by appositional bone growth, giving rise to narrowed vascular canals surrounded by lamellae typical of osteons. H&E, paraffin, × 100.

The cartilage model

Growth of the ribs, long bones, and vertebrae is achieved by forming a miniature but enlarging cartilage model, which is gradually replaced by bone, normally in a precise manner. The rudimentary limb buds of mesenchyme in embryos are formed at about 6 weeks of development, the timing being variable from bone to bone. Mesenchymal cells proliferate and differentiate into chondroblasts, producing a cartilage model that resembles the adult bone shape; this is genetically determined (Fig 10.19). When this model is replaced by bone, the shape is influenced by muscular tensions, mechanical loading, gravity, and internal remodeling. In adult life, the latter process is vital for normal bone metabolism but may be compromised in situations of prolonged inactivity, such as confinement to bed or in the microgravity of space flight.

The cartilage model increases in bulk and length by chondrocyte proliferation and maturation, together with formation of matrix (with type II collagen), and it reaches a size at which distribution of nutrients by diffusion becomes limited since cartilage is avascular. In the center the oldest cells hypertrophy, switch their synthesis to type X collagen, attract blood vessels and chondroclasts, and direct the mineralization of the surrounding cartilage matrix. This represents the future site at which bone deposition takes place—the primary ossification center (Fig 10.20a & b).

The first sign of ossification

Inner perichondral cells of the shaft of the cartilage model develop into osteoblasts, a process governed by hypertrophic chondrocytes. Thus in the mid-section a cylindrical collar of bone is formed, penetrated by the

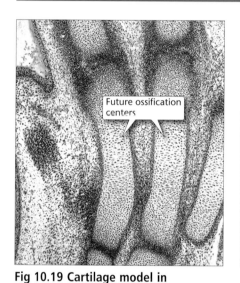

Fig 10.19 Cartilage model in endochondral ossification. In the developing limb, mesenchymal condensations differentiate into miniature cartilage models of the definitive adult bones. This is directed by gene activity and is an early phase of endochondral ossification, although no bone is yet formed. Note sites of future joints, and the enlargement and dispersal of chondrocytes at the midpoint of the cartilage model. This is the site where ossification will commence. H&E, paraffin, × 12.

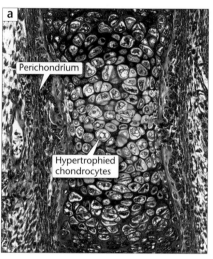

▲ **Fig 10.20a Preparation for ossification.** Chondrocytes in the midpoint of this developing cartilage model of a long bone have hypertrophied and secreted a matrix, which surrounds them. The hypertrophic chondrocytes mineralize the cartilage. The perichondrium is highly cellular and appears to be invading the cartilage at the narrowest width of the model. This is the site at which (i) a bone collar will be formed and (ii) the primary ossification center will soon appear. PAS/H&E, acrylic resin, × 70.

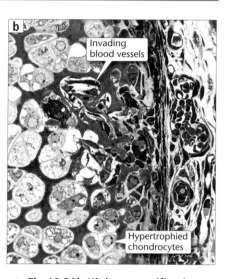

▲ **Fig 10.20b Higher magnification of the waist region of the cartilage model.** Blood vessels are invading the calcified cartilage matrix, bringing with them cells that differentiate into chondro/osteoclasts, osteoprogenitor cells, and hemopoietic precursors. The hypertrophic chondrocytes will die by apoptosis and be removed by the clast-lineage cells. Cartilage matrix is gradually resorbed and this creates larger spaces, with osteoblasts depositing new bone on the remnants of the eroded calcified cartilage. It is at this location that perichondral cells will differentiate into osteoblasts that produce a midsection bone collar or subperiosteal shell for the cartilage model. Toluidine blue, araldite, × 350.

nutrient artery of the developing bone. The superficial layer of this bone collar is the periosteum (Fig 10.21). Hypertrophic chondrocytes then die by apoptosis. Ramification of the nutrient artery into the cartilage model is followed by a hollowing-out process (the formative marrow space) through gradual resorption of the cartilage by chondroclasts. Infiltration of osteogenic precursor cells (supplied via the blood vessels) deposits new bone matrix that is rich in type I collagen, eventually forming a recognizable primary center of ossification. This new bone matrix is the primary spongiosa. Most fetal long bones reach this stage by about 2 months. This process is termed endochondral ossification.

Growth in length and width

Newly formed central cancellous woven bone is partly resorbed, leaving a medullary cavity for hemopoietic tissue. The shaft, or diaphysis, of the model is gradually replaced by bone and marrow, but

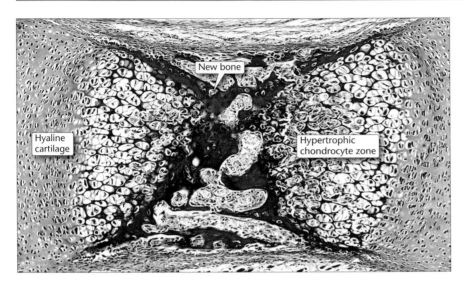

◀ **Fig 10.21 Primary ossification center.** The calcified cartilage has been replaced with new bone growing into trabeculae and resembling an early cancellous/spongy bone morphology; the spaces in between will be occupied by bone marrow. The two ends of the model remain as hyaline cartilage, with a wide zone of hypertrophic chondrocytes, which produce a scaffold of cartilage matrix. Chondrocytes can proliferate and contribute to long axis growth of the model. Bone tissue cannot grow from within, as its cells—the osteocytes—are non-proliferative. Bone matrix is deposited on the slowly but continuously produced cartilage scaffold. H&E, paraffin, × 75.

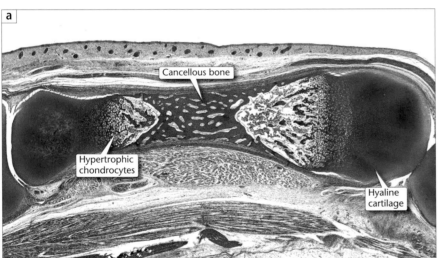

◀ **Fig 10.22a Growth in length.** A later phase of endochondral ossification in a human fetal finger. The two epiphyseal ends, still hyaline cartilage, have grown apart, and the presumptive diaphysis is filling with cancellous-type bone, which is being deposited on the cartilage scaffolds that form in the region of the future metaphysis. The region between the epiphysis and metaphysis is occupied by hypertrophic chondrocytes, which supply the scaffolds of calcified cartilage, and thus these cells are essential for gradual growth in length of the bone. H&E/alcian blue, paraffin, × 15.

the two ends, still made entirely of cartilage, become the epiphyses. In short bones such as a phalanx (Fig 10.22a & b), where the bone of the shaft meets a region of epiphyseal cartilage, a special zone of hyaline cartilage is formed; this contains the chondrocytes that produce cartilage matrix. This zone is responsible for linear bone growth by making a continuous supply of cartilage matrix, which is in turn replaced by bone as the diaphysis extends longitudinally (see below). New woven bone is deposited on the already calcified cartilage matrix at the metaphysis, which is between the diaphysis and the epiphysis. Bone grows in width by deposition of new bone on the periosteum and its removal on the endosteum to maintain appropriate cortical width.

In the epiphyses of longer bones, chondrocytes proliferate and centrally placed cells eventually come to be beyond the limits of nutrient diffusion. They undergo programmed hypertrophy and cell death and are replaced by new bone formation initiated by invasions of blood vessels (also called cartilage canals; Fig 10.23) and osteogenic cells, forming a secondary center of ossification usually shortly after birth. Regions of cartilage persist on the bone ends to become the articular surface. The transverse disk/plate of cartilage retained between the epiphyseal and the diaphyseal centers of ossification is called the epiphyseal growth plate. As new chondrocytes are added to the plate and older cells are eliminated, the growth plate becomes critically important for longitudinal growth of the shaft

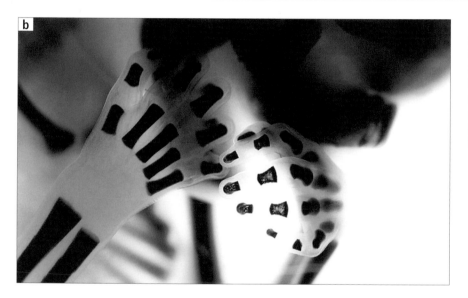

◀ **Fig 10.22b Growing fetal hands**, stained with alizarin dye to show regions of ossification. Metacarpals and phalanges are seen as cylinders of bone. Gaps between them and in the carpal region are not stained because these regions are cartilaginous. Each cylinder of bone is the diaphysis with rudimentary metaphyses at the ends.

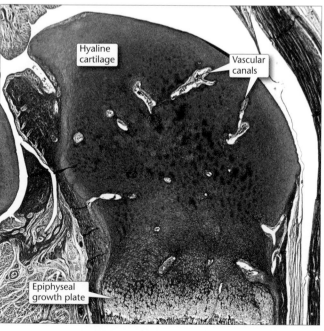

◀ **Fig 10.23 Epiphyseal cartilage.** A growing long bone, showing the penetration of vascular canals from perichondral vessels into the epiphysis. A canal typically contains an arteriole, venule, and capillaries, and delivers osteoprogenitor cells, which form the basis for establishing a secondary center of ossification. H&E/alcian blue, paraffin, × 12.

of the longer bones. The biology of the growth plate is discussed next. Eventually growth plates disappear when bones stop growing in late adolescence. Endochondral ossification is summarized in Fig 10.24.

Tip: Development of bone requires osteoblasts to produce osteoid (a "pre-bone" matrix) and then to direct its mineralization. In the axial skeleton and long bones, cartilage formation antedates ossification, because chondrocyte proliferation results in tissue growth and the cartilage matrix is replaced with osteoblast-derived bone. Bone tissue in the shaft of developing long bones cannot grow in length. Elongation can be achieved only at the growing ends (epiphyses) by the proliferation, maturation, and death of chondrocytes in the growth plates.

Epiphyseal growth plate

In the growth plate, chondrocytes align into columns and represent the functional units of longitudinal bone growth (Fig 10.25a–c).

Four layers of cells are described:

- Resting zone—reserve chondrocytes, which merge with epiphyseal cartilage
- Proliferative zone—chondrocytes proliferate and orient into columns
- Maturation zone—chondrocytes enlarge and calcify the adjacent cartilage matrix
- Hypertrophic zone—chondrocytes complete mineralization of the cartilage and prepare for programmed cell death.

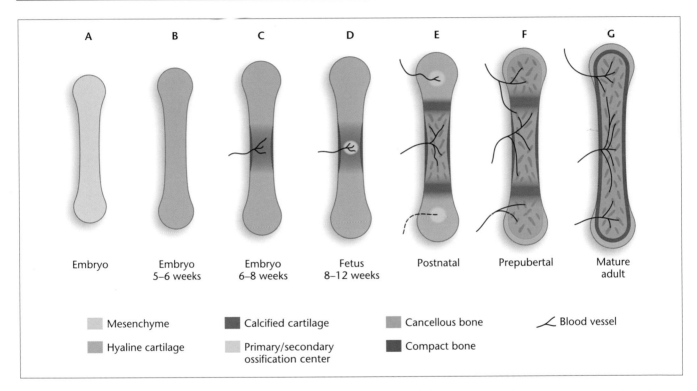

| A | B | C | D | E | F | G |

Embryo   Embryo 5–6 weeks   Embryo 6–8 weeks   Fetus 8–12 weeks   Postnatal   Prepubertal   Mature adult

■ Mesenchyme   ■ Calcified cartilage   ■ Cancellous bone   ∠ Blood vessel

■ Hyaline cartilage   ■ Primary/secondary ossification center   ■ Compact bone

▲ **Fig 10.24 Development of a long bone by endochondral ossification.** Diagrammatic representation of the transformation of an embryonic bone into the adult form. In **A** and **B**, the initial cartilage model resembles a miniature version of the definitive bone. In **C**, the collar of periosteal bone appears in the shaft and buds of periosteal vessels appear. In **D**, cartilage cells enlarge, and in the center the matrix becomes calcified; a nutrient artery penetrates the bony collar, ramifies, and supplies osteogenic precursor cells, which begin to deposit bone that will form the primary ossification center.

In **E**, the medulla becomes cancellous bone, and the cartilage forms epiphyseal growth plates that recede away from the mid-zone of the bone (via continuous cell proliferation and degeneration), allowing elongation. Secondary centers of ossification develop in the epiphyses at or after birth. In **F**, the growth plates remain active and continue to move apart according to the required length of each particular bone. In **G**, the epiphyseal growth plates become fully calcified, are replaced by bone, and disappear; the articular surfaces retain a covering of hyaline articular cartilage.

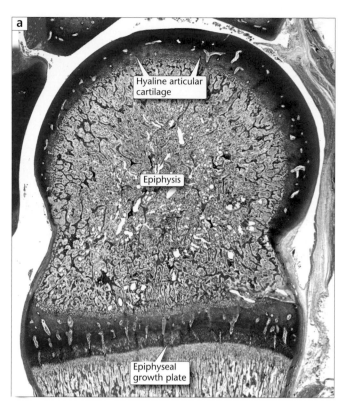

◀ **Fig 10.25a Epiphyseal growth plate.** Histologic section of a growing long bone associated with a synovial joint. Hyaline cartilage is stained blue; cancellous bone is red, together with bone marrow. A substantial region of hyaline articular cartilage covers the end of the bone facing the joint space. Deep to it is the epiphysis, its cancellous bone being formed earlier from a secondary ossification center. The epiphyseal growth plate separates the epiphysis above from the metaphysis below. The function of the growth plate is essential for normal growth of the bone in its longitudinal axis. It achieves this by supplying new chondrocytes that proliferate from reserve chondrogenic stem cells found in the growth plate, and produce calcifying cartilage matrix on the metaphyseal aspect. Production of cartilage is accompanied by the death of the chondrocytes facing the metaphysis. Continued addition above, and elimination from below, of cells of the growth plate results in slow migration of the plate upwardly allowing a trail of newly formed bone spicules to develop inferior to it. The bone gradually increases in length. H&E/alcian blue, paraffin, × 6.

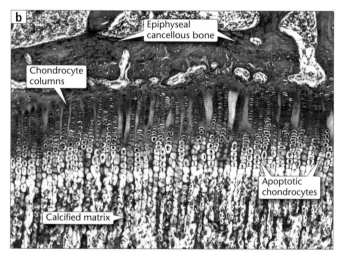

◀ **Fig 10.25b A wide growth plate of a fast-growing bone** consists of columns of chondrocytes and the matrix they secrete. Reserve or resting zone cells are adjacent with and anchored by matrix to the bone of the epiphysis. From these stem-like cells, chondrocytes proliferate, their flattened shape resembling stacks of coins. Between them is the cartilage matrix that assists in maintaining their longitudinal orientation. Following proliferation, the cells mature and then enlarge; termed hypertrophic chondrocytes, they (i) mineralize the surrounding cartilage matrix and (ii) undergo programmed cell death, possibly assisted by their isolation from nutrient supply. Note the shrunken chondrocyte nuclei in the center of their lacunae. Calcified matrix extensions into the metaphysis remain as the surface upon which newly produced bone matrix will be deposited by invading osteoblasts delivered by the metaphyseal capillaries. Masson's trichrome, paraffin, × 60.

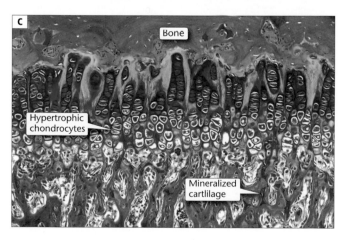

◀ **Fig 10.25c Epiphyseal growth plate from a slow-growing bone** exhibits shorter columns of chondrocytes, which tend to be elongated clusters rather than the tall columns typical of faster-growing bones. Reserve zone chondrocytes are apposed to epiphyseal bone by interdigitation. The deep-blue-stained matrix surrounding chondrocytes represents the high concentrations of proteoglycans embedded in collagen, both of which are produced by these cells. After the hypertrophic chondrocytes die, the cartilage matrix that they have mineralized is retained as many irregular extensions, stained blue in the lower half of the micrograph. The red-stained material that surrounds these structures is new bone matrix laid down by osteoblasts that originate from capillaries in the spaces between. This bone is immature, non-lamellar bone which will ultimately be the trabeculae of cancellous bone typical of the medullary cavity. H&E/alcian blue, paraffin, × 75.

A further layer, sometimes called the ossification zone (Fig 10.26), is located at the metaphysis, where capillaries deliver osteogenic cells to deposit osteoid on the columns of calcified cartilage. This is gradually replaced by bone matrix during remodeling.

The extensions of calcified cartilage provide a suitable surface upon which bone is deposited (Fig 10.27). Epiphyseal growth plates allow the epiphyses to be pushed apart without being replaced by new bone. When chondrocytes stop dividing, the growth plate is converted into bone, and in adult bones it may be visible on radiographs as an indistinct line in the region of the previous growth plate.

Signaling pathways

The growth plate is the engine of bone elongation during postnatal life. Three of many mechanisms that ensure this are:

- Alignment of cells into columns parallel to the long axis of the bone
- Entry, progression, and exit of cells
- The crucial role of hypertrophic chondrocytes.

Each of these parameters is complexly interrelated and relies upon expression of gradient-dependent signaling proteins (morphogens), which act as paracrine factors within the growth plate. Resting zone cartilage contains stem cells that generate the clones of proliferative

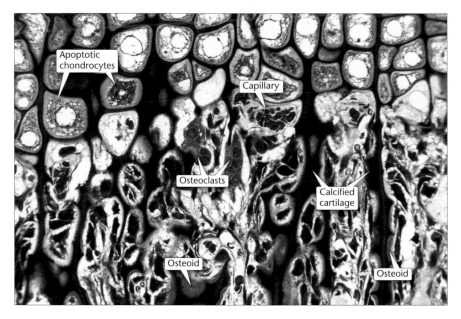

◀ **Fig 10.26 Ossification zone.**
High-magnification view of the region of the growth plate where new bone is forming. Elongated and scallop-shaped extensions of calcified cartilage alternate with invading capillaries, which end as loops adjacent to the hypertrophic and apoptotic chondrocytes. The vessels deliver (i) nutrients, (ii) osteoclasts/chondroclasts, which partly resorb cartilage, and (iii) osteoblasts, which begin to deposit osteoid on the irregular surfaces of cartilage. Over time the cartilage is replaced with bone matrix and both are mineralized under the direction of the osteoblasts. Full mineralization and growth of the spicules of bone will form cancellous bone trabeculae. Toluidine blue, araldite, × 420.

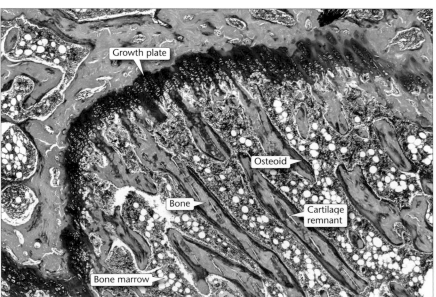

◀ **Fig 10.27 New bone deposition.**
Spicules contain a core of calcified cartilage remnants (stained deep blue) and slender lamellae of new bone (green) with entombed osteocytes. Superficial seams of osteoid (red) cover the spicules (i.e. unmineralized pre-bone containing collagen, proteoglycan, and other non-collagenous proteins). Osteoid is mineralized to form bone; the cartilage cores are replaced by bone. Spaces between the bone spicules are occupied by bone marrow with extracted fat cells. Chondrocytes in the growth plate degenerate to leave a scaffold of cartilage for bone deposition on the spicules. Masson's trichrome, paraffin, × 50.

chondrocytes. When a segment of resting zone cartilage is surgically excised, rotated 90°, and reinserted to bring it lateral and adjacent to the proliferative zone, new chondrocytes arising in the proliferative zone reorientate by 90°. The morphogens involved (and no doubt others) are parathyroid hormone related protein (PTHrP) and Indian hedgehog (Ihh); respectively, these diffuse from perichondral cells into cartilage, and from cartilage cells into perichondral cells and differentiating chondrocytes. Hypertrophic chondrocytes are key cells in the growth plate, not only for producing a calcified cartilage matrix but also as the source of Ihh, which establishes an Ihh/PTHrP negative feedback loop (Fig 10.28). Together these signaling proteins direct chondrocyte and osteoblast differentiation, the height of the growth plate (by entry and exit of cells), and the formation of the early bone collar.

Endocrine regulation

Longitudinal growth is dependent upon a balance between chondrocyte proliferation and differentiation, and is regulated by hormones and growth factors that act in both endocrine and autocrine/paracrine situations. These include growth hormone, insulin-like growth factor, thyroid hormone, estrogen, androgen, leptin, and vitamin D. Nutrition, genetic factors, and environment also influence growth. In postnatal life there are three phases of development that modulate growth velocity (GV). The fetus shows rapid GV, which quickly decelerates in the infantile phase up to three years of age. In the childhood phase GV gradually decelerates until puberty. In the pubertal phase GV again accelerates, reaching a peak about two years after initiation, followed by a rapid decrease in GV until it stops. About 20% of final height is gained during puberty (the pubertal growth spurt) and occurs before closure of the growth plates.

Growth during puberty

Acceleration of longitudinal bone growth shows sexual dimorphism, with maximum GV in girls occurring earlier than in boys. Gender differences in the growth spurt are mainly attributable to increased secretion of estrogens and androgens, and to the associated responses of the growth plates. The source of estrogen in females is the ovary and in males is the aromatization of testosterone and androstenedione to estrogen. Before puberty, peripheral estradiol levels in boys and girls is below 10–20 pmol/L but become elevated above 100–200 pmol/L during middle (girls) or late (boys) puberty. It has become clear that in both sexes, estrogen is essential for initiation of the growth spurt and for fusion of the growth plates in early adult life.

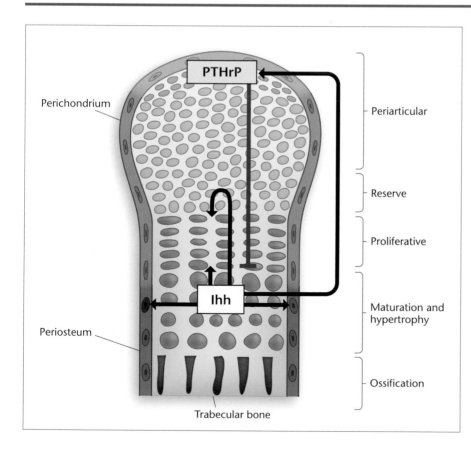

◀ **Fig 10.28 Local regulation of the growth plate.** The structure of a developing long bone at the fetal stage is used to illustrate how the PTHrP/Ihh feedback loop controls the entry and exit of chondrocytes in the growth plate. PTHrP is produced by perichondrial cells and chondrocytes at the ends of the growing bone. PTHrP acts on chondrocytes to keep them dividing, and to delay their differentiation into mature/hypertrophic cells. The length of the chondrocyte column is dependent on the rate of chondrocyte proliferation, differentiation, and hypertrophy. When chondrocytes stop dividing, they differentiate into prehypertrophic and hypertrophic chondrocytes, both of which synthesize Ihh. Ihh secretion acts on the bone end to increase the synthesis of PTHrP, thus establishing a negative feedback loop by regulating the onset of chondrocyte hypertrophy. Ihh also increases proliferation of local chondrocytes and stimulates perichondrial cells to differentiate into osteoblasts.

Estrogen receptors

The exact mechanisms of estrogen action and the identity of the target cell types remain unclear when considering sex differences, species investigated, and the levels of circulating estrogens. From studies of a few rare individuals with disturbances of the estrogen receptor (ER) or natural estrogen deficiency, together with extensive animal studies, it is known that the growth plate expresses mRNA and/or protein for three ERs (ERα, ERβ, and membrane-bound ER). The role of these ERs in stimulating or inhibiting chondrocyte proliferation and differentiation in the growth plate is incompletely understood. To some extent this is confounded by rodent studies, in which estrogen levels compared with those of humans are roughly 10 times lower; also, mice and rats do not exhibit a pubertal growth spurt nor do they show growth plate fusion.

It has been suggested that in humans activation of ERα by early elevation of estrogen increases endochondral ossification, with later and peak estrogen levels (100 versus 10 pmol/L) activating ERβ receptors, which results in growth plate fusion. The roles of non-ER-dependent pathways that affect the growth plate (growth hormone, insulin-like growth factor, glucocorticoids) remain to be determined.

> **Tip:** An important fact about chondrocytes in the growth plate is that these cells do not move down the plate; rather they stay fixed in place. The chondrocytes at the top of the columns proliferate and make the plate taller, while chondrocytes at the bottom die and are replaced with bone. The net result is that the width of the plate remains the same, but it and the epiphysis move away from the metaphysis–diaphysis, thus lengthening the bone.

Growth of cancellous bone

The sequence of events for endochondral development of cancellous bone is shown in Figure 10.29a–d. The

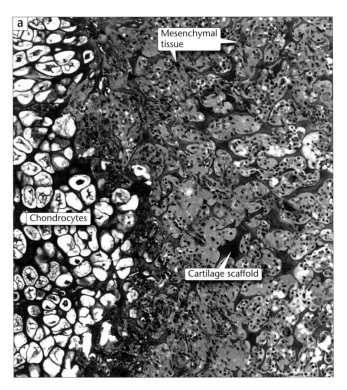

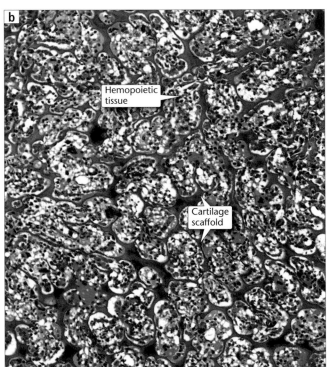

▲ **Fig 10.29a Growth of cancellous bone.** Developing rib is shown here and in Figures 10.29b, c, and d. Through the endochondral-type process, hypertrophic chondrocytes have produced a cartilagenous scaffold surrounded by vascularized mesenchymal tissue. H&E/alcian blue, paraffin, × 120.

▲ **Fig 10.29b With further development**, the calcified cartilaginous framework is thin and the early marrow space is now highly vascular and cellular, containing hemopoietic precursors together with osteoprogenitor cells and differentiating osteoclasts. H&E/alcian blue, paraffin, × 120.

cartilage anlage defines the shape and location of the model that will determine the morphology of the specific bone. As hypertrophic chondrocytes die and leave scaffolds of calcified cartilage, the intervening mesenchymal tissue is a source of osteogenic and hemopoietic cells and blood vessels. Osteoblasts produce new bone matrix, which is added as layers to the cartilage framework—a process that by appositional growth gradually increases the width of the scaffolds to form trabeculae with scattered osteocytes. The trabecular core is calcified cartilage that progressively diminishes as it is replaced with newly mineralized bone. In the presumptive marrow spaces, many vessels are noted that in time will coexist with the cells of the hemopoietic system. Continued addition of bone to the trabeculae establishes their coalescence into the typical architecture of cancellous bone.

REMODELING OF BONE

Remodeling is defined as removal and replacement of bone tissue without alteration of its overall shape. It is a process of bone reconstruction. Modeling refers to a construction process with changes in shape and size of bone by appositional formation of new bone in the periosteum and endosteum. It occurs without previous bone resorption.

Formation of primary (first-generation) osteons is a consequence of the ability of new woven bone to form ridges and crests. But bone is not a static organ and throughout life osteons are partially replaced by secondary and higher orders (up to 10 generations) of new osteons. Elimination of bone tissue and the rebuilding process are usually in balance and referred to as bone remodeling. This is achieved by resorption canals which cut tunnels through the pre-existing bone to be refilled with bone, thus forming

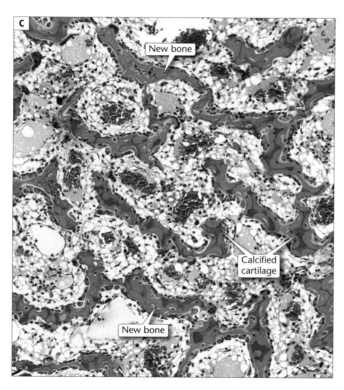

▲ **Fig 10.29c Later stage of growth** showing early formation of bony trabeculae with central cores of calcified cartilage. The trabecular surface is covered with many cells representing osteoblasts and osteoclasts. The future marrow space is richly supplied with vessels. H&E/alcian blue, paraffin, × 120.

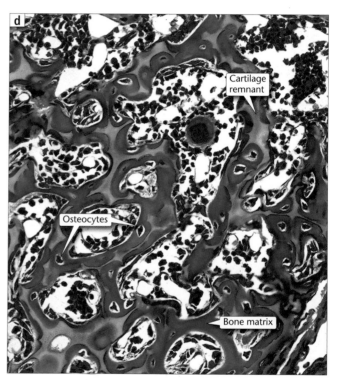

▲ **Fig 10.29d With continued deposition of bone** in layers on the existing trabecular surfaces, the struts and bridges of trabeculae begin to resemble the structure of cancellous bone, being thicker and united to form the familiar honeycomb-type morphology. Remnants of cartilage are seen in the core of the bone tissue. H&E/alcian blue, paraffin, × 250.

new osteons (Fig 10.30a–d). The blood vessels that deliver cells and nutrients to the core of the tunnel are gradually narrowed and will ultimately occupy the Haversian canal. The bone-remodeling cavity and the new osteon into which it evolves are occupied by the BMU, comprising the osteoclasts, osteoblasts, and osteocytes. A mixture of old and new bone is recognized histologically by angular lamellae (partly excavated by a previous resorption canal) in between circular, fully formed osteons (Fig 10.31a & b). Cancellous bone is similarly resorbed and replaced by BMUs, except that in this case cavities

are excavated and new lamellae are deposited to fill them in.

THE SYNOVIAL JOINT AND ARTICULAR CARTILAGE

The chief tissues of synovial joints (Fig 10.32) are:
- Articular cartilage covering the bone ends
- Synovial membrane protruding partly into the joint space
- Capsule with ligament thickenings strategically placed.

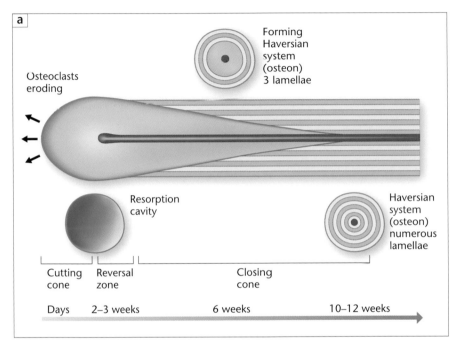

◀ **Fig 10.30a Bone remodeling (reconstruction).** Diagram of the basic multicellular unit (BMU) in the resorption and restoration of compact bone. Osteoclasts cut a tunnel through the bone (the cutting cone). In the reversal zone, osteoblasts are introduced from the central vascular tissue and produce consecutive layers of new bone from the periphery toward the center. Successive lamellae of bone reconstruct a new osteon in the closing cone, so-named because the layers of new bone close in toward the central vasculature.

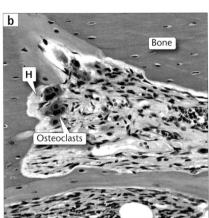

▲ **Fig 10.30b Resorption.** Resorption of bone is achieved by osteoclasts forming the leading edge of a cutting cone that bores a tunnel through bone. Howship's lacunae (**H**) represent sites where osteoclasts release acid and lysosomes, which dissolve bone mineral and degrade collagen and proteoglycans. The resorption canal contains vascularized connective tissue. H&E, paraffin, × 175.

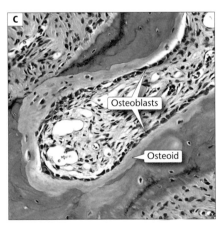

▲ **Fig 10.30c Vessels in the reversal zone** contain perivascular cells, which differentiate into osteoblasts that line the wall of the tunnel and begin to deposit osteoid seams. As osteoid becomes mineralized, new lamellar bone surrounds the osteoblasts, which then are recognized as osteocytes. H&E, paraffin, × 175.

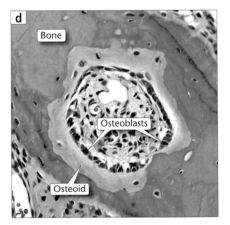

▲ **Fig 10.30d Transverse section of a closing cone,** showing a vascularized connective tissue core, osteoblasts and a ring of osteoid. Mineralization of the latter over 8–10 days forms a ring of lamellar bone. Addition of further lamellae inward gives rise to a new osteon or Haversian system. H&E, paraffin, × 175.

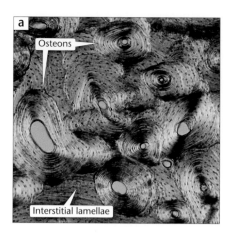

a

Osteons

Interstitial lamellae

◀ **Fig 10.31a Successive generations of osteons.** Unstained ground section of compact bone viewed with partly polarized light. Different generations of osteons partly overlap and obliterate other osteons. Intact osteons—those that are complete circles or irregularly elliptical—have been formed later than those that they partly obscure. Most of these osteons are therefore second generation or older. Note the interstitial lamellae between osteons. × 100.

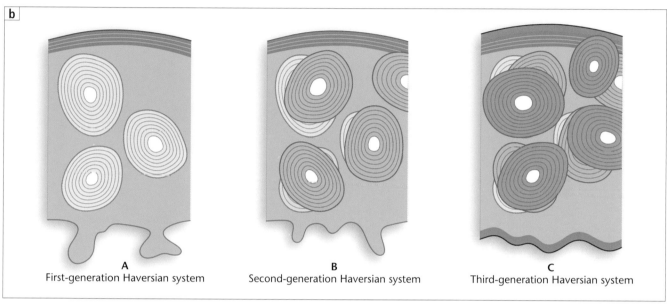

b

A	B	C
First-generation Haversian system	Second-generation Haversian system	Third-generation Haversian system

▲ **Fig 10.31b Haversian systems.** Diagrams illustrating the formation of Haversian systems of osteons in compact bone with increasing age. Degree of color represents first (light), second (medium), and third generation (dark) osteons. In **A**, primary osteons lie in lamellar bone and the cortical surface shows a strip of circumferential lamellae. In **B**, at a later time, four new osteons have developed from tunnels, or resorption canals, that have bored through the preexisting bone. These tunnels are filled progressively with concentric layers of newly deposited bony lamellae to form secondary osteons. The latter show thickened, peripheral cement lines (unlike the primary osteons), so contributing to the irregular or angular regions of interstitial lamellae. In **C**, a third generation of osteons is shown. The outer circumferential lamellae form new layers as the bone grows in width and the inner trabeculae have been partly resorbed and replaced with thin inner circumferential lamellae facing the medullary cavity.

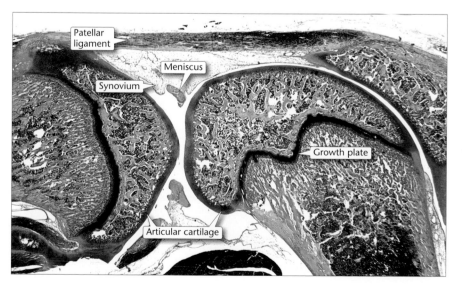

Patellar ligament

Meniscus

Synovium

Growth plate

Articular cartilage

◀ **Fig 10.32 Synovial joint.** Histologic section of adult rodent knee joint. The femur and tibia both show growth plates that indicate continued elongation of bone. Articular cartilage caps the ends of the bones facing the joint cavity. Part of the fibrocartilage of the menisci is shown, together with synovium. The patellar ligament (quadriceps tendon) is attached to the patella and forms part of the anterior capsule of the joint. Masson's trichrome, paraffin, × 8.

251

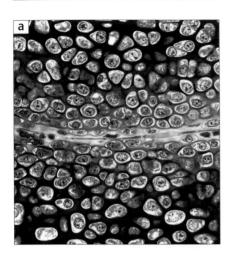

◀ Fig 10.33a Articular cartilage.
Histologic section of a developing synovial joint in the fetus, showing the chondrocytes that will form articular hyaline cartilage. The boundary is a split between the cartilage models where chondrocytes have degenerated. This is the future joint space. Chondrocytes are densely packed and separated by cartilage matrix. PAS/H&E, acrylic resin, × 95.

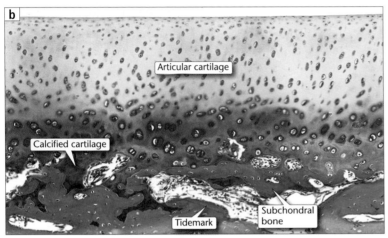

◀ Fig 10.33b Articular cartilage. Articular surfaces of joints are lined by a special hyaline cartilage, where the expected perichondrium is absent but replaced with a very thin layer of collagen running parallel to the surface; no cells occur in this layer. In the deepest layer, chondrocytes abut subchondral bone. The tidemark represents a line of calcification where a mineralization front is present. Articular cartilage is avascular and non-renewable and it has a high (70%) water content. H&E/alcian blue, paraffin, × 70.

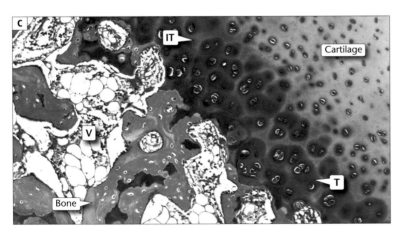

◀ Fig 10.33c Cartilage–bone interface. Where hyaline cartilage meets with bone the cartilage becomes calcified. The calcified cartilage is devoid of cells and originates from a zone of cartilage containing single or paired chondrocytes (chondrons). A deep-staining territorial matrix (**T**), which is rich in aggrecan, surrounds each chondron; the interterritorial matrix (**IT**) contains collagen and proteoglycans of low molecular weight. Vascular (**V**) and hemopoietic tissues are noted. H&E/alcian blue, paraffin, × 150.

Articular cartilage

Articular cartilage covers the weight-bearing bony ends of synovial joints and is firmly anchored to the subchondral bone plate, which supports the cartilage for transmitting load to the cortical bone via underlying trabeculae (Fig 10.33a–c). Varying in thickness from 1 mm to 7 mm, articular cartilage is an avascular tissue that receives nutrients by diffusion from the subchondral bone and from the synovial fluid in the joint cavity. Lubrication by synovial fluid provides almost frictionless movement of the apposed articulating cartilage surfaces. The most superficial aspect of articular cartilage contains no cells; rather it is a thin layer of collagen fibrils with several deeper zones of chondrocytes and matrix. This matrix consists of collagen for tensile strength and a mesh of proteoglycans, which attract and retain water. In adult bones, a layer of calcified cartilage is interposed between articular cartilage and subchondral bone. A distinct border, or "tidemark," represents the mineralization front between the articular and calcified cartilage. The high content of water in articular cartilage matrix resists compression. When cartilage is indented by mechanical load, it extrudes water. Upon removal of the compressive force, water is osmotically reabsorbed by proteoglycans and the cartilage returns to its former shape. If damaged or diseased, articular cartilage cannot repair itself.

Synovial membrane and capsule

The synovial membrane lines internal, non-articular joint surfaces and consists of folds of vascularized connective tissue (Fig 10.34). Cells on its surface resemble macrophages and fibroblast-type cells, the latter possibly contributing to the proteins found in the synovial fluid. Synovial fluid is mainly a filtrate of plasma from blood vessels mixed with hyaluronan and glycoproteins secreted by synovial cells. The fluid acts as a lubricant and a nutrient supply for articular cartilage.

The fibrous capsule enclosing most synovial joints is continuous with the periosteum, forming a joint capsule that internally is lined with synovial membrane. Nerves supplying the joint are found in the capsule and may be accompanied by sensory receptors such as Pacinian corpuscles and Ruffini endings.

THE VERTEBRAL COLUMN

Bones of the vertebral column are separated by cartilaginous joints classified as symphyses, in which the articular hyaline cartilages covering the superior and inferior surfaces of the vertebral bodies are separated by a central disk of fibrocartilage. The hyaline cartilages adjacent to the intervertebral disk are remnants of the epiphyses of the developing

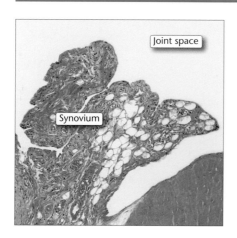

Joint space

Synovium

◀ **Fig 10.34 Synovial membrane.**
Lining the inside of the capsule of synovial joints, the synovial membrane may protrude a little into the joint space. Its surface, sometimes called an intima, is lined with cells but these do not form an epithelium as there is no basal lamina. The core is loose fibro-fatty connective tissue, the vessels of which supply a dialysate of blood that, together with proteins secreted by intimal cells, contributes to the formation of synovial fluid. Synovial fluid is a viscous lubricant containing hyaluronan and glucosamine, and may partly infiltrate into articular cartilage. H&E, paraffin, × 70.

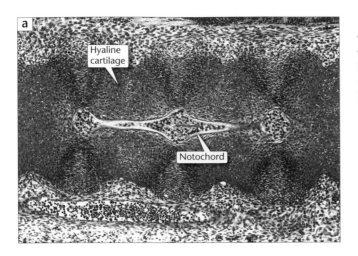

◀ **Fig 10.35a Vertebral column.** Early development of the vertebral column, showing formation of blocks of hyaline cartilage, which will contribute to the endochondral ossification of vertebral bodies. The notochord passes centrally and contains cells of mesenchymal origin. Between the cartilages, the notochord extends into the mesenchymal tissue. H&E/alcian blue, paraffin, × 120.

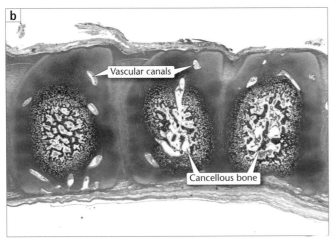

◀ **Fig 10.35b Primitive vertebral bodies** have formed showing central ossification into cancellous-type bone. Vascular canals penetrating the cartilage supply nutrients, bone-forming cells and precursors of the hemopoietic lineage. Gaps between the developing vertebral bodies are sites where the intervertebral disks will form. H&E/alcian blue, paraffin, × 15.

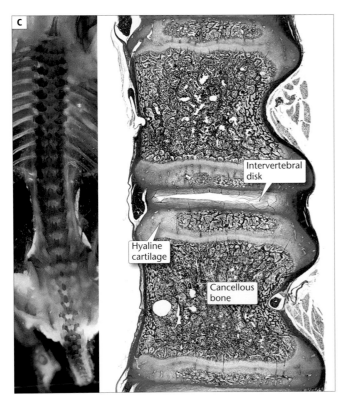

◀ **Fig 10.35c Vertebral column.** *Left:* Early postnatal rodent skeleton stained with alizarin and alcian blue. Vertebral bodies show regions stained red for bone, and blue for cartilage. Alizarin/alcian blue, × 4. *Right:* Histologic section of vertebral column. Cancellous bone occupies the medulla of each vertebral body with superior and inferior surfaces covered with hyaline articular cartilage. An intervertebral disk is seen between the vertebral bodies. Its core appears empty due to extraction during tissue processing. H&E/alcian blue, paraffin, × 6.

vertebral bodies and lock into the osseus vertebral end plates (Fig 10.35a–c). Disks consist of an outer annulus fibrosus, made of 15–25 concentric rings of fibrocartilage, and an inner nucleus pulposus—a soft gelatinous core derived from the notochord (Fig 10.36a & b). Disk thickness increases from cranial to caudal locations.

Collagen surrounding the annulus extends to and unites with the rim of the vertebral body and with the anterior and posterior longitudinal ligaments that hold the intervertebral disk in position. In humans, notochordal (mesenchymal) cells in the nucleus pulposus normally disappear early in childhood. Intervertebral disks act as shock absorbers to resist the compressive forces transmitted through the vertebral column, but they also allow movement and flexibility in what would be an otherwise rigid spine. The proteoglycan molecule aggrecan is a major component of the disk and its natural swelling pressure by retention of water counteracts compression. Tensile strength and load distribution is achieved by the highly organized sheets of type I fibrillar collagen in the lamellae. Disk degeneration with age and herniation are commonly associated with local and/or referred pain.

DISORDERS OF THE SKELETON
Fracture repair

The resistance to fracture of adult bone is due not only to its great tensile and compressive strength but also to its flexibility. When bending forces are applied, bone acts more like a bundle of straws than a solid stick. The latter snaps with a lower bending load than the former, in which each straw slips slightly relative to its neighbors. Similarly, the lamellae within osteons can slip relative to each other, conferring flexibility to the bone before it breaks or cracks ("stress fracture") under excessive load. When fractured, bone can repair itself in two different ways.

Primary fracture repair occurs with rigid surgical fixation of cortical bone and heals by osteonal regrowth with little endochondral bone formation. Fractured bone ends are dead, but after 3 weeks end-to-end bone union is achieved by osteoclasts removing dead bone, which is replaced with new living lamellar bone. Thus the bone ends are "welded" together without the formation of an external fracture callus. Periosteal osteoblasts lay down woven bone at about 4–5 weeks, forming an internal fracture gap callus that is hard but still not safe for weight bearing. Mineralization of the new lamellar matrix proceeds, but development of strong osteons takes months to occur.

Secondary fracture repair occurs when there is minimal movement of fracture ends, forming an external callus around and between the fractured bone ends. The callus contains cartilage and bone, and the former is gradually replaced by the latter in a process similar to that of endochondral ossification. The callus attains maximum size within 3 weeks. With bone remodeling, the former fracture site is normally completely repaired as compact and cancellous bone.

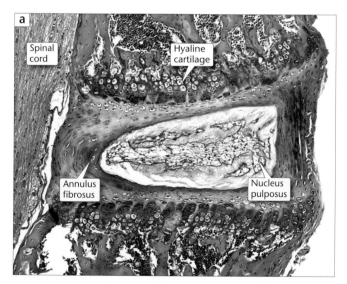

▲ **Fig 10.36a Intervertebral disk.** In immature animals the histology of the disk shows a central nucleus pulposus and peripheral annulus fibrosus. The nucleus pulposus is a remnant of the notochord—the midline rod of mesenchymal tissue in the embryo that defines the axial skeleton. It has a few cells, collagen fibers, and a gel-like matrix of proteoglycans; in the first decade of life the nucleus pulposus becomes less gelatinous and more fibrous. The annulus consists of concentric rings of fibrocartilage, which resist compression but allow limited multiaxial movements of the vertebral column. H&E/alcian blue, paraffin, × 30.

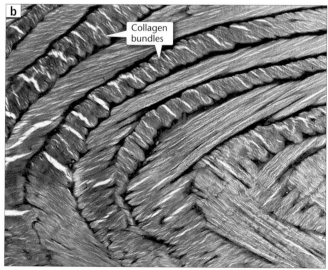

▲ **Fig 10.36b Fibrocartilage.** The concentric lamellae of fibrocartilage of the annulus fibrosus have abundant collagen fibers oriented in orthogonal patterns, which facilitate resistance to load bearing through tensile strength. But this arrangement also allows flexibility of the spine when subject to bending and shear forces. H&E/alcian blue, paraffin, × 80.

Disorders of bone development

Rickets (in children) or osteomalacia (in adults) occurs when bone is poorly calcified and growth plates fail to calcify; this often leads to bowing of long bones owing to the effects of gravity. Bone weakness is due to dietary vitamin D deficiency, lack of exposure of the skin to ultraviolet light (which normally stimulates vitamin D synthesis), or both.

Achondroplasia presents as limb shortness or dwarfism. It is due to a deficiency of growth hormone, as a result of which the epiphyseal plate fails to grow.

Metabolic bone disorders

Metabolic bone disorders are also numerous. Paget's disease is associated with bone weakness and fractures because of abnormal remodeling in which woven bone is excessive and trabeculae are disordered. The condition is thought to be due to viral infection of osteoblasts.

Osteoporosis (bone fragility), synonymous with low bone-mineral density, is common in the elderly of both sexes, although women are more likely to exhibit rapid bone loss at and after menopause. It is related to a declining estrogen level, which normally inhibits bone resorption by osteoclasts. Hormone replacement therapy, exercise, and dietary calcium counteract further bone loss, but may not necessarily rebuild bone to its earlier, denser condition.

Arthritis and arthrosis

Collectively these terms refer to abnormalities of joints and represent an imbalance between the synthesis and degeneration of cartilage and bone. Arthritis, or joint inflammation, has different forms. Infective osteoarthritis occurs in response to local infectious organisms that cause inflammation, release of lytic enzymes, and removal of proteoglycans.

Osteoarthrosis is a non-infective condition and is very common with advancing age; there may be limited inflammation or no inflammation at all, but loss of articular cartilage occurs because of diminishing proteoglycan and the erosion of collagen matrix; abnormal bone spurs (osteophytes growing at the joint margins) and fragments may occupy the joint cavity.

In rheumatoid arthritis, chronic inflammation of numerous joints may occur. This initially involves the synovial membrane, which develops a fibrous ingrowth into the joint. This body (or pannus) erodes cartilage and bone and ultimately may fill the joint cavity and calcify. The joint may become stiff, difficult to move, and painful. The disease may be an autoimmune reaction involving antigen–antibody complexes.

Gout is a disorder of metabolism characterized by excess uric acid production or decreased clearance (possibly associated with renal failure), leading to the accumulation of uric acid in blood. Crystals of sodium urate may precipitate from the blood, eliciting an acute and painful inflammatory reaction often in the first metatarsophalangeal joint of the big toe, the fibrocartilage of the ear, or the interphalangeal joints of the digits.

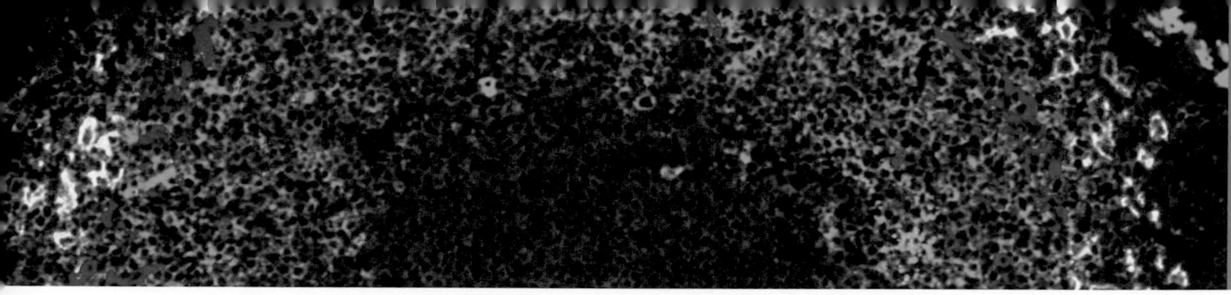

Immune system

Most, and possibly all, multicellular organisms have some sort of immunity to infection. With increasing complexity of cells and tissues among invertebrate and vertebrate animals, the immunological defense system has evolved to protect and defend the organism from foreign organisms or substances (antigens). The immune system protects against infection by pathogens, the four main types being viruses, bacteria, protozoa, and parasites; it heals physical damage such as wounding, and may oppose the development of some tumors. An immune response is shown against all material that is recognized as foreign or "non-self" (e.g. an organ transplant or non-matching blood transfusion), but the immune system exhibits tolerance to self tissues and so normally does not attack the organism it serves to protect.

Although it is important to recognize the histology of lymphoid tissues, together with their common and unique subcomponents, much of what is occurring in these tissues cannot be seen and must, importantly, be imagined and conceptualized. The emphasis in this chapter is to integrate function and concepts with morphology; the morphology is used to illustrate the function. Figure 11.1 summarizes the main activities of the immune system.

BASIC DEFENSE SYSTEMS

The cells, tissues, and organs of the immune system are constantly faced with challenges from foreign molecules, many of which are harmless, but others not. When exposed to a microbe, the immune system must decide whether or not to respond. If a response is required, it must decide what type of defense to initiate. Depending on the pathogen, a defining feature of the immune system is its ability to use sophisticated and highly specific mechanisms to counteract infection and prevent disease.

The repertoire of defense mechanisms may be broadly defined as (i) the primitive or innate immune system established in simple multicellular organisms and (ii) the emergence of the specific or adaptive immune system found in vertebrates such as mammals including humans, but extending back to the cartilaginous fishes such as rays and sharks. A characteristic feature of the mammalian immune system is the ability to initiate qualitatively different types of responses directed against different pathogens. To detect, combat, and destroy or disable the myriad harmful and rapidly evolving/mutating pathogens, the immune system arsenal versus infectious agents has been likened to a military arms race. The system

What happens	Where	When
Foreign substance (antigen) enters the body.	Skin, epithelial surfaces	Constantly
Immediate response by innate immune system (phagocytic cells, especially dendritic cells). Phagocytosis and intracellular destruction. Digestion of foreign microbial proteins into small pieces (peptides) that are displayed on the surface of "antigen-presenting cells," especially dendritic cells, which move to local lymph nodes.	Site of entry	Seconds to minutes
Antigen-presenting cells activate "resting" or "naïve" T cells that have not previously encountered antigen, by binding to specific receptors on the T-cell surface. B cells are activated by the combined action of antigen, which binds to their surface receptors, and direct cell–cell contact with activated T cells. This results in the differentiation of the B cells into plasma cells which secrete antibody into the blood.	Nearby lymph nodes	1–3 days
Antibodies circulate throughout the body via the blood and lymph. Lymphocytes (especially T cells) circulate through the body and fight infections by inducing inflammation, activating phagocytic cells, and killing infected cells.	Throughout the body	Days to weeks to years

▲ **Fig 11.1** The activities of the immune response.

of immunological defenses relies upon many and varied specialist units equipped to deal with threats of many types.

- The innate immune system launches immediately available responses largely made up of cells with phagocytic functions (but including physical barriers and soluble factors). Innate immune mechanisms are a "first-line" defense that contains and limits the spread of infection. Although it is mainly a non-specific defense mechanism, a growing body of evidence indicates that the innate system uses a few dozen "hard-wired" recognition systems, such as the Toll-like receptors (TRLs) that recognize molecular motifs that are found in infectious agents but are absent from multicellular organisms. The innate system can be activated within seconds to minutes but does not have memory of infection.

- The adaptive immune system is slower-reacting (over a period of days) but is infinitely more flexible, with highly specific and effective responses. It allows each individual to respond and remember (i.e. "adapt") to particular microbial challenges for many years, and often for a lifetime. Adaptive immunity is mediated by lymphocytes, which can be classified as T (thymus derived) and B (bone-marrow derived). After activation by antigen, and with help from T cells, B cells differentiate into plasma cells which secrete proteins known as antibodies into the blood. This is sometimes known as "humoral" immunity because antibodies travel in bodily fluids, especially blood. In contrast, T cells generally work by direct cell–cell contact, by killing infected cells and helping B cells make antibodies.

Comparing innate versus adaptive systems

Unlike the innate immune system, the adaptive system can discriminate between an almost infinite variety of antigens. It relies upon a complex system of genes encoding cell surface receptors, and these genes are rearranged in many different ways in individual cells. This is known as the clonal selection theory, and is reviewed later. Another unique feature of the adaptive system is retention of immunological memory of its first encounter with a particular antigen, such that a second encounter gives rise to a "secondary response" that is more rapid, stronger, and longer lasting. This ability is the basis for immunity after infection and immunization.

Older textbooks refer to "cell-mediated immunity" and "humoral immunity." The former refers to the activities of T cells working by direct contact with other cells. In contrast, humoral immunity refers to immunity that is intrinsic to body fluids, notably blood, and is mediated by antibodies. These terms are somewhat misleading, because all proteins, including antibodies, are made by cells. Strictly speaking, all immune responses are cell-mediated; but these terms are hallowed by long usage.

The major features of the innate and adaptive immune systems are summarized in Figure 11.2. Both systems are essential for survival. They form an integrated defense system, analogous to the army and the navy. We will see that the innate and adaptive systems interact synergistically, both at the induction of immune responses when antigen first enters the body, and at the "effector phases" where antigen is destroyed (Fig 11.3).

Feature	Innate	Adaptive
Speed of response	Seconds to minutes	Days, weeks, years
Ability to recognize a diverse range of antigens	Limited to a few dozen "hard-wired" patterns	Almost infinitely flexible, and capable of responding to proteins that differ from "self" by as little as a single amino acid
Memory	No memory	Second encounter with the same antigen results in a faster, stronger and longer response, often lasting a lifetime.
Cellular actions	Phagocytosis and intracellular destruction	B cells secrete antibodies into the blood and lymph. Antibodies bind tightly to antigens, neutralizing them and facilitating their phagocytosis and intracellular destruction. T cells kill infected cells, limiting spread of infection, and help B cells make antibodies. They also activate phagocytes.

▲ **Fig 11.2** The major features of the innate and adaptive immune systems.

Initiation of immune response	Execution of immune response
Antigen is taken up by dendritic cells and broken into small fragments that are displayed on the cell surface, where they activate T cells.	Antibodies bind tightly to antigens, and the antigen–antibody complexes attach to the surface of phagocytic cells and are taken into the cell and destroyed.

▲ **Fig 11.3** Interactions between the innate and adaptive immune systems.

Self, non-self, specificity, and tolerance

The immune system is continually required to make decisions. The most important of these is the ability to distinguish between self and non-self. What is self? The simplest definition is that self is what is present in the body all the time—i.e. self is the sum total of all of the normal components of the body. Non-self has two essential characteristics. Firstly, it is structurally different from self at the biochemical level, for example by virtue of minor differences in the amino acid sequence of a particular protein. A single amino acid difference is sufficient to provoke an immune response. Secondly, non-self is not present all the time, but comes into the body at unexpected times as a result of infection or tissue transplantation.

The immune system must make an even more subtle distinction, although one that is still incompletely understood. The cells, tissues, and organs of the immune system are constantly faced with challenges from foreign molecules. But in the case of microorganisms, how does the immune system defend against pathogenic bacteria, yet tolerate enteric host–bacteria symbiosis? We still do not have a clear understanding of how the body can distinguish between pathogens and harmless commensal organisms.

The ability to make these distinctions is known as specificity, a defining feature of the immune system. Specificity is determined by a complex set of molecular recognition mechanisms involving receptor proteins that can bind to other molecules and deliver "friend or foe" signals to the cells of the immune system.

An immune response will usually occur against all material that is recognized as foreign or non-self (e.g. microbes, transplanted organs, or non-matching blood transfusions). However, the immune system does not normally respond to self. This failure to respond to self is known as immunological tolerance. Self-tolerance is not encoded in the germ line, and is learned as the immune system develops in each individual. Occasionally, for reasons that are poorly understood, self-tolerance breaks down and the immune system attacks normal components of the body as if they were foreign, resulting in auto-immune disease. Examples include insulin-dependent diabetes mellitus, and some forms of arthritis and thyroid disease.

The immune system as a military machine

Under the microscope, all lymphocytes look much the same: small, round cells with round nuclei and a thin rim of cytoplasm, densely packed into deep-blue-staining cell clusters. That their morphology is so featureless reflects the fact that the vast majority of lymphocytes are in stand-by mode, like sentries on guard and waiting for trouble. When trouble does strike, the clonal selection theory indicates that only 1 lymphocyte in 1,000—or even only 1 in 10,000—will respond. This means that the immune system goes about its work with minimal morphological changes.

Trouble, in the form of infection, can strike any part of the body. Accordingly, all parts of the body (with the exception of the brain) contain many millions of lymphocytes, ready to be challenged by antigens. Their ability to discriminate between friend and foe allows them to attack and destroy virtually any foreign substance.

No defense system is perfect. Defense forces are large and expensive to maintain, and require multiple components, such as the army, navy, and air force, as well as multiple weapons to fight different types of enemies. Rarely, the troops may mutiny. Certain parallels may be drawn between the attributes of the immune system and military defense (Parham P. Nature 1990; 344:709–11):

1. Its function is selective destruction.
2. It is large, complicated and elaborate.
3. It is expensive.
4. It is wasteful.
5. It has distinct components performing apparently identical functions.
6. It is slow to react.
7. It is prepared for events that never happen.
8. It fights today's problems with the solutions of past problems.
9. It is susceptible to corruption.
10. It can destroy that which it protects.

INNATE IMMUNITY

The innate immune system is phylogenetically old and found in simple animals such as *Porifera* (sponges) and echinoderms (starfish, sea urchins). It is immediately available to combat threats (and may persist for days), but is of limited flexibility and mainly relies upon phagocytic cells. In higher vertebrates the main phagocytic cells are macrophages and neutrophils, which are assisted by physical barriers and chemical secretions. Innate defenses may be effective against various microbes, recognized as foreign by their surface molecules, which have remained largely unchanged in the course of evolution. The innate system provides little protection against novel types of pathogens (particularly those that mutate), and innate responses do not lead to immunological memory. Thus the response cannot change how the system will react to the same threat upon successive exposures. Importantly, the innate immune system does not attack the host.

The components associated with both innate and adaptive immunity are reviewed in relation to vertebrates in the following sections.

Barrier protection

Barriers against entry into the body are physical and chemical. The former includes skin, mucous membranes (epithelia), and cilia. Chemical barriers include mucus, the acidic properties of skin (sebum from sebaceous glands), and acid secretion by the gastric mucosa. Body fluids contain antibacterial proteins, such as defensins, and lysozyme in tears and saliva, which is an enzyme that causes lysis of some bacteria, although its importance as a defense mechanism is uncertain.

Complement system

The complement system comprises a group of plasma proteins, produced mainly by the liver, that form a triggered enzyme system that defends against microbes. Complement refers to the ability of these proteins to assist, or complement, the antimicrobial activity of antibodies of the adaptive immune system. When activated by antibodies (or directly by bacteria), enzymatic cascade reactions produce bioactive molecules that facilitate osmotic lysis of bacteria, opsonization (rendering the target they coat susceptible to phagocytosis), and attraction of phagocytes to the sites where foreign materials have initiated the complement reaction. The last effect is associated with acute inflammatory responses and with mast cells, producing mediators of vascular permeability, together with the generation of chemotactic factors promoting cell migration that arise from leukocytes, plasma enzyme systems, and injured tissue.

Intracellular killing

Intracellular killing of microbes is carried out by macrophages and neutrophils, both products of the myeloid lineage in bone marrow. Macrophages belong to the mononuclear phagocyte system and derive from circulating monocytes, which become distributed in tissues as resident or wandering macrophages that survive for weeks or months (Fig 11.4a & b). Macrophages or macrophage-type cells are found in virtually all tissues, especially in connective tissues, lung, liver (as Kupffer cells), bone (as osteoclasts), lymphoid organs, kidney (as mesangial cells), and brain (as microglial cells).

Neutrophils survive for several days only, and thus the marrow produces them in vast numbers. They comprise about 60% of circulating white blood cells (Fig 11.5). The killing activity of neutrophils is primarily mediated through release of activated proteases, which destroy bacteria.

Recognition of threats by cells of the innate immune system relies upon detection of common structures called pathogen-associated molecular patterns, or PAMPs. Examples are bacterial cell walls, viral nucleic acids (single-stranded or unmethylated DNA), and bacterial endotoxins. These are recognised by the Toll-like receptors (TLRs), transmembrane proteins on the cell surface or within endosomes. The Toll gene was discovered in *Drosophila* and directs the prototypic dorsal–ventral body axis. TLRs activate inflammatory and immune responses to destroy invaders, and provide a link between innate and adaptive immunity, particularly by activating antigen-presenting cells.

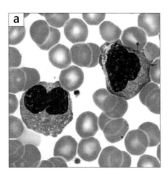

▲ **Fig 11.4a Monocytes and macrophages.**
Monocytes in circulating blood, identified by their large size, eccentric, indented nucleus, and very small cytoplasmic granules. Monocytes circulate for perhaps a day, then enter tissues and serous cavities and mature into macrophages. Wright's stain, × 650.

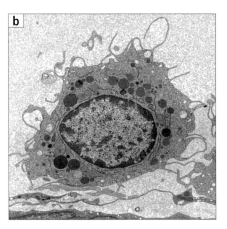

▲ **Fig 11.4b Ultrastructure of a tissue macrophage,** showing many cytoplasmic extensions indicative of their active movement, and numerous lysosomes involved with destruction of phagocytosed materials. Macrophages are antigen-presenting cells for lymphocytes and secrete cytokines that activate many elements of the adaptive immune system. × 3,800.

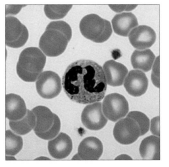

▲ **Fig 11.5 Neutrophil.**
These cells primarily destroy bacteria and other pathogens by phagocytosis. They are the most abundant of the leukocytes (60%) with a life span of only several days in blood. At sites of tissue injury, activated neutrophils are very common in inflammatory responses. Wright's stain, × 700.

Phagocytes contain a large arsenal of lysosomal and microbiocidal proteins, which destroy engulfed bacteria, cellular debris, or foreign particulate matter, but there are important differences between neutrophils and macrophages. Neutrophils die after disposing of their target, whereas macrophages can produce new lysosomes to prolong the killing process, and may survive to continue with recurrent episodes of engulfment and destruction of foreign material. Activated macrophages are an important component of the immune system, since they affect the lymphocytes of the adaptive immune response in two ways:

- They secrete potent peptides, termed cytokines, that control lymphocyte proliferation and differentiation.
- They process and present antigen in a form that can be recognized and responded to by lymphocytes.

Extracellular killing

Extracellular killing mechanisms provide additional protection against microorganisms, served by natural killer (NK) cells, and eosinophils (Fig 11.6a & b). NK cells are large, granular lymphocytes comprising about 10% of the lymphocyte population. They attach to virus-infected cells and some tumor cells, and kill by releasing their granules, which form pores in the target cell membrane followed by apoptotic death. NK cells also activate macrophages to kill phagocytosed microbes. Eosinophils contain granules with cytotoxic proteins and, in conjunction with the production of active oxygen metabolites, these cells are thought to attack parasites too large to be phagocytosed.

Basophils and mast cells also contribute to rapid, first-line responses as part of the innate immune system. Basophils often are considered as progenitors of mast cells, but the relationship between these cells remains controversial. There is evidence in the mouse for a bipotent basophil–mast cell progenitor, and also separate basophil and mast cell progenitors in bone marrow. Basophils are thought to be fully developed in the bone marrow and exit this tissue fully matured, where they are seen in blood. Basophils have a lifespan of only several days and are rarely found in tissues, whereas mast cells may be found in many tissues and survive for weeks or months. Commonly associated with allergic reactions due to the release of very many compounds, including those stored in their characteristic cytoplasmic granules (Fig 11.7a & b), the activated basophils/mast cells are responsible for local irritations, anaphylaxis, and provocation of asthma attacks by increasing vascular

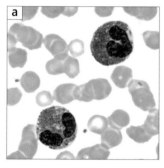

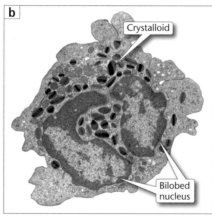

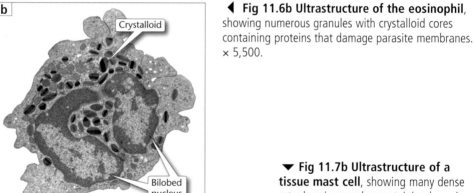

▲ **Fig 11.6a Eosinophils.** These are bilobed granulocytes with prominent cytoplasmic granules containing enzymes and proteins that, when released, attack parasites. Wright's stain, × 650.

◀ **Fig 11.6b Ultrastructure of the eosinophil,** showing numerous granules with crystalloid cores containing proteins that damage parasite membranes. × 5,500.

▼ **Fig 11.7b Ultrastructure of a tissue mast cell,** showing many dense cytoplasmic granules containing heparin, histamine, proteases, and cytokines that are released when the cell is activated, a process termed degranulation. Mast cells defend against parasites such as worms, and mediate allergic reactions. × 5,400.

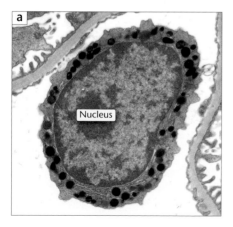

◀ **Fig 11.7a Basophils and mast cells.** Ultrastructure of a circulating basophil, showing its characteristic granules, which are the source of pro-inflammatory molecules, vasoactive amines, and cytokines. Basophils initiate immunoglobulin E (IgE) – mediated chronic allergic inflammatory reactions by recruitment of eosinophils and neutrophils. × 5,500.

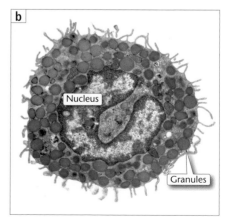

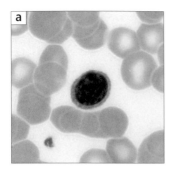

◀ **Fig 11.8a Lymphocytes.** In blood, most lymphocytes are small, similar in size to erythrocytes, and are the second most common leukocyte in blood (20%–30%). The identity of circulating lymphocytes (B or T cells) cannot be determined by their cytology alone and requires labeling with CD markers. Wright's stain, × 750.

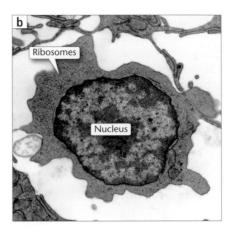

▲ **Fig 11.8b Ultrastructure of a lymphocyte.** There are no characteristic structural features that allow its classification as a B cell or a T cell. Free ribosomes are abundant in the cytoplasm, but other organelles are few in number. × 8,500.

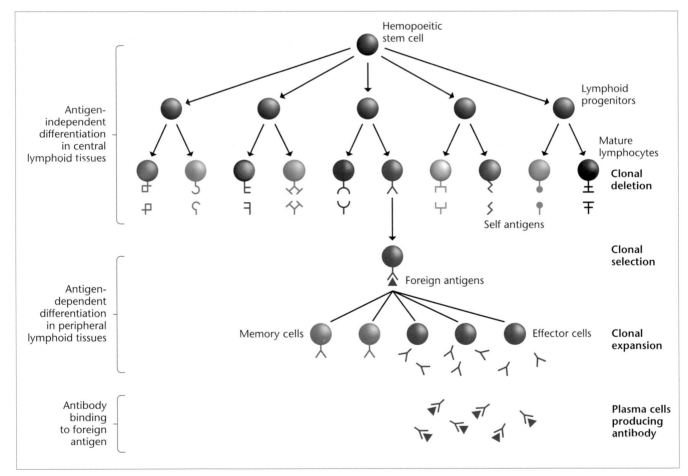

▲ **Fig 11.9 Clonal selection.** This shows the development of lymphocytes, using B cells as an example. In the bone marrow, pluripotent hemopoietic stem cells produce myeloid and lymphoid progenitor cells; the latter differentiate into lymphocytes. Independent of exposure to foreign antigens that will be encountered outside the bone marrow during the life of an individual, many millions of mature but virgin lymphocytes are produced, each with a unique surface receptor capable of binding to a specific antigen. By mechanisms that remain incompletely understood, developing lymphocytes that are defective or capable of reacting against self antigens are deleted. In lymphoid tissues, binding of antigen to a specific lymphocyte clone stimulates antigen-dependent differentiation; the selected type thus proliferates into clones of effector cells (in this case plasma cells) and memory cells. The secreted antibodies are thus available to bind to the same antigenic determinant originally responsible for their production; a variety of effector immune responses eliminates the antigen.

permeability and bronchoconstriction. But these cells also have beneficial effects: their secretory products defend against bacteria, parasites, and toxic peptides, and, by activating inflammatory reactions, attract neutrophils to sites of infection. Among the large range of potent biologically active mediators secreted by mast cells are histamine, heparin, proteases, leukotrienes, cytokines (tumor necrosis factor), chemokines, and various factors that mediate for or against inflammatory and immunoregulatory effects. Basophils and mast cells therefore link the innate and adaptive immune responses.

Neutrophils also participate in extracellular killing by releasing antimicrobial peptides and enzymes embedded in an extracellular fibrous network of chromatin DNA and histones. This complex is known as a neutrophil extracellular trap (NET); it is part of the innate immune system because it traps and kills pathogens.

ADAPTIVE IMMUNITY

The adaptive immune system, which is phylogenetically new (confined to vertebrates), is slow-reacting but highly flexible in its ability to respond to an almost infinite range of different organisms. This results from a complex genetic system for receptor molecules that can recognize foreign substances (i.e. antigens). The key effector cells of the adaptive responses are the lymphocytes, small round cells (mostly 7–10 µm in diameter) with little cytoplasm (Fig 11.8a & b). They originate from bone marrow in adults and from the liver in the early fetus, and make up 20%–30% of circulating leukocytes. Their structure illustrates their function—most of the time they are like policemen, standing around waiting for trouble, apparently doing little but actually serving a crucial role: surveillance. When activated by antigens they enlarge and divide, and subsequently acquire their effector functions (see below).

T lymphocytes mature in the thymus gland, having previously entered this organ, via the blood, as non-functional precursors from the bone marrow. B lymphocytes are made in the bone marrow. Both T cells and B cells are made throughout life, and migrate via the blood to lymphoid tissues; they may return to the blood via lymphatic vessels. Lymphocytes have a lifetime that ranges from a few days to many months or years. Although lymphocytes all appear much the same, they are all different. Each lymphocyte has a unique receptor for antigen, so there are many millions of different lymphocytes (at least 10^{11}), each pre-programmed to recognize a particular antigen. The fully activated, effector B cells secrete antibodies that may act locally or far away; effector T cells act at short range by direct cell–cell contact, for example in the case of killer (cytotoxic) T cells.

Clonal selection theory

The clonal selection theory, and other theories developed from it, provides a generally accepted explanation of how the immune system is equipped to recognize and respond specifically to a whole universe of potential foreign substances, whether or not the body has encountered them at any time in life (Fig 11.9).

In the immune system a lymphocyte clone refers to a family of identical cells that derive from a common progenitor. The theory supposes the following:

- Lymphocytes are made continuously, with each cell having surface receptors with individual specificity for antigen.
- All surface receptors on any one cell have the same binding specificity.
- For each antigen, only a tiny fraction of the whole pool of lymphocytes carry surface receptors to which it can bind. Specificity for antigen is clonally distributed and its genetic mechanisms are discussed below.
- Lymphocytes must be non-reactive to self antigens. This is known as tolerance.

For B cells, the membrane surface receptor called the B cell receptor complex (BCR) is a modified antibody held in the plasma membrane. Antibodies whose specificity is unknown are often referred to as immunoglobulins (Ig) or the older term gamma globulins. The antibody is the secretory Ig product of antigen-activated B cells, and the pool of antibodies in blood constitutes about 20% of the total serum proteins. For T cells, the receptor (TCR) for antigen occurs only in the surface membrane and is never secreted. The TCR shares structural similarities with Ig but is encoded in a separate family of genes.

The binding of an antigen to a lymphocyte selectively activates the cell to proliferate and differentiate, that is, the antigen selects from a huge pool of lymphocytes those capable of recognizing its epitopes (small parts of an antigen—most antigens present multiple epitopes). Activation results in clones of lymphocytes; each clone derives from the same ancestor and all members have the same receptor. B cells and T cells thus comprise vast numbers of clones, each of which is committed to the synthesis of the same surface receptor as the original lymphocyte.

> **Tip:** Selective binding of antigen only with a particular antibody can be likened to buying a new suit that fits. The options are (i) go to the tailor and get a suit made to measure, or (ii) go to a department store and try on lots of suits until you find one that fits. The immune system uses a selection method similar to the second option.

B cells and antibodies

The function of B lymphocytes in adaptive immunity is to provide defense mechanisms against specific antigens that are recognized and disposed of through the production of antibodies.

Development of B cells occurs initially in the bone marrow, followed by further differentiation in the peripheral lymphoid tissues. In the absence of being activated by encounter with a particular antigen, newly minted B cells (also known as naïve or unprimed B cells) in the peripheral circulation die within days. In contrast, antigen-induced activation of B cells stimulates their differentiation into plasma cells, which are the source of antibodies that neutralize or eliminate the antigen. Activated B cells also form long-lived memory B cells poised to vigorously respond to a second encounter with antigen.

B cell maturation

The microenvironment provided by bone marrow stromal cells supports the generation of naïve/immunocompetent B cells in the absence of antigen. This antigen-independent process produces B cells expressing surface immunoglobulins, with each cell having a different antigen-binding specificity. There are about 100,000 membrane-bound immunoglobulin (Ig) molecules on each B cell, acting as receptors for antigen. Those newly minted B cells that are defective or potentially harmful (reactive to self) are usually deleted by apoptosis, or exhibit anergy (inability to be functionally activated). Anergy can also occur in the peripheral lymphoid tissues. Only a small minority of all new B cells survive these culling mechanisms.

Diversity among immunoglobulins (and therefore among B cells, as each cell expresses a unique immunoglobulin) is enormous and thought to be represented as 10^{11} different antigen-combining sites. This huge variation among these proteins far exceeds the current estimated number of 25,000 protein-coding genes in the human genome. How is antibody diversity generated? One fundamental mechanism is the random rearrangement of immunoglobulin gene segments, which takes place early in the development of each lymphocyte. In theory, millions of different peptides are assembled to make an essentially infinite array of different antibody molecules.

This repertoire of unique BCRs on specific B cell clones made in the bone marrow is additionally expanded with changes in nucleotide sequences occurring by the variable joining of gene segments, and quasi-random pairing of the polypeptide heavy (H) and light (L) chains characteristic of antibody molecules. Genes coding for antigen receptors on lymphocytes are designated as variable (V), diversity (D), and joining (J) gene segments. Rearrangement of immunoglobulin V, D, and J gene fragments is an ancient trait of jawed vertebrates, developed approximately 500 million years ago. For each clone, the antibody genes are rearranged in different ways, by reshuffling, joining, and random insertions of nucleotides. The result is that each lymphocyte is committed to a different specificity.

The antibody H and L chains form the two pairs of arms of the Y-shaped Ig molecule, and the stem is formed by one pair of H chains. The N-terminal ends of the arms (fragment of antigen binding [Fab] region) of each Ig molecule are identical sites for binding to a specific epitope or antigen. The C-terminal end of the stem (Fc region) determines the class of Ig and its biological activity (Fig 11.10).

> **Tip:** The antigen binding sites of different Ig classes use their valency (combining property) to cross-link antigen. For example, IgG is divalent so it can cross-link to two antigen sites; IgM has a pentameric structure, so it has 10 binding sites. Even if each binding site is weak, overall binding is strong. By analogy, Velcro® nylon has many individual weak interactions for each of its filaments, but when all are combined they contribute to strong binding.

B cell activation

After naïve/immunocompetent B cells leave the bone marrow and pass into the circulation, they are said to enter the antigen-dependent phase of their development. At this time, B cells may encounter and bind to antigen, which results in proliferation and differentiation into memory B cells and effector cells. Activation of B cells into effector cells produces

Class	Percent serum immunoglobulin	Function
IgM	10	Ancestral Ig; activates complement; produced first and secreted early.
IgA	15–20	In fluids and mucosal surfaces; complexes viruses and bacteria.
IgE	Trace	Binds to basophils, mast cells; allergic inflammation.
IgD	1	Mostly bound on resting B cells; possible B cell trigger.
IgG	70	Major Ig of secondary response; opsonizes antigen; enters fetus from placenta.

▲ **Fig 11.10** Classes and functions of immunoglobulins.

plasmablasts, which continue differentiation into plasma cells (Fig 11.11a–c), which secrete antibody (humoral immunity). While B cells are programmed to synthesize the membrane form of immunoglobulin, plasma cells produce secretory immunoglobulins but retain the same antigen-recognition specificity as the surface immunoglobulin receptors.

Antigen-induced activation of B cells occurs in the peripheral lymphoid tissues (spleen, lymph nodes, mucosa-associated lymphoid tissues [MALTs]) and specifically within their germinal centers. B cells can be activated directly by certain antigens that are intact or soluble, or by repetitive epitopes, such as surface polysaccharides on pneumococci and streptococci. However, these immune responses are mostly restricted to IgM antibodies and generally fail to produce memory B cells. Reinfection might not be prevented.

For most other antigens (e.g. proteins), B-cell activation requires assistance from helper T cells, which themselves are activated when presented with the same antigen(s). In turn, the T cells bind to the B cell and secrete hormone-like molecules (cytokines) that specifically stimulate the B cell. T-cell-dependent stimulation of B cells enhances antibody secretion and results in vigorous immune responses (e.g. activation of phagocytes and complement reaction), local fixation of antibody–antigen complexes, and switching from IgM to IgG, IgA, and IgE, and production of memory B cells.

The collaboration between B cells and T cells ensures that, in response to antigens, specific or selected types of activated B cells proliferate to form clones of antibody-secreting plasma cells together with memory B cells. In the case of a second challenge by the same antigen, and during the second phase of antibody response after primary infection and immunization, the immune response provided by memory cells is faster, of greater magnitude, and longer lasting, and involves antibodies with higher affinity for the antigen.

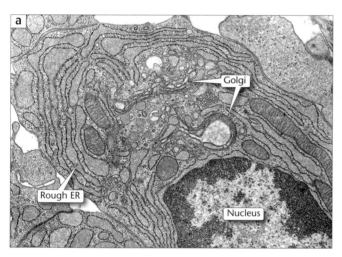

▲ **Fig 11.11a Plasma cells.** Ultrastructure of a plasmablast-type cell in an advanced stage of differentiation toward a mature plasma cell. Note the central Golgi complexes with associated vesicles, and the abundant rough endoplasmic reticulum (ER) with regions of dilatation due to synthesis and accumulation of proteins. × 8,000.

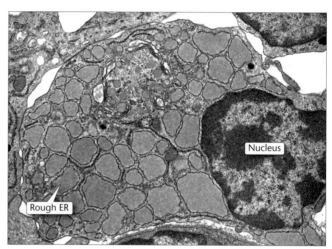

▲ **Fig 11.11b Mature plasma cell** identified by many dilated cisternae of rough ER filled with particulate material representing immunoglobulins. The large proportion of heterochromatin in the nucleus is not indicative of inactivity, since a small fraction of the genome in the euchromatin is highly active in the synthesis of many thousands of copies of a single antibody. × 8,000.

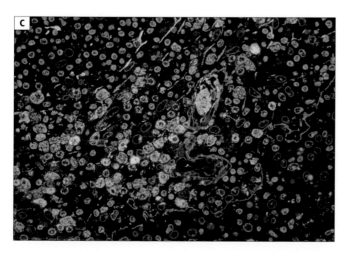

◄ **Fig 11.11c Immunofluorescence labeling of plasma cells in the tonsil.** Immunoglobulins with kappa (κ) light chains are labeled red with the fluorochrome Alexa 488 (about 60% of all antibodies). Plasma cells with lambda (λ) light chains are labeled green with fluorochrome Cy-3. (Courtesy J. Zbaeren, Inselspital, Bern, Switzerland.) × 300.

The antibodies produced in response to encounter with antigen are further "fine-tuned" during the immune response, in which antibody gene segments mutate. Nucleotide mutations among the VDJ gene segments occur at about 1 in every 1,000 base pairs per cell generation. This is about 100,000 times more frequent than the spontaneous mutation rate in other genes. Clones of activated and mutated B cells with greater antigen specificity are preferentially expanded and produce antibody with higher affinity. This process is called somatic hypermutation and is an adaptive response that leads to affinity maturation. It takes place in germinal centers (see later). In other words, B cells compete for antigen, and those with a stronger molecular "match" or "fit" with an antigen are preferentially selected for survival because of their greater ability to bind to the antigen.

The biological activity of such antibodies is also modified to dispose of immunogens by changing the class of antibody synthesis and secretion while retaining specificity for the antigen. Resting B cells produce IgM and IgD surface receptors. Following activation, H chain synthesis changes to produce mostly IgG or IgA (with some IgE), an event called class switching. This allows particular Ig classes to engage distinct pathways of effector mechanisms (e.g. neutralization, opsonization, phagocytosis) in specific locations (mucous membranes, body fluids, lymphoid tissues) to defend the host against infection (Fig 11.12).

T cells and cell-mediated responses

T lymphocytes do not produce classic antibodies, but have surface receptors for antigens, commonly designated as T cell receptor (TCR) complexes, which are related to antibodies. A T cell may have about 10,000 TCRs. The TCR has two peptide chains with variable and constant regions homologous to immunoglobulin regions. Unlike antibodies, TCR chains are anchored in the plasma membrane, are not secreted, and do not undergo somatic hypermutation, affinity maturation, or class switching. Each T cell (and its clones) is different from the next one (and its clones), in that their specificity for an antigen is unique. About 75% of peripheral blood mononuclear leukocytes are T cells.

There is a fundamental difference between T cells and B cells in how they "see" antigens. B cells are capable of binding soluble or free antigens, but T cells don't "see" naked antigens. T cells detect and bind antigens only if they are displayed on the surface of self cells such as antigen-presenting (dendritic) cells, virus-infected cells, some cancer cells, and tissue or organ transplants. This component of the immune system has evolved to attack and eliminate structures that are identified as "altered self."

Diversity among T cells

During T cell maturation in the thymus, random rearrangement of TCR genes in individual clones defines the T cell commitment and selection for specificity to antigen. In addition, T cells "learn" to discriminate between self and non-self. Through a complex process of editing and selection of maturing T cells, the possible number of TCR specificities is estimated to be 10^{12} or greater. The TCR is associated with surface marker molecular complexes termed cluster of designation markers (CD markers, numbering in the hundreds, determined by binding of groups of monoclonal antibodies, largely confined

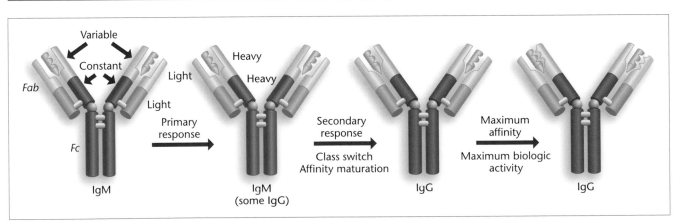

▲ **Fig 11.12 Modification of immunoglobulin (antibody) in response to antigen.** The Ig molecule consists of two arms, the Fab (fragment of antigen binding) regions, and a stem or Fc (fragment crystallizable) region. Polypeptide heavy and light chains have large and smaller molecular weights, parts of which are constant for a particular class of Ig, and parts which are variable to allow for recognition of a particular antigen. During the initial antigenic challenge or immunization, antigen binding is of low relative affinity, and IgM is the major antibody class. For a secondary antigen challenge, the antibodies produced are mainly IgG and, via alterations in the variable segment region, antigen–antibody "fit" or affinity is greatly enhanced. This process is driven by antigen, as variants or mutated forms of the Fab region are selected for when the B cells exhibit intense proliferation of antibody-bearing clones.

to leukocytes); CD3 and CD28 molecules are both required for signal transduction as the TCR binds antigen. More than 95% of T cells maturing in the thymus do not survive the selection process (reviewed later under *Thymus*); those that do form distinct subpopulations.

Cell types

T cells that emerge from the thymus are composed of two major subpopulations, defined by surface expression of CD4 or CD8, and functionally divided into two main classes (Fig 11.13):

- CD4 are helper T cells (Th, CD4$^+$) that secrete cytokines to activate other cells (e.g. 'help' B cells make antibody).
- CD8 are killer (cytotoxic) T cells (Tc, CD8$^+$) that kill foreign and virally infected cells and foreign grafts by direct contact.

Regulatory T cells (Tr) of several types are CD4$^+$ and suppressor T cells (Ts) are CD8$^+$; these cells possibly antagonize or redirect immune responses. The correlations between CD markers and T cell function(s) are not absolute. About 5%–10% of circulating T cells are CD4$^-$ and CD8$^-$ and—unlike CD4$^+$ or CD8$^+$ cell types, which bind peptide antigen fragments—these lymphocytes can recognize carbohydrate or lipid antigens associated with certain bacteria.

How do Th cells "help"?

When activated, the cytokines produced by Th cells are critical for activation of Tc cells, B cells, and a variety of non-lymphocyte cells. Th cells also may differentiate into specialized Th1 and Th2 cells that release their own cytokines involved with defense against intracellular viruses and bacteria and, with

B cell activation, help respond against allergens, fungi and parasites such as worms.

How do Tc cells kill?

Cytotoxic T cells destroy their targets by releasing special secretory lysosomes, called lytic granules, at the immunological synapse that forms between the Tc cell and the target. Granules contain a pore-forming protein called perforin, and proteases called granzymes, the latter entering the cell to be killed through the pores made in its plasma membrane. After contact with the target, the microtubule organizing center of the Tc cells is polarized toward the immunological synapse, mobilizing the granules toward the centrosome, which now establishes contact with the synapse. Lytic granules are thus directed precisely to the corresponding plasma membrane of the target cell.

Antigen processing and presentation

Since T cells cannot recognize "naked" or intact antigen, the activation of T cells requires that antigen must be captured, broken down, or processed into short peptide fragments (usually 8–25 amino acids), and specially presented on the surface of cells to enable the T cell to recognize the antigen as foreign. Presentation or display of antigen can be performed by almost every cell type, but is especially efficient in a range of leukocytes, designated as antigen-presenting cells (APCs).

Peptide fragments are held in the groove of the major histocompatability complex (MHC) proteins, which are surface proteins encoded by the genetic region known to be responsible for immune responses that result in rejection of organ and tissue allografts

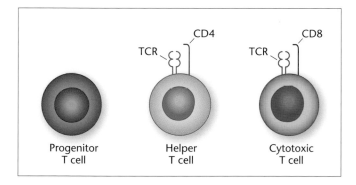

▲ **Fig 11.13 Major types of T lymphocytes.** Progenitors of T cells are bone-marrow-derived cells that circulate in blood and home to the thymus. They do not express surface membrane proteins found on differentiated T cells. Immunocompetent/naïve T cells that leave the thymus are of two main types, helper T cells (Th) and cytotoxic T cells (Tc). Both types express T cell receptors (TCRs) in the surface membrane, comprising α and β peptide chains with variable and constant domains similar to the immunoglobulins of B cells. Each T cell may have 10,000 identical TCRs. The number of different T cells, each with unique TCRs, is estimated to be 10^{12} and

up to 10^{15}. TCRs are antigen-specific receptors that bind antigen only in combination with antigen presented by major histocompatability complex (MHC) molecules. A small minority of T cells (5%), called intraepithelial T cells, found in the gut and its lamina propria express γδ TCRs. Mature lymphocytes also display accessory surface proteins designated as cluster of differentiation (CD) markers, CD4 on helper T cells, and CD8 on cytotoxic T cells. About two-thirds of peripheral T cells are CD4 and one-third are CD8. CD markers act as co-receptors for the interaction between the TCR and the MHC.

(Fig 11.14). The definitive features of the MHC are the "transplantation antigens" that it encodes (i.e. class I and class II MHC molecules). In humans, MHC proteins are called human leukocyte-associated (HLA) antigens. Unlike blood group antigens A, B, and O, which are relatively simple (and do not elicit T cell responses), MHC proteins are derived from genes with hundreds of alleles and show extreme polymorphism. It is very unlikely that two unrelated individuals will have the same set of MHC molecules. This explains the high incidence of transplant rejection.

Grafts and transplantations don't occur in nature. An exception is the implantation in the uterus of a conceptus, which is protected from immune-based rejection. So, what is the purpose of MHC molecules? The physiologic function of the MHC is to act as a "platform" or a "cradle" that allows T cells (i.e. the TCR complex) to "see" antigens presented in association with self MHC molecules; in other words, T cells see antigen as "modified self." The evolution of MHC diversity among individuals in an outbred population virtually guarantees that there will always be a few members that can present specific microbial antigens for activation of an immune response directed against such challenges.

Function of MHC molecules

Recall that B cells mediate humoral immunity by producing antibodies that enter blood and mucosal fluids. Here they neutralize and eliminate microbes and their toxins outside of host cells, and prevent such pathogens from colonizing and infecting otherwise healthy cells. But many microbes get inside cells, proliferate, and exploit the cell's function for their own survival. In these cases, the pathogen can be considered "invisible" and in a sense is hidden inside

the cells that it subverts. The function of the MHC is to allow T cells to detect this intracellular mischief (e.g. viral infection) and deal with it by killing the cell, a process called cell-mediated immunity.

> **Tip:** In effect, invading pathogens located outside of cells are opposed by B cells, and those sheltered within cells are revealed by MHC molecules and attacked by T cells; there is nowhere to hide!

Class I MHC proteins

CD8+ killer T cells (Tc) only see antigen when it is in the MHC I groove.

Class I MHC proteins are found on most nucleated cells, although hepatocytes, muscle cells, fibroblasts and neurons in the CNS have very low levels. Class I MHC binds peptides of about 8–10 amino acids that are endogenous or synthesized inside the cell, and originate from virus-infected cells, intracellular bacteria, mutant cells (such as tumor cells), grafted cells, or transplanted organs. Tc cells kill their targets by direct contact. Transplanted organs are seen as foreign by T cells: since their MHC is different, the MHC groove of transplanted cells contains a different mixture of peptides to that in the self MHC. T cells probably recognize foreign graft cells as being infected with viruses and deal with such "perceived infection" by killing the cells.

Class II MHC proteins

CD4+ helper T cells (Th) only see antigen when it is in the MHC II groove.

Class II MHC proteins occur on APCs, mainly monocytes and macrophages, B cells, and dendritic cells; the last are found predominantly within lymphoid tissues and, in terms of antigen capture and

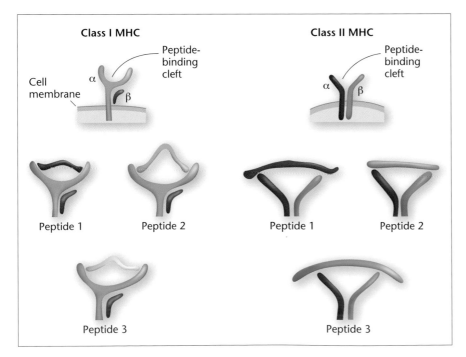

Class I MHC — Peptide-binding cleft — Cell membrane — α — β — Peptide 1, Peptide 2, Peptide 3

Class II MHC — Peptide-binding cleft — α — β — Peptide 1, Peptide 2, Peptide 3

◀ **Fig 11.14 MHC binding sites.**
Schematic representation of the MHC proteins and how they bind peptides. Many hundreds of alleles of each class I and class II gene exist. Class I MHC molecules have an α chain with a binding groove and a β chain that has no peptide-binding function or attachment to the cell surface. A wide range of peptides, 8–10 amino acids in length, can be held in the groove because only the ends are anchored and the central residues protrude out of the groove. Class II molecules have α and β chains with an open-ended binding groove that in most cases allows binding of longer peptides of 13–18 amino acids, with other residues extending beyond the ends of the binding groove. Although there is a high degree of MHC polymorphism in human populations, any individual has a maximum of 6 different class I MHC molecules and 12 different class II MHC molecules.

presentation, are the most potent type of APC. MHC class II presents antigen that comes from outside the cell. The exogenous antigenic proteins are endocytosed or phagocytosed, cut into fragments commonly 13–14 amino acids in length, and displayed in the groove of the MHC II protein. Exogenous antigens include most bacteria and/or their toxins, parasites, and virus particles released from infected cells. CD4+ Th cells secrete cytokines that act on B cells, Tc cells, and macrophages, and activated T cells produce memory T cells.

> **Tip:** Although an MHC molecule presents only one peptide because there is only one groove, the floor of the groove anchors just a few residues and therefore can bind many different peptides. This is important for displaying many different antigens. When the extreme polymorphism (within each class) of MHC molecules between individuals is added to how antigens are displayed, it is therefore very difficult to find perfect MHC matches between unrelated individuals for transplants.

Dendritic cells and immune responses

Located in most tissues, dendritic cells (DCs) are antigen-presenting cells that initiate and regulate much of the adaptive immune response served by B and T lymphocytes. They are not easily seen in conventional hematoxylin and eosin (H&E) stained sections, and require specialized techniques such as immunofluoresence or immunoperoxidase to be revealed. Most, but not all, DCs arise from the bone marrow myeloid lineage; some may arise from monocytes or, in the mouse, from the lymphoid lineage; others may develop locally within lymphoid tissues. DCs capture and process antigens and display large amounts of MHC–peptide complexes on their surface. The DCs that carry out immunosurveillance in tissues are said to be immature because when activated, they mature into stellate-type cells with an extensive membrane surface area that presents antigen fragments and interacts with lymphocytes (Fig 11.15).

Categories of dendritic cells

Plasmacytoid DCs circulate through blood and lymphoid tissues. They are produced in the bone marrow and migrate to lymph nodes, MALT and the spleen, driven mainly by inflammatory stimuli. Plasmacytoid DCs might not initiate immune responses but may specialize in modulating the activities of NK, T, and B cell immune responses.

Conventional DCs are found in the thymus, spleen and lymph nodes. On the basis of the paths they take to access these organs, these DCs form two groups:

- Migratory DCs arise from precursors in peripheral tissues and reach local lymph nodes via afferent lymphatics; they include the Langerhans DCs that migrate from skin epidermis (Fig 11.16a & b). Migratory DCs make up about 50% of all lymph node DCs.

◀ **Fig 11.15 Dendritic cells.** Cultured dendritic cells show irregular shapes reflecting a state of maturation that has followed their activation by antigen. The many long, dynamic surface extensions in vivo act as a mesh for detecting pathogens. Class II MHC molecules are expressed on the cell surface, labeled red. Nuclei are blue. Confocal fluorescence microscopy. (Courtesy J Villadangos, Immunology Division, Walter and Eliza Hall Institute, Melbourne, Australia.) × 1,600.

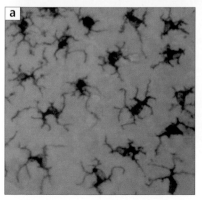

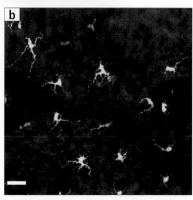

◀ **Fig 11.16 Langerhans cells.**
a Immunohistochemistry of Langerhans cells in skin expressing MHC II (red). **b** Two-photon image of Langerhans cells of a transgenic mouse expressing an enhanced yellow fluorescent protein driven by the CD11c promoter. (Courtesy L Cavanagh, W Weninger, Centenary Institute, Sydney, Australia; from Immunol Cell Biol 2008; 86:428–38.) Bar = 25 μm.

- Resident DCs make up the other 50% of lymph node DCs (sometimes referred to as follicular DCs) and all of those found in the thymus and spleen. These DCs originate from bone marrow precursors within the lymphoid organs and do not pass through peripheral tissues.

When fluorescent-labeled DCs are examined in vivo with two-photon microscopy, they show extensive networks tethered to the fibroreticular supporting tissue. The tips of their dendritic processes are motile, touching adjacent DCs, and their ruffled surface membranes extend and retract, suggesting a probing function. In this way each DC can present MHC-bound antigen to thousands of wandering lymphocytes that pass by a DC every hour.

The function of dendritic/antigen-presenting cells in the initiation of adaptive immune responses that activate T and B cells is summarized in Figure 11.17.

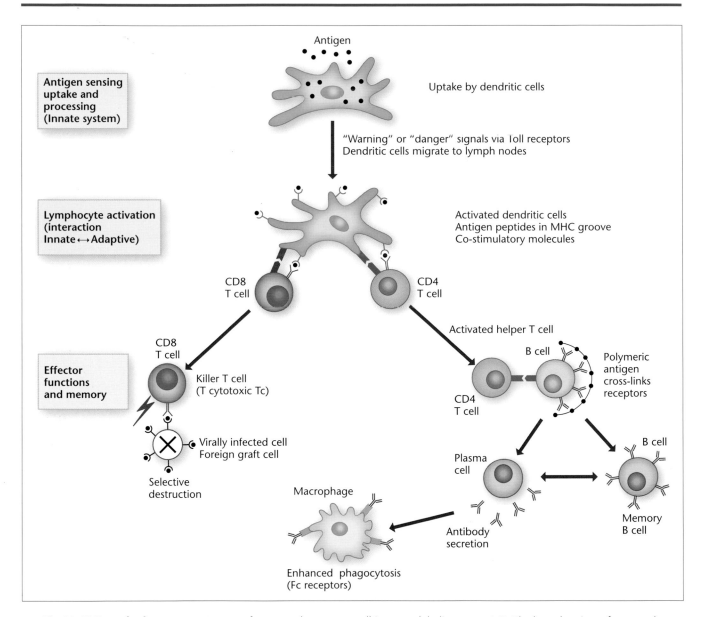

▲ Fig 11.17 How the immune system works: general concepts of some of the major events occurring in and between the innate and adaptive immune responses, with details in the text. Note: (i) Interaction between the helper T cell and the B cell has been simplified but involves interactions between helper TCR and MHC II on the B cell, and between CD40 co-receptors on both cells. (ii) Elimination of pathogens via antibody production (humoral response) from plasma cells occurs when antigen–antibody complexes are bound to Fc receptors on phagocytes such as macrophages. Fc receptors can bind to the Fc region of all immunoglobulins except IgD. The bound antigen, for example a bacterium, is not shown. The macrophage physically eliminates the antigen–antibody complexes by internalization and destruction. (iii) Interaction between a CD8 cytotoxic T cell and the class I MHC on dendritic cells is an example of cross-presentation, where antigen derived from extracellular sources is captured and presented by the MHC. Cross-presentation to the cytotoxic T cell population enables the dendritic cell to initiate an immune response against a virus even if the dendritic cell itself is not infected. (Courtesy J Goding, Monash University, Melbourne, Australia.)

LYMPHOID TISSUES

The immune system is compartmentalized into organs and tissues that are functionally unified via blood and lymph vascular systems that allow trafficking and recirculation of lymphocytes between the sites of lymphoid aggregations and the vasculature. **Primary lymphoid organs** are sites where lymphocytes are made—B cells in bone marrow and T cells in the thymus. These sites produce naïve/immunocompetent lymphocytes, which

- are capable of recognizing antigen;
- localize in appropriate parts of the body where they concentrate in lymphoid tissues.

Moving via blood, the lymphocytes are distributed to the **secondary lymphoid organs** (or peripheral lymphoid tissues), which consist of the lymph nodes and spleen, and to numerous sites associated with gut, lungs, and other mucosal sites collectively termed mucosa-associated lymphoid tissues (MALT). Secondary lymphoid tissues are sites where lymphocytes and antigen interact and thereby initiate immune responses.

Bone marrow

Bone marrow is the major hemopoietic organ in most mammals, and is primarily found in cancellous (spongy) bone (Fig 11.18). It is a highly cellular tissue that produces all blood cell types except mature T cells. It contains numerous arterial, venous, and sinusoidal blood vessels, and a reticular stroma with macrophages, extracellular matrix, and a high proportion of fat cells (yellow marrow), easily identified in contrast to the red marrow, the location for common precursor hemopoietic stem cells (HSCs; reviewed in Chapter 2). HSCs are found near endosteum and vascular sinusoids. Here they associate with stromal cells thought to create HSC niches, where they self-renew and differentiate.

Cells of the lymphoid lineage account for less than 10% of all cells in bone marrow. Perhaps only 5% of the B cells produced each day in bone marrow reach maturity. The remainder undergo apoptosis due to self-reactivity or non-productive receptor gene rearrangements. Naïve/immunocompetent B cells that leave the bone marrow are IgM^+IgD^+.

Thymus

The thymus is located deep to the manubrium of the sternum, overlaying the great vessels of the heart. Within the thymus, T cells exhibit several phases of maturation, and following their release into the circulation may be activated in peripheral lymphoid tissues. Unlike B cells, T lymphocytes do not produce antibodies; these cells differentiate into various types of T cells that form the basis of cell-mediated immunity. Prominent at birth, the thymic mass enlarges up to puberty, but thereafter reduces in size and is replaced progressively with adipose tissue. After middle age there is a relatively slower loss of thymic tissue that continues into old age.

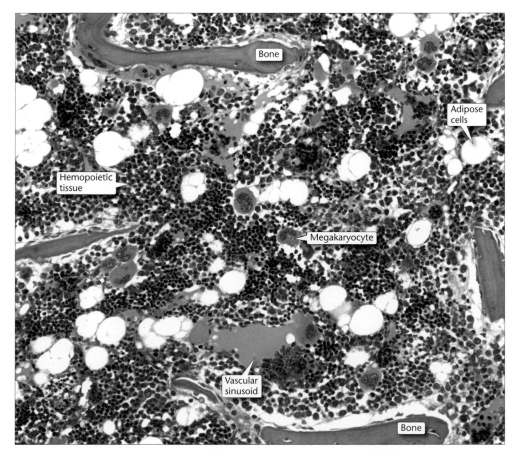

◀ **Fig 11.18 Bone marrow.** Red marrow is the site of hemopoiesis and the home of hemopoietic stem cells (HSCs). The hemopoietic compartment is dispersed through the stromal tissue, consisting of a fibroreticular network, vascular sinusoids, adipose cells, and nerves. HSCs are not identified in routine histologic sections but are known to occur in niches. Niches are defined as microenvironments that maintain stem cell self-renewal. HSCs occur in (i) endosteal/osteoblastic niches on the surface of trabecular bone where osteoblasts regulate HSC activity or quiescence, and (ii) vascular sinusoidal niches to which HSCs are attracted for differentiation and proliferation and eventual mobilization through the sinusoidal endothelium into the circulation. H&E, paraffin, × 150.

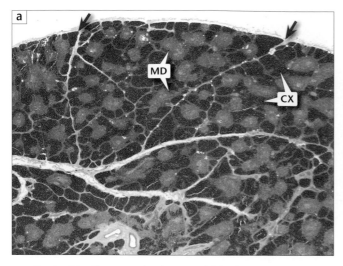

▲ **Fig 11.19a Thymus.** The thymus is bilobed, surrounded by a connective tissue capsule and extending septa (**arrows**) inward to form lobules that show a densely staining cortex (**CX**) and pale medulla (**MD**). Precursor lymphocytes from the bone marrow enter the thymus through capsular and septal blood vessels, and these cells may be termed thymocytes. The thymic stroma is a framework of connective tissue elements and specialized epithelial cells together with macrophages and antigen-presenting cells. Thymocytes proliferate and mature in the thymus, but only a very small fraction (about 1%–3%) survive the selection processes that allow immunocompetent T cells to enter the peripheral circulation. H&E, paraffin, × 8.

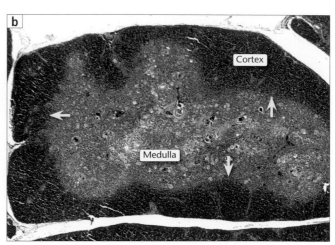

▲ **Fig 11.19b Thymic cortex.** The cortex is densely stained with many developing T cells, giving a mottled or "starry-sky" appearance because of macrophages that eliminate T cells with inappropriate T cell receptors (TCRs). The medulla contains fewer T cells, but numerous epithelial and dendritic cells, some macrophages, and capillaries and venules that drain via septa into the capsule. A distinct corticomedullary junction (**arrows**) is rich in blood vessels from the septa, and contains a concentration of dendritic cells (special antigen-presenting cells), which are also scattered throughout the thymus. The cortex, medulla, and junction between them all participate in T cell maturation, elimination, and selection. H&E, paraffin, × 25.

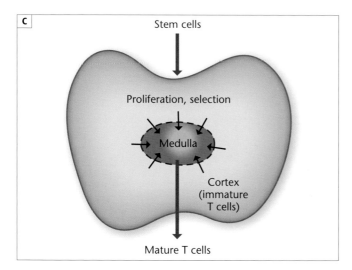

▲ **Fig 11.19c Concept of thymus function.** Marrow-derived T cell progenitors are stem-type cells that enter the thymus in the cortex, where they commence a complex phase of proliferation and maturation into T cells. As T cells mature, the vast majority do not survive the thymic selection processes, but those that do migrate to the medulla, undergo further selection tests and development, and exit the thymus as CD4 helper or CD8 cytotoxic T cells.

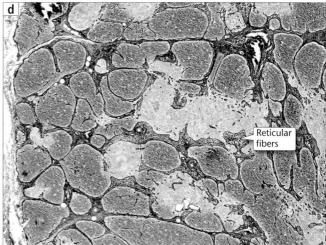

▲ **Fig 11.19d Supporting tissue framework in the thymus** consists of two components. Reticular fibers (type III collagen) are noted in the trabeculae, the septa, and vessel adventitia but are absent from the cortical lobules and in the central medulla. The other supporting network in the lymphoid regions of the thymus is a reticulum of epithelial cells unique to the tissue. Reticulin stain, paraffin, × 15.

The two lobes of the thymus consist of many lobules separated by connective tissue septa. Lobules show a lymphocyte-dense outer cortex and an inner, lighter-staining medulla, usually confluent within adjacent lobules. Together, the cortex and medulla "educate" multipotent T cell precursors that arrive from the bone marrow. Subsequently these cells, also known as thymocytes, mature into competent T cells that are released into the peripheral circulation (Fig 11.19a–f). In addition to the crowded, developing T cells in the cortex, this region and the medulla contain specialized epithelial cells, DC, and macrophages that form the stromal framework for the tissue together with collagen, extracellular matrix network, and blood vessels. Some efferent lymphatics are present, but afferent vessels are absent.

The roles of the epithelial, dendritic and macrophage cells are, in general, to allow T cell development to proceed, subject to the differentiating cells passing stringent tests of their suitability for export to other regions of the body.

The thymus "educates" T cells

The critical role of the thymus is to create a diverse population of T cells capable of responding to non-self or foreign antigens in the context of self MHC, but not to self antigen alone. Inevitably the random generation of newly forming T cells with a vast repertoire of antigen specificities will include T cells with (i) receptors for non-self (useful), (ii) receptors for self (potentially harmful), and (iii) useless T cells with no receptor at all. Deletion of potentially harmful

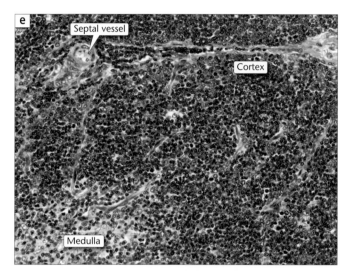

◀ **Fig 11.19e The thymic cortex** is seeded with immature thymocytes, which enter via vessels in the septa that terminate near the medulla. The outer cortex is a site for intense thymocyte proliferation. A variety of epithelial cells positively select T cells that weakly recognize MHC II (and some MHC I) on the epithelial cell surface. Non-selected or negatively selected (high affinity with self MHC or self MHC + self antigen) T cells undergo apoptosis and macrophage phagocytosis. As T cells move toward the medulla, dendritic cells with MHC-antigens negatively select those T cells that are auto- or self-reactive. These die by apoptosis and/or are eliminated by macrophages; survivors may be further selected in the medulla. H&E, paraffin, × 120.

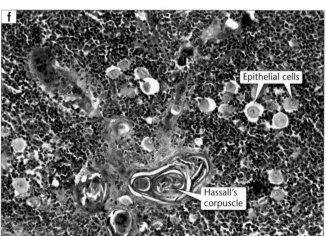

◀ **Fig 11.19f Thymic medulla.** Medullary thymic epithelial cells have a rounded shape with processes that support the numerous T cells, and predominantly express MHC I molecules. These cells can promote positive selection of MHC I restricted cells (CD8+ or T cytotoxic [Tc] cell precursors) and MHC II restricted cells (CD4+ or T helper [Th] precursors), and their expression of autoantigens can induce negative selection of autoreactive cells that may have escaped deletion in the cortex. Whorls of epithelial cells form Hassall's corpuscles, prominent in primates but less obvious in rodents. These epithelial complexes coordinate dendritic cell-mediated central tolerance to generate CD4+CD25+ regulatory T cells. H&E, paraffin, × 120.

self-reactive T cells in the thymus is termed "central tolerance." Education of T cells in the thymus is achieved by a series of selection "tests" that determine the survival or death of T cells (Fig 11.20). These processes are referred to as:

- **positive selection** of T cells (i.e. the TCR) that weakly recognize self MHC;
- **negative selection**—subsequent elimination of those T cells that interact too strongly with self MHC, or self MHC + self antigen.

In essence, the developing T cells actively sample numerous antigen-presenting thymic stromal cells. This increases the probability of encountering rare negatively selecting ligands that are essential for central tolerance.

New progenitor cells from the bone marrow enter the thymus at the cortico-medullary junction. They are thought not to be T-lineage committed, although this notion is controversial. Thus they do not express CD4 or CD8 co-receptors or the TCRs that characterize most T cells, and are described as CD4⁻CD8⁻ double-negative (DN) cells. Once inside the thymus, DN cells undergo massive proliferation, start rearranging and expressing TCR genes, and are subject to an orderly, stringent differentiation and selection repertoire resulting in around only 1%–2% of them finally surviving as immunocompetent, single-positive (SP) cells, that is, CD4⁺ or CD8⁺ T cells (Fig 11.21).

The journey taken by thymocytes (a broad term covering all intrathymic T cells or their progenitors) through the thymic cortex and medulla has been estimated to require 3–4 weeks (Fig 11.22).

The scale of T-cell proliferation and cell death is astounding: even though only a tiny fraction of T cells survive their "education in the university of the thymus," many billions of single-positive T cells with different TCRs survive.

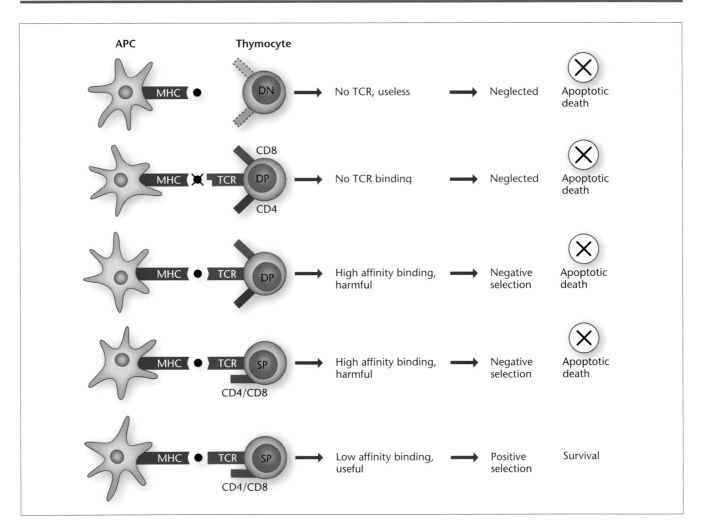

▲ **Fig 11.20 T cell selection processes in the thymus.**
Entering the thymus from the bone marrow, undifferentiated T cell progenitors are referred to as thymocytes. These cells do not express the typical surface molecules found on T cells, such as the T cell receptor for antigen (TCR) or CD4/CD8 co-receptors, and are referred to as double-negative (**DN**) cells. The sequence of selection steps is shown from the top downward. Interactions occur between the TCR and a peptide fragment of self antigen (**black dots**) held by the MHC on an antigen-presenting cell. Double-positive thymocytes (**DP**) express CD4 and CD8 co-receptors. Differentiation of single-positive (**SP**) thymocytes express either CD4 or CD8. Only SP thymocytes with weak affinity for self antigens survive the selection process; these are said to be positively selected and leave the thymus as mature, immunocompetent T cells.

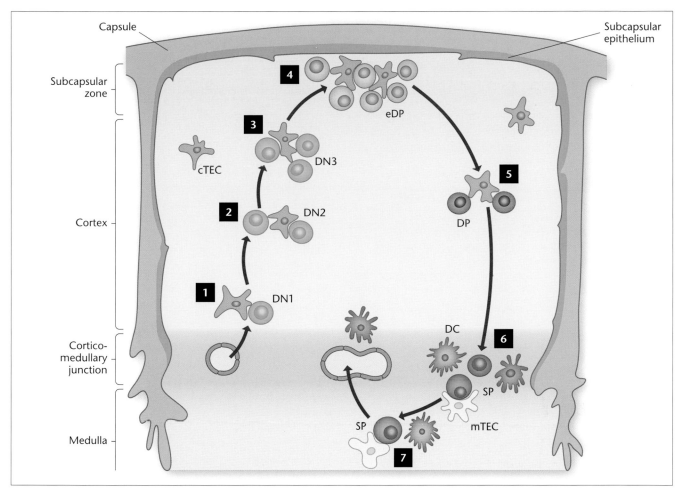

▲ **Fig 11.21 Development of T cells in the thymus.**
Pathways taken and interactions experienced by developing T cells that pass through the cortex and medulla, in which T cell receptor (TCR) genes are rearranged to produce competent CD4+ and CD8+ cells: **1** Incoming double-negative (**DN**) progenitors from bone marrow enter via capsule or septa; **2–3** Association with cortical thymic epithelial cells (**cTEC**) with thymocyte proliferation;

4 Greatly increased proliferation and differentiation into early double-positive (**eDP**) thymocytes; **5** Selection and differentiation of DP thymocytes; **6** Migration to medulla and differentiation into single-positive (**SP**) thymocytes with interactions and further selection in association with dendritic cells (**DC**) and medullary thymic epithelial cells (**mTEC**); **7** Completion of maturation and export into venous system.

Thymic region	Thymocyte type	Time of residence	Developmental events
1 Cortico-medullary junction	Double-negative	10 days	Recruitment of bone marrow T-cell progenitors Significant proliferative expansion
2 Inner cortex	Double-negative	2 days	Migration toward capsule via stromal signals Proliferation and early thymic imprinting by TCR gene rearrangement
3 Outer cortex	Double-negative	2 days	Migration and proliferation TCR gene rearrangement and absolute T-lineage commitment
4 Subcapsular zone	Early double-positive	1 day	Immature/pre-TCR expression; death of faulty TCR cells Significant proliferation creates multicellularity Acquistion of CD4 and CD8 expression
5 Cortex	Double-positive	2 days	Proliferation inhibited; ongoing TCR development Positive selection and survival by self MHC on epithelial cells; MHC restriction CD4 and CD8 lineage divergence
6 Outer medulla	Single-positive	5 days	Negative selection and death by self MHC or self antigen + self MHC on dendritic/epithelial cells or macrophages Self-tolerance
7 Central medulla	Single-positive	5 days	Retention for full functional capacity Tolerance induction Export

▲ **Fig 11.22 Timeline for migration of thymocytes** through the thymic microenvironments. Numbered regions correspond to those in Figure 11.21. (Based on data in Petrie HT and Zuniga-Pflucker JC, Annu Rev Immunol 2007; 25:649–79.)

In creating lymphocyte diversity in the bone marrow and thymus, lymphocytes "learn" to discriminate self from non-self. Are all self antigens expressed in these formative organs? This seems unlikely, and therefore central tolerance may not be absolute and autoreactive B cells and T cells persist in normal individuals. Various mechanisms of peripheral tolerance eliminate or silence these cells. Breakdown of these mechanisms may lead to organ-specific or systemic autoimmune diseases.

> **Tip:** Immature progenitor cells enter the thymus, and through proliferation, differentiation, and selection steps generate immunocompetent T cells for export to the circulation. As they pass through the thymus, maturing T cells "run the gauntlet" of tests that determine their fate. The T cell repertoire is self-tolerant and binds self MHC with low affinity. "The thymus selects the useful, neglects the useless and destroys the harmful" (von Boehmer H et al. Immunol Today 1989; 10:57–61).

Secondary lymphoid organs

Secondary lymphoid organs include the spleen, lymph nodes, and MALT. In histologic sections they are identified as darkly staining areas densely packed with small round cells, and contain spherical structures called "primary follicles." These are mostly composed of B cells and specialized follicular dendritic cells (FDCs). Areas between the follicles contain predominantly T cells and epithelial dendritic cells. Following antigenic stimulation, primary follicles undergo massive expansion into secondary follicles containing morphologically identifiable germinal centers.

The lymphoid stroma

Lymphoid tissue architecture is supported by a three-dimensional meshwork of stromal cells and reticular fibers (Fig 11.23). Stromal cells include follicular dendritic cells in B-cell follicles, and fibroblastic reticular cells in T-cell zones that produce the collagen-rich reticular fibers and extracellular matrix. Together these cells form a maze of stromal channels that guides and supports lymphocyte migration within lymph nodes and the spleen, facilitating their interactions with APCs. The directed trafficking of lymphocytes through the stroma is achieved by stromal cell expression of cytokines, chemokines, and adhesion molecules. Lymphocyte movement within lymphoid tissues may be studied in real-time with live imaging two-photon microscopy.

Lymph nodes

Lymph nodes are ovoid-shaped organs of variable size ranging from barely visible when quiescent to a centimeter or more when activated in immune responses. They receive lymph from lymphatic vessels that drain tissue spaces, and thus are strategically positioned to detect and counteract infectious agents and pathogens that invade tissues. In response to tissue injury or local or systemic infection, lymph nodes may enlarge ("swollen glands") and become palpable in, for example, the cervical, axillary, or inguinal regions. Enlargement is due to increased leukocyte populations. Each node is a physical and biological filter, trapping microbes and antigen that arrive in afferent lymph and releasing lymphocytes into the efferent lymphatics, which ultimately enter

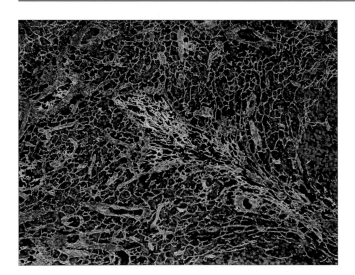

▲ **Fig 11.23 Lymphoid organ stroma.** Part of the supporting stromal network of reticular fibres in a lymph node. The fibers show an extraordinary three-dimensional mesh-type morphology that provides structural integrity to the lymphoid tissues and produces many factors for the migration and survival of immune cells. Reticulin stain, darkfield microscopy, paraffin, × 90.

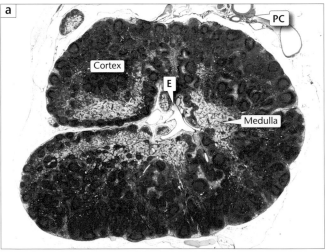

▲ **Fig 11.24a Lymph node.** Architecture of a lymph node, showing pericapsular connective tissues (**PC**) with minor blood vessels and afferent lymphatics; the latter bringing lymph, draining from tissues, into the lymph node, which acts as a filter. Afferent lymph percolates through the cortex, which contains numerous ovoid lymphoid follicles, then into the medulla, which has a meshwork-like morphology, and exits through efferent lymphatics (**E**), located at the hilum. Most of the blood supply enters and exits the node through the hilum. H&E, paraffin, × 5.

the venous blood via the major lymphatic ducts. Supported by connective tissue trabeculae from its capsule, the nodes show an outer cortex with lymphoid follicles rich in B cells and specialized APCs, and a deeper paracortex with T cells and macrophages (Fig 11.24a–d). In the center is the medulla, comprised of medullary cords (lymphocytes, macrophages, and plasma cells) surrounded by medullary sinuses that are continuous with the efferent lymphatics that exit the lymph node. Lymph percolates through these regions,

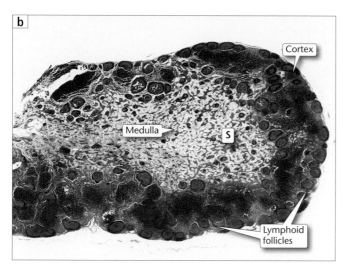

▲ **Fig 11.24b Section of lymph node**, showing the histologic separation of the cortex and the inner medulla. The latter consists of an irregular meshwork of dense medullary cords and sinuses (**S**) that contains lymph. The cords are ramifying processes of lymphoid tissues, with lymphocytes, macrophages, and plasma cells supported by a framework of reticular tissue and associated with blood vessels. Circulating lymphocytes enter the node via high endothelial venules that specifically attract these cells into the paracortex, populated by T cells and antigen-presenting dendritic cells. Lymphoid follicles are the source of B cell development. H&E, paraffin, × 5.

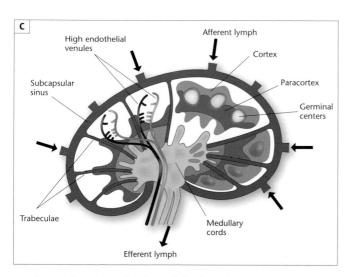

▲ **Fig 11.24c Organization of the lymph node.** Antigens and some lymphocytes and dendritic cells in afferent lymph enter the subcapsular sinus. Circulating lymphocytes and dendritic cells enter the paracortex, containing mostly T cells, via high endothelial venules. The cortex, rich in B cells, contains primary lymphoid follicles that form secondary follicles with germinal centers when antigen activates specific B cells. Filtered lymph that contains plasma cells, antibodies, and lymphocytes passes through sinuses between medullary cords, rich in lymphocytes, plasma cells and macrophages, and exits in the efferent lymph. Trabeculae provide anchorage for a fine reticular network throughout the node. Antigen-presenting cells in (para) cortical regions capture antigen; macrophages of the medulla scavenge particulate antigen.

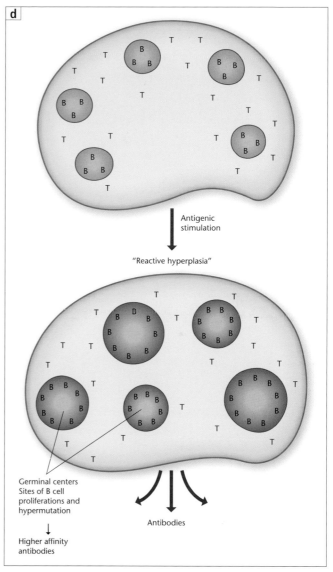

▲ **Fig 11.24d Concept of lymph node function**, showing (top) the unstimulated state with lymphoid follicles in the cortex containing B cells and T cells scattered in the paracortex. If a node reacts to antigen, it initiates an active immune response, resulting in B-cell proliferation and differentiation in germinal centers and enlargement of the node. Reactive lymph nodes may enlarge to a centimeter or more. Reactive hyperplasia of lymph nodes is associated with tissue injury or infection.

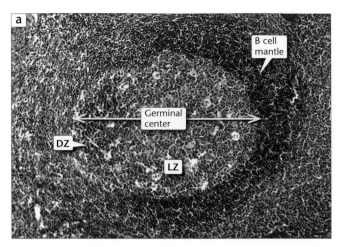

a

B cell mantle

Germinal center

DZ

LZ

◀ **Fig 11.25a Germinal center.** Secondary follicle with inner germinal center, in which antigen-activated B cells mature, and a rim, or mantle, of resting and memory B cells. Activated B-blasts proliferate into centroblasts at one pole (the dark zone, **DZ**) and express little surface immunoglobulin (Ig). Centroblasts proliferate, re-express surface Ig, with class-switching, to form centrocytes of the light zone (**LZ**). Cells with low-affinity Ig become apoptotic and are phagocytosed by macrophages. Surviving clones become plasma cells that migrate to the medullary sinuses. B-cell maturation depends upon antigen–antibody complexes presented by follicular dendritic cells and germinal center dendritic cells, which activate resident T cells to assist B-cell differentiation. H&E, paraffin, × 75.

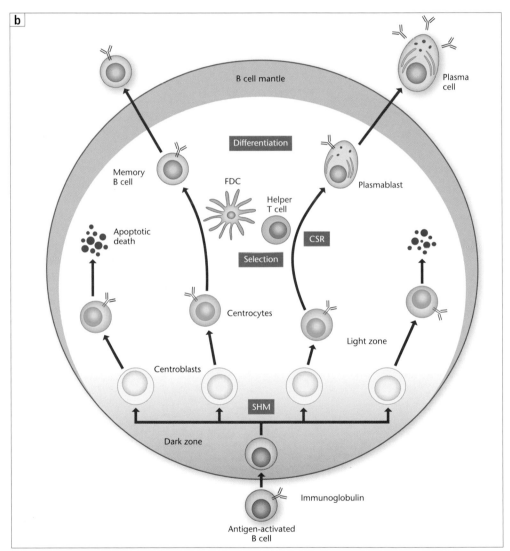

b

▲ **Fig 11.25b Concept of B-cell maturation in the germinal center.** Antigen-activated B cells differentiate into centroblasts in the dark zone and undergo clonal expansion and somatic hypermutation (**SHM**), involving the rearrangement and diversification of genes encoding the immunoglobulins. Passing into the light zone, centroblasts differentiate into non-dividing centrocytes (B cells expressing antibody), which are selected for improved antigen binding by interactions with immune complexes on follicular dendritic cells (**FDC**) with assistance from T helper cells. Failure to produce high-affinity antigen binding marks a centrocyte for apoptosis and destruction by tingible body macrophages. Some centrocytes undergo class switching recombination (**CSR**) and ultimately differentiate into memory B cells or plasma cells, or recycle to the start of the process for further expansion, diversification, and selection. (Redrawn and modified from Klein U and Dalla-Favera R, Nat Rev Immunol 2008; 8:22–33.)

usually passing along a series or chain of lymph nodes, each of which responds to antigenic challenges by collection and processing of antigen, activation of T cells and B cells, and release of lymphocytes and antibodies into efferent lymphatics or the hilar vein.

Follicles and germinal centers

Follicles are zones rich in B cells and are of two types:
- Primary follicles have recirculating B cells within a network of follicular dendritic cells (FDC).
- Secondary follicles arise from primary follicles when they are colonized by activated B cells as part of an immune response, and are easily recognized by the presence of a lighter-staining germinal center (GC).

Naïve/immunocompetent B cells enter the lymph node and migrate to the paracortex, encountering and interacting with dendritic cells and T helper cells. If activated, the B cells either develop directly into antibody-secreting cells in the medullary cords, or colonize a primary follicle to establish a germinal center (Fig 11.25a & b). In this location B cells rapidly proliferate and displace the recirculating B cells to form a mantle around the GC, which now consists of a dark zone of densely packed dividing B cells called centroblasts, and a light zone of their non-dividing progeny, the centrocytes, which are surrounded by FDCs, T cells, and macrophages. Centroblasts and centrocytes represent the sequence of proliferation and differentiation that produces memory and effector B cells (i.e. somatic hypermutation, selection, Ig class switching and production of memory B cells and plasma cells).

Germinal centers remain active for about 4 weeks, after which they involute and disappear.

T cells in lymph nodes

T cells enter lymph nodes by binding to high endothelial venules (HEV) that are characterized by cuboidal-type endothelial cells in contrast to conventional squamous-type endothelium. HEVs are found in all secondary lymphoid tissues except for the spleen. Bound lymphocytes are then attracted to the paracortex by chemokines. Killer T cells (Tc, CD8+) are activated in lymph nodes. In response to infection mediated, for example, by viruses, T cells migrate from the paracortex to the subcapsular sinus, where they are activated by interactions with antigen-bearing DCs. Following this they exit the node through efferent lymphatic vessels to attack virally infected targets.

Spleen

The spleen, about the size of a fist, has the consistency of a dense sponge. It comprises a connective tissue framework and branching arterial vessels that end in a blood-filled venous sinusoidal system making up the red pulp. Randomly scattered lymphoid tissue and follicles (gray in color to the naked eye) form the white pulp (Fig 11.26a & b). Supported by connective tissue trabeculae originating from the fibrous capsule, this rich vascular supply filters blood, surveys it for antigen or circulating pathogens, and removes aged platelets and erythrocytes with recovery of iron. Major functions of the spleen include antibody

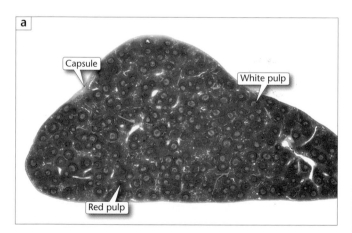

▲ **Fig 11.26a Spleen.** Transverse section showing a sharp border with a capsule that extends inward as profiles of branching and cuff-shaped trabeculae that provide basic framework support and blood vessels (originating from the hilum, not shown). Red pulp for blood filtration surrounds many rounded areas of white pulp which consists of aggregated lymphoid cells. H&E, paraffin, × 5.

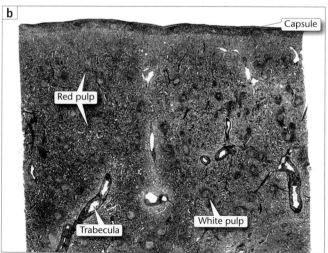

▲ **Fig 11.26b** Red pulp is sponge-like and consists of blood sinuses and cords of reticular meshwork with plasma cells, and macrophages that eliminate aged and abnormal erythrocytes and platelets, distributed via blood vessels that enter from trabeculae. Blood supplies the white pulp (weakly stained here) with antigens and lymphocytes. Trichrome, paraffin, × 8.

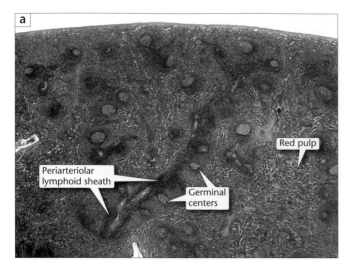

▲ Fig 11.27a Splenic lymphoid tissues. Segments of branched trabeculae with arterial supply are associated with variable-sized cuffs of white pulp that form periarteriolar lymphoid sheaths (PALS) and germinal centers of B cells within them. Becoming divested of white pulp, the arterioles narrow and, with branching into capillaries, supply the red pulp cords and sinuses, probably by opening into extracellular spaces. This permits erythrocytes, particles, antigens, lymphocytes, and antibodies to be scrutinized in the red pulp; they are either retained or enter the pulp and trabecular veins. H&E, paraffin, × 15.

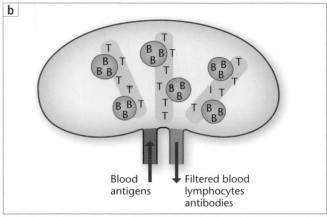

▲ Fig 11.27b Simple model of splenic organization. White pulp is lymphoid tissue associated with arterioles that form segments or sheaths of T cells, with B cells organized into primary lymphoid follicles. Due to the curvature of the vessels, long sectors of sheaths are not commonly seen in thin histologic sections. The surrounding red pulp, the largest compartment within the spleen, is a network of vascular sinusoids for filtration of blood.

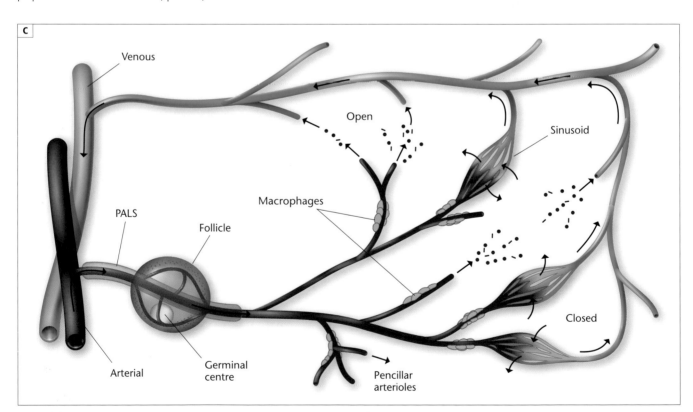

▲ Fig 11.27c Concept of splenic vasculature and lymphoid tissue. Blood entering via branches from trabecular arteries passes through regions of white pulp consisting of T-cell-rich white pulp PALS, and red pulp that fills in the surrounding regions (not illustrated). After exposure to the tissues of the red and white pulp, including the macrophage population, the filtered blood is collected in trabecular veins. Antigens within blood may stimulate resting primary follicles of B cells to form germinal centers. These secondary lymphoid follicles produce plasma cells and antibodies, which pass into vascular sinusoids along with formed elements of blood, particulate matter, and plasma. Circulation in the red pulp may be closed (blood remains in vessels) or open as blood percolates through cords and then sinusoids.

defense against blood-borne bacteria and phagocytosis of opsonized particles. As the arterioles pass through the spleen, they are invested with short sleeves or cylinders, chiefly of T cells, called periarteriolar lymphatic sheaths (PALS), at intervals associated with lymphoid follicles rich in B cells (Fig 11.27a–c). Functionally, the white pulp responds to antigenic challenge, producing antibodies and lymphocytes, most of which are transported from the venous side of the red pulp into the peripheral circulation.

Red pulp

The arterial system terminates in the cords of the red pulp (reticular fibers/fibroblasts, macrophages, blood cells in transit) as open capillaries with discontinuous endothelium (Fig 11.28). Blood then passes into venous sinuses of the red pulp and ultimately into the splenic vein. The endothelium of the venous sinuses has slit-like gaps that act as a selective barrier for blood cells leaving the red pulp cords (Fig 11.29a & b). Destruction of aged erythrocytes by macrophages yields a source of iron from the degradation of hemoglobin. Red pulp macrophages store iron as ferritin, visible as dense granular cytoplasmic deposits. Many plasmablasts and plasma cells are found in red pulp, the latter producing antibodies for entry into the venous system.

White pulp

The lymphoid component of the spleen—the white pulp—is arranged as sheaths around the branching blood vessels. The sheaths have T- and B-cell

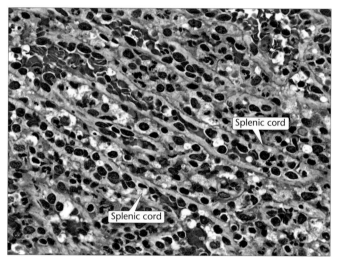

▲ **Fig 11.28 Red pulp tissue.** The regions in between and at the termination of blood vessels are highly cellular and are occasionally referred to as splenic cords, due to their linear and branching arrangement. The cords are in fact like a honeycomb permeated by the vessels, and contain fibroblasts, macrophages, erythrocytes, and granulocytes. H&E, acrylic resin, × 300.

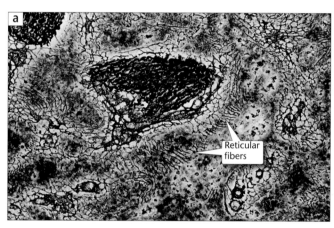

▲ **Fig 11.29a Venous sinuses in splenic red pulp.** Red pulp region in which the section was stained with silver salts to reveal the patterns of reticular fibers. Blood sinuses are at times noted as clear areas, but in other sinuses parallel fibers from the parenchymal (cord) tissue form rings around the endothelium. Blood cells exit or enter the venous sinuses through the rings and gaps between the endothelial cells. Reticulin stain, paraffin, × 250.

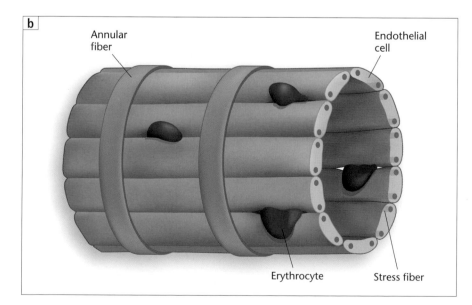

◄ **Fig 11.29b Blood enters the sinus from the splenic cords.** The sinus consists of parallel endothelial cells connected by stress fibers to annular arrangements of fibroreticular fibers. Stress fibers are composed of actin- and myosin-type filaments that contract and form slits between the endothelial cells. Aging erythrocytes, with stiffened membranes, are unable to pass through the slits and are phagocytosed by red pulp macrophages. (Redrawn from Mebius R and Kraal G, Nature Rev Immunol 2005; 5:606–16.)

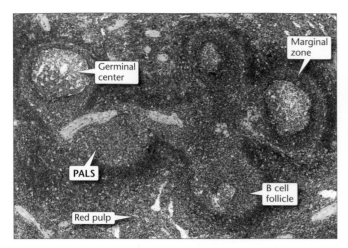

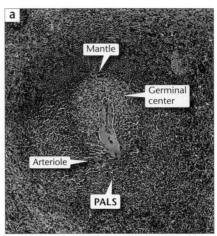

▲ **Fig 11.30 White pulp.** Ovoid areas of white pulp seen here are cross and longitudinal sections of sheaths of diffuse and follicular lymphocytes; the former are called periarteriolar lymphoid sheaths (**PALS**) and consist of T cells associated with central arterioles derived from trabecular arteries; the latter are B-cell-rich follicles, many with germinal centers that arise in the PALS. The marginal zone is shown and red pulp surrounds this lymphoid tissue. Afferent blood, with lymphocytes and antigens, thus passes through these B- and T-cell regions before reaching the red pulp, and may stimulate immune responses. H&E, paraffin, × 40.

▲ **Fig 11.31a Splenic lymphoid follicles.** A germinal center, associated with a central arteriole, contains differentiating B cells together with dendritic, phagocytic, and T helper cells, similar to germinal centers in lymph nodes. A mantle of resting B cells lies opposite the bulk of T cells of the periarteriolar lymphoid sheaths. In response to blood-borne antigen, T cells (activated by antigen-capturing dendritic cells) probably migrate toward antigen-specific B cells in resting follicles. The B cells then are activated to form founder B-blasts, from which germinal centers arise. H&E, paraffin, × 60.

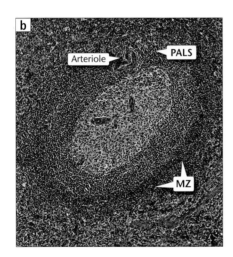

▲ **Fig.11.31b Germinal center and mantle of B cells**, partly surrounded by a (uniquely splenic) marginal zone of dendritic cells, macrophages, B cells, and some T cells. On the outside is red pulp. Blood-borne antigens, and circulating lymphocytes, enter the white pulp initially through the marginal zone (**MZ**) via capillary branches derived from the central arteriole. Thus, the outer periarteriolar lymphoid sheath (**PALS**) region is the initial site of antigen-specific B cell selection, activation, and deletion. Recirculating lymphocytes may cross the white pulp into red pulp via channels, or discontinuities, in the PALS. H&E, paraffin, × 60.

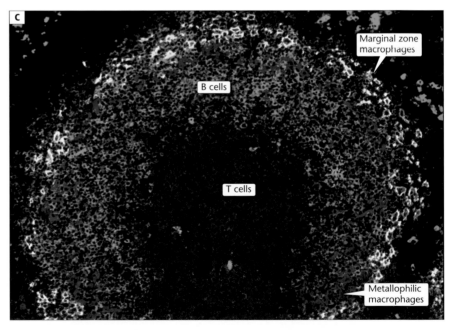

▲ **Fig 11.31c Immunofluorescence staining of a white pulp unit in the mouse spleen.** T cells surround the arteriole; B cells localize around the T cell area. Metallophilic macrophages and a more peripheral layer of marginal zone macrophages are shown. The marginal zone is located between these two layers of macrophages. (Courtesy J Kearney, University of Alabama at Birmingham, USA.) × 180.

compartments, attracted to particular domains by chemokines (Fig 11.30). The PALS are rich in T cells, whereas the B-cells are aggregated into B cell follicles that undergo the same proliferative and differentiation steps as those associated with lymph node follicles. A collection of cells known as the marginal zone (MZ) in rodent spleens surrounds the splenic follicles and PALS, and is supported by a framework of reticular fibroblasts (Fig 11.31a–c). The MZ is separated from the white pulp by marginal sinuses that receive blood from open, terminal arterioles. In addition to dendritic cells and leukocytes, the MZ contains a unique subset of B cells, and inner and outer rings of specialized macrophages, all of which are exposed to incoming blood-borne antigens. Marginal zone B cells shuttle

back and forth between the MZ and follicles, and thereby capture and transport antigen from the blood to follicular dendritic cells. In the human spleen, immunocytochemical analysis has shown that the B-cell regions equivalent to the rodent MZ are restricted to peripheral aspects of follicles and appear to be absent from the PALS.

Mucosa-associated lymphoid tissue

The MALT consists of populations of immune cells in the mucosa of many epithelial tissues, organized into discrete lymphoid follicles such as the tonsils, appendix, or Peyer's patches of the ileum (Fig 11.32a–c). These cells also form a diffuse immune system, scattered widely in various mucosae as large numbers

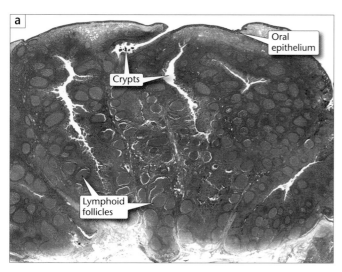

▲ **Fig 11.32a Mucosal lymphoid follicles.** Section of a palatine tonsil, a concentrated mass of partly encapsulated lymphoid tissue in the submucosa of the oropharynx, constituting an example of mucosa-associated lymphoid tissue (MALT). Note three characteristic features—smooth surface of oral epithelium, penetrating crypts derived from the surface, and many lymphoid follicles, mostly with germinal centers. The function of tonsils is to detect and respond to pathogens in the oral cavity; the crypts provide the necessary surface area for antigen sampling, and the follicles serve the immune response reactions. H&F, paraffin, × 12.

▲ **Fig 11.32b Peyer's patches** (gut-associated lymphoid tissue). These are organized aggregations of lymphoid follicles in the submucosa and lamina propria of the gut, mainly the ileum. The brown staining shows proliferating cells. The associated epithelium contains modified enterocytes called M (microfold) cells, which sample antigens and microbes from the lumen. Lymphocytes, macrophages and dendritic cells beneath M cells process and/or present antigen to the underlying follicles. This triggers production of IgA by B cells, some of which enter the lymph and lymph nodes, become further activated, and re-enter the systemic circulation to home back to wider areas of gut and confer immune protection. Immunocytochemical reaction for proliferating nuclear cell antigen, paraffin, × 30.

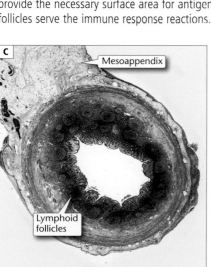

◀ **Fig 11.32c Appendix.** The irregular, scalloped lumen is lined by a mucosa similar to that of the colon. Lymphoid follicles occur in the lamina propria and submucosa; the former is associated with epithelial specializations similar to Peyer's patches. In this way, lumenal contents are sampled for pathogens. The function of the appendix is uncertain, but probably contributes to regional mucosal immunity. Neutrophilic and eosinophilic infiltration of mucosa, submucosa and muscularis externa usually characterize acute appendicitis. At birth, few or no lymphoid follicles are present, but their numbers increase in children and then decline with age. H&E, paraffin. × 8.

of lymphocytes, plasma cells, and macrophages, for example in the small and large intestine (Fig 11.33a & b). The MALT is specialized for sampling and collection of antigen across mucosal epithelia. Mucosal surfaces contain locally adapted dendritic cells that serve this purpose. Antigen stimulates the induction of secretory immunity, and the secreted antibodies (usually IgA) serve to protect the mucosa against pathogens, particularly microorganisms. The MALT may be subdivided into bronchus-associated lymphoid tissues of the lungs and gut-associated lymphoid tissues in the gastrointestinal tract. Quantitative estimates of comparisons of total lymphoid tissues, gut histology and lymphocyte numbers are available in different mammalian species (mouse, pig, macaque, human). It is widely believed that most of the lymphocytes and plasma cells of the body are found in the gut mucosa.

MEDICAL IMPORTANCE OF THE IMMUNE SYSTEM
Transplantation
Rejection of transplanted organs results from immune reactions, with three forms of graft rejection:
- **Hyperacute.** Occurs when the recipient already has antibodies against a graft and thus alloantigens (graft antigens detected as non-self) are recognized

rapidly. Occurs within seconds to minutes. Rapid thrombosis and death of the graft. Irreversible.
- **Acute.** Arises when T cells encounter graft alloantigens and cause intensified inflammation and tissue destruction. Occurs within hours to days. Massive infiltration with lymphocytes; sometimes the graft can be saved by treatment with immunosuppressive drugs.
- **Chronic.** Associated with a balance between rejection and tissue repair, and leading to pathologic tissue remodeling. Occurs within weeks, months, and years. Slow destruction of graft, with fibrosis and lymphoid infiltration.

Recognition of allograft tissues (organ/tissue grafts between non-identical individuals) is the function of MHC molecules. Alloantigens generally consist of small differences in amino acid sequences of donor versus recipient proteins. They can be:
- Graft-derived peptides bound by self MHCs on recipient APCs
- Graft-derived peptides bound by graft MHC molecules
- Recipient peptides bound by graft MHCs on donor APCs.

Although cytotoxic T cells have long been accepted as the primary effectors of graft rejection, some emerging evidence suggests that cytokines may induce inflammatory responses in which Th cells

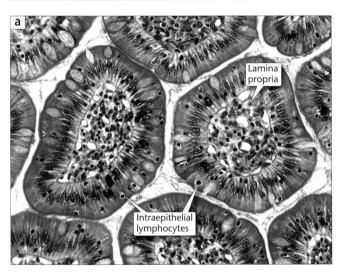

▲ **Fig 11.33a Mucosal lymphocytes.** Transverse section of villi, in which the core of lamina propria contains mostly T cells, and plasma cells secreting IgA across the epithelium. Numerous intra-epithelial T cells (IEL) have γδ T cell receptors (TCRs; most T cells have αβ TCRs), and home to the gut from bone marrow, perhaps bypassing the thymus. IELs are located between the antigen-rich gut lumen and the lymphocyte-rich lamina propria. They may activate and coordinate innate responses (monocytes, neutrophils) and adaptive responses (T cells and B cells), and respond to cell stress and injured epithelium, an appropriate function for mucosal surfaces. H&E, paraffin, × 190.

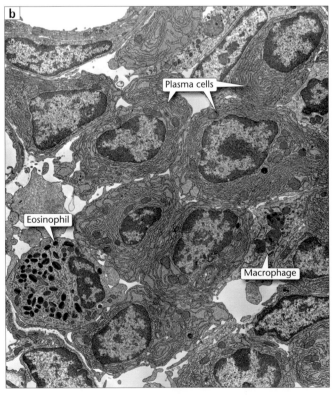

▲ **Fig 11.33b Ultrastructure of the lamina propria core of a villus**, showing the abundance of immune cells. The lamina propria is filled with plasma cells that secrete up to 5 g of IgA into the gut lumen each day. The considerable proportion of loose connective tissue within the gut, especially in the small bowel, suggests that the gastrointestinal system holds a population of leukocytes that exceeds the numbers of these cells in the remainder of the tissues and organs that comprise the immune system. × 3,700.

may participate in graft rejection. The mechanism of tissue damage is unclear. In the treatment of certain malignances that require bone marrow transplantation, the immune system of the recipient is suppressed, which increases the risk of an immune attack on recipient cells by the transplanted bone marrow (i.e. graft-versus-host disease [GVHD]). This reaction remains a significant barrier to marrow and stem-cell transplantation, but is partly offset by the development of bone marrow registries to increase the identification of MHC-matched donors.

Allergic reactions

Allergic rhinitis, allergic asthma, and anaphylaxis are associated with immediate hypersensitivity reactions, activated by antigen-induced cross-linking of specific IgE bound to Fc receptors on mast cells and/or basophils. The released mediators act upon the vasculature, leukocytes, and also various glands, which results in physiologic effects. Late-phase reactions that involve skin may lead to local swelling and also affect the nasal passages and respiratory tract. Hypersensitivity reactions may arise in response to food allergens, particularly in infants, (e.g. milk, eggs, wheat), but this declines with age. Such reactions, if IgE-mediated, may develop within minutes or hours and involve the oropharynx, gut, lungs, nose, and eyes, and in severe cases cardiovascular shock (anaphylaxis) may occur, and is potentially fatal. This reaction in sensitive individuals is often associated with ingestion of peanuts, fish, and shellfish. Cationic proteins from activated eosinophils may be associated with allergic diseases that cause damage to the respiratory mucosa and local edema.

Immunopharmacology

Traditional forms of immunopharmacotherapy are aimed at immune suppression to modify disease processes, but newer forms of immunomodulation are constantly under development and are directed at specific cells or cytokines associated with immune responses. Some strategies are designed to enhance immunity against malignancies, and the opportunistic infections that arise in association with these and other disorders. Selected treatment categories are given below:

- Cytotoxic agents (ionizing radiation, methotrexate, cyclophosphamide), which inhibit or disrupt deoxyribonucleic acid (DNA) repair and/or synthesis, are used in transplantation, GVHD, and autoimmune disorders.
- Fungus-derived drugs (e.g. cyclosporine) are immunosuppressive, and block T-cell activation for organ transplantation or GVHD.
- Monoclonal antibodies (anti-CD, anticytokine agents) are used in the treatment of autoimmune diseases, graft rejection, and rheumatoid arthritis.
- Immune-enhancing agents (interferons and interleukins) stimulate Tc and Th lymphocytes or

macrophages for the treatment of malignancies and/or tumors, hepatitis, and Kaposi's sarcoma related to acquired immunodeficiency syndrome.
- Gene therapies to correct inherited or acquired gene defects or modify cell function are currently under development for the treatment of immune deficiencies and genetic inborn errors. There have been some spectacular successes, but also some disastrous outcomes, including development of leukemia after gene replacement therapy.

Immunization

Active immunization is the procedure of antigen administration to induce antibody production, or to provide protective immunity. The basic principle is to administer an attenuated or inactivated antigen to induce active immunity without causing symptoms of the disease. Most vaccines fall into one of three categories:

- Killed viruses or bacteria in which surface molecules stimulate antibody production (e.g. Salk poliovirus vaccine)
- Live, attenuated (weakened) organisms, which are infective and stimulate immunity but do not cause disease (e.g. Sabin poliovirus vaccine)
- Inactivated bacterial toxins (toxoids), which are harmless but stimulate immune responses (e.g. diphtheria and tetanus vaccines).

Live vaccines, although attenuated, replicate in the body and produce much antigen from a single treatment, whereas killed vaccines may require several treatments to induce long-term immunity. The risks of vaccination are exceedingly small (contamination, virus mutation), but the risks of disease and suffering from non-vaccination are far higher. Passive immunization involves the administration of exogenous antibodies, and gives immediate short-term protection over a few months. Passive immunization relies upon three approaches:

- Human immunoglobulin, mostly IgG, used to prevent hepatitis A
- Specific human immunoglobulin, commonly used against hepatitis B
- Animal-derived antibodies or antitoxins (in use for over a century, usually generating horse antiserum), such as snake and spider antivenom, and tetanus immunoglobulin.

Experimental vaccines based on DNA plasmid vectors are currently being explored. The DNA is taken up by host cells, in which the introduced gene for pathogen antigen produces endogenously created antigen processed through MHC I molecules, and stimulates cell-mediated and/or Tc immune responses. This approach has been shown to be effective against influenza viruses in animal models, and DNA vaccine development potentially may enhance immune responses in chronically infected patients with hepatitis C, human immunodeficiency viruses, malaria, or herpes simplex viruses.

Respiratory system

The lungs are the site of respiratory gas exchange and can be considered as a large assembly of thin-walled sacs that must be kept at least partially inflated. This is achieved by the rigidity of the chest wall, which resists the inherent tendency for the lungs to collapse. This results in a slightly subatmospheric pressure between the outer surface of the lung and the inner wall of the thorax. A thin film of fluid coats these surfaces, or pleural membranes, to allow movement of the lungs within the thoracic cavity.

DIVISIONS OF THE RESPIRATORY TRACT
Respiratory passages

The pathway taken by inspired air from the mouth and nose to the gas-exchanging region of the lungs makes up the respiratory passages. The respiratory passages constitute the conducting zone of the lungs because their purpose is to deliver inspired air to the gas-exchanging (or respiratory) zone of the lungs. The conducting zone is made up of the nasal passages, pharynx, larynx, trachea, bronchi, and most of the bronchioles as far as the terminal bronchioles.

The respiratory zone

Exchange of gases between the air and blood commences in the respiratory zone proper (i.e. the lung acinus), which is made up of the respiratory bronchioles, alveolar ducts, and definitive alveoli.

Anatomic divisions of the respiratory tract

An alternative system of describing the respiratory passages is based upon anatomic and clinical considerations:
- The upper respiratory tract, extending down to and including the larynx
- The lower respiratory tract, made up of the trachea, the lungs, and the respiratory tree.

The main emphasis of this chapter is on the structure and function of the nasal passages, the trachea, and the intrapulmonary portion of the respiratory tract.

UPPER RESPIRATORY TRACT

Most of the nasal passages are lined by pseudostratified ciliated columnar epithelium (i.e. respiratory-type epithelium) except for the vestibule, which shows keratinizing stratified squamous epithelium.

It is important to point out that the name "respiratory-type epithelium" refers to structural rather than functional attributes, since respiration or gas exchange occurs only in the lung acini (see below).

The distribution of respiratory epithelium in the upper respiratory tract can be variable, particularly in the nasopharynx, where it coexists with regions of stratified squamous epithelium. Except for the oropharynx, the vocal cords, and the anterior margin of the epiglottis (which all have stratified squamous epithelium), respiratory epithelium predominates in the upper respiratory regions.

The functions of this mucosa are the following:
- To warm and humidify inspired air
- To provide an immunologic defense and a ciliary clearing mechanism against infective and inert particles
- To provide the sense of smell (via the olfactory epithelium).

In the nasal cavity, the warming and humidifying function is enhanced by the presence of projecting scrolls of bone—the conchae—on the lateral nasal wall (Fig 12.1a–c). Because the mucous membrane here is often contiguous with the underlying bone, the term mucoperiosteum is sometimes used. In this location the respiratory mucosa is modified in that the subepithelial tissues in the lamina propria contain fibrous and elastic tissue together with seromucous glands and dilatable vascular sinuses that assist with warming the air—hence the increased tendency for nosebleeds.

Secretions from the glands and the epithelium itself contain mucus together with antimicrobial substances. Mucus is a viscous fluid containing glycoproteins. It lines the respiratory tract as a thin layer as far as the ends of the bronchi. The action of the cilia moves the mucus continuously toward the pharynx, where it is usually swallowed or expectorated. The serous component of the secretions contains immunoglobulins, lysozyme, and enzymes directed against bacteria.

In a small area on the roof of each nasal cavity is the olfactory epithelium of tall, pseudostratified columnar cells with intercalated bipolar neurons acting as sensory receptors. The structure and function of this tissue is discussed in Chapter 20.

The nasopharynx (behind the nose and above the soft palate) shows a variable distribution of columnar

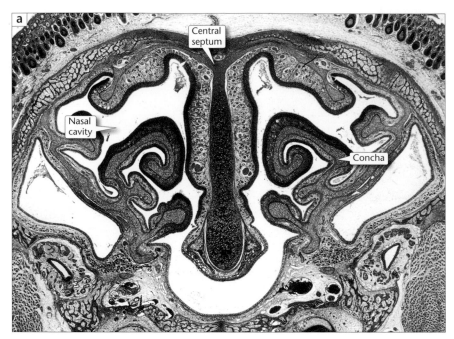

▲ **Fig 12.1a Nasal passages.** Vertical section through the nasal cavity taken from a late fetal guinea pig. The oral cavity is below the micrograph. The central nasal septum and lateral pairs of conchae are shown and at this age have cores of cartilage that will later be partly or fully replaced with bone. The large mucosal surface area provides for humidification, temperature adjustment, and cleansing of inspired air. Most of the mucosa is pseudostratified columnar epithelium. Hematoxylin & eosin (H&E), alcian blue, paraffin, × 10.

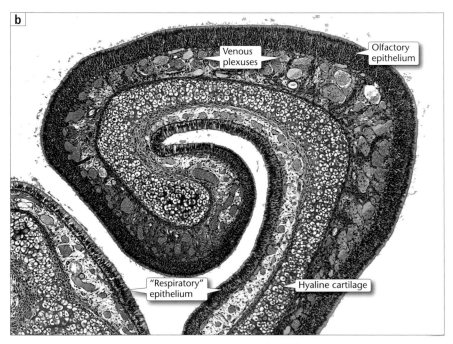

▲ **Fig 12.1b Concha and mucosa.** Detail of a concha with a core of hyaline cartilage and the mucosa with segments of "respiratory" and olfactory epithelium. The submucosa has many loops of venous plexuses resembling those in erectile tissue. Acting as a countercurrent exchange by flowing in the opposite direction to inspired air, the blood acts as a heat exchanger. The "respiratory" epithelium purifies the air, and pollutants are trapped in the superficial mucus. H&E, alcian blue, paraffin, × 50.

and stratified squamous epithelium and scattered seromucous glands. Extending down to the epiglottic region, the oropharynx exhibits stratified squamous epithelium. Lymphoid tissue makes an important contribution to the defense mechanisms of the upper respiratory tract and is seen as individual cells of the lymphoid series and as focal collections of lymphoid follicles. The functional histology of the tonsils and the soft palate is considered in Chapter 13.

The larynx (Fig 12.2), which is continuous below with the trachea, is a hollow, muscular tube reinforced with cartilage; its upper end forms the spoon-shaped epiglottis, which acts as a flap to direct food and fluids away from the glottis and into the esophagus. Projecting into the lumen of the larynx are the vocal cords (also known as the vocal folds). These are covered by stratified squamous epithelium, which is also seen on the anterior (lingual) and upper part of the posterior (laryngeal) surfaces of the epiglottis. The remaining surfaces show pseudostratified ciliated columnar epithelium. Elastic cartilage, perforated by occasional foramina produced by seromucous glands, forms the core of the epiglottis and provides elastic recoil of the organ after swallowing.

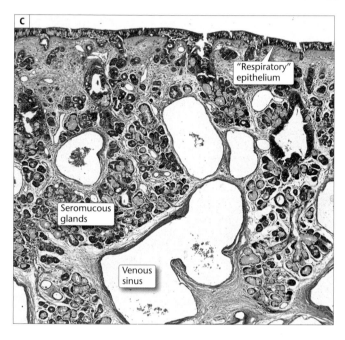

◀ **Fig 12.1c Detail of the nasal "respiratory" mucosa**, showing mucous cells in the epithelium and many seromucous glands in the submucosa. Large venous sinuses are plentiful, forming the cavernous plexus of the concha. If engorged the mucosa swells, giving a "blocked" or "stuffy" nose. The veins give off heat to the inspired air. H&E, paraffin, × 15.

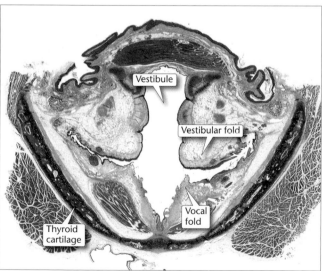

◀ **Fig 12.2 Larynx.** Horizontal section of the larynx showing the thyroid cartilage, vestibular fold, laryngeal vestibule, and vocal fold. The thicker epithelial surfaces are "respiratory" type, and the thinner regions are stratified squamous. H&E, alcian blue, paraffin, × 5.

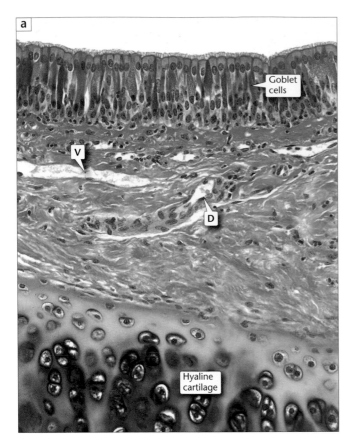

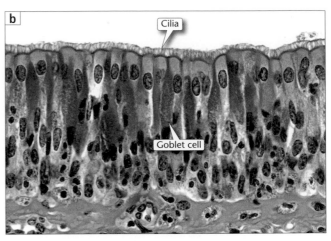

▲ **Fig 12.3b Detail of the tracheal "respiratory" epithelium**, which is a ciliated, pseudostratified columnar epithelium with goblet cells that secrete mucus onto the mucosa surface. Nuclei appear at many different levels, but the cytoplasm of all cells is in contact with the basal lamina. Although gas exchange does not occur in "respiratory" epithelium, the designation is used because it occurs in conducting airways down to the start of the bronchioles. H&E, alcian blue, paraffin, × 370.

▲ **Fig 12.3a Trachea.** Medium magnification of the wall of the trachea with pseudostratified columnar epithelium containing numerous mucus-secreting cells (goblet cells). The submucosa is wide and shows part of a duct (**D**) and some blood vessels (**V**). Deep to the submucosa is part of the hyaline cartilage, which forms complete or, more commonly, partial rings that provide structural support and patency of the trachea. H&E, alcian blue, paraffin, × 180.

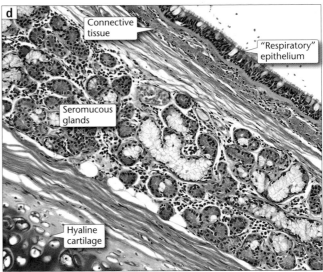

▲ **Fig 12.3d Trachea wall.** The thick wall of the trachea shows irregular clusters of seromucous glands in the submucosa, flanked by inner and outer layers of irregular connective tissues. The rings of hyaline cartilage (only the edge seen here) form C-shaped structures, deficient posteriorly but united by fibrous tissue and bands of smooth muscle. Rings of cartilage provide support for the trachea, preventing its collapse, in much the same way that the rings of a vacuum cleaner hose keep the tube open. H&E, alcian blue, paraffin, × 135.

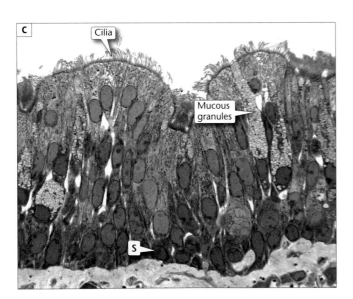

▲ **Fig 12.3c Tracheal epithelium.** Thin epoxy resin section of tracheal epithelium, showing cilia, mucous cells, non-ciliated cells or brush cells, and basal or stem cells (**S**). Brush cells (small microvilli) may be variants of the ciliated cells. Basal cells are probably precursors of the above types, but also include scattered neuroendocrine cells, or amine precursor uptake and decarboxylation (APUD) cells, which secrete regulatory peptides in response to either neural stimulation or exogenous chemical stimuli. Toluidine blue, araldite, × 450.

TRACHEA

Incomplete rings of hyaline cartilage provide an important structural role in keeping open much of the system of airways. In the trachea their posterior ends are related to strips of smooth muscle that complete the encirclement of the lumen, itself shaped like a D. Fibroelastic tissues located between the cartilages assist the smooth muscle in allowing tracheal diameter and length to vary slightly during forced respiration.

Tracheal epithelium

Because the tracheal mucosa is so often considered as the archetypal "respiratory" epithelium, it is worth mentioning its major features (Fig 12.3a–d). All the cells are in contact with the basal lamina, which is unusually thick. Ciliated columnar cells predominate, and there are also numerous mucus-secreting goblet cells. There are slender brush cells with apical microvilli, and roundish basal cells represent either stem cells or cells with a local neuroendocrine function. Wandering and focal sites of lymphoid cells occupy the lamina propria, with the submucosa showing mucous glands and serous demilunes, together with elastic fibers.

Although the "respiratory" epithelium of the trachea has no role in gas exchange, its important function down to the level of the commencement of the bronchioles is to coat the surface with a viscous film produced by goblet cells and excreted by ducts emptying the submucous glands (Fig 12.4a & b). This sticky layer contains mucins, immunoglobulins, lysozyme, and antiproteases, which disable bacterial functions. Inhaled particles, liquids, microorganisms, and sloughed-off epithelial cells within the viscous

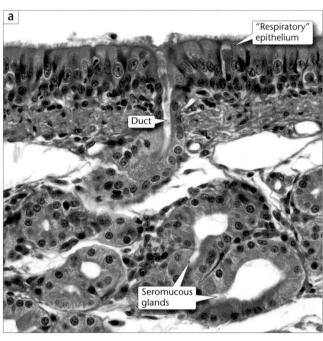

▲ **Fig 12.4a Tracheal secretions.** The respiratory epithelium is ciliated, pseudostratified columnar with mucous cells that discharge mucus. A mixed serous–mucoid secretion is added to the mucus; this reaches the lumen via ducts from glands in the submucosa. The population of basal cells in the epithelium comprises reserve stem cells and some neuroendocrine cells. The glands are more prevalent in the dorsal aspect of the trachea and secrete via secretomotor nerves in response to ventilation and noxious insults or inflammation. H&E, paraffin, × 220.

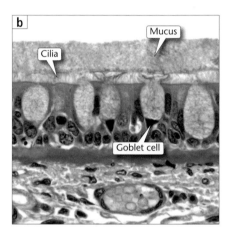

▲ **Fig 12.4b Detail of the tracheal epithelium**, showing the discharge of mucus from goblet-type cells. On the epithelial surface just above the cilia, the mucus forms a protective coat that traps particulate matter. The rhythmic beating of the cilia moves the mucus blanket upward toward the oral cavity. H&E, paraffin, × 360.

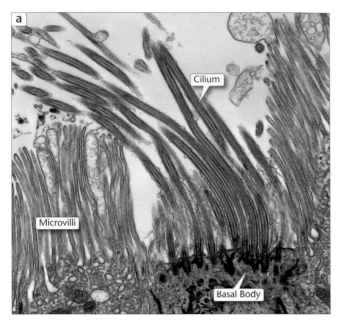

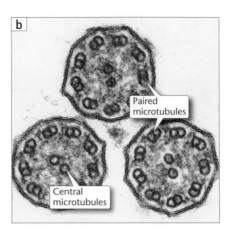

▲ **Fig 12.5b Ultrastructure of cross sections of cilia**, showing the axoneme comprising 2 central and 9 paired microtubules. Short hook-shaped dynein arms extend from the latter and these are responsible for the sliding of the microtubules that results in bending of the cilia. × 54,000. (Courtesy Pavelka M and Roth J. Functional ultrastructure. Vienna: Springer-Verlag, 2005.)

▲ **Fig 12.5a Ultrastructure of the cilia of the trachea.** The cilia may be up to 5 μm in length and are anchored to the apical cell cytoplasm by dense basal bodies that are modified centrioles. In their core the cilia contain a 9 + 2 arrangement of axonemal microtubules, giving them coordinated motility for movement of surface particles, mucus, and cell debris. Adjacent cells show slender microvilli of the tracheal brush cells. × 7,000.

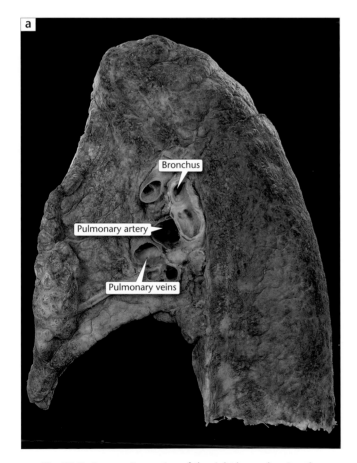

▲ **Fig 12.6a Lungs.** Prosection of the right lung, showing the mediastinal surface and the root of the lung. The main bronchus, pulmonary and bronchial vessels, and nerves and lymphatics enter and exit the lung through the lung root. The surface of the lung is relatively smooth, with an external layer of adherent visceral pleura.

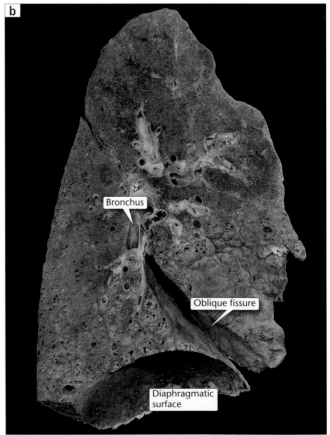

▲ **Fig 12.6b Branches of respiratory tree.** A sagittal section through the left lung, showing profiles of the branches of the respiratory tree. The left lung has an oblique fissure separating the superior and inferior lobes. Smaller branches of the bronchial tree are evident from the numerous and varied cavities upon the cut surface.

layer are moved via ciliary action toward the pharynx (Fig 12.5a & b). Main or primary bronchi are formed where the trachea bifurcates; their structure is similar to that of the trachea.

> **Tip:** "Respiratory" epithelium is not associated with respiration, but is involved with humidifying, cleansing, and warming inspired air before it enters the lungs. True respiratory epithelium occurs in the thin walls of the alveoli.

LOWER RESPIRATORY TRACT (INTRAPULMONARY AIRWAYS)

At the macroscopic level, the roots of the lungs (Figure 12.6a–e) show the pulmonary vessels and the main bronchi, with the bronchial tree demonstrated with radiological techniques. With a gradual reduction in diameter and multiple branching, the conducting airways of the bronchi and bronchioles of the lung give rise to the clusters of alveoli. Depending

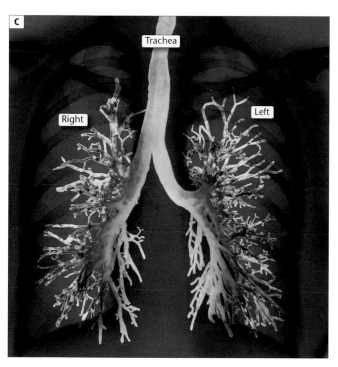

▲ **Fig 12.6c Bronchial tree.** Anteroposterior radiograph of the thorax after the introduction of a contrast medium into the trachea. The contrast passes into the bronchial tree to reveal its branching to the level of the segmental bronchi. Note that as the trachea bifurcates into the principal bronchi, the right bronchus is at a steeper angle compared with the left bronchus.

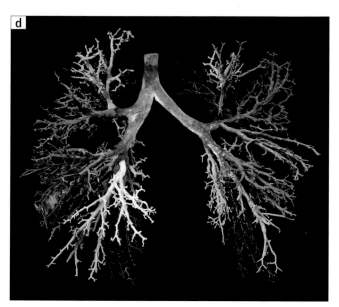

▲ **Fig 12.6d Bronchopulmonary segments.** Resin cast of human lungs, anterior view, showing bronchopulmonary segments. *Right lung*—superior lobe, apical = yellow; inferior lobe, anterior basal = pale blue and posterior basal = red. *Left lung*—superior lobe, superior lingual = deep blue; inferior lobe, lateral basal = pale blue.

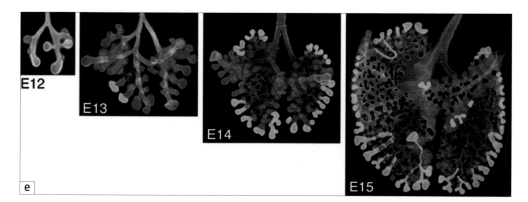

▲ **Fig 12.6e Branching morphogenesis of bronchial tree.** Whole-mount mouse lungs at the embryonic day indicated, showing the patterns of branching morphogenesis of the bronchial tree. Added pseudocolors blue (domain branching in rows like a bottlebrush), green (planar branching by splitting of a branch tip into two), and red (orthogonal branching with 90° rotation forming rosettes). Domain branches form the basic scaffold in a lobe; planar branching forms the thin edges of lobes, and orthogonal branches create surfaces and fills in the interior. (Courtesy R Metzger, Stanford University/University of California, San Francisco USA; from Metzger R, et al. Nature 2008; 453:745–50.)

upon the particular location, there may be between 8 and 23 generations of branching in the bronchial tree. In average adults, the two lungs combined have a volume of around 2.5 liters at rest (expandable to about 6 liters with maximum inspiration); an initial assessment of lung histology with low magnification microscopy confirms its sponge-like structure (Fig 12.7), in which the volume of all blood vessels and bronchial tree amounts to only 10% of total lung volume. The remaining parenchyma is dedicated to respiratory function.

There are a large number of histologic "facts" that apply to the lung, but these can be reduced to a more manageable form by following a systematic plan, commencing with the bronchus and ending at the alveolus. The following are key markers for describing lung histology:
- Bronchi—contain cartilage in their walls
- Bronchioles—lack cartilage, but have smooth muscle in their walls
- Blood vessels—identified by their inner lining, which is squamous endothelium

- Respiratory bronchioles—show outpocketings of alveoli
- Alveoli—clusters of sacs or arranged along respiratory bronchioles.

The epithelial lining of the bronchial tree follows a general pattern of simplification and reduction in height, culminating in a predominantly thin squamous lining in the alveoli.

The bronchus

Arising left and right from the trachea, which itself is about 18 mm in diameter, the bronchi occur in the first four generations of branching. The larger bronchi diminish in diameter to about 4 mm; the smaller bronchi of generations 5–11 are 3–1 mm in diameter. The bronchus, by definition, is supported by islands or cusps of hyaline cartilage, and the mucosa is of the respiratory type, similar to that of the trachea (Fig 12.8a–c). Between the cartilage and the mucosa is smooth muscle, which becomes more prominent as the bronchi branch and become smaller and as the

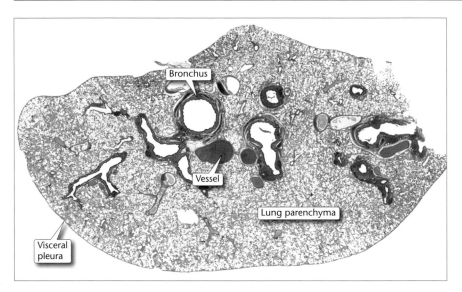

▲ **Fig 12.7 Lung architecture.** Section through the lung, illustrating its largely sponge-type appearance, together with pulmonary blood vessels and airways. Airways appear empty, containing air in vivo, have thick walls, and show branching. Bronchi are associated with cartilage, whereas the smaller bronchioles lack this feature. Vessels usually retain their erythrocytes and hence stain pink or red. The entire pulmonary vasculature contains up to 500 mL of blood, or 40% of the weight of the lung. The respiratory tree terminates in many millions of alveoli, and the lung surface is bordered by visceral pleura that consist of an outer mesothelium resting on an inner, thicker layer of fibrous connective tissue. H&E, paraffin, × 6.

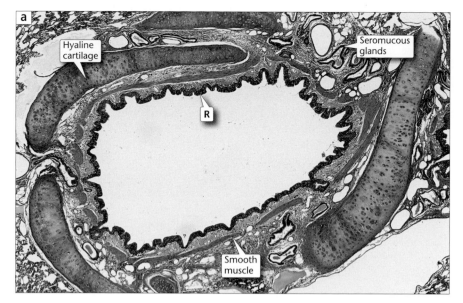

◀ Fig 12.8a Bronchus. Bronchi are large-diameter airways characterized by crescent or U-shaped plates of hyaline cartilage in their walls. Bronchi enter lobes and, with branching, supply bronchopulmonary segments. The cartilage gradually diminishes and finally disappears with the formation of bronchioles. The cartilage prevents the bronchi from collapsing. Respiratory mucosa (**R**) lines the bronchus, with smooth muscle and seromucous glands in the submucosa. H&E, alcian blue, paraffin, × 70.

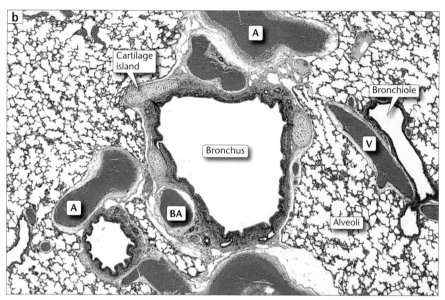

◀ Fig 12.8b Bronchus. A bronchus is shown with cartilage reduced to islands, supported by collagenous tissues containing numerous glands. Note that bronchioles lack cartilage and show a thinner epithelium, which reduces in depth from the tall respiratory epithelium in bronchi to simple columnar in bronchioles. The mucosa is kept moist by seromucous secretions from the glands, mucus-secreting cells in the respiratory epithelium, and water vapor in the humidified air. Extensive vascular supply is noted by pulmonary arteries (**A**) and veins (**V**), together with bronchial arteries (**BA**) supplying the bronchial tree. H&E, paraffin, × 40.

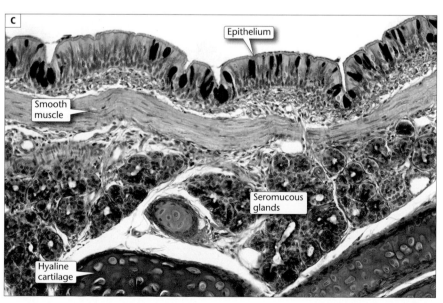

◀ Fig 12.8c Detail of the bronchus, showing a tall, ciliated, pseudostratified columnar epithelium, smooth muscle deep to the lamina propria, numerous seromucous glands, and plates of hyaline cartilage. Bronchial secretions from the epithelium and glands contain water, mucins, serum proteins, lysozyme (which destroys bacteria), and antiproteases (which inactivate bacterial enzymes). Together with lymphocytes in the connective tissues, the glands produce secretory immunoglobulins, especially immunoglobulin A, which enhances the antimicrobiological activities of neutrophils and macrophages. PAS stain, paraffin, × 150.

cartilage gradually diminishes. Elastic fibers occupy the lamina propria and, in the submucosa, seromucous glands empty their secretions onto the bronchial epithelium via collecting ducts. On the epithelium, these secretions mix with the mucin secreted from the epithelial goblet cells. The mucoid layer thus produced consists of a gel and a sol component, and it contains immunoglobulins and antibacterial substances. It serves to keep the mucosa wet and to trap particulate matter. Lymphoid cells, both free and in small follicles, occur in the lamina propria and the submucosa.

Bronchioles

The bronchioles within the twelfth to fourteenth generations of branching are usually less than 1 mm in diameter and lack cartilage and submucosal glands. Rather, incomplete bundles of smooth muscle form a circle around the mucosa, supported by elastic fibers (Fig 12.9). This arrangement holds the air passageways open, in much the same way as the ropes attached to a tent. The epithelial lining is now simple columnar in type, gradually becoming cuboidal as the bronchioles decrease in caliber. Ciliated cells persist, but the goblet cells disappear at the level of the terminal bronchioles. Clara cells emerge within the terminal bronchioles. They are non-ciliated elements with a domed apical surface. It is believed that the function of the Clara cells is to secrete surfactant proteins that reduce the stickiness of the mucus produced by larger diameter airways, and to produce lysozyme and immunoglobulins. Clara cells may also be precursors of the epithelial cells.

Owing to their very small size and lack of cartilaginous support, individual bronchioles are vulnerable to blockage or closure. This may occur because of hypersecretion of mucus in chronic bronchitis; hyperplasia and contraction of the smooth muscle (in obstructive airway diseases such as asthma) can reduce airflow, with possibly fatal consequences.

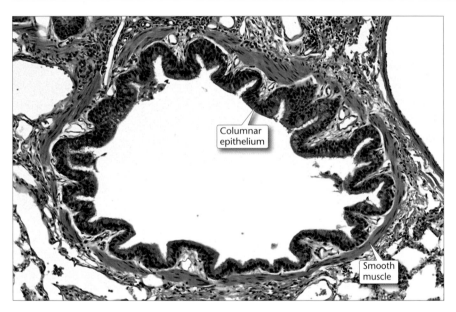

Columnar epithelium

Smooth muscle

▲ **Fig 12.9 Bronchiole.** Because they pass through the lung parenchyma (areas of alveoli), bronchioles do not require supporting cartilage, since the lung is opened up and expanded by the movements of breathing. The walls of bronchioles contain smooth muscle (which controls bronchiolar diameter and hence airflow) responding to parasympathetic stimuli, circulating bronchoactive agents, and local factors such as histamine release from mast cells. Asthmatic attacks, allergic reactions, and cough reflexes may thus constrict bronchioles. The mucosa shows a low columnar or cuboidal epithelium, with ciliated and non-ciliated cells but few mucous cells. Occasional neuroendocrine cells (neuroepithelial bodies) release biogenic amines. Clara cells occur in terminal or respiratory bronchioles. Their secretions may be involved with xenobiotic metabolism of carcinogens and lung toxicants. H&E, alcian blue, paraffin, × 120.

Acini

The parenchyma of the lung consists of a complex honeycomb-type morphology, representing alveoli together with scattered and fewer hollow tubular structures of blood vessels and bronchioles (Fig 12.10). The acinus is the chief unit of lung function. In physiologic terms, it includes all components capable of facilitating gas exchange. It consists of respiratory bronchioles, alveolar ducts and alveoli.

Respiratory bronchioles, about generations 16–18 (Fig 12.11), are about 0.4 mm in diameter, are said to be "transitional airways" because they conduct air (and so are bronchiolar-like), and also participate in gas exchange and thus are alveolar-like (Fig 12.12a & b). Lined by a cuboidal epithelium containing Clara cells, they have smooth muscle and elastic fibers that allow them to expand and contract. Occasional or numerous alveoli are distributed along their length. An increasing abundance of the alveoli forms the alveolar

duct, a tube-like structure identified by its branching and termination into one or more sacs lined only by alveoli. Alveolar ducts occur in generations 19–22 of branching. Both the duct and the sacs are made up of alveoli, with small amounts of smooth muscle present in some walls of the ducts, but not beyond. The epithelium of the respiratory tree down to the alveolar ducts contains cells of the diffuse neuroendocrine system termed neuroepithelial bodies or Kulchitsky cells derived from the neural crest. These cells have granules containing various hormones such as serotonin, dopamine, norepinephrine, and peptide. It is thought that these agents act locally on smooth muscle, and the cells may have a chemoreceptor role.

Tip: Bronchi are identified by hyaline cartilage in their walls; bronchioles are characterized by no cartilage but have smooth muscle in the wall.

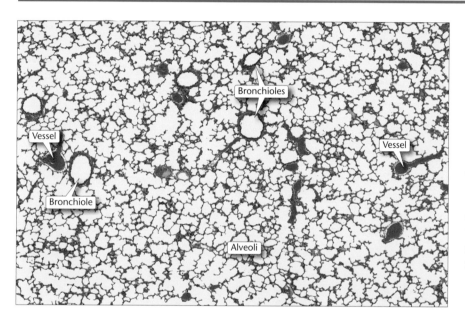

◀ Fig 12.10 Lung parenchyma. Among the many alveoli are pulmonary vessels and bronchioles. The lung provides ventilation of air, diffusion of gases, and perfusion of blood. Alveoli are thin-walled, with squamous cells and associated capillaries. They expand during inspiration, but their collapse during expiration is prevented by their surfactant production (which reduces surface tension), together with intrinsic recoil via elastic fibers. The lung has no inherent rhythmicity or motor system for ventilation; it expands in response to forces transmitted from the chest wall via the pleura. Expansion is limited by the inherent "stiffness" of its delicate connective tissues. H&E, paraffin, × 40.

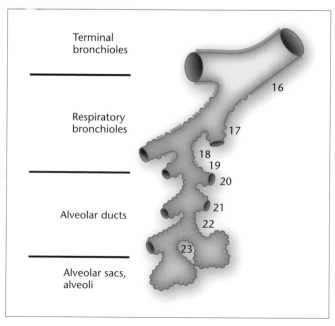

◀ Fig 12.11 Bronchial tree. Diagram of the termination of the respiratory tree, showing the respiratory zone, which commences with the respiratory bronchioles and ends in alveoli (i.e. the lung acinus). The numbers indicate the generations of dichotomous branchings, which begin with the bifurcation of the trachea into the left and right main bronchi. Assuming, in this model, 23 generations of branches, about 8 million alveolar sacs would be derived from an earlier small bronchus. Orange strips indicate smooth muscle, which is absent as the alveolar ducts branch into alveolar sacs.

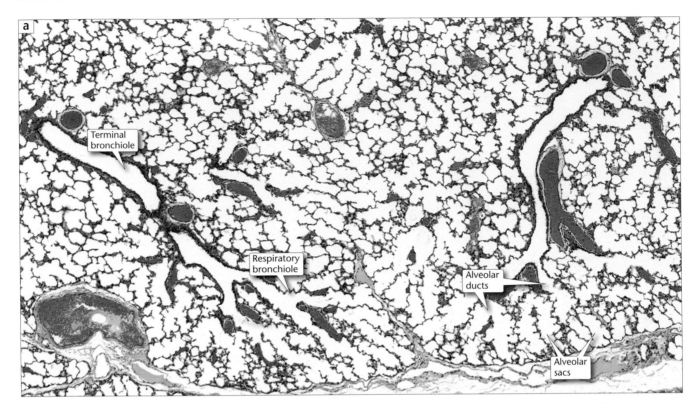

▲ **Fig 12.12a Acinar airways.** Terminal bronchioles lead to the acini, or gas exchange zones, which are marked by the appearance of alveoli. Airways for gas exchange consist of respiratory bronchioles, alveolar ducts, sacs, and, finally, the alveoli. At rest, atmospheric pressure (P_{atm}) equals alveolar pressure (P_{alv}), and hence there is no air flow. With inspiration $P_{atm} > P_{alv}$, and hence air enters the lung; at the end of inspiration, $P_{atm} = P_{alv}$ again, and hence there is no air flow. In expiration, $P_{alv} > P_{atm}$, and hence air flows out. H&E, paraffin, × 65.

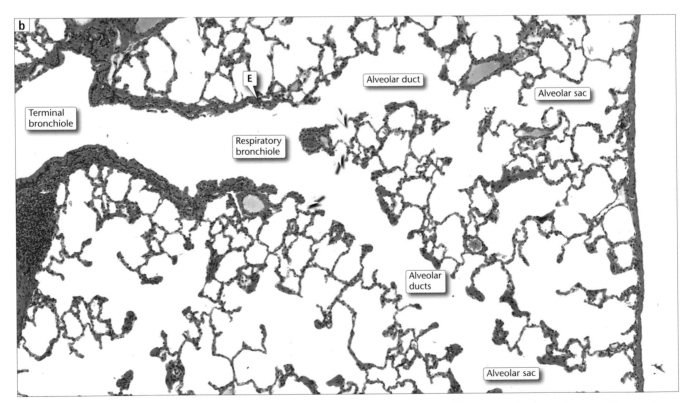

▲ **Fig 12.12b Acinar airways.** A terminal bronchiole branches into respiratory bronchioles with acquisition of alveoli (**arrows**) and the cuboidal epithelium (**E**) becoming squamous. Alveolar ducts lead to alveolar sacs, whose walls contain the alveoli and their capillary networks. When the thorax expands, alveolar air pressure falls, allowing the sacs to fill with air. Alveolar surfactant surface tension is reduced in proportion to alveolar radius, thus ensuring equalization of alveolar pressures in alveoli of different sizes and maintenance of stability throughout the lung. H&E, paraffin, × 275.

ALVEOLI AND THE BLOOD–AIR BARRIER

The alveoli that form the limits of the alveolar sacs are so numerous that paraffin sections show a honeycomb-type arrangement of empty spaces bordered by thin walls, forming open sacs or closed polygons. This shape applies to the expanded lung, but during expiration the alveoli are smaller and flatter: they unfold and stretch when filling with inspired air. Alveoli are 200–250 μm in diameter (Fig 12.13).

Small openings of about 5–10 μm in diameter—the pores of Kohn—provide a potential route for communication between alveoli, but whether these remain open in breathing is controversial. Alveolar air pressure is equivalent to atmospheric pressure, so that the only way more air can fill the alveoli is for the whole lung to expand in volume, thereby decreasing alveolar pressure to allow more air to be inspired.

Within the septa of adjacent alveolar walls are abundant capillaries of the pulmonary circulation, supported by collagen and elastic fibers (Fig 12.14) and containing wandering lymphoid cells and macrophages. In two adult human lungs there are, on average, around 500 million or more alveoli with a surface area variously estimated at 80 to 140 m^2, depending on body size and also on whether the morphometric analysis is performed on fluid-filled or air-filled fixed tissue. (For the sake of comparison, the area of a singles tennis court is 196 m^2.)

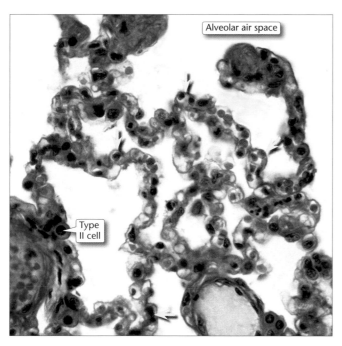

▲ **Fig 12.13 Alveoli.** Partly collapsed due to fixation and processing, the alveoli resemble a honeycomb structure. They are composed of squamous type I alveolar cells, which occupy 90% of the surface area but make up less than 10% of cell numbers; their function is to allow gas exchange with capillaries of the alveolar wall. Type II alveolar cells are cuboidal; they occupy 10% of the surface area and their chief functions are production and clearance of surfactant, and differentiation into type I cells. Numerous macrophages line the alveolar surface, but these cannot readily be identified in sections. The alveolar interstitium carries the capillaries, which are the source of monocytes and lymphocytes (although these are few in number), fibroblasts, collagen, and elastic fibers. Gas exchange occurs across the blood–air barrier (**arrows**) (i.e. capillary endothelium, fused basal laminas, and type I attenuated cytoplasm). Endothelial cells convert angiotensin I to angiotensin II, which regulates renal salt balance and blood pressure. Toluidine blue, araldite, × 380.

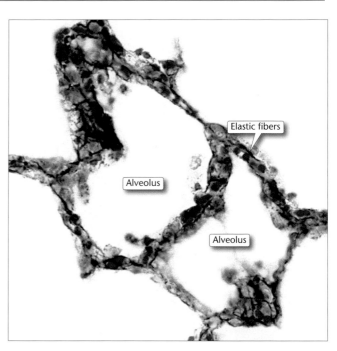

▲ **Fig 12.14 Alveolar elastin.** The alveoli have a network of elastic fibers in their walls, here stained black. Elastin is important for the regulation of alveolar shape and size as the lung expands and contracts, requiring elastic recoil of the tissue. Elastin is produced locally by fibroblast-type cells that are numerous in the alveolar septa. Van Gieson's, paraffin, × 500.

Diffusion of gases between the air and the blood across the alveolar septa is facilitated by the extraordinary richness of capillaries (Fig 12.15). These capillaries have an estimated total length of 1,600 km but contain only about 200 mL of blood. This volume is therefore spread extremely thinly over the total alveolar surface, and this allows very rapid exchange of gases.

The histology of the alveolar epithelium is simple, since it comprises only three cell types:
- Type I alveolar cells, which are squamous and cover most of the alveolar wall
- Type II alveolar cells, which are cuboidal in shape but account for a small fraction of the alveolar surface area
- Macrophages.

Type I alveolar cells

Type I alveolar cells, which may be formed from type II cells, have an extremely thin cytoplasm (0.15 μm thick) stretched over and conforming to the shape of the capillaries that invest the alveolus (Fig 12.16a & b). These cells comprise under half of the alveolar cell population but occupy 90% of its surface area. The very close apposition between the thin alveolar walls and the thin endothelium of capillaries constitutes the blood–air barrier. Sandwiched between the two cell processes at their thinnest part is the basal lamina of each cell type, which is fused into a single layer. Oxygen and carbon dioxide thus diffuse across a barrier consisting of the basal lamina and four plasma membranes (i.e. two membranes for each endothelial cell and type I alveolar cell). Water and most other molecules do not diffuse across the blood–air barrier. Alcohol and other organic compounds are exceptions.

Type II alveolar cells

Type II alveolar cells occupy only 10% of the alveolar surface area and are usually seen in the alveolar niches. The major function of type II alveolar cells is to secrete surfactant (surface active agent), which is a mixture of lipids and proteins. Surfactant forms a monolayer on the inner alveolar surface; it reduces surface tension, and this prevents collapse of alveoli during exhalation, thereby facilitating alveolar expansion during the inspiratory phase of breathing. The surfactant molecules synthesized by type II cells are stored in secretory granules called multilamellar bodies. Upon secretion, surfactant coats the inner surface of the alveolus as a monolayer of phospholipids. The first few breaths taken by a newborn baby require that the previously fluid-filled lungs contain adequate surfactant to counteract alveolar surface tension, allowing the lungs to remain expanded and reducing the energy expenditure imposed by breathing. Type II alveolar cells are stem cells and may replace type I cells after injury.

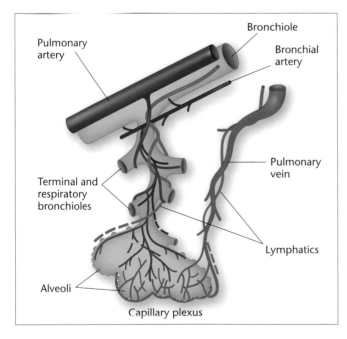

◀ **Fig 12.15 Vascular supply.** Diagram showing the relationship between the airways and vascular supply. Note that the pulmonary arterial system accompanies the bronchial tree. It leads to a dense capillary network in the alveolar walls. Oxygenated blood is collected in tributaries of the pulmonary veins, which are separate from the distal bronchial tree, and enter interlobular septa. Pulmonary veins become associated with the bronchial system as they leave the lung lobules. Bronchial arteries supply the bronchial tree down to the lung acini, and they supply visceral pleura. Lymphatic capillaries do not occur in interalveolar walls but arise nearby in the alveolar interstitium, forming vessels at the level of the respiratory bronchioles.

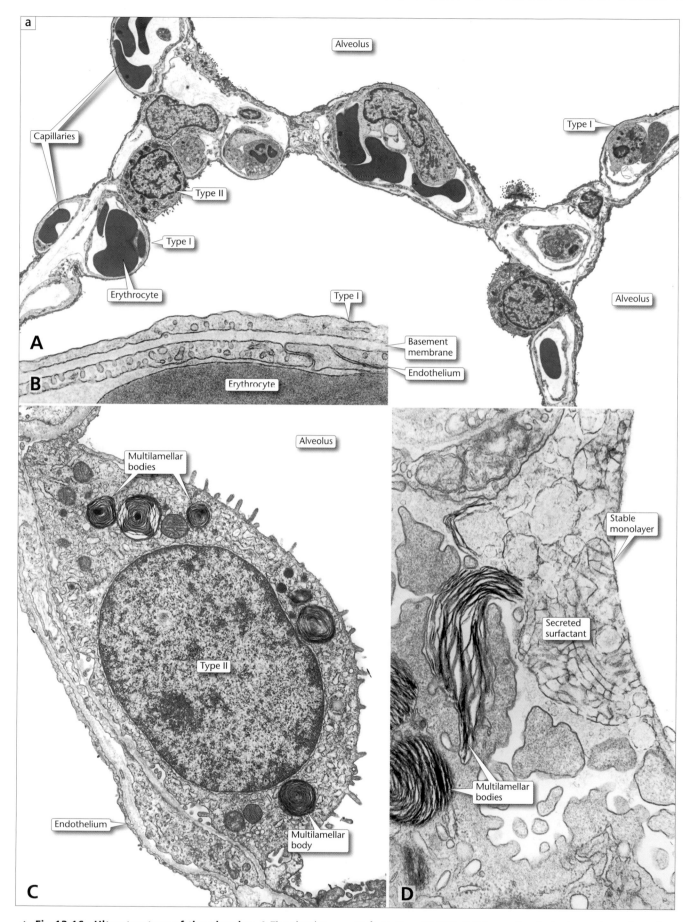

▲ **Fig 12.16a Ultrastructure of the alveolus. A** The alveolar wall is very thin where capillaries interface with air and are separated only by the attenuated cytoplasm of type I cells. × 2,200. **B** Note fusion of basal lamina of type I and endothelium that is the blood–air barrier. × 48,000. **C** Type II cell with lamellar bodies containing surfactants. × 10,200. **D** Release of surfactant onto the surface of the alveolus, spreading as a monolayer of phospholipids. × 36,000. (From Pavelka M and Roth J. Functional ultrastructure. Vienna: Springer-Verlag, 2005. With permission.)

Macrophages

Macrophages are present in large numbers within the alveoli and to a lesser extent in the septa, where they are derived from monocytes circulating in the blood. These cells are wandering cells, and their phagocytic activities are directed against irritants, particulate matter, and microorganisms. Pulmonary macrophages also partly ingest surfactant. Constantly replenished in the lung, they are removed by passing into the bronchial tree or by coughing, sneezing, or swallowing, or they may return to the lymphatics that commence at the alveolar ducts.

PLEURA

The pleura are serous membranes covering the surfaces of the lung, called visceral pleura (except at the hilum), and the inner aspect of the thorax, called parietal pleura. On the surface are squamous or cuboidal mesothelial cells, deep to which is supporting tissue with elastic fibers and abundant blood vessels. The so-called "pleural space" is a potential space, as it contains a watery exudate enabling the two membranes to slide over each other but resists their separation, or peeling apart. At rest, after quiet expiration, intrapleural pressure is about 5 mmHg

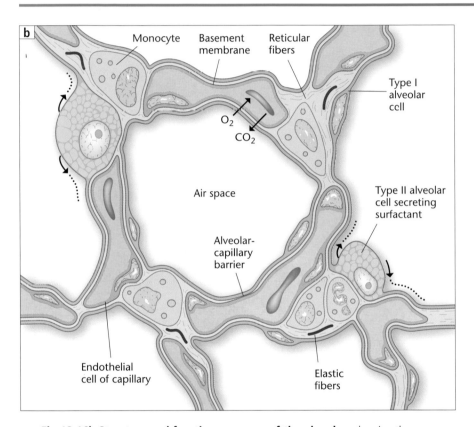

▲ **Fig 12.16b Structure and function summary of the alveolus**, showing the relationships of its walls to capillaries. Type I alveolar cells are interrupted only by type II alveolar cells with macrophages adherent to the walls (not shown). Macrophages arise from monocytes in the alveolar interstitium. Gas exchange (**arrows**) occurs across the blood–air barrier, which is about 0.2 μm thick. Erythrocytes spend less than 1 second in the alveolar capillaries, sufficient for the rapid exchange of oxygen and carbon dioxide. The capillaries bulge into the air space and are literally suspended in air; their endothelial cells provide adhesion for leukocytes, produce coagulant and anticoagulant molecules, and synthesize prostaglandins for regulation of vascular tone. Surfactant is mostly phospholipid with surfactant-specific proteins. It is secreted by type II cells as lamellar bodies that unfold and disperse along the alveolar wall as a thin film, thereby reducing surface tension by limiting the attractive forces of water molecules that cover the alveolar membranes. Surfactant is constantly secreted and recycled by type II cells, and its production in the fetal lung before birth is critical for the prevention of alveolar collapse. Macrophages, resident for months or years, kill foreign organisms, trap particles, present antigen to T cells, recruit other leukocytes, and may activate all classes of inflammatory cells in response to infection or lung damage.

below barometric pressure (760 mmHg). The visceral pleura contribute to the elastic recoil of the lungs. The elephant is the only mammal in which the pleural space is replaced with loose connective tissues; this prevents rupture of pleural blood vessels and excessive transudation when this animal is submerged in lakes or rivers and uses the trunk as a snorkel.

> **Tip:** The function of the pleura and the "pleural sac" can be likened to two apposed glass histology slides with a few drops of water between them. The two slides are almost impossible to separate by peeling them apart but they easily slide over each other. The latter is similar to the action of the two pleural membranes.

RESPIRATORY DISORDERS AND INFECTIONS

Asthma

Asthma is a common respiratory disorder. It presents with wheezing, difficulty in breathing, and possibly chronic cough. In the industrialized nations it kills thousands of children every year. Impairment of breathing occurs because of bronchiolar constriction associated with contraction and hyperplasia/hypertrophy of airway smooth muscle, excess mucus production, and narrowing of the airways with mucosal thickening. Asthma attacks may arise from non-specific stimuli such as particulate matter or cold air, or they may be an allergic reaction accompanied by mast cell degranulation. Asthma is sometimes familial.

Treatment is aimed at reducing or eliminating suspected environmental factors and at reversing or limiting the airway constriction. Medications such as inhaled bronchodilators and administration of anti-inflammatory substances such as cortisone provide significant benefits.

Cystic fibrosis

Cystic fibrosis (CF), an inherited disorder affecting about one in every 1,600 newborn children, may cause airway obstruction because of excessive and hyperviscous mucus secretion. This commonly leads to chronic lung infection. CF is usually a mutation in the transmembrane conductance regulator (CFTR) gene, in which there is impaired chloride ion secretion causing dehydration and mucous plugs.

Emphysema

Emphysema is a destructive disease of the respiratory acinus (which becomes enlarged) and is associated with narrowing (inflammation) of the smaller bronchioles. Emphysema may also destroy alveoli. The condition is commonly associated with smoking.

Bronchitis

Bronchitis results from overproduction of mucus. Its acute presentations are inflammatory and may be caused by viral infection. Chronic cases are often associated with prolonged exposure to irritants, particularly tobacco smoke, and they may be related to mucous gland enlargement. The incidence of this form of airway disease is significant, affecting millions and killing tens of thousands each year.

Embolism

An embolism may cause respiratory dysfunction via the passage and lodgement of a blood clot within a pulmonary arterial vessel. A common type is the thromboembolism, in which the thrombus detaches from a distal vein or the right side of the heart. Depending on the size and nature of the embolism, there may be no symptoms; however, massive or multiple emboli may be fatal within seconds, hours, or days.

Abnormalities of development

Respiratory distress syndrome occurs in the newly born when the alveoli are deficient in producing surfactant. This is usually a result of immaturity of the type II cells or of insufficient numbers of type II cells following preterm birth. Gas exchange is compromised because alveoli do not remain expanded. Survival of preterm neonates is heavily dependent on surfactant production, which is initiated at about 20 weeks' gestation. By 24–26 weeks' gestation, sufficient numbers of alveoli and surfactant-secreting type II cells give preterm babies a realistic, albeit low, chance of survival. Full-term babies have less than 10% of the adult numbers of alveoli. A form of the respiratory distress syndrome may occasionally occur in adults (adult respiratory distress syndrome).

Kartagener's syndrome (or immotile cilia syndrome) is a rare congenital abnormality associated with respiratory problems caused by the accumulation of airway mucus. The cilia show total or partial loss of the dynein arms attached to the outer microtubule doublets, resulting in impairment of ciliary movement. Chronic infections of the lungs and upper airways is common in this syndrome, which may also be associated with infertility resulting from immotile sperm and possible ciliary dysfunction in the oviducts.

Inflammation and infection

Croup is a common viral infection in children and presents as a persistent, rasping cough. The larynx is inflamed and treatment is directed at relieving symptoms.

Diphtheria, a bacterial infection prevalent in infants, is associated with chronic coughing spasms. Usually the upper respiratory tract is affected by toxic necrosis of the pharyngeal or tonsillar regions. Prevention is available by immunization and is usually offered as a component of the triple vaccine (diphtheria, tetanus, and pertussis).

Whooping cough (pertussis), another bacterial infection with potentially serious effects in children, causes local tissue damage in the upper respiratory tract and inflammation of the bronchial tree. Symptoms, which may last for weeks, include nasal obstruction and coughing fits; they gradually subside.

Pneumonia, or inflammation of the lung parenchyma, may develop from bacterial or viral infections. Histologically the lung contains inflammatory exudates and may include fibrosis and alveolar destruction. In otherwise healthy people, the condition normally resolves and, when indicated, antibiotics assist this process. It is of interest that a form of pneumonia was associated with the Black Death and the Great Plague of the fourteenth and sixteenth centuries.

Pleurisy (inflammation of the pleura) is often a secondary infection associated with pneumonia or, in particular, tuberculosis. An exudate is formed, which may be fibrous and cause discomfort and restriction of lung movement.

Tuberculosis is a major cause of mortality in developing countries. It is caused by inhalation of a bacterium. The lungs become inflamed and show granulomas, fibrosis, and necrosis, but in healthy people the condition usually abates before this stage is reached.

Sinusitis, an infection of the nasal passages, presents as nasal discharge, facial discomfort, and blockage of the sinuses. It is caused by viral infection leading to edema and subsequent infection with bacteria.

Similarly, rhinitis may result from a wide variety of viral infections all contributing to the common cold. Rhinitis and sinusitis may occur simultaneously with hay fever, which is an allergic reaction to pollen, flowers, animal hair, or dust; it is not a fever and most sufferers are not exposed to hay.

Tumors

Lung cancer commonly develops from bronchi and may metastasize to any other tissue of the body, usually via the bloodstream. Generally the tumors are squamous-type or adenocarcinomas. Smoking, exposure to asbestos, and excessive radioactivity are implicated as causative factors.

Mesothelioma is a malignant tumor of the pleura often, but not always, associated with a history of exposure to asbestos dust. The tumor spreads throughout the pleural membranes and between the lobes of the lung, and it may completely surround the organ. Treatment of lung tumors may involve radiotherapy or chemotherapy together with surgery.

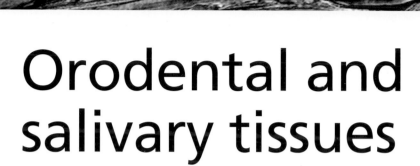

Orodental and salivary tissues

The oral cavity consists of two unequal parts—the vestibule lying between the lips and cheeks superficially and the teeth and gingivae, and an inner, larger buccal cavity extending between the arches of the teeth and the oropharynx. Posteriorly, the buccal cavity is bounded by the soft palate above and the epiglottis below. It may seem obvious that the functions of the oral cavity include mechanical and chemical breakdown of food and swallowing, but there are numerous other functions. These include speech and taste, lubrication of food, defense against infections, maintenance of a moist environment and irrigation, providing a fluid seal for sucking and suckling, and response to tactile stimuli.

TONGUE

The tongue consists mostly of intrinsic skeletal muscle arranged in longitudinal, transverse, and vertical bundles that frequently appear to intersect in histologic section (Fig 13.1a–c). Its surface is covered by the

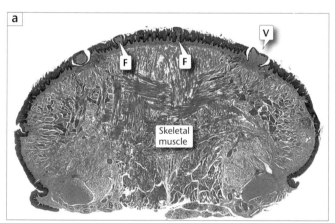

▲ **Fig 13.1a General histology of the tongue.** Transverse section of tongue through the sulcus terminalis region, showing skeletal muscle fascicles with the lateral and dorsal surfaces covered by mucosa of stratified squamous epithelium with variable keratinization. Upward projections of the lamina propria form the many lingual papillae, mostly of filiform type together with fungiform (**F**) and large vallate papillae (**V**). The latter are surrounded by a trough and "walled in" by adjacent mucosa. Hematoxylin & eosin (H&E), paraffin, × 5.

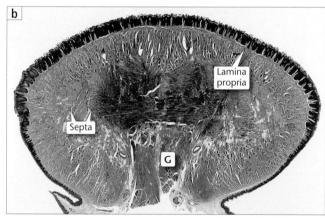

▲ **Fig 13.1b Arrangement of skeletal muscle fibers** in the tongue showing the central genioglossus (**G**), which is extrinsic, and the many intrinsic muscles that lie above and lateral to it. Lower lateral muscles are parts of other extrinsic muscles such as the glossus and hyoid groups. Note the many septa that partition the muscle fibers. Trichrome, paraffin, × 4.

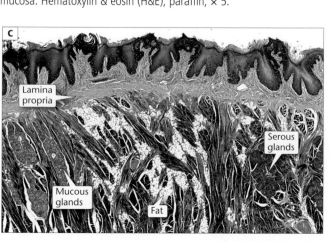

◀ **Fig 13.1c Detail of intrinsic lingual skeletal muscles** in longitudinal, vertical, and transverse orientations, which together alter the shape of the tongue. Deep to the surface epithelium the dense connective tissue of the lamina propria extends between the muscle fascicles, allowing the distribution of blood and lymph vessels, and nerves. The sensory innervation serves not only for general and gustatory sensation, but also has the proprioceptive function of protecting the tongue from being bitten. Serous and mucous glands, and fat tissue are indicated. Trichrome, paraffin, × 25.

lingual mucosa (Fig 13.2). On the dorsum (superior part) it is partly or fully keratinized stratified squamous epithelium; on the ventral surface, it is non-keratinized, similar to the remainder of the oral mucosa, which is also incompletely cornified.

The dorsal surface of the tongue shows numerous specializations related to the oral (anterior) and pharyngeal (posterior or root) regions, which are separated macroscopically by the V-shaped sulcus terminalis—the oral region that displays many elevated lingual papillae (giving a roughened appearance), with the pharyngeal part exhibiting smoother, although still numerous, undulations of the mucosa.

Specialized mucosa

The components of the tongue that are of histologic interest are the papillae, taste buds, lingual glands, and lingual tonsils. Papillae serve the functions of sensory perception (temperature, texture), of increasing friction between the lingual mucosa and food, and of the detection of taste. In accordance with their shape, four types of papillae are described (Fig 13.3a–d):
- Filiform are the most numerous on the dorsum and are pointed, conical projections.
- Fungiform are occasionally found among the filiform papillae and resemble a short blunt projection of the mucosa.

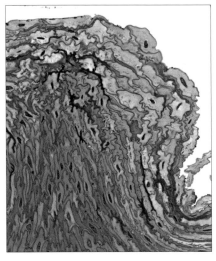

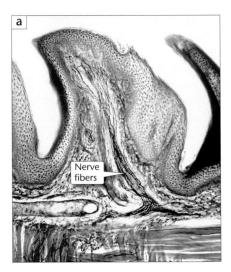

▲ **Fig 13.2 Tongue epithelium.** The inferior surface of the tongue is stratified squamous epithelium with little or no keratin, which is also found in regions of the oral cavity not subjected to significant abrasion, such as the floor of the mouth and the cheek. Unlike skin, there is no stratum corneum. Toluidine blue, araldite, × 400.

◀ **Fig 13.3a Filiform papilla.** Filiform papilla projecting from the dorsal surface of the tongue, showing an irregular conical specialization, which is partly keratinized. Other surfaces are partly keratinized or show no stratum corneum. Filiform papillae are abundant on the anterior two-thirds of the tongue and have no taste buds. Nerve fibers of the lamina propria are branches of the lingual nerve for general sensory function. Gold stain, paraffin, × 100.

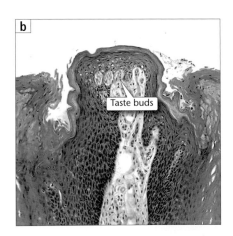

▲ **Fig 13.3b Fungiform papilla** shows a flattened, dome-shaped projection slightly higher than the adjacent surface. The core is associated with several taste buds. H&E, paraffin, × 40.

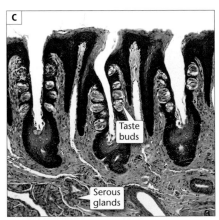

▲ **Fig 13.3c Foliate papillae** show alternating clefts and ridges, with taste buds on the lateral margins. Serous glands empty into the base of the clefts. Trichrome, paraffin, × 50.

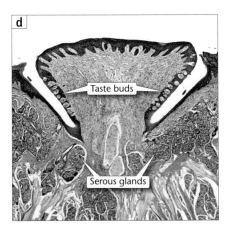

▲ **Fig 13.3d Vallate papilla** resembles a mushroom shape with taste buds on the stalk region. Deeper serous glands of von Ebner empty their watery secretions into the furrow or sulcus that surrounds the papilla. This assists the distribution of substances that stimulate the taste receptors. H&E, paraffin, × 25.

- Foliate papillae may be found along the posterior margins of the tongue and are blunt and leaf-shaped.
- Vallate or circumvallate papillae are large and dome-shaped, flanked by a furrow and circumferential mucosal wall. About 6 to 12 in number, they occur in front of the sulcus terminalis.

Taste buds are concentrated on the lateral aspects of most papillae (particularly the vallate type), except for the filiform type. Individual taste buds may occur elsewhere on the dorsum and sides of the tongue, the epiglottis, and the soft palate. The function of taste buds is discussed further in Chapter 20.

Lingual glands are serous, mucous, and mixed seromucous. Serous glands (of von Ebner) are associated with aggregations of taste buds, notably emptying into the sulcus of vallate papillae, where their flushing secretions distribute food particles and thus assist with taste perception. Serous and mucous gland acini occur in the anterior core of the tongue (Fig 13.4), emptying on the inferior surface; mucous acini are abundant in the pharyngeal region where they serve to lubricate masticated food boluses before swallowing.

Abundant lymphoid follicles occur in the submucosa of the pharyngeal region of the tongue and together form the lingual tonsil. Clusters of nodules occur around crypt-like invaginations of the surface mucosa, which itself is infiltrated by lymphocytes (Fig 13.5).

SALIVARY GLANDS
Functions of saliva

Production of saliva is essential for oral health. It is formed by the major and minor salivary glands and from fluid from the gingival sulcus. Saliva has many functions:

- Protection of the oral mucosa by lubrication; secretion of IgA (from the parotid gland), which aggregates microorganisms, allowing these to be swallowed
- Digestion of starch compounds via enzymatic breakdown
- Acting as a solvent for ingested molecules that are dispersed among the taste buds, chiefly in the tongue
- Protection of teeth by its high ion content, especially calcium, which acts as a buffer against acid demineralization of enamel
- Supplying growth factors that assist wound healing.

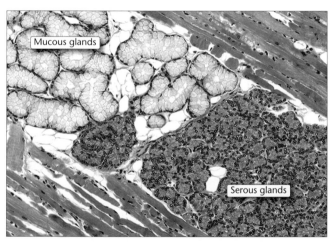

▲ **Fig 13.4 Lingual glands.** Mucus-secreting glands are identified as tubuloalveolar collections of pyramid-shaped cells with pale-staining granular cytoplasm and nuclei dispersed basally. A central lumen is often seen. Adipose cells usually extracted and empty in appearance are noted. Serum-secreting glands may be mixed with some mucus-secreting glands. Note the alveolar-type shape of clusters of secretory cells, with spherical nuclei and eosinophilic cytoplasm representing stored secretory vesicles that contain digestive enzymes, which contribute to saliva. H&E, paraffin, × 85.

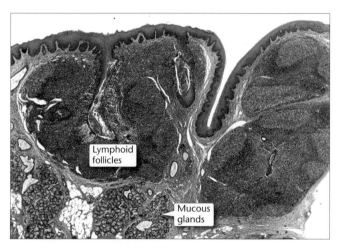

▲ **Fig 13.5 Lingual tonsils.** Lymphoid follicles gathered around mucosal crypts in the pharyngeal region are lingual tonsils, showing germinal centers surrounded by many other lymphoid cells, particularly lymphocytes. These cells migrate across the surface epithelium to participate in immune reactions within the oral cavity, chiefly by forming plasma cells, which secrete antibodies in response to antigenic challenge. Mucus secreted by the deeper mucus-secreting glands tends to cleanse the crypts and minimize tissue infections. H&E, paraffin, × 25.

Major and minor salivary glands

The major salivary glands are the parotid, submandibular, and sublingual glands; minor salivary glands consist of those within the tongue (lingual) and labial, buccal, and palatal glands. Minor salivary glands of the oral cavity secrete a mainly mucous product. Their histology is as described for the major salivary glands. Although minor salivary glands secrete only 10% of the total volume of saliva (about 500 mL per day), they contribute most of the mucus secreted.

With the exception of the parotid gland, which contains only serous-secreting acini together with adipose tissue that increases in quantity with age, the submandibular and sublingual glands are composed of a mixture of serous, mucous, and combined seromucous secretory units. In histologic sections, salivary glands thus show heterogeneous morphology, which also varies between species; sexual dimorphism is present in the submandibular glands of some rodents, pigs, and insectivores. For this reason, the terms serous, mucous, and seromucous are somewhat loosely applied according to the various proportions of each type of secretory cell. All salivary glands are lobulated, with the secretory units organized into branches that terminate as "end-pieces." The latter may be tubular, acinar, or tubuloacinar if they are intermediate between elongate and spheroidal shape. Mucous end-pieces tend to be tubular; serous end-pieces are typically acinar (Fig 13.6).

Differences between serous and mucous cells

When examining stained sections of salivary glands, particularly if the precise identity is not known, it is useful to be aware of the basic structural differences between serous-secreting and mucous-secreting cells.

Serous cells secrete a watery solution rich in proteins. They are pyramidal, cuboidal, or crescent-shaped, with spherical nuclei. The basal cytoplasm stains with hematoxylin, whereas the apical cytoplasm stains with eosin and numerous small zymogen granules may be visible. The parotid gland acini are purely serous-secreting in humans (Fig 13.7).

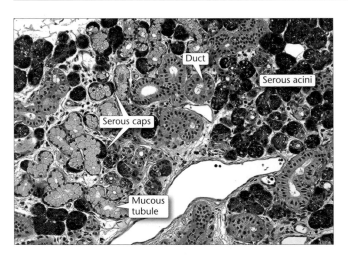

◀ **Fig 13.6 Salivary gland secretory units.** Serum-secreting cells (stained deep blue with H&E), contain sialoglycoproteins and some digestive enzymes in secretory vesicles. Serous units occur as acini and/or serous caps or end-pieces at the ends of mucous units. Mucus-secreting cells, always extracted, contain mucins (carbohydrate-rich glycoproteins) and, depending on the plane of section, occur as branched glands. Serous secretions are watery; mucous secretions are viscous. Note the scattered ducts. H&E, paraffin, × 85.

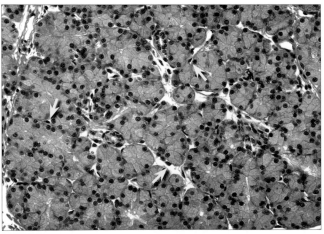

◀ **Fig 13.7 Parotid gland.** The largest of the main salivary glands, the parotid is a serous exocrine gland secreting a watery solution containing electrolytes and the enzyme amylase. Shown here are the so-called secretory end-pieces (as distinct from ducts), typically acinar or alveolar in shape, containing cuboidal or pyramidal exocrine cells with spherical nuclei and cytoplasmic secretory vesicles. Myoepithelial (contractile) cells surround acini (**arrows**). The major salivary glands are supplied by parasympathetic and sympathetic secretomotor fibers, the former increasing and the latter decreasing the rate of secretion. H&E, paraffin, × 150.

Mucous cells secrete mucus (a viscous mixture of glycoproteins) and are poorly stained with hematoxylin and eosin (H&E), the mucoid droplets giving a foamy appearance to the cytoplasm, with the nucleus displaced or flattened at the base of the cell. Most of the acini in the sublingual gland are mucous-secreting (Fig 13.8).

Serous demilunes are components of mixed acini, which occur in the submandibular glands (mostly serous, some mucous acini) and sublingual glands (mostly mucous, some serous acini). Demilunes show a crescent or cap of serous cells covering the mucous end-pieces (Fig 13.9a & b).

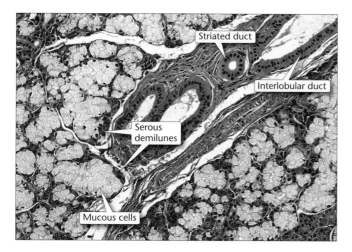

◀ **Fig 13.8 Sublingual gland.** Mucus-secreting cells predominate with a minor proportion of serous demilunes. A striated duct is noted together with larger interlobular ducts. Sublingual gland secretions contribute less than 10% of the volume of saliva, most of which (about two-thirds) comes from the submandibular glands. H&E, paraffin, × 85.

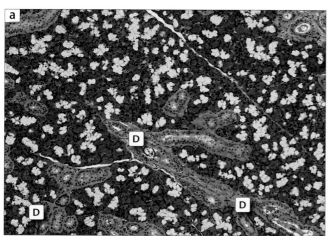

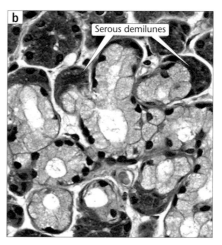

▲ **Fig 13.9a Submandibular gland.** Characteristic histologic features are a predominance of serum-secreting component (deeply stained) compared with the mucus-secreting portions (partly extracted and pale), and the extensive duct system (**D**), mostly of the intercalated or initial part of the branching ducts. Connective tissue supports all these elements and contains blood vessels, nerves, ganglia, and plasma cells contributing secretory IgA to the saliva. H&E, paraffin, × 60.

▲ **Fig 13.9b Submandibular gland.** Typical mixed secretory end-pieces of the submandibular gland, showing tubular mucus-secreting glands capped with crescent-shaped serous cells, termed serous demilunes. Serous secretions (enzyme-rich secretory vesicles) reach the lumen by narrow channels or intercellular canaliculi between serum-secreting and mucus-secreting cells, hence the primary saliva contains mucins and digestive enzymes. Hematoxylin/PAS, paraffin, × 350.

Salivary secretion and the duct system

After secretion of saliva by the secretory units—a process that is aided by associated myoepithelial cells and regulated chiefly by parasympathetic nerve fibers—the saliva passes through a duct system (Fig 13.10a & b). Here, the luminal contents are modified with reabsorption of sodium (actively) and chloride ions (passively) across the ductal epithelium, resulting in the release of hypotonic salivary fluid into the oral cavity. Structural specializations matching this physiologic data are provided by the presence of striated ducts located between the intercalated and excretory ducts; these ducts have in-folded basolateral plasma membranes and many mitochondria which, together, extract sodium ions from the primary saliva. The duct system is also secretory, adding IgA, proteases, and bicarbonate ions to the saliva.

Tip: The correct identification of salivary glands is based upon the different morphology of secretory units. Serous glands are normally more densely stained than mucous glands because of their enzyme-rich granules and rough endoplasmic reticulum. Mucous-secreting glands are commonly branched and always weakly stained with H&E, with a foam-type cytoplasm and flat, basal nuclei. Salivary glands cannot be confused with the exocrine pancreas because the latter has duct nuclei of centroacinar cells that lie in the middle of the secretory acini.

TEETH

The adult human has 32 permanent teeth (16 in each of the upper and lower dental arches), but because teeth need to be accommodated in the small, growing jaws of children, the permanent teeth are preceded by 20 deciduous teeth. These are progressively shed

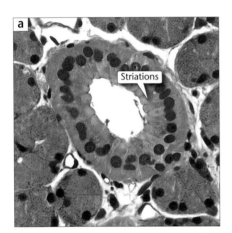

◀ **Fig 13.10a Salivary gland ducts.**
A striated duct in the parotid is shown with columnar epithelium and parallel striations of mitochondria and in-folded basal membranes. Extraction of sodium ions renders the saliva hypotonic. Growth factors and enzymes are secreted by striated ducts. H&E, paraffin, × 400.

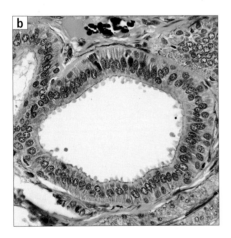

◀ **Fig 13.10b Salivary gland ducts.**
Interlobular ducts have wide lumens and pseudostratified columnar epithelium, which becomes stratified squamous near the oral mucosa. The chief function is to transport saliva, but the cells may undergo metaplasia or neoplasia in pathologic disorders. Trichrome, paraffin, × 200.

and replaced during the sixth to about the twentieth year. Teeth are not rigidly attached to bone, but are suspended in a socket of bone by a dense connective tissue called the periodontal ligament. They are grouped according to differences in their shape into four classes—from the front to the back of the jaw, incisors, canines, premolars, and molars (Fig 13.11).

To study adult teeth using conventional paraffin sections, the teeth must first be decalcified to remove hard, mineralized tissue. The procedure dissolves almost all the constituents of the enamel; therefore, in paraffin sections, enamel is usually studied in developing teeth before full mineralization. In thin ground sections of adult teeth, cellular detail is mostly lost, but mineralized substances including enamel and dentin remain, and their highly ordered arrangements of mineralized elements may be displayed to advantage using polarized light microscopy (Fig 13.12a–c).

An individual tooth consists of a crown and a root, which is comprised mostly of dentin—an avascular and strictly acellular but living connective tissue, similar to bone but harder. The crown projects

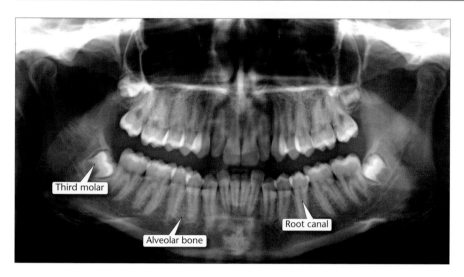

◀ **Fig 13.11 Teeth in situ.**
Panoramic radiograph of the dentition (orthopantomogram) at 17 years of age. Enamel is more radiopaque than dentin and the pulp is seen as a central radiolucent region in the roots. Note that the third molars have not yet erupted. The faint, honeycomb-type pattern around the teeth is the alveolar bone.

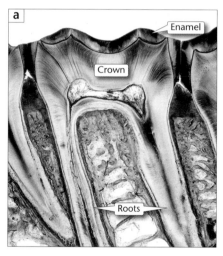
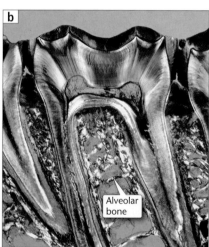
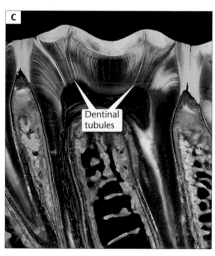

▲ **Fig 13.12 Adult teeth, unstained sections.**
a Thin ground section viewed with brightfield microscopy, showing the enamel (of reduced depth due to wear), the dentin forming roots extending into alveolar bone sockets, and bony septal bridges between sockets. The pulp is connective tissue, seen here in part. It is nutritive and sensory for the dentin. **b** Cross-polarized light microscopy shows many different colors as a result of the changing orientations and absorptive properties of mineralized hard tissues in relation to the vibration plane of the polarized light. In dentin it is the dentinal tubules and in alveolar bone the collagen fibers that give the color tints. **c** Diffracted light contrast microscopy, a variant of the darkfield technique, showing to advantage the dentinal tubules of the tooth crown. All × 3.

from the gingivae and is covered with enamel, a heavily mineralized cell secretion that is the hardest substance in the body, consisting of 96–98% by weight hydroxyapatite crystals. Most of the tooth is made up of the root, suspended in and anchored by the periodontal ligament in a socket of alveolar bone (Fig 13.13a & b). The root is covered by a thin layer of bone-like tissue called cementum, which contains cells and extracellular matrix. Enamel and cementum usually meet at the gingival crevice. The tooth contains a central pulp cavity of loose connective tissue, narrowed in the deeper root(s) to form a pulp or root canal, which, via a small foramen at the tip of each root, is continuous with the periodontal ligament and allows vessels and nerves to enter the pulp cavity. The gingivae or gums are specialized regions of oral mucosa that consist of parakeratinized stratified squamous epithelium attached to adjacent bone at the neck or cervical margin of the teeth. Collectively, the gingivae, periodontal ligament, alveolar bone, and cementum are called the periodontium. Inflammation and the consequential breakdown of this complex is a major cause of tooth loss over the age of 40 years.

Enamel

Enamel is the hardest tissue in the body. Originating during tooth development from ameloblasts (see below), enamel extends from the underlying core of dentin to a maximum thickness of about 2.5 mm, and consists of very closely packed enamel prisms or rods, each shaped in cross section like a keyhole or fish-scale. Prisms are about 5 µm in width and contain flat, overlapping ribbons of hydroxyapatite crystals of extreme hardness. Each prism is demarcated from its neighbors by a thin zone where enamel crystals in adjacent prisms pack together poorly, allowing some organic matrix to remain. When fully formed, enamel is not renewable, which means that damaged enamel cannot regenerate. Calcium and phosphate in the saliva can assist with remineralization of enamel and saliva may neutralize the acids that cause cariogenic lesions of enamel.

Dentin

Dentin is hard tissue in the body of the tooth. It is produced slowly throughout life and provides firm attachment to the enamel by the intermingling of hydroxyapatite crystals. The important difference between bone and dentin is that in dentin the forming cells are *external* to the hard tissue. The mineralized component of dentin is responsible for up to 80% of its mass, forming near-parallel dentinal tubules that radiate out from the pulp chamber. The latter is covered by a layer of pre-dentin (non-mineralized matrix) secreted by odontoblasts, which form a pseudostratified layer lining the pulp. Each dentinal tubule contains a long cytoplasmic process of an odontoblast cell, with an external collar of dentin (Fig 13.14a & b). Covering the dental roots, the avascular layer of cementum contains cementocytes (analogous to osteocytes), and the outermost layer consists of cementoblasts (similar to osteoblasts). Bundles of collagen fibers, termed Sharpey's fibers, are embedded in the cementum; beyond this interface, bundles of interlacing collagen fibers extend outward and constitute the principal fiber component of the periodontal ligament, which anchors into adjacent alveolar bone (Fig 13.15a–c).

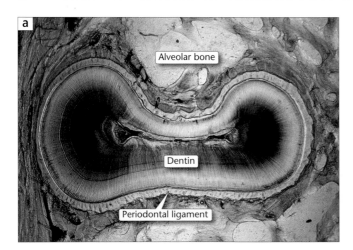

▲ **Fig 13.13a Teeth in situ within the alveolus.** Horizontal section of a mandibular molar tooth, showing its dumbbell-shaped root that consists of dentin formed from radially arranged dentinal tubules. The dentin is surrounded by a collar of periodontal ligament, which anchors the tooth to the bony tooth socket (alveolus). Unstained ground section, × 8.

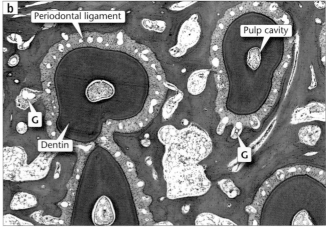

▲ **Fig 13.13b Forming teeth.** Horizontal section of forming teeth near the deepest (apical) part of the roots showing the pulp cavity, and an annulus of dentin. Glomerulus-like (**G**) pockets of bone around the periodontal ligament convey blood and lymphatic vessels and nerves, the latter with proprioceptive endings. These sensory receptors detect pressure overload on the teeth, and pain reflexes protect against biting hard on dense particles. H&E, paraffin, × 8.

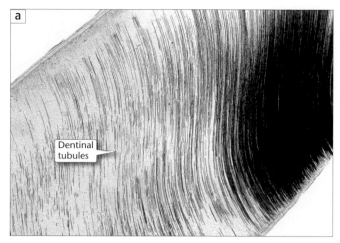

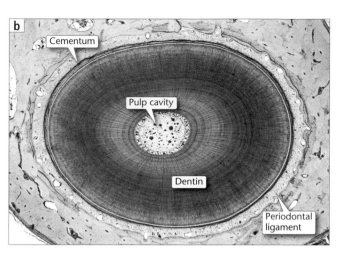

▲ **Fig 13.14a Dentin.** Unstained ground section of a tooth root, showing many curved dark lines representing dentinal tubules. Tubules contain very thin, tapered cytoplasmic processes of odontoblasts, the cells that secrete collagen and other proteins that are essential organic components mixed in with the hard mineralized dentin matrix of hydroxyapatite and other minerals. The S-shaped curves represent the path taken by the progressive inward migration of odontoblasts during tooth formation. × 100.

▲ **Fig 13.14b Dentin.** Cross section through the root of a tooth in a decalcified section showing many concentric lines perpendicular to the radial dentinal tubules. These lines are the imbrication lines of von Ebner, indicating incremental deposition of dentin, believed to be deposited at a rate of 4–8 μm per day. Surrounding the dentin is cementum, a thin layer of calcified tissue that provides attachment of the tooth with the outer periodontal ligament. H&E, paraffin, × 30.

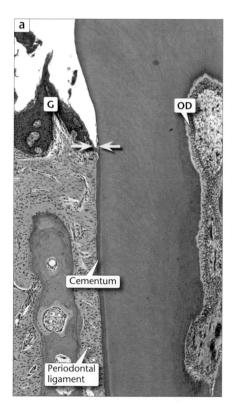

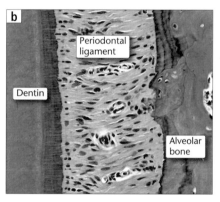

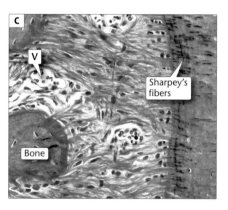

▲ **Fig 13.15b Periodontal ligament** extends between the cementum layer of the tooth (covering the dentin) and the alveolar bone, which shows mineralization fronts. Collagen of the periodontal ligament attaches to cementum and bone via Sharpey's fibers. The periodontal ligament allows for natural or orthodontic tooth movement and gradually diminishes in width with age. H&E, paraffin, × 150.

▲ **Fig 13.15c Developing periodontal ligament** between alveolar bone and the outer cementum and cementoblasts covering the root of the tooth. Bundles of collagen insert into bone and cementum, forming Sharpey's fibers, but the wave-like collagen does not extend uninterrupted between tooth and bone, thus allowing movement during tooth growth. Numerous blood vessels (**V**) indicate high metabolic activity of the tissue. Trichrome, paraffin, × 160.

▲ **Fig 13.15a Periodontal ligament.** Adult tooth, decalcified section. The crown and root consist of living dentin tissue with a core or pulp cavity containing vessels, nerves (which enter through the deep apical foramen, not shown), and odontoblasts (**OD**). The root is covered by cementum, which terminates at a point (**arrows**) near the gingival epithelium (**G**). The periodontal ligament attaches the tooth to a socket of alveolar bone. H&E, paraffin, × 20.

Tooth development

Teeth form through a complex series of epithelial–mesenchymal interactions that are similar to the formation of hair follicles of the skin. It takes about 14 months for a tooth to develop. Tooth formation is referred to as odontogenesis. The process begins with the formation of 20 primary tooth germs that grow and expand. The tooth germs contain differentiated

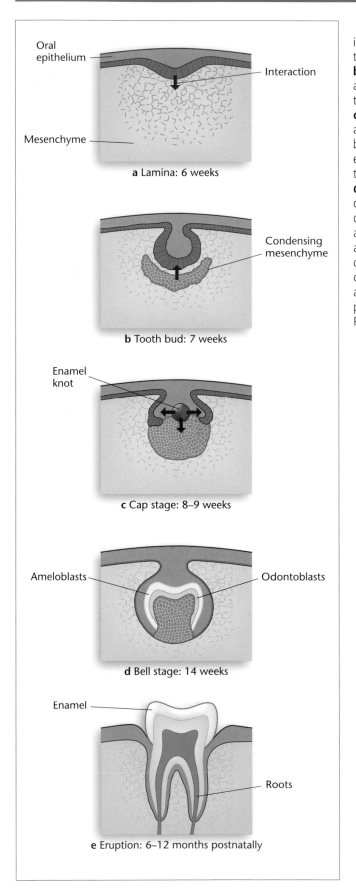

◀ **Fig 13.16 The formation of a tooth. a** During the sixth week in utero at sites for the future alveolar processes, the oral epithelium thickens, elongates into a lamina, and signals the mesenchyme. **b** The induced mesenchyme produces its own signals, condensing around the protrusion to form a tooth bud by about 7 weeks. The tooth bud is known as the enamel organ because it will form enamel. **c** Further specialization of the epithelium during weeks 8–9 forms a cap over the mesenchyme, the latter termed the dental papilla because it will form the dentin and pulp of the tooth root. The enamel knot at the center of the cap is a source of signals directing the growth and morphogenesis of epithelial and mesenchymal cells. **d** The bell stage reached by 14 weeks is associated with formation of presumptive ameloblasts from the enamel organ, and odontoblast development from the mesenchyme. Odontoblasts form pre-dentin and when this has been mineralized, ameloblasts are differentiated and will then form the enamel. **e** Eruption of the tooth occurs as a consequence of growth of the root/s, pushing the enamel-covered crown through the oral epithelium. Deciduous (baby) teeth mostly appear by 12 months of age and are progressively replaced by the permanent teeth from about 7 years of age until the early 20s. Primordia of permanent teeth are found in the fetus.

cells that later will form the mineralized tissues. These formative cells contribute to the production of dentin during the phase of dentinogenesis, which is followed by the development of enamel, called amelogenesis (Fig 13.16).

Thickening of the oral epithelium

Initially, in the 6-week embryo, the oral mucosa over the future dental arches thickens and is called the dental lamina stage (Fig 13.17). Gene activity in its cells produces signals that act on the underlying mesenchymal tissue. Occasionally this tissue is called ectomesenchyme because the mesenchyme is derived from the neural crest, which is of ectodermal origin.

Bud stage: early definitive tooth

The dental lamina invaginates to form a rounded, localized growth bud surrounded by a condensation of ectomesenchymal cells that aggregate in response to their own signaling molecules. Proliferation of oral epithelial cells in the bud form the so-called enamel organ (Fig 13.17).

Cap stage: the tooth germ

When the enamel organ is at the cap stage, the epithelial cells gain a concave surface (Fig 13.18). This shape is directed by signals from the epithelial cells. Mesenchyme partially surrounded by the growing cap-shaped enamel organ is called the dental papilla. Cells flanking the papilla and those outside the enamel organ grow to form the dental follicle. The enamel organ forms enamel; the papilla will form the dentin and pulp; the follicle forms the cementum, periodontal ligament, and adjacent alveolar bone. The epithelium on the underside of the cap is the inner enamel epithelium (IEE) and consists of the presumptive ameloblasts that will later form enamel.

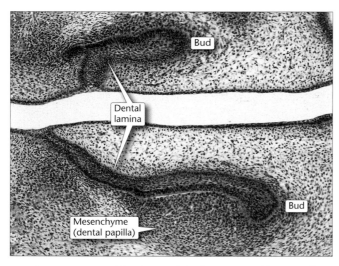

▲ **Fig 13.17 Dental lamina and bud stage.** Proliferation of the oral epithelium forms a process that invades the mesenchyme. This is called the dental lamina and has a stem and two arms like an inverted Y. One arm will eventually become the buccal sulcus; the other, elongating further, will become the growing tooth. The thickening epithelium is the source of a secreted signal (fibroblast growth factor, FGF) that induces differentiation of the adjacent mesenchyme. The invading epithelium proliferates at its end, forming a discrete bud. Epithelial cells will eventually form enamel, and the condensing ectomesenchyme will become the dentin and pulp. The mesenchyme secretes bone morphogenetic protein (BMP) that reciprocally acts on the epithelial cells. The positions of tooth formation separated by gaps are controlled by the antagonistic signaling of BMP and FGF in regions between the developing teeth. H&E, paraffin, × 100.

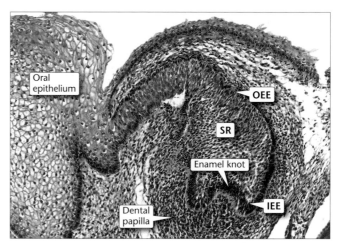

▲ **Fig 13.18 Cap stage.** The epithelium, now responding to BMP signals, forms the enamel knot. In turn the knot secretes FGF to promote epithelial proliferation, resulting in a concave undersurface that resembles a cap overlying the mesenchyme. Note the continuity of the earlier dental lamina with the cap tissue. Differentiated epithelial cells close to the mesenchyme are termed cells of the inner enamel epithelium (**IEE**) and are presumptive ameloblasts. The outer enamel epithelium (**OEE**) is shown. Cells of the stellate reticulum (**SR**) secrete extracellular materials. H&E, paraffin, × 120.

Bell stage: defining the future crown

The outer cell layer of the enamel organ is the outer enamel epithelium (OEE). The stroma of the enamel organ has star-shaped cells bound together by desmosomes; these cells are called stellate reticulum and secrete much extracellular material (Fig 13.19a & b). IEE induces the nearby dental papillae cells to become odontoblasts, which eventually form the dentin. Interactions between the IEE and the differentiating odontoblasts map out the future shape of the enamel–dentine junction and thus the tooth crown.

Dentinogenesis

Late in the bell stage, hard tissues (dentin, and then enamel) begin to form (Fig 13.20). The early shape of the "bell" is made permanent by secretion of pre-dentin by odontoblasts and its subsequent mineralization. The mineralization of dentin is believed to signal the transition of the IEE into young ameloblasts. Breakdown of the basal lamina lying between the IEE and the forming ameloblasts is essential for hard-tissue formation. Removal of the basement membrane results in a tight bond between the enamel and dentin at the dento-enamel junction (Fig 13.21). Odontoblasts are

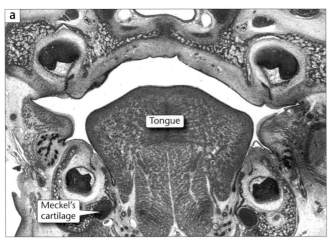

▲ **Fig 13.19a Bell stage.** Coronal section of a fetal head (rabbit), showing teeth forming in the developing maxilla and mandible. Enamel organs resemble the shape of a bell adjacent to the more deeply stained dental papillae. Meckel's cartilage is noted, this being the remnant of first arch cartilage derived from neural crest cells. H&E/alcian blue, paraffin, × 9.

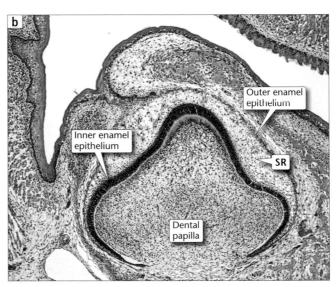

▲ **Fig 13.19b Bell stage.** The shape of the future crown is being defined by the outline between the IEE and the dental papilla. Induction of odontoblast cells by the IEE is associated with early formation of pre-dentin, which, when mineralized, signals the IEE to develop into ameloblasts. Blood vessels near the OEE bring nutrients to the stellate reticulum (**SR**) supporting future enamel synthesis by ameloblasts. H&E/alcian blue, paraffin, × 100.

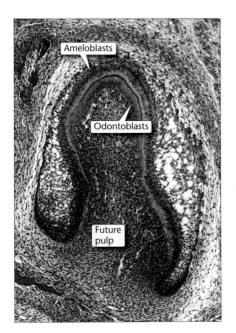

◀ **Fig 13.20 Dentinogenesis.** Late bell stage, showing the core of the tooth root, which will become progressively smaller to form the pulp. Odontoblasts and ameloblasts face each other with opposite cell polarity. Separation of these cells is the early sign of the formation of enamel and the adjacent dentin. H&E/alcian blue, paraffin, × 130.

tall columnar cells that project a single, long process into the dentin, which is the mineralized matrix laid down by these cells. Dentinal tubules make up the matrix between the odontoblastic processes (Fig 13.22). Dentin is a very porous tissue and microorganisms that cross the dentoenamel junction have direct access to the tooth pulp.

Amelogenesis

Ameloblasts do not form until after dentin has been mineralized. These cells are tall columnar, with the elongated cytoplasm adjacent to the odontoblasts and their secreted dentin forming a tapered shape called a Tomes' process. It is through this process that primary enamel is secreted and subsequently

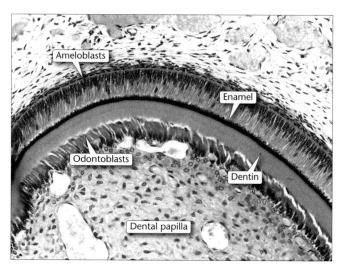

◀ **Fig 13.21 Dento-enamel junction.** The ameloblasts are responsible for enamel development. Odontoblasts regulate formation of pre-dentin, which, when mineralized, becomes mature dentin. In earlier stages of tooth development, the presumptive ameloblasts and odontoblasts were separated by a basal lamina between the epithelium and the mesenchyme. This basal lamina must break down to allow the formation of a bond between the hard tissues of enamel and dentin, called the dento-enamel junction. This process is regulated by numerous local-acting growth factors that diffuse between the layers. H&E/alcian blue, paraffin, × 220.

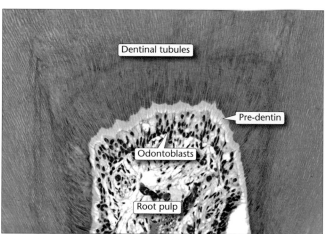

◀ **Fig 13.22 Dentinal tubules.** Part of the dentin adjacent to the root pulp. Odontoblasts are seen, together with a zone of pre-dentin that initially is not mineralized. Odontoblasts create a local environment in the pre-dentin that promotes mineralization. Thin odontoblastic cell processes extend apically into the dentin tissue within cylinders called dentinal tubules. Tubules are tapered and branched. Dentin nearest the tubules is hypermineralized and lacks collagen; dentin deposition continues as long as the pulp remains viable and is slowly turned over in association with healthy odontoblasts. H&E, paraffin, × 150.

mineralized (Fig 13.23a & b). Enamel rods or prisms are formed into columns of enamel matrix that resemble a mineralized trail as the ameloblasts migrate outward during amelogenesis. Ameloblast cells degenerate at the conclusion of enamel formation; ameloblasts, stellate reticulum, and the OEE become fused into a single epithelial sheath that covers the formed enamel of the fully formed crown. The sheath persists until the tooth erupts.

The dental papilla and surrounding follicle form the dental root(s), cementum, and periodontal ligament.

Tip: Dentin must first be formed and mineralized before cells of the inner enamel epithelium become young ameloblasts. Dentin is similar in composition to bone and is innervated, but unlike bone, dentin has no trapped cells or blood vessels. Dentin has limited capacity for repair. Enamel is highly mineralized tissue but, unlike bone, has no collagen.

TONSILS

Aggregations of lymphoid tissues in the oral cavity are called tonsils, namely pharyngeal, palatine, and lingual. The latter have been discussed in relation to the tongue. The tonsils collectively form an annulus (ring of Waldeyer) of lymphoid masses, with numerous nodules or follicles that have germinal centers of lymphocyte proliferation. Although the tonsils have efferent lymphatic vessels that drain them, they do not have afferent lymphatic vessels.

Pharyngeal tonsil

When enlarged, the pharyngeal tonsil is referred to as the adenoids. It is a single midline lymphoid mass in the wall of the nasopharynx covered by respiratory-type epithelium. The mucosa is folded but lacks crypts, and this tonsil may extend to the auditory tube, where it is called the tubal tonsil.

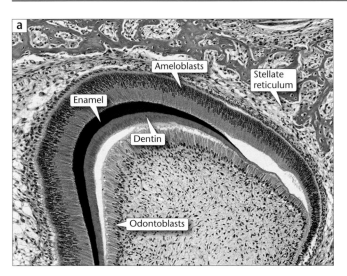

◀ **Fig 13.23a Enamel formation.** The polarized ameloblasts are secreting the organic matrix that becomes mineralized. Over time the ameloblasts migrate away from the enamel they produce. Simultaneously, the stellate reticulum slowly collapses as it loses its intercellular substances. The ameloblasts are supplied by nutrients derived from the stellate reticulum and the follicular capillary vessels near the outer enamel epithelium. Columns of enamel matrix are called enamel rods or prisms. Note the position of odontoblasts, dentin, and artifact spaces produced during tissue preparation. H&E/alcian blue, paraffin, × 80.

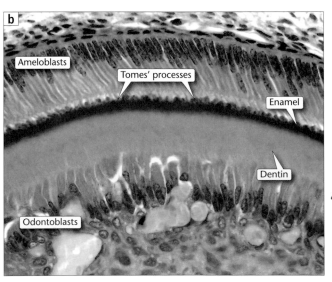

◀ **Fig 13.23b Higher magnification of the dento-enamel junction.** The irregular apices of the ameloblasts represent Tomes' processes, through which proteins, chiefly amelogenin, are secreted to form new enamel. Mineralization occurs with the addition of hydroxyapatite crystals, which contribute to a three-dimensional matrix characteristic of the developing enamel rods or prisms. Following the disassembly of the basal lamina between the growing enamel and dentin, the dento-enamel junction forms a tight mechanical bond with a scalloped interface. Dentin is less brittle than enamel and dissipates force applied to the tooth. Masson's trichrome, paraffin, × 500.

Palatine tonsils

Commonly referred to as simply "the tonsils," these are larger than the pharyngeal tonsil. Each of the two palatine tonsils is located in the lateral oropharynx, behind the third molar tooth and covered by stratified squamous epithelium that characteristically forms tonsillar crypts (Fig 13.24a–c). In childhood these tonsils frequently become inflamed (tonsillitis), perhaps in part because of the lack of flushing action by saliva of foreign materials that lodge in the crypts. This may lead to bacterial infection, chronic inflammation, and ill health.

Lingual tonsils

These are found on the posterior third of the tongue, from the circumvallate papillae to the epiglottis, and their surface epithelium is similar to that of the oral mucosa. Numerous crypts are noted between the lymphoid follicles and an incomplete capsule is seen on the deep aspect (see Fig 13.5).

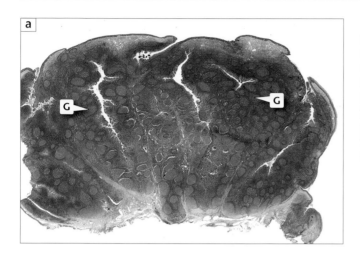

◀ **Fig 13.24a Palatine tonsil.** Low magnification of a palatine tonsil, consisting of in-foldings and crypts of the oral mucosa associated with lymphoid follicles, most of which show a germinal center (**G**) with differentiating lymphocytes. The outer corona contains B lymphocytes, with T lymphocytes in the interfollicular regions. Connective tissue septa are noted in continuity with a deep, fibrous capsule, facilitating surgical removal in tonsillectomy. The palatine tonsils are part of Waldeyer's ring, an annulus of lymphoid tissues that consists of lingual, pharyngeal, and tubal tonsils in the oropharynx. H&E, paraffin, × 5.

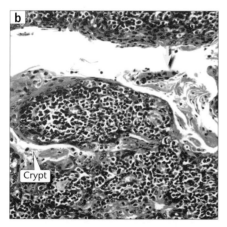

◀ **Fig 13.24b Higher magnification of a tonsillar crypt**, showing the non-keratinized surface epithelium highly folded and extending bulbous processes into the crypt lumen, forming secondary crypts. The junction between lymphoid tissue and the squamous epithelial cells lining the crypt is often difficult to distinguish. The lymphoid tissues contain lymphocytes, plasma cells, and neutrophils, and with migration toward the surface are exfoliated, together with epithelial debris, into the lumen (**arrow**). Palatine tonsils are variable in size and are often infected in childhood, the inflammatory change resulting in hypertrophy of the tissue. H&E, paraffin, × 150.

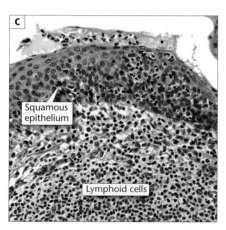

◀ **Fig 13.24c Tonsillar crypt.** Lymphocytes, neutrophils, and plasma cells are shown passing across the squamous epithelium of the tonsillar crypt and emerging onto the luminal surface. The lumen contains commensal bacteria, mucous material, and residual debris of ingested foods. The epithelium also contains dendritic cells (best identified with silver stains), which present antigen to the lymphocytes, assisting with initiation of immune responses. Foreign antigens from the oral cavity (there are no afferent lymphatic vessels to tonsils) stimulate B lymphocytes to produce antibodies, an important role in the immune defense function of the oral cavity. H&E, paraffin, × 180.

SOFT PALATE, EPIGLOTTIS

As a posterior extension of the hard palate, the soft palate is a mobile mucosa-covered fold that assists with voice tone and prevents regurgitation into the nasal cavity during swallowing. Its histology is simple, but diverse (Fig 13.25). On the upper (pharyngeal) surface the epithelium is ciliated, pseudostratified columnar with goblet cells; on the inferior (oral) surface this changes to stratified squamous epithelium. The core of the soft palate contains an aponeurosis (similar to a tendon) and skeletal muscle, derived from the palatine musculature, together with occasional lymphoid aggregations and abundant mucous glands.

During swallowing, fluid and food are deflected from the entrance to the larynx and trachea by the cartilagenous epiglottis (Fig 13.26a & b), which is shaped like a leaf or spoon. Its lingual surface and apical part of the pharyngeal surface are covered by stratified squamous epithelium, which changes to a typical respiratory-type epithelium lower down. The core of the epiglottis consists of a plate of elastic cartilage, occasionally interrupted by perforations or small islands of connective tissue and adipose cells. Beneath the surface epithelium, the lamina propria contains some mucous glands.

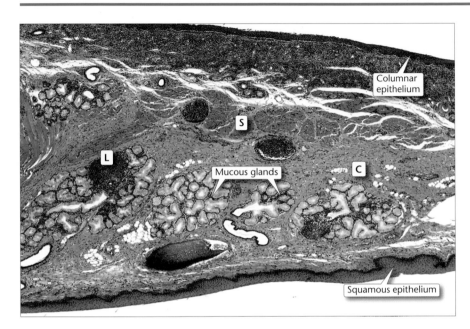

◀ **Fig 13.25 Soft palate.** This is a posterior, muscular extension of the hard palate which, during swallowing, is elevated to prevent food or fluid from entering the nasal cavity. Accordingly, the upper nasal surface is pseudostratified columnar epithelium with stratified squamous epithelium on the oral aspect. Note mucus-secreting glands and duct, skeletal muscle (**S**), lymphoid tissue (**L**), and dense connective tissue (**C**). H&E, paraffin, × 15.

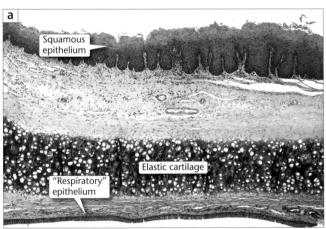

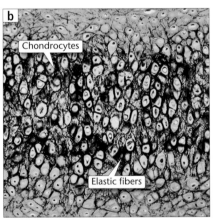

▲ **Fig 13.26a Epiglottis.** Extending upwards from the larynx into the oropharynx, the epiglottis shows a core of elastic cartilage, lamina propria, and stratified squamous epithelium on its lingual and upper laryngeal sides, but respiratory-type epithelium on the lower, posterior surface. During swallowing, the epiglottis retroverts partially to deflect a bolus from entering the respiratory pathway. Closure of the glottis chiefly prevents food from entering the trachea. H&E, paraffin, × 40.

▲ **Fig 13.26b Elastic cartilage of the epiglottis** contains chondrocytes in lacunae, embedded in a matrix abundantly supplied with elastic fibers, giving more intense staining compared with hyaline cartilage. This tissue withstands repetitive bending. Occasionally, the cartilage plate is interrupted by discontinuities or collections of adipose tissue. Gomori trichrome, paraffin, × 150.

ABNORMAL CONDITIONS AND CLINICAL FEATURES

Disorders of the constituent parts of the oral cavity can be considered to be either infrequent or universal in occurrence. In the former case, infections of the oral mucosa, including the tongue, lymphoid tissues, and the salivary glands, are comparatively uncommon, given the presence of microorganisms. On the other hand, dental caries (tooth decay) and periodontal diseases, including gingivitis, are among the most common diseases affecting humans.

Oral mucosa and tongue

Small ulcers of the oral mucosa such as aphthous stomatitis may be painful, solitary, or multiple, and possibly recurrent. The etiologic factors are diverse and include bacteria, viruses, abrasions, and hypersensitivity. Normally the lesions heal with no scarring. Herpes simplex virus (type I) infection may cause cold sores, blisters, or ulcers, affecting the gingiva, oral mucosa, or lips. The ulcers usually heal spontaneously with no scar formation. Oral candidiasis is a fungal infection of the oral mucosa by *Candida albicans*, a common inhabitant of the mouth. Lesions are typically white patches containing fungal hyphae, often found in patients with poorly fitting dentures and in immunocompromized or diabetic patients. Topical antifungal treatments usually eradicate the fungus. A biofilm is a thin layer coating the surfaces of the oral cavity and is inhabited by bacteria. There are many hundreds of different species of microorganisms in the human mouth, many of which are preferentially associated with the tongue or the teeth (Fig 13.27). The microbial milieu of the tongue contributes to halitosis (bad breath).

Geographic tongue (erythema migrans) is a non-infectious inflammatory condition presenting as irregular, reddish patches with yellow–white borders in which filiform papillae are absent and neutrophilic accumulation is excessive. The oral mucosa may be affected, and the lesion changes shape and location. Although the cause(s) is unknown, the condition may represent a hypersensitivity reaction. Leukoplakia is a clinical, not a histologic, term and refers to single or multiple white patches with distinct borders, occurring at any oral site. Most patches show some epithelial abnormality including thickening, hyperkeratosis, or dysplastic changes, and up to 10% of cases are thought to undergo malignant transformation. Etiologic factors are diverse and include tobacco, alcohol, and chewing betel nuts. Squamous cell carcinoma is the most common malignant tumor of the oral mucosa and the predisposing factors are similar to those for leukoplakia.

Salivary glands

All the salivary glands are susceptible to inflammation or infection or to the development of neoplasms. A common and acute viral disease of the parotid glands is mumps (paramyxovirus), which is spread by infected saliva. The pancreas and testes may also be affected, showing inflammation. The gland is infiltrated with lymphocytes, plasma cells, and macrophages, with epithelial degeneration. Mumps occurs most often in young children, but treatment with measles–mumps–rubella (MMR) vaccine, in compliance with recognized immunization schedules, greatly reduces the incidence.

Most tumors of salivary glands are benign, composed of mixtures of ductal and myoepithelial cells, and are termed "pleomorphic salivary adenoma."

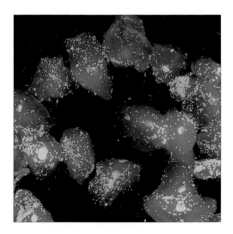

◀ **Fig 13.27 Microorganisms in mouth.** Fluorescence micrograph of buccal epithelial cells, obtained by gently scraping the mucosa of the cheek with a toothpick and smearing the tissue onto a slide. The epithelial cells show a central nucleus. Many bacteria are noted clinging to the surface of the cells, their high RNA content fluorescing orange. Acridine orange, × 400.

Single-cell tumors derived from ductal epithelium, such as Warthin's tumor, contain cells called oncocytes. These tumors may be cystic and are benign. Malignant tumors may arise in any of the salivary glands, but in proportion to tumor incidence in each type of gland, are more common in the minor glands and are, in general, carcinomas.

Dental caries and periodontal diseases

Tooth decay, or dental caries, is a result of the interaction of several factors and is the most prevalent chronic disease of the calcified component of the teeth. Tooth decay is the destruction of the mineralized enamel by acid and may progress to cause decalcification of dentine and, ultimately, invasion of the pulp by microorganisms, causing inflammation, infection, pulpal necrosis, and cyst formation.

Dental caries is an infectious disease of bacterial origin, in which the bacterial colonies in the oral biofilm coalesce with salivary glycoproteins and food debris to form dental plaque, which clings to the tooth surface. Bacteria such as *Streptococcus mutans* metabolize the carbohydrates, especially sucrose, producing organic acids that demineralize enamel. Saliva helps to neutralize the acids and shows bactericidal properties. Raw or natural foods (but not processed products) cleanse the teeth rather than adhere to the crown, reducing plaque accumulation. Fluoride added to the water supply forms fluoroapatite in the enamel, especially in growing teeth; fluoroapatite is less acid-soluble than enamel apatite. Progressive lesions, involving cavitation, may reach the dentin and, if these are untreated, microorganisms may cause inflammatory reactions in the pulp, resulting in pain. Necrosis of the pulp and abscess or cyst formation require root canal or endodontic therapy (debridement and obturation with inert material) or extraction.

Calcification of plaque forms calculus, or tartar, which, if wedged between tooth and gingiva, allows bacterial invasion, leading to gingivitis and periodontitis; extension of the infection to alveolar bone causes osteomyelitis. Periodontitis accounts for the loss of more adult teeth than any other disease, including caries. Weakened by inflammation and damaged by direct or indirect attack by toxins, endotoxins, and proteolytic enzymes, the disrupted periodontal tissues cause loosening and eventual loss of teeth. Vitamin C deficiency (scurvy) results in the production of defective collagen and loss of teeth due to progressive loss of the collagen-rich periodontal ligament.

Tonsils and epiglottis

Tonsillitis and pharyngitis frequently occur together, affecting mainly children, in whom multiple attacks are not uncommon. The causative agents are not clearly identified and may be viral or bacterial, or the latter superimposed on the former. Typically, the presentation is of enlarged, reddened tonsils with an infiltration of neutrophils and exudate (pus) in the tonsillar crypts. Lymphoid follicles are characteristically large and show lymphoblast proliferation. Treatment is normally directed at relieving the symptoms because tonsillitis usually subsides spontaneously, but in repeated attacks, tonsillectomy may be indicated. Infectious mononucleosis (glandular fever), caused by infection with Epstein-Barr virus, may also cause tonsillitis.

"Adenoids" is a term that refers to chronic inflammatory hyperplasia of the pharyngeal lymphoid tissue and, if untreated, may cause sleep apnea or middle-ear infections from blocked Eustachian tubes.

Epiglottitis, usually caused by influenza virus, can occur in children in whom the swollen, inflamed tissue may obstruct airflow, and thus is a serious disorder with potentially fatal effects.

Gastrointestinal tract

From the esophagus to the anal canal, the gut is basically a hollow, muscular tube with an internal mucosa that shows regional histological and functional differences. Despite some similarity in structure throughout its length, the key to recognizing its component parts and understanding what functions they perform is systematic microscopic study, supplemented by detailed regional investigation, rather than the reverse approach. Students are often confused about gastrointestinal histology, not realizing that each named region has unique and/or distinctive histological features.

The gastrointestinal tract has four main layers, as shown in Fig 14.1.

Starting from the lumen and working outward, the layers are:

- Mucous membrane or mucosa, composed of epithelium, connective tissue, and thin, smooth muscle

- Submucosa, a region of connective and supporting tissue
- Muscularis externa, composed of two thick layers of smooth muscle
- Adventitia or serosa, a thin, outer covering of connective and epithelial tissue.

The essential regional differences in histology superimposed on this plan and the basic features of each of the four layers and their modifications along the length of the gut are given below. The entire gut, from the oral cavity to the rectum, secretes and absorbs considerable quantities of fluid. The total volume of ingested fluid plus gut and gut-associated glandular secretions is approximately 8–9 liters a day. The small intestine absorbs most of this, allowing about 1.5 liters to pass to the colon. The colon absorbs all but 100 mL, an amount that contributes to the volume of excreted feces. During an average lifetime the gastrointestinal tract processes approximately 100 tons of food.

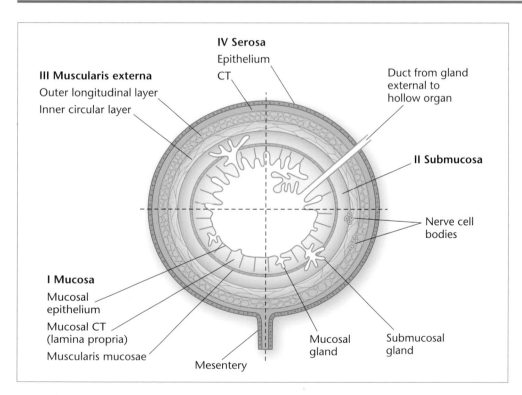

▲ **Fig 14.1 General organization of the gastrointestinal tract.** Epithelium of the mucosa is usually folded and contains cell types characteristic of particular regions. An autonomic nerve plexus is found in the submucosa and in the muscularis externa. The layers of smooth muscle regulate local contraction–relaxation cycles, including peristalsis. Mesothelium and thin connective tissue comprise the serosa. Intramural or extramural glands empty their secretions into the lumen via ducts. (From Telser AG. Elsevier's integrated histology. Philadelphia: Mosby/Elsevier, 2007. With permission.)

GENERAL ORGANIZATION
Basic architecture

The histology of the esophagus, stomach, and small and large intestines shows characteristic features that are modifications of the following components.

Mucous membrane or mucosa

This includes the tissues facing the lumen and extending outwards (i.e. deeper to) a thin, circumferential layer of smooth muscle.

Surface epithelium

A surface epithelium rests on a basal lamina, the main variations of which are shown in Figure 14.2a–d. Except for the esophagus and anal canal, the gut epithelium is simple columnar with recognizable regional specializations. The epithelium serves as a selective barrier that has absorptive and secretory roles, and importantly also functions in immune surveillance.

Gut epithelium is a highly dynamic structure; it is renewed every 5–6 days from a population of stem cells that give rise to all the differentiated cell types, including various absorptive, secretory, enteroendocrine, Paneth and M cells. Immune cells, such as resident or transient lymphocytes, are common in the gut epithelium and are derived from the vasculature and/or associated lymphoid-rich connective tissue. Absorptive cells are most abundant in the epithelium of the small and large bowel and participate in digestive functions. Secretion takes many forms in the gut and is particularly high in the stomach and small bowel. The population of enteroendocrine cells comprises several dozen cell types in the epithelium of the stomach and intestines and is said to represent the largest collection of hormone-producing cells in the body. Paneth cells and M cells are discussed later.

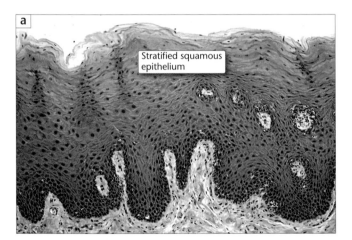

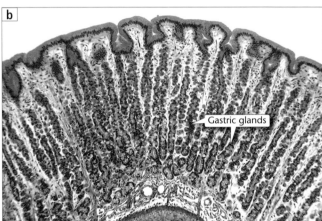

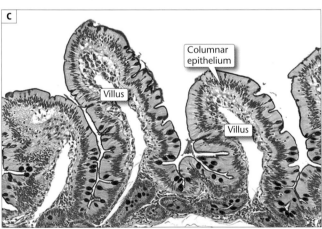

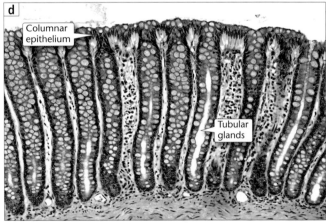

▲ **Fig 14.2 Variations of gut epithelium. a** *Barrier* structure for protection; stratified squamous epithelium is found in the esophagus and anal canal. Hematoxylin & eosin (H&E), paraffin, × 120. **b** *Secretory epithelium of the stomach*, showing surface pits and long gastric glands secreting acid, mucus, and digestive enzymes. H&E, paraffin, × 75. **c** *Absorptive epithelium of the small bowel*, expanded in surface area by finger-like villous projections. H&E/periodic acid–Schiff (PAS), paraffin, × 110. **d** *Absorptive epithelium of the large bowel*, modified to extract water and electrolytes with secretion of mucus. H&E, acrylic resin, × 100.

Lamina propria

Adjacent to the surface epithelium is the lamina propria, a supporting tissue containing abundant neurovascular supply and cells of the immune system (Fig 14.3). Often overlooked merely as connective tissue that "fills in the gaps," the subepithelial fibroblasts and mesenchymal cells play vital roles as mechanosensory receptors. They make contact with capillaries, sensory and motor neurons, smooth muscle, and the adjacent epithelium, and release adenosine triphosphate (ATP) and cytokines such as transforming growth factor (TGF) and tumor necrosis factor (TNF). In addition to synthesizing components of the basal lamina, lamina propria fibroblasts are thought to contribute to migration, proliferation, permeability,

and secretory properties of epithelial cells, and to the regulation of injury and inflammatory responses in the mucosa. The lamina propria of the intestine is filled with antibody-producing plasma cells, which each day secrete several grams of IgA immunoglobulin into the gut lumen.

Muscularis mucosae

This thin, double layer of smooth muscle may be flat/linear or folded to follow the contour of the epithelium and its glands (Fig 14.4a & b). In the stomach and small bowel, muscle bundles extend into the lamina propria. Contraction or relaxation of this smooth muscle, governed by the enteric nervous system (see below), assists with modifying the shape

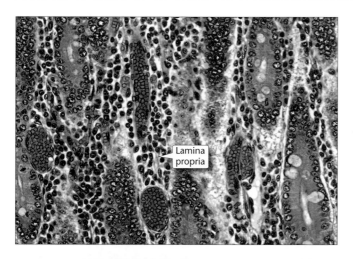

◀ **Fig 14.3 Lamina propria.** Supporting the gastrointestinal epithelium, the lamina propria is loose connective tissue with neurovascular elements and a high concentration of immune cells, especially plasma cells and lymphocytes. These cells are vital for immune surveillance to protect the thin epithelium of the stomach and intestine. Mesenchymal cells and fibroblasts in the lamina propria regulate epithelial function by local signaling, and also influence vascular and neural function in the mucosa. H&E, paraffin, × 200.

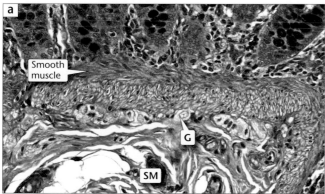

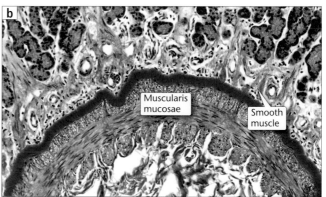

▲ **Fig 14.4a Muscularis mucosae.** Thin layers of smooth muscle are noted, marking the deep limit of the mucosa. Occasionally ganglia of the submucosa are seen that are part of Meissner's nerve plexus. This plexus regulates the activity of the muscularis mucosae to alter the shape of the mucosa necessary for peristalsis and mixing of luminal contents. Meissner's plexus is noted as small ganglia (**G**) in the submucosa (**SM**). This ganglionated plexus has fewer neurons than the myenteric plexus of Auerbach found in the outermost muscle layers. Meissner's plexus is two interconnected plexuses— one nearest to the mucosa (true Meissner's) and another nearest the circular muscle of the muscularis externa (the plexus of Henle). Although anatomically distinct, they act as a single functional unit. Peristalsis of the gut involving Meissner's and Auerbach's plexuses is initiated by special pacemaker cells associated with the muscularis externa, by mechanosensitive mucosal cells termed enteroendocrine and enterochromaffin cells, or by extrinsic innervation. The submucosal plexus influences both the mucosa and the myenteric plexus. H&E/alcian blue, paraffin, × 180.

▲ **Fig 14.4b Muscularis mucosae.** In the proximal region of the porcine stomach several layers of its muscularis mucosae are found with an innermost oblique layer added to the circular longitudinal layers. The extra layer diminishes toward the stomach antrum. Its prominence in the fundus perhaps facilitates the storage function of the proximal stomach. Smooth muscle fibers of the muscularis mucosae are shown extending into the lamina propria. H&E/alcian blue, paraffin, × 155.

of the mucosa, thus facilitating the mixing of luminal contents. In certain parts of the gut the muscularis mucosae may be interrupted by glands, ducts, or lymphoid aggregations.

Submucosa

This is a zone of variable width formed of fibroelastic loose connective tissue with blood vessels, lymphatics, and, depending on the exact region, nerves of the submucosal plexus (Fig 14.5a & b). Wandering leukocytes and variable quantities of fat also are found. In certain regions, such as the duodenum, glands are prominent.

Muscularis externa

Making up the usually thick, outermost wall of the gut, the external muscle layer comprises two (in some regions three, as for the stomach) layers of smooth muscle (Fig 14.6). The inner layer is circular, with the cells organized as tight spirals, and serves to constrict

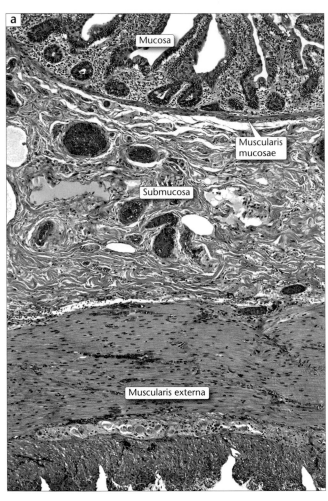

▲ **Fig 14.5a Submucosa.** The submucosa is a zone of connective tissue immediately deep to the mucosa. It shows variations in width, and its cellular and extracellular composition ranges from loose to dense irregular bundles of collagen fibers. Often this variation is caused by variable fixation and artifactual separation of the mucosa and the muscularis externa. Note the abundant blood supply. The submucosa has extensive nerve plexuses not readily visible at low magnification in routine paraffin sections. H&E/alcian blue, paraffin, × 25.

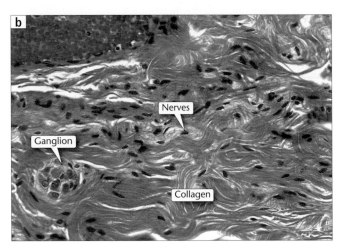

▲ **Fig 14.5b Detail of submucosa**, showing complex multidirectional collagen bundles, a ganglion of Meissner's/Henle's plexus, and fibers of unmyelinated nerves. H&E, paraffin, × 400.

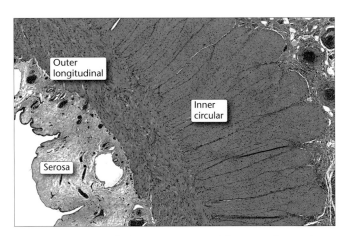

▲ **Fig 14.6 Muscularis externa.** Part of the external smooth muscle wall of the colon, showing the inner circular and outer longitudinal layer. The ganglia of the myenteric plexus, located between the two layers, is not visible at this magnification. Covering the muscle is a wide layer of serosa that comprises fibroelastic/areolar tissue with blood vessels associated with the arterial supply and venous drainage of the bowel. The outer margin is a thin mesothelium that faces the peritoneum. H&E, paraffin, × 20.

the gut lumen. The outer layer shows longitudinal fibers, with a more elongated spiral pattern than the inner layer, which regulate the length of the gut tube. Between the layers is the myenteric nerve plexus, which controls, for example, intestinal motility and sphincter function.

Serosa

This is the outermost tissue layer. If the gut wall is free and mobile, this layer consists of irregular, fibroelastic connective tissue covered with mesothelium and is termed the serosa. It is continuous with the mesentery and conveys the neurovascular structures that enter and leave the gut (Fig 14.7a & b). A thin, outer layer of loose connective tissue, if continuous with an adjacent organ or tissue such as those parts of the gut that are retroperitoneal, is termed the adventitia.

Enteric nervous system— largely autonomous

The gastrointestinal tract has an extensive intrinsic nerve supply, consisting of ganglia and plexuses capable of functioning independently of central control. The enteric nerve system has neurons that synapse with one another to reflexly regulate muscle activity, epithelial absorption and secretion, and blood flow. This intramural nerve system interacts with control centers in the brain and spinal cord via nerve trunks that connect with the gut for both motor and sensory innervation. Extramural (external) nerves exist in two systems that act separately. Craniosacral innervation (parasympathetic; increases secretion and gut motility) comprises the vagus nerve, which supplies the stomach via the esophageal plexus and down to the mid-colon indirectly through abdominal ganglia (Fig 14.8). Sacral nerves supply the distal colon. Thoracolumbar supply (sympathetic; decreases secretion and motility) by the splanchnic nerves innervates much of the gut through the celiac, mesenteric, and hypogastric ganglia.

The intramural, or enteric, nervous system is represented by two major ganglionated plexuses. The myenteric plexus (also called Auerbach's plexus) lies between the circular and longitudinal layers of the muscularis externa and is a continuous network from the esophagus to the internal anal sphincter. Essentially it floats in a loose, collagenous stroma and the polygonal, mesh-like arrangement of its nerve

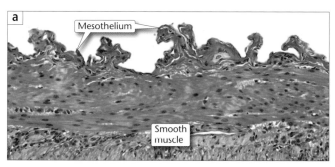

▲ **Fig 14.7a Serosa.** For much of the gut, the outermost coat, or serosa, consists of a thin mesothelial layer and supporting loose connective tissue. The thoracic part of the esophagus has no serosa but is covered by a thin layer of fascia. H&E, paraffin, × 150.

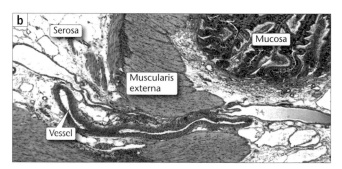

▲ **Fig 14.7b Serosa.** The serosa is penetrated by the blood vessels and nerves supplying the gut, and at these frequent entry points it is a continuity of the mesenteries that suspend much of the gastrointestinal tract. H&E/PAS, paraffin, × 20.

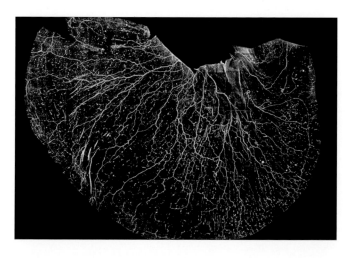

◀ **Fig 14.8 Extrinsic nerve supply.** This shows the vagal afferent (sensory) innervation of the stomach. Nerve fibers enter from the esophageal region at upper right, radiating toward the greater curvature. In the antral region (upper left) gastric branches of the vagus supply the pylorus. Silver stain, darkfield microscopy, whole mount, × 1.5. (Courtesy T Powley, Psychological Sciences, Purdue University, USA.)

fibers enables it to alter in shape in concert with the movements of the gut. The ganglia are readily seen in clusters or nodes (Fig 14.9a–c).

Accompanying the myenteric plexus and within the circular component of the muscularis externa is a population of stellate, myoid-type cells known as the interstitial cells of Cajal (ICC). Coupled to smooth muscle cells via gap junctions and to myenteric nerve varicosities via synapse-type junctions, these cells act as pacemakers, generating spontaneous electrical slow waves along the gut wall. ICC regulate the frequency and propagation of peristaltic contractions.

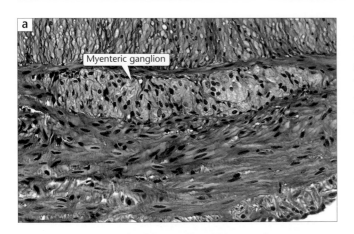

◀ Fig 14.9a Ganglion of myenteric plexus. A ganglion of the myenteric (Auerbach's) plexus is shown between the two smooth muscle layers of the muscularis externa. Ganglia are of variable size, comprising several or dozens of nerve cell bodies, or more. They are found along the gastrointestinal tract from the esophagus to the anorectal junction and, in addition to nerve cell bodies, show unmyelinated processes (not seen in routine sections), sparse connective tissue, but no blood vessels. Mixed in with the cell bodies are the pacemaker interstitial cells of Cajal, only visible with, for example, immunocytochemical methods for c-Kit (a receptor tyrosine kinase). Cells of Cajal are also found in the smooth muscle of the urinary and reproductive tracts and of the vascular system. The myenteric plexus is connected to and may be regulated by the CNS via extrinsic sympathetic/parasympathetic nerves serving both motor and sensory functions. H&E, paraffin, × 290.

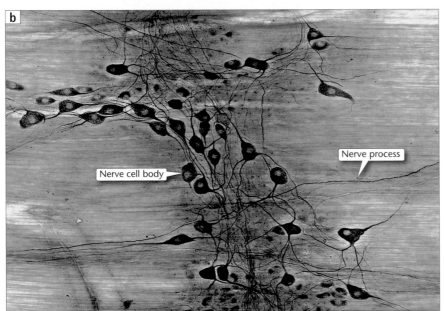

◀ Fig 14.9b Ganglion of myenteric plexus. Thin whole mount of the external muscle layer of the small bowel, revealing a ganglion of the myenteric plexus. The processes of dendrites and axons make up a network that extends to other ganglia, forming a two-dimensional rhomboidal mesh ideally suited to the stretching of the gut. Gold stain, × 450.

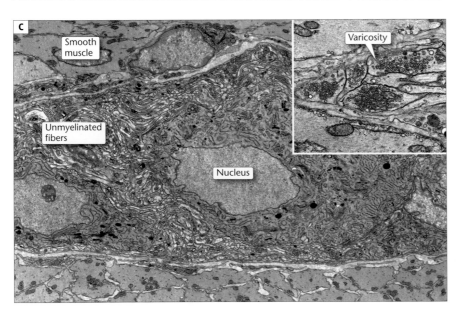

◀ Fig 14.9c Ultrastructure of part of a ganglion of the myenteric plexus, showing nerve cell bodies surrounded by unmyelinated fibers. Points of neurotransmitter release (seen as varicosities in the inset), innervate the smooth muscle or contact other cell bodies and are specializations of plexus fibers that may be hundreds of micrometers in length. One axon may thus supply many cell bodies. Nitric oxide mediates muscle relaxation, and acetylcholine and other neurotransmitters mediate contraction. Serotonin from enteroendocrine cells also regulates increased/decreased motility, depending on the receptor type on the enteric neurons. × 3,200.

Although the primary target of the myenteric plexus is the muscularis externa, nerve fibers of the plexus extend widely and are connected to the submucosal plexus, a second continuous network of small ganglia in the submucosa of the small and large bowel (see Fig 14.4). This consists of two components; the inner, close to the muscularis mucosae, is known as Meissner's plexus and the outer is the plexus of Henle. Respectively, these plexuses regulate the mucosa and its blood vessels, and also contribute to the motility of the external muscle. Nerve fibers from the submucosal plexus extend into the lamina propria. The stomach lacks an organized submucosal plexus and contains only a few scattered ganglia in this region.

Motility—important for food processing

Contraction of the gastrointestinal tract can be described in several ways. Tonic contractions are continuous and of low pressure, and occur in storage regions such as the rectum. In sphincters tonic activity is necessarily of high pressure. Transient and rhythmic contractions include peristalsis, whereby constriction followed by relaxation forces luminal contents distally, as occurs in the esophagus down

to the small bowel and particularly vigorously in the stomach during gastric churning. Contraction of circular muscle of the small bowel provides mixing of contents without propagation, but in the colon, mass movement of segmented pockets of forming feces is due to a proximal–distal longitudinal contraction that stimulates defecation.

Tip: The cellular lining of the intestine is characterized by the most rapid turnover of epithelial cells in the body, yet for the majority of its length (the small bowel) it rarely gives rise to benign or malignant tumors. In contrast the epithelium of the colon and rectum are common sites for primary neoplasms. Why uncontrolled cell division (acquired or inherited mutations in DNA sequences) is prevalent in the large bowel remains uncertain.

ESOPHAGUS

The esophagus is readily identified by two features—a non-keratinized stratified squamous epithelium showing numerous folds, which gives the empty esophageal lumen a stellate shape, and a prominent muscularis mucosae following the sinusoidal shape of the mucosal folds (Fig 14.10a & b). Small, infrequent groups of mucous glands occupy the submucosa and

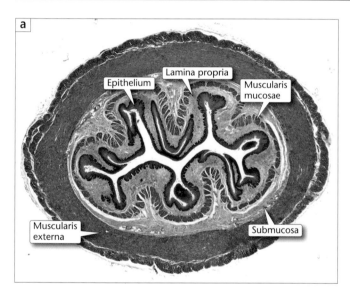

▲ **Fig 14.10a Esophagus.** When relaxed, the esophageal lumen is highly irregular in transverse section, but becomes distended with the peristaltic movement of a bolus of swallowed food. Note the inner surface epithelium, lamina propria, muscularis mucosae, submucosa, and two layers of smooth muscle forming the muscularis externa. In the upper regions of the esophagus, the muscularis is chiefly skeletal muscle, which is replaced with smooth muscle from the middle third downward. The mucosal surface is kept moist by secretions of glands located in the supporting connective tissues. H&E, paraffin, × 12.

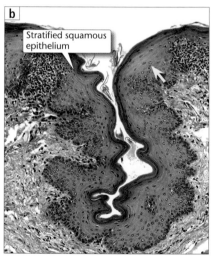

▲ **Fig 14.10b Esophagus.** The luminal surface of the esophagus is non-keratinized stratified squamous epithelium, similar to much of the epithelial lining of the oral cavity. The most superficial layers of stratum corneum are only several cells thick, and the nuclei are retained with little or no transformation into plaques of keratin. Individual lymphocytes are noted in the epithelium (**arrow**) and at intervals in the subjacent lamina propria. In the relaxed esophagus the mucosa is folded as indicated here, but these folds are momentarily flattened as food passes down the tube. Contraction and relaxation of the esophagus are regulated by the vagus nerve. H&E, paraffin, × 75.

their secreted mucus lubricates the surface epithelium for the passage of food (Fig 14.11). Peristaltic contractions of the muscularis externa, coordinated by nerve plexuses within it and the submucosa, propel each bolus of food toward the stomach.

STOMACH

The chief functions of the stomach are to mix or churn food into a soft, fluid consistency (called chyme) and to carry out preliminary digestion via the secretions of digestive enzymes. A third layer of smooth muscle in the stomach wall facilitates mixing and dispersal of ingested food. In the pyloric region, the circular muscle is thickened to form a sphincter that allows only semi-liquid material to enter the duodenum. Anatomically, the stomach shows three histologically distinct regions of the gastric mucosa (Fig 14.12)—the cardia, corpus, and pylorus.

Gastric mucosa

The macroscopic appearance of the mucosa shows deformable folds, or rugae (Fig 14.13). Macroscopically these present either an irregular, honeycomb appearance or longitudinal ridges. Most rugae are not permanent features and flatten with gastric filling, but mucosal folds are always found at the proximal and distal orifices of the stomach. The gastric mucosa shows a simple columnar surface epithelium of mucus-secreting cells that is invaginated downward to form gastric pits; this arrangement is similar throughout the stomach. Gastric pits open into long, single or often branched gastric glands that extend down to the muscularis mucosae (Fig 14.14a & b). Distinctive variations in the size and shape of the glands and their cell types are evident in the following anatomical regions of the stomach: the cardia (near the esophagus), the body (or corpus, including the fundus), and the pyloric region (antrum and canal) leading to the duodenum.

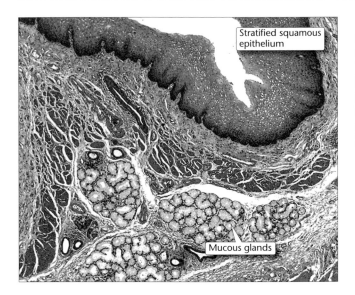

Stratified squamous epithelium

Mucous glands

◀ **Fig 14.11 Glands of the esophagus.** The surface of the esophageal epithelium is kept moist and lubricated by a thin layer of mucus secreted by tubuloacinar glands located in the submucosa. The mucus minimizes abrasion and assists in the smooth passage of food along the length of the esophagus. Near the commencement and termination of the esophagus, additional mucus-secreting glands may be found in the lamina propria. The duodenum is the only other segment of the gut to contain glandular elements in the submucosa. H&E, paraffin, × 50.

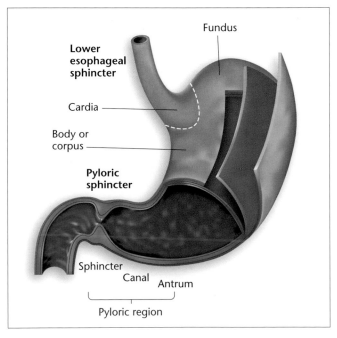

Fundus

Lower esophageal sphincter

Cardia

Body or corpus

Pyloric sphincter

Sphincter

Canal   Antrum

Pyloric region

◀ **Fig 14.12 Regions of the stomach.** The histologically distinct regions are the cardia, corpus, and pylorus. The lower esophageal sphincter is a physiological sphincter with no structural specialization, whereas the pyloric sphincter is a thickening of the circular muscle in the muscularis externa. The muscularis externa may show three layers: the inner oblique (distal half of stomach), the middle circular (whole stomach), and the outer longitudinal layer (upper two-thirds of stomach).

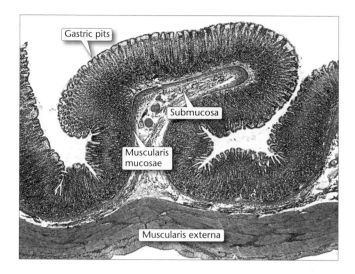

◀ **Fig 14.13 Structure of the stomach.** The gastric mucosa is folded into rugae, which form irregular longitudinal ridges in the empty stomach. The luminal surface displays many shallow invaginations, which represent gastric pits leading downward to the gastric glands and extending almost to the muscularis mucosae. The submucosa of supporting tissue is prominent, and the thick muscularis externa of smooth muscle forms outer longitudinal and inner circular layers, with an occasional oblique layer adjacent to the submucosa. The gastric mucosa secretes gastric juice (acid and digestive enzymes), mucus, and hormones such as gastrin. H&E, paraffin, × 15.

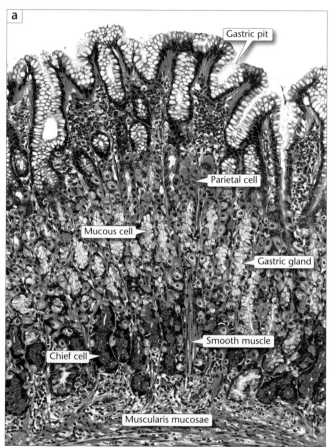

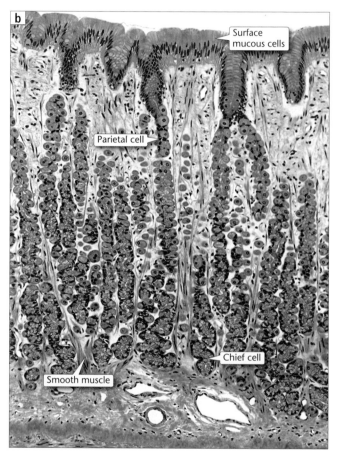

▲ **Fig 14.14a Typical gastric mucosa.** Basic features of the human gastric mucosa show surface pits lined with mucous cells. These open into deep, highly cellular gastric glands, between which are vertical strands of smooth muscle arising from the muscularis mucosae. The glands present with three recognizable cell types: Cells with halo-type cytoplasm (acid-secreting), cells with foam-type cytoplasm (mucous cells), and deep eosinophilic cells (enzyme-secreting). H&E, paraffin, × 120.

▲ **Fig 14.14b Gastric mucosa from a primate.** The histology is similar to that in a human, although the gastric glands are well defined with eosinophilic parietal cells (acid production) and granulated chief cells (enzyme production). Thin strands of smooth muscle from the muscularis mucosae extend superficially in the lamina propria toward the surface mucous cells. H&E, acrylic resin, × 110.

331

The gastric mucosa is populated with numerous cells of the immune system, comprising plasma cells and lymphocytes, seen in the lamina propria and epithelium, together with occasional lymphoid follicles in the pyloric region, rich in lymphocytes (see the discussion of the ileum below). Surface mucous cells line all gastric pits, and those at the narrow junction with the gastric glands (the neck) are termed mucous neck cells. From this zone, stem cells are believed to produce new mucus-secreting cells that constantly replace those on the surface, which survive for about 3 days (Fig 14.15). Mucus secretion lubricates the surface epithelium and protects the cells from the acidic and enzymatic properties of gastric juices and the potentially toxic substances introduced by ingestion.

Cardia

Here the gastric pits occupy a third of the depth of the mucosa, but the distinguishing feature is the glands, which are short, coiled, and branched. They have mucous-type cells, and the glandular tubular lumen is open (Fig 14.16a & b).

Corpus, or body

The long, narrow gastric glands are the dominant feature of the corpus, and several may empty into a gastric pit (Fig 14.17a–c). Each gland has several different cell types—mucous cells, stem cells, parietal (oxyntic) cells, chief (zymogenic) cells, and enteroendocrine cells. The stem cells for the surface epithelium and glands have traditionally been

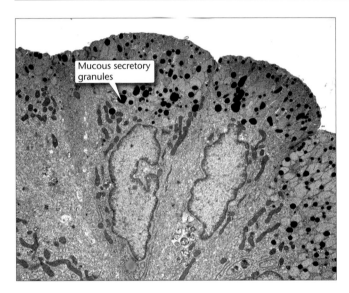

◀ **Fig 14.15 Surface mucous cells.** Ultrastructure showing many mucous secretory granules subjacent to the lumen of the stomach. Unlike mucus-secreting goblet cells of the intestinal epithelium, gastric surface mucous cells remain columnar in shape and do not bulge laterally. Mucus in surface cells is a neutral glycoprotein and, when released to form a gel-like layer, it protects the epithelium from acid and digestive enzymes and mechanical trauma. × 3,800.

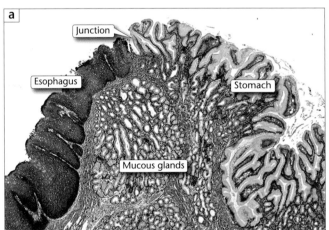

▲ **Fig 14.16a Cardia of stomach.** The esophagogastric junction is marked by an abrupt change of the epithelium from stratified squamous to columnar, the latter representing the cardia of the stomach. At this junction, cardiac mucus-type glands of the esophagus are similar to those deep to the gastric pits. During development of the gut, mesenchymal cells induce regional specialization of the gut endoderm to differentiate into specific epithelial types. A balance between local transcription factors and blocking proteins is thought to regulate this tissue development. H&E, paraffin, × 40. (Specimen courtesy P de Permentier, Anatomy Department, University of New South Wales, Sydney.)

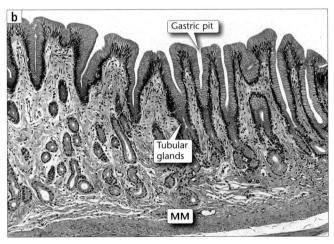

▲ **Fig 14.16b The surface epithelium of the cardia region** shows invaginations or gastric pits that branch into tortuous, loosely packed tubular glands. Most of the lining epithelium is columnar and secretes mucus. The muscularis mucosae (**MM**) is indicated. The cardiac mucosa is just distal to the lower end of the esophagus and is usually only 1–2 cm in width. H&E, paraffin, × 95.

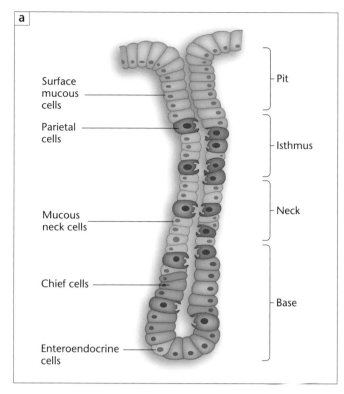

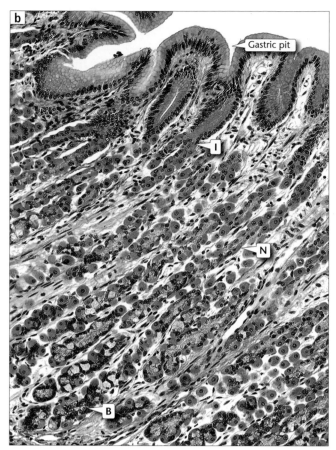

▲ Fig 14.17a Corpus, or body, of stomach. Cellular composition of a typical cardiac gland arising from a gastric pit. One to several long, tubular structures resemble blind-ending tunnels whose cellular walls surround a narrow secretory lumen. Each gland is divided into three regions—isthmus, neck, and base. The five main cell types are mucous neck cells, stem cells, parietal (or oxyntic) cells, chief cells, and enteroendocrine cells. The isthmus is traditionally considered to be the region where stem cells divide to maintain their numbers and differentiate into the cells that populate the surface epithelium and glandular epithelium by upward or downward migration. Recent research in mice has proposed that the stem cells may be located at the base of the gland.

▲ Fig 14.17b Body of gastric mucosa shows gastric pits and glands consisting of the isthmus (**I**), neck (**N**), and base (**B**). Parietal cells are eosinophilic (stained pink), chief cells are basophilic (stained blue-purple), and mucous cells have a foam-type cytoplasm. The supporting tissue of the lamina propria contains a loose network of collagen and reticular fibers, wandering cells of the immune system, capillaries, and strands of smooth muscle extending vertically from the deeper muscularis mucosae. H&E, paraffin, × 180.

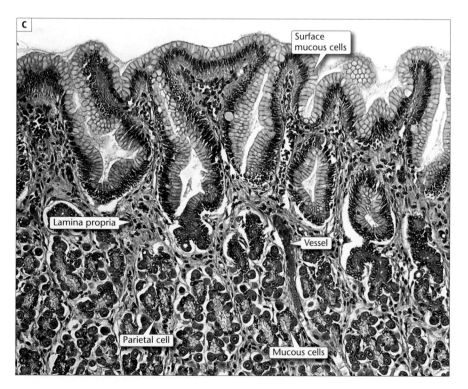

◀ Fig 14.17c Surface mucous cells. The entire surface of the gastric mucosa is lined by simple columnar epithelial cells that extend into the gastric pits. Surface mucous cells resemble goblet cells of the intestine in that the apical cytoplasm is eosinophilic with H&E stains, resulting from the high content of mucous granules. These give a lightly stained cytoplasm. The secreted mucus contains mucins—that is, glycoproteins that form a viscous gel layer that is resistant to pepsin (enzymatic) degradation. Mucus is produced via mechanical irritation and in response to stimulation of the vagus nerve. Mucin also coats luminal contents, assisting slippage through the stomach. Gastric glands cut in oblique planes show prominent eosinophilic parietal cells and mucous neck cells with foam-type cytoplasm. H&E, paraffin, × 200.

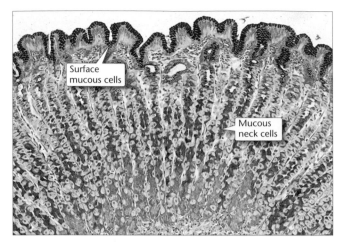

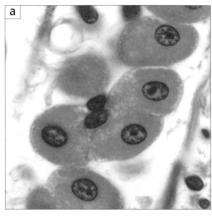

▲ **Fig 14.18 Types of mucous cells.** With the PAS-staining technique, the full extent of mucus-containing cells in the gastric mucosa is well demonstrated by the distribution and abundance of the magenta-stained cells. Surface and pit mucous cells stain intensely and contain insoluble, neutral glycoproteins that provide cell protection. These cells are replaced every 1–3 days. Mucous neck cells within the glands contain soluble acidic glycoproteins (mucous granules are less dense) and are thought to play a role in lubrication of the semi-solid chyme. Pale pink circular cells are parietal cells; deep in the glands chief cells stain weakly. Hematoxylin/PAS, paraffin, × 75.

▲ **Fig 14.19a Parietal cells.** In paraffin sections, parietal cells are eosinophilic with a central nucleus and some clear areas throughout the cytoplasm. This mottled appearance represents a mixture of mitochondria and an extensive array of smooth membranes that assist with the production of HCl. In addition to secreting acid, parietal cells simultaneously secrete bicarbonate (HCO_3^-) ions into nearby capillaries, transporting HCO_3^- ions toward the surface mucous cells. This "alkaline tide" helps to neutralize any back-diffusion of hydrogen ions from the gastric lumen. H&E, paraffin, × 700.

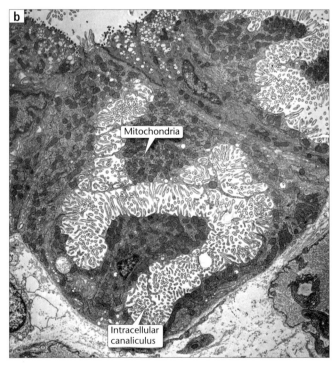

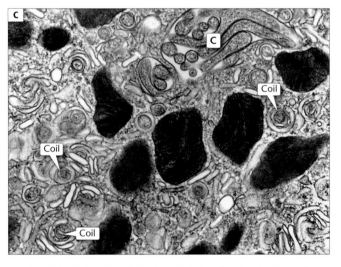

▲ **Fig 14.19c Unstimulated parietal cell.** Ultrastructure of a freeze-fixed/freeze-substituted unstimulated parietal cell, showing helical coils of tubular membranes and stacked cisternae, which contain the proton pump enzyme. When the cell secretes acid, the tubules and cisternae with their enzymes are recruited to join the apical membrane surface of the canaliculus (**C**). Tubulovesicles, commonly seen in chemically fixed parietal cells, are not seen after rapid-freeze fixation. The dense bodies are mitochondria. × 13,000. (Courtesy The Company of Biologists Ltd; from Petitt JM et al. J Cell Science 1995; 108:1127–41.)

▲ **Fig 14.19b Stimulated parietal cell.** Ultrastructure of a stimulated parietal cell, showing the extensive intracellular canaliculus with many projecting microvilli. The canaliculus is fused with the apical cell membrane and connects with the lumen of the gastric gland (not seen in this micrograph). Canalicular membranes and microvilli contain H^+, K^+-ATPase proton pumps secreting H^+ into the lumen. A chloride channel transports Cl^- into the lumen to form HCl. To provide this energy, the parietal cell cytoplasm is 40% occupied with mitochondria, which in three dimensions form an extensive reticular network. × 3,100.

considered to reside in the isthmus–neck region, but recent research has suggested they originate from the bottom of the glands. Mucous-type cells and enteroendocrine cells are found scattered throughout the gastric glands (Fig 14.18).

Parietal cells tend to be most abundant in the mid- to upper region of the glands and are readily identified in H&E sections by their intense pink (eosinophilic) color. They secrete hydrochloric acid, which provides an acidic environment (about pH 1) for enzymatic breakdown of proteins in the chyme (Fig 14.19a–c).

Chief cells are numerous in the deeper aspect of the gastric gland; they are moderately bluish (basophilic after H&E staining) and produce pepsin, a proteolytic enzyme activated by acid secretions (Fig 14.20a & b).

There are many different types of enteroendocrine cells scattered through the gastric mucosa. They are physiologically important as the source of local hormonal stimuli in the mucosa. These cells are also discussed in the section on endocrine tissues. Enteroendocrine cells are classified as open types, where the apical cytoplasm reaches the lumen and is believed to respond to its environment, and closed types confined to the basal region of the epithelium (Fig 14.21). Major enteroedocrine cells of the stomach include: G cells (open type) secreting gastrin, which stimulates acid secretion from parietal cells; D cells (closed type), secreting somatostatin, which is generally inhibitory for other epithelial cell secretions and for blood flow; and ghrelin-secreting cells that stimulate appetite by the action of blood-borne ghrelin on the hypothalamus. Ghrelin counteracts the action of leptin, a hormone of adipose tissue origin that reduces the hunger drive.

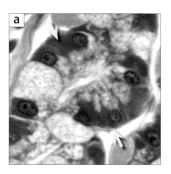

▲ **Fig 14.20a Chief cells.** The lower regions of gastric glands contain enzyme-secreting chief cells with a basophilic cytoplasm (**arrows**) and secretory (zymogen) granules at the apical aspect facing the lumen. Chief cells are protein-secreting exocrine cells, and their membranes of rough endoplasmic reticulum account for the blue staining in H&E preparations. The digestive enzymes are proteases, which are stored and secreted as proenzymes called pepsinogens. Zymogen granules, released into the lumen by exocytosis, enable the acid environment to convert the inactive pepsinogens into pepsins, which partly hydrolyze proteins by cleaving peptide bonds, forming smaller peptides available for digestion to amino acids in the small bowel. Chief cells are stimulated by the parasympathetic nervous system (vagus) and by local factors produced by enteroendrocrine cells (gastrin, histamine). H&E, paraffin, × 300.

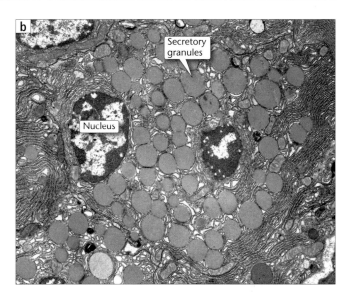

▲ **Fig 14.20b Ultrastructure of a chief cell**, showing many pepsinogen-containing secretory (zymogen) granules and rough endoplasmic reticulum. Acid secretion by parietal cells converts the inactive pepsinogen precursor into the enzyme pepsin. Leptin is also found in chief cells (and in the enteroendocrine cells) and is released into the gastric juice to exert its effects in the small bowel, where it regulates absorption of nutrients. × 4,300.

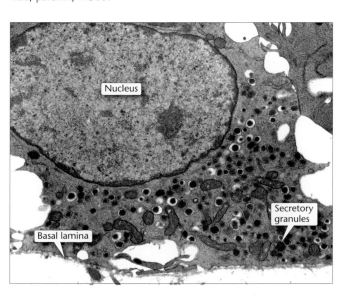

◀ **Fig 14.21 Enteroendocrine cell.** Ultrastructure of an endocrine cell from a gastric gland. Note the basal location of secretory granules and the proximity to the lamina propria, via which the granules are released into the blood. Endocrine cells in the stomach include G cells, located mainly in pyloric glands and glands of the antrum. Granules within G cells contain the protein hormone gastrin, which is released into the blood and distributed to the wider gastric mucosa, where it stimulates acid secretion and gastric motility. D cells secrete somatostatin, which is inhibitory for both gastric secretion and other enteroendocrine cells. × 8,000.

Pylorus

The pylorus region is characterized by deeper gastric pits (about half mucosal depth) leading to the glands. The pits may be branched or coiled and show mostly mucous-type cells, together with parietal and enteroendocrine cells (Fig 14.22a & b).

SMALL INTESTINE

In passing from the pylorus to the intestine, the mucosa changes from pits and glands typical of the stomach to the villi and crypts typical of the small intestine.

The three anatomical segments of the small intestine—the duodenum, jejunum, and ileum—each exhibit characteristic histologic features that can readily be identified using light microscopy at low-to-medium magnification. The following descriptions concentrate on these features. For detailed discussion of the cell and molecular biology, and physiology of the intestines, a formal gastroenterology text should be consulted.

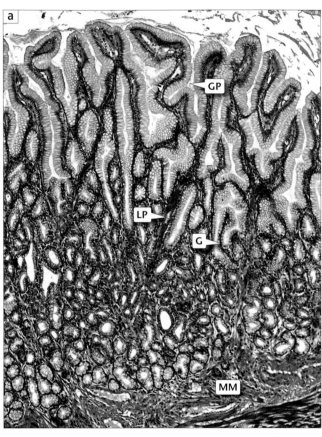

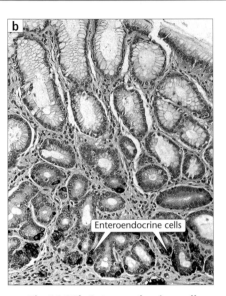

▲ **Fig 14.22b Enteroendocrine cells of the pyloric region** are located deep in the gastric pits, as indicated by their specific labeling with an antibody to chromogranin. Chromogranin is a protein associated with secretory vesicles in neuroendocrine cells and enterochromaffin cells. Immunocytochemistry, paraffin, × 150.

▲ **Fig 14.22a Pyloric mucosa.** In the pyloric region of the stomach, the characteristic feature is the deep, penetrating nature of the gastric pits (**GP**), which are often branched and extend down through at least half the depth of the gastric mucosa. The glands (**G**) have relatively wide lumina and may show short branches. Most of the cells lining the pits and glands are mucous-type secretory cells, although these cells are typically columnar near the surface and become more cuboidal in the glands. Within the lamina propria (**LP**) there may be numerous wandering immune cells, occasionally forming lymphoid follicles. Upward extensions of smooth muscle arise from the muscularis mucosae (**MM**). Small numbers of parietal cells occur in the pyloric mucosa, and enteroendocrine cells are also present, but neither cell type is easily observed in H&E preparations. A major function of the pyloric glands is to secrete mucus, which protects the mucosa from acid and enzyme attack and lubricates the stomach contents en route to the duodenum. H&E, paraffin, × 110.

Mucosa

Common features

Throughout most of its length the small intestine shares common histologic elements. The mucosal surface forms permanent transverse ridges, termed the plicae circulares or valves of Kerckring (Fig 14.23a–d). Enormous numbers of finger-type projections of the mucosa form the villi, between which tubular glands or crypts of Lieberkühn extend down to or occasionally beyond the muscularis mucosae. The mucosal epithelium is simple columnar in type, composed of mucus-secreting goblet cells and many absorptive cells or enterocytes (Fig 14.24). Enterocytes have thousands of surface microvilli, often referred to as the brush border or striated border. Microvilli greatly increase the cell surface area, facilitating absorptive and special secretory activities. For the whole small intestine the surface area of the mucous membrane exposed to the lumen is about 250 m², similar to the area of a doubles tennis court. The epithelial cells of the villi are short-lived, constantly being exfoliated or phagocytosed. Billions of cells are lost and replaced every day. Stem cells are found near the base of the crypts and, by proliferation and differentiation, give rise to all cell types of the small intestinal epithelium.

Important immune functions

Throughout the gastrointestinal tract the mucosa is abundantly supplied with cells of the immune system. Lymphocytes, mostly T cells, reside in the surface epithelium and are referred to as intraepithelial lymphocytes (Fig 14.25). These cells provide for immune surveillance, including the detection of abnormal epithelial cells. Dendritic cells, which sample foreign antigens and microorganisms, are also present in the epithelium but are identified only with immunocytochemical techniques. The underlying lamina propria is richly supplied with a wide range of dispersed immune cells, 60% of which are T cells. Aggregation of lymphocytes in the form of thousands of non-encapsulated lymphoid follicles occurs throughout the gut mucosa. Together with the dispersed component, these immune cells constitute the gut-associated lymphoid tissue (GALT). Their functional histology is reviewed in more detail in the section on the immune system.

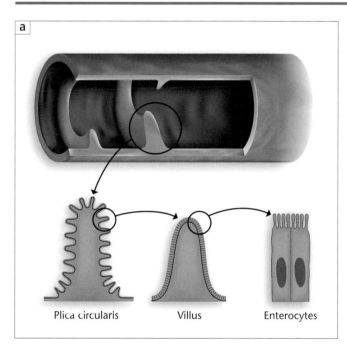

Plica circularis   Villus   Enterocytes

◀ **Fig 14.23a Intestinal mucosa.** To fulfill its role in digestion, the small bowel depends on a large surface area. Permanent transverse folds of the mucosa, the plicae circulares, are themselves amplified in surface area by the multitude of villi projecting into the lumen. In turn the villi each have thousands of microscopic, finger-type extensions, which add to the absorptive surface area. It is estimated that in comparison with a simple hollow tube, these specializations collectively increase epithelial surface area by a factor of 600.

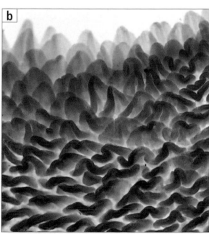

◀ **Fig 14.23b Surface morphology of the mucosa of the small bowel**, showing the microfolds, ridges, and leaf-shaped villi that together greatly increase the surface area available for absorption and secretion across the intestinal epithelium. Unstained formalin-fixed, × 15.

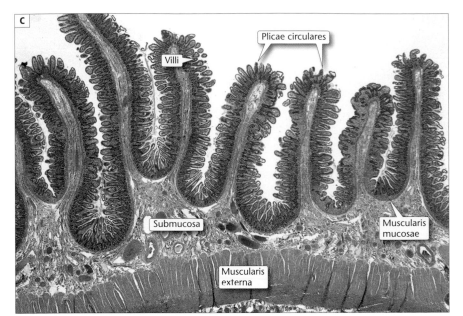

c

◀ **Fig 14.23c Intestinal mucosa folds.** Human jejunum at low magnification, showing the full thickness of the bowel with numerous regular folds of the mucosa, termed plicae circulares. Many villi project into the lumen. The internal contour of each fold is bordered by the smooth muscle of the muscularis mucosae. Contraction and relaxation of this, together with the external muscle layers, are regulated by the enteric nervous system to induce peristalsis and local segmentation. H&E, paraffin, × 12.

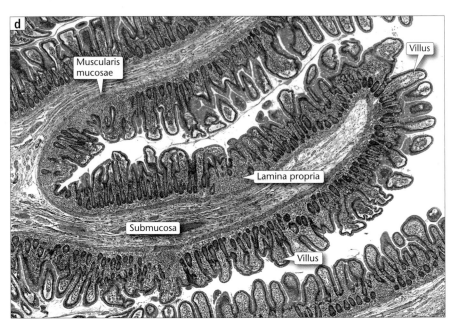

◀ **Fig 14.23d Plica circularis.** Detail of a jejunal plica circularis, with a core of submucosa containing connective tissue and blood vessels. The muscularis mucosae follows the mucosa, which shows many finger-type villi; the base of each of these extends deep into the crypts of Lieberkühn. The cellular density of the lamina propria is indicative of the abundant supply of diffuse immune cells. H&E, paraffin, × 35.

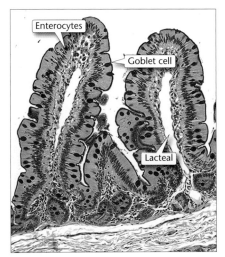

◀ **Fig 14.24 Villus epithelium.** Enterocytes are primarily absorptive in function and form a columnar epithelium interspersed with mucus-secreting goblet cells. The luminal surface is stained magenta, similar to the goblet cells, indicating the glycoproteins and enzymes associated with the submicroscopic microvilli. In the core of the villus, the empty gap represents an expanded lymph vessel, or lacteal, that collects lipoprotein complexes for export to the lymphatic circulation. Hematoxylin/PAS, paraffin, × 120.

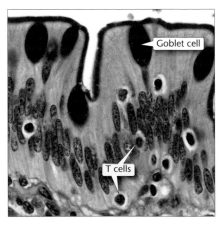

▲ **Fig 14.25 Intestinal epithelial immune cells.** Throughout the intestine some wandering but mostly resident immune cells, notably T lymphocytes, are found at various levels within the epithelium. These cells are called intraepithelial lymphocytes (IEL) and regulate epithelial homeostasis via production of cytokines that kill infected target cells. Hematoxylin/PAS, paraffin, × 490.

Duodenum

The distinctive feature of the duodenum is the submucosal Brunner's glands (Fig 14.26a–c), which diminish in the distal half of the duodenum. The cells are mostly mucous-type; their alkaline mucoid secretion empties into the crypts of Lieberkühn, neutralizing the acidic chyme and protecting the surface epithelial cells against enzymatic digestion and acid-induced injury.

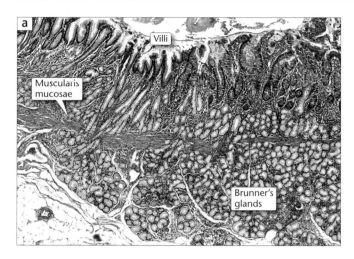

◀ **Fig 14.26a Duodenum.** The duodenum shows many surface villi. Aggregations of Brunner's glands in the submucosa are a distinctive feature of the duodenum. Some of these glands are located above the muscularis mucosae and send their ducts into the recesses or crypts at the bases of the villi. Brunner's glands diminish in number along the length of the duodenum. Their chief function is to secrete an alkaline mucus-type fluid (about 200 mL/day) that counteracts the acidity of chyme discharged from the stomach. Cholecystokinin (CCK) is an important hormonal regulator of the digestive process. CCK cells occur mainly in the villi of the duodenum and proximal jejunum. These enteroendocrine cells secrete CCK in response to food entering the small intestine. CCK released into blood vessels stimulates pancreatic secretion, gall bladder contraction, and intestinal peristalsis, but inhibits gastric acid secretion and induces satiety. H&E, paraffin, × 40.

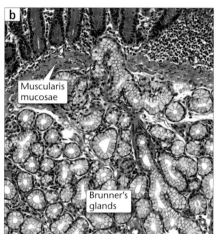

◀ **Fig 14.26b Cells of Brunner's glands** show a morphology typical of mucus-secreting cells, with a nucleus flattened near the base of the cell and a light-staining cytoplasm filled with mucus droplets. Ducts convey the viscous, mucoid secretions into the crypts of Lieberkühn. Scattered endocrine cells may occur in the glands, and peptidergic nerves with locally acting neuroendocrine factors probably function to control glandular secretion. H&E, paraffin, × 140.

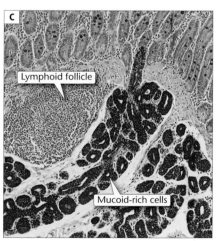

◀ **Fig 14.26c Brunner's glands** stained with the PAS reaction reveal the high concentration of carbohydrates and mucoid substances, which appear magenta. Secretion of bicarbonate ions by Brunner's glands assists the alkaline mucus to protect the duodenal mucosa from erosion by acid from the stomach and by the digestive activities of the enzymes discharged into the duodenal lumen from the pancreas. The cluster of small cells represents a single lymphoid follicle. Hematoxylin/PAS, paraffin, × 80.

339

Jejunum

The jejunum is recognizable by having the tallest villi, which extend from the surface of the permanent circular folds of the mucosa and submucosa (plicae circulares). Brunner's glands are not seen, and single lymphoid follicles spanning the lamina propria and submucosa are infrequent.

The villus and intestinal glands

The crypts of Lieberkühn (intestinal glands) play a vital role in the small bowel; they are the source of the epithelial cells that line the crypts and the surface of the villi (Fig 14.27a & b). Most of these epithelial cells only survive for a week and therefore are continuously replaced. In mice—the species most thoroughly studied—the prevailing view is that there are 4–6 stem cells per crypt located just above the crypt base and forming an irregular annulus around the crypt circumference. Dividing about once per day (in the lifetime of a mouse or human perhaps 1,000 and 5,000 divisions respectively), each stem cell produces two daughter cells, one of which enters a dividing

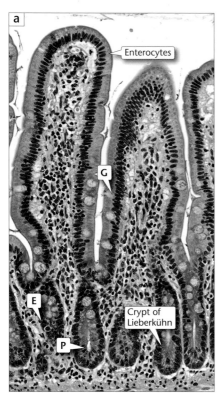

▲ **Fig 14.27a Villi and crypts.** Vertical section through villi and the deeper folds of the epithelium that form crypts of Lieberkühn. Most of the epithelium consists of enterocytes, but in routine sections they have no distinguishing features to suggest stages of differentiation. Several differentiated cells are noted—goblet cells (**G**), enteroendocrine cells (**E**), and Paneth cells (**P**). H&E, paraffin, × 130.

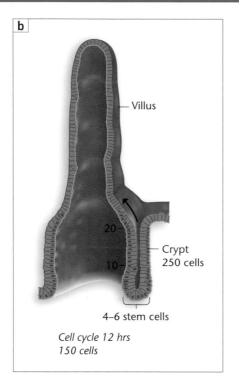

▲ **Fig 14.27b Diagram of a villus and a flask-shaped crypt.** In the mouse it is thought that there are four to six ancestral stem cells scattered around the circumference of the crypt, at an average cell position 4 above the base. An alternate view based upon expression of the *Lgr5* gene (leucine-rich G-protein-coupled receptor 5), a target of the Wnt glycoprotein family, suggests that crypt stem cells are located at the bottom of crypts. Within the crypt, up to cell position 20, there are 100 or more rapidly dividing transit cells and a total of 250–300 in a crypt. Cell lines committed to differentiation pathways migrate up the villus similarly to an ascending escalator, and in several days reach the vicinity of the tip and are lost by apoptosis. In contrast, Paneth cells remain at the base of the crypt.

transit cell population (Fig 14.28a–c). Through further mitoses that amplify their numbers, these cells produce the various lineages committed to the differentiation pathways that characterize the range of gut epithelial cells. Recent studies of the expression of stem cell markers related to Wnt signals (the glycoproteins

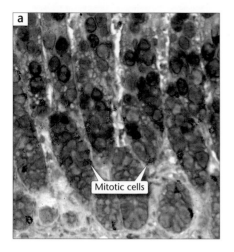

◀ Fig 14.28a Detecting proliferative cells. Autoradiograph of dividing transit cells in crypts of the large bowel detected by silver grains representing incorporation of ³H-thymidine into replicating DNA. The radiolabeled thymidine was given 1 hour before tissue sampling and shows that most cell proliferation (i.e. expansion of cell numbers) occurs in the zone above the base of the crypt. Hematoxylin/PAS, paraffin, × 100.

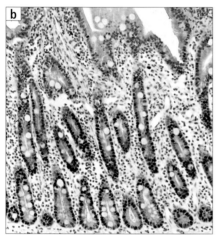

◀ Fig 14.28b Localization of proliferative crypt cells. Proliferative cell nuclear antigen (PCNA) labels as dark brown cells in pre- or S-phase of mitosis. Some cells are positive in the base and many more are positive in the walls of the crypts, where they amplify the epithelial population into several cell lineages destined for migration into the villi. Hematoxylin/PCNA immunocytochemistry, paraffin, × 70.

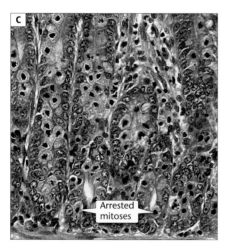

◀ Fig 14.28c Detecting mitosis. Stathmokinetic technique for detecting mitosis. In these colonic crypts, mitosis has been arrested at metaphase by prior treatment with colchicine to disrupt the mitotic spindle. The "metaphase-arrested" cells are clearly seen and occupy positions corresponding to the dividing transit cells. H&E, paraffin, × 100.

that govern crypt biology) suggest that the crypt stem cells occupy a position at the very base of the crypt. Mesenchymal and myofibroblast cells in the villus core (Fig 14.29a–c) interact with the stem cell niche and the epithelium derived from it to regulate mitosis, differentiation, and apoptosis along the crypt–villus axis. Wnt signaling (wingless integrated glycoprotein) plays a dominant role in these interactions.

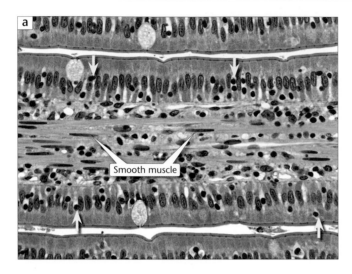

◀ **Fig 14.29a Villus core—longitudinal view.** The core is filled with loose connective tissue of the lamina propria, containing many free cells of the immune system, particularly plasma cells and lymphocytes with a rich vascular and muscular framework. Strips of smooth muscle originating from the muscularis mucosae run the length of the villus core and provide motility for each villus. Numerous lymphocytes appear in the mucosal epithelium (**arrows**), having migrated across the basement membrane from the lamina propria. H&E, paraffin, × 300.

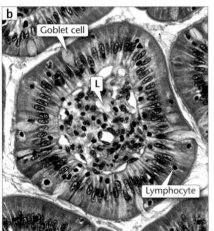

◀ **Fig 14.29b Villus core—transverse view.** When viewed in transverse section, the villus core displays a central lymphatic capillary (**L**) surrounded by cells of connective tissue and a variety of leukocytes. The blood vessels are located just deep to the epithelium and represent either capillaries or postcapillary vessels that form from the branching of one or more arterioles supplying the villus. Goblet cells and intraepithelial lymphocytes are indicated in the mucosal epithelium. H&E, paraffin, × 300.

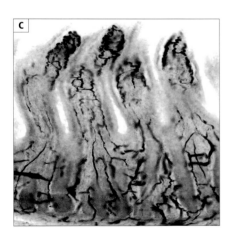

◀ **Fig 14.29c Villus core—blood vessels.** Injection of a colloid dye into the abdominal aorta reveals the fine blood vessels of the villus core, concentrated as capillary loops near the tips. This arrangement reflects the metabolic activities of enterocyte absorption/secretion and the requirement for immune defense mechanisms involving exchange of macromolecules and cells between the epithelium and the lamina propria. Colloid perfusion, paraffin, × 85.

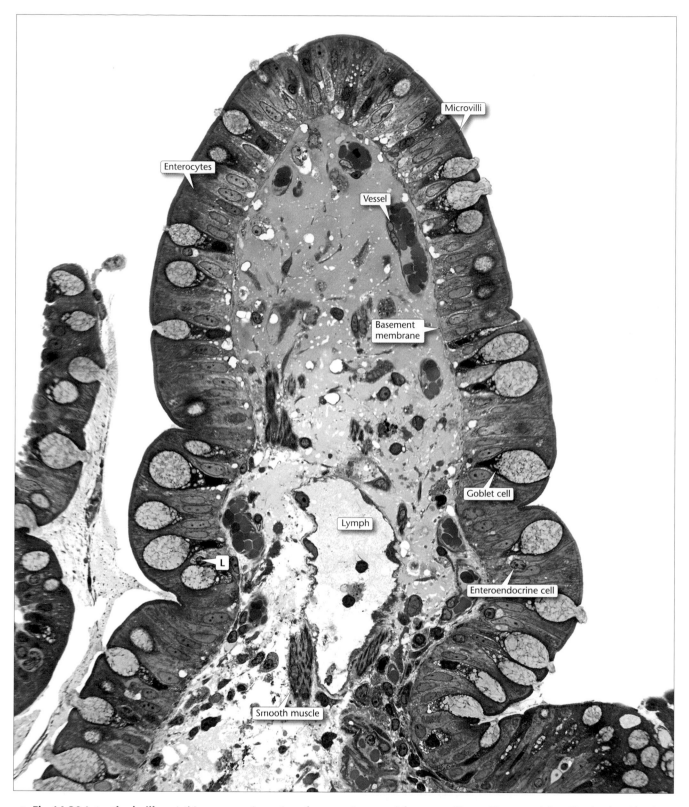

▲ **Fig 14.30 Intestinal villus.** A thin, epoxy resin section of an intestinal villus from the ileum shows its simple columnar epithelium, which consists of numerous absorptive cells or enterocytes, scattered goblet cells secreting mucus, and occasional enteroendocrine cells serving local stimulatory or inhibitory functions. The luminal surface exhibits a brush or striated border, consisting of microvilli that greatly increase the surface area. Wandering or intraepithelial lymphocytes (**L**) are noted between enterocytes, and these cells provide local immune defense surveillance. The core of the villus (outlined by the basement membrane) displays blood and lymphatic vessels, a mixture of smooth muscle, connective tissue cells and matrix, and various cells of the immune system. The villus core, or lamina propria, is an extension of the deeper supporting tissue above the muscularis mucosae, and thus provides vascular, neural, and immunological components that interact with the intestinal epithelium. Toluidine blue, araldite, × 500.

Cells of the crypt–villus axis

The cytology of a villus typical of the small bowel is shown in Figure 14.30. Enterocytes are the most abundant cell type, forming an epithelial barrier, with each cell joined to its neighbors by apical junctional complexes. The apical microvilli increase the surface area of the mucosa 600-fold compared with the effect of a simple tube (Fig 14.31a & b). It is common knowledge that the small bowel is absorptive, but for absorption to occur the enterocytes must also secrete

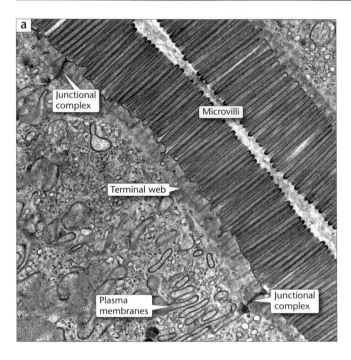

◀ **Fig 14.31a Surface of the villus epithelium.** Ultrastructure of the brush border of microvilli lining the surface of the intestinal absorptive cells. Note the diffuse appearance of the terminal web, containing filaments of actin. The lateral plasma membranes of adjacent cells interdigitate extensively and contain ion pumps, which facilitate transport of fluids and absorbed nutrients into the intracellular space that opens up during periods of intestinal absorption. The contents flow into capillaries in the lamina propria and then into the portal system en route to the liver. Adjacent cells are joined by junctional complexes that prevent intercellular transport (see Ch 1 for details). × 11,000.

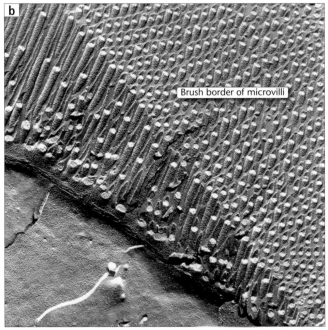

◀ **Fig 14.31b Freeze-fracture ultrastructure of the microvilli**, showing their remarkable density on the villus surface. × 15,000. (Courtesy L Orci, University of Geneva, Switzerland.)

fluid to maintain a fluid environment for mixing food with digestive enzymes. In diseases such as cholera, excessive secretion results in secretory diarrhea.

Enzymes on the surface of the microvilli and within the enterocytes are essential for digestion of dietary sugars, peptides, fats, vitamins, and minerals (Fig 14.32a & b).

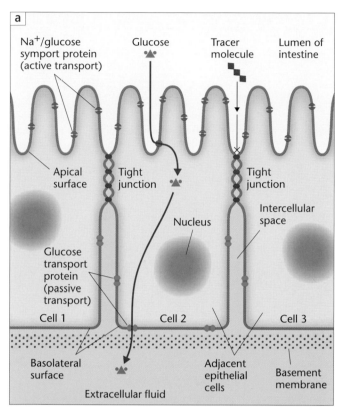

◀ **Fig 14.32a Transcellular transport.** Diagram of the mechanism by which enterocytes absorb a nutrient such as glucose. The apical membrane contains symport carrier proteins that actively pump glucose and Na⁺ ions simultaneously. A high glucose concentration is established in the enterocyte cytoplasm. Glucose passes out of the cell down its concentration gradient via passive transport through a second type of carrier protein in the basolateral cell membrane. The tight junctions not only serve to bind adjacent cells, but also restrict the entry of large-molecular-weight substances from entering the cell. Junctions also maintain enterocyte polarity by confining specific membrane proteins to apical or basolateral domains.

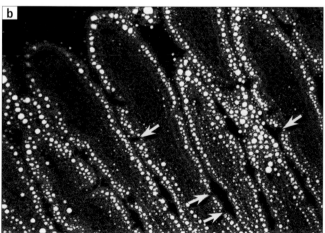

◀ **Fig 14.32b Uptake by enterocytes of fluoresterol** (fluorescent cholesterol analog). Fluoresterol was given orally by liquid diet and 2 hours later a sample of jejunum was analyzed. Fluoresterol is noted in absorptive epithelial cells (but not within goblet cells; **arrows**) and is packaged into lipoprotein particles known as chylomicrons seen in the villus core. Chylomicrons enter the lacteals, which transport them to the efferent lymphatics and ultimately to the blood. Frozen section, confocal microscopy, × 120. (Courtesy C Sparrow, Merck Research Laboratories, Rahway, New Jersey, USA.)

Goblet cells increase in abundance from the duodenum to the ileum, their mucus secretion serving to lubricate the epithelial surface by creating an unstirred layer of mucous gel. This barrier protects against surface shearing injury and traps microorganisms for antibody binding (Fig 14.33a & b).

Paneth cells are a subset of differentiated secretory cells found in the base of intestinal crypts and survive for about 3 weeks. They secrete antimicrobial agents such as defensins or cryptdins, phospholipase, and lysozyme (Fig 14.34).

Enteroendocrine cells of the "open" or "closed" type

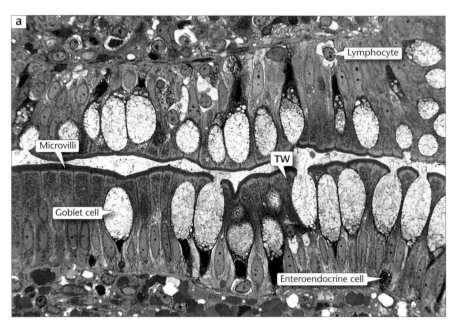

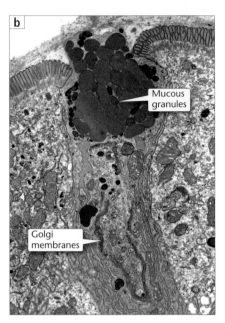

▲ **Fig 14.33a Goblet cells.** Thin epoxy resin section of surface epithelium of two villi from the human jejunum. Goblet cells with mucous granules are seen, some releasing onto the surface of the microvilli. The precise role of mucus in the small bowel is unknown, but it may provide barrier protection for the epithelium against harmful agents (microorganisms or toxins), envelop exfoliated cells and clear them by distal transport, or stabilize immunoglobulins directed against bacteria or viruses. Tall columnar absorptive cells (enterocytes) display a clear zone or terminal web (**TW**) subjacent to the brush border, representing an anchoring site for the core of microvilli. Lymphocytes are usually T-suppressor/cytotoxic cells serving as an immunological defense. Basal epithelial cells with granules represent enteroendocrine cells. Toluidine blue, araldite, × 620.

▲ **Fig 14.33b Ultrastructure of a goblet cell**, showing dense mucous granules for release into the intestinal lumen, where they contribute to a viscous hydrated gel of polydispersed glycoproteins composed of about 80% carbohydrate. Close to the microvilli the gel is unstirred, but within the lumen it shows more convection in concert with the turbulent flow in the gastrointestinal tract. The amino acid threonine is an important component in the synthesis of mucin, and goblet cell secretion is influenced by the enteric nervous system and dietary fiber. × 6,000.

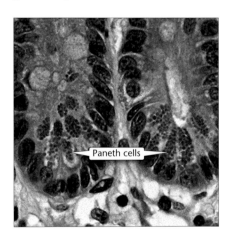

◀ **Fig 14.34 Paneth cells.** Located at the base of intestinal crypts, Paneth cells are pyramidal in shape and show distinctive granules. Granules contain antimicrobial peptides such as defensins or cryptdins (crypt defensins). Defensins are also produced by neutrophils, the kidney, and infected skin. Together with lysozyme, Paneth cells effectively kill bacteria and contribute to the remarkably low abundance of microbes in the human small bowel. Degranulation of Paneth cells (see Fig 14.35a) is stimulated by bacteria and cholinergic signals from the lamina propria. H&E, paraffin, × 600.

are scattered throughout the epithelium (Fig 14.35a & b). Comprising many different types, all with secretory granules, their identity cannot be ascertained in routine histology sections; identification requires immunocytochemistry, in situ hybridization, or ultrastructural analysis. Many enteroedocrine cells contain more than a single hormone and most contain serotonin (5-hydroxytryptamine); their hormones may act locally or enter the blood. Examples of small bowel-derived peptide hormones include secretin (stimulates pancreatic secretion; inhibits acid secretion), cholecystokinin (decreases food intake; increases pancreatic secretion), somatostatin (inhibitory for other enteroendocrine cells), and motilin (triggers peristalsis; increases pepsin secretion).

Tip: The source of intestinal epithelial cells is multipotent stem cells at or near the bottom of crypts, where new cells migrate upward to supply the crypt and villus. A villus may receive epithelial cells from several crypts. Proliferation stops at the crypt–villus junction. Paneth cells also arise from the stem cells and remain at the base of crypts. The health of the epithelium is maintained by a balance between bidirectional proliferation, differentiation, migration, and cell death.

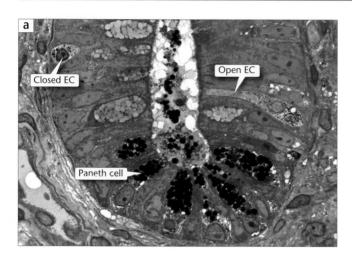

◀ **Fig 14.35a Enteroendocrine cells.** There are numerous types of enteroendocrine cells (ECs) that secrete a variety of peptides or amines performing local stimulatory or inhibitory functions to regulate secretory or absorptive activities of the mucosa. ECs of the "closed" or "open" types are recognized, the latter extending cytoplasm to the crypt lumen. Their granules are mostly confined to the basal cytoplasm. In the past ECs were classified as amine precursor uptake and decarboxylation (APUD) cells, which provided protein or biogenic amine hormones acting locally. It was thought that ECs were derived from the neural crest, but their true origin is from stem cells within the crypts and not modified migrant neurons. Paneth cells are seen discharging their granules into the crypt lumen to attack microorganisms. Toluidine blue, araldite, × 620.

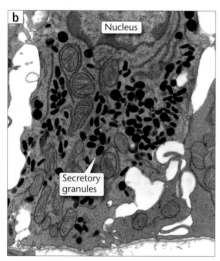

◀ **Fig 14.35b Ultrastructure of an enteroendocrine cell** with many small secretory granules in the basal cytoplasm. Granules are released by exocytosis across the basal lamina, enter nearby capillaries, and access their target cells elsewhere in the gut or other organs. × 11,000.

Ileum

The ileum is characterized by shorter and less abundant villi and distally by aggregated lymphoid follicles (or nodules), called Peyer's patches. Patches are located in the submucosa and often breach the muscularis mucosae extending into the lamina propria (Fig 14.36a–c). The follicle-associated epithelium (Fig 14.37) that overlies the nodules contains membranous or microfold

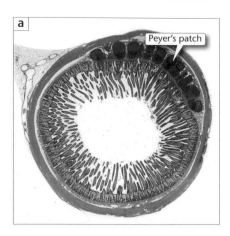

▲ **Fig 14.36a Ileum and Peyer's patches.** A rat ileum in cross section shows lymphoid follicles aggregated in the submucosa forming a Peyer's patch, which, specifically in the ileum, is usually located opposite the attachment of the mesentery. Lymphoid follicles are abundant in the ileum, providing immune defense functions to combat lumenal antigens and microorganisms. The villi, crypts of Lieberkühn, muscularis mucosae, and the outer wall of the muscularis externa are similar to the duodenum and jejunum. The ileum absorbs fluid, electrolytes, amino acids, fats, bile salts, and vitamin B$_{12}$. H&E, paraffin, × 10.

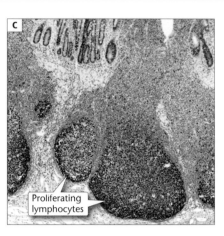

▲ **Fig 14.36c Peyer's patches—lymphoid cells proliferating.** Peyer's patches stained by PCNA immunocytochemistry, showing many lymphoid cells preparing for or in the process of proliferation. Activated lymphoid cells include T- and B-cell blasts that have responded to antigen captured and presented to the follicles by dendritic cells and macrophages in the lamina propria. Hematoxylin/immunocytochemistry, paraffin, × 75.

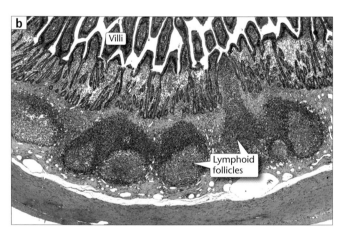

▲ **Fig 14.36b Peyer's patches.** The largest collection of aggregated and diffuse lymphoid tissue is represented by the gut-associated lymphoid tissue (GALT). The lymphoid nodules/cells provide effective mechanisms that exclude toxic, infectious, and antigenic material from entering the body via the gut. Peyer's patches are aggregated lymphoid follicles in the small intestine and occur mostly in the ileum. Each patch may contain very small or very large numbers (from five to hundreds) of lymphoid follicles per patch, and the number of patches in young adults may exceed 200, declining with increasing age. In the mature adult the number is around 40. Note extension of the lymphoid mass toward the lumen. H&E, paraffin, × 75.

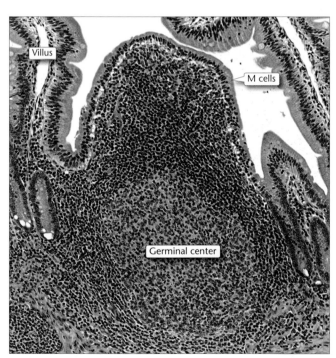

▲ **Fig 14.37 M cells.** Lymphoid tissue of Peyer's patches extend to the surface epithelium, which is termed follicle-associated epithelium. It contains specialized M cells (microfold or membranous cells). M cells take up material continuously from the lumen. Selected antigens encounter antigen-presenting cells, which enables naïve lymphocytes to recognize the luminal antigen. A local immune response may be triggered, as evidenced by the pale-staining blast cells in the lymphoid follicle. Migrating away from this region, activated lymphocytes enter afferent lymphatics and eventually pass to the systemic circulation. These immune cells subsequently home back to the site of the original antigenic challenge and to other mucosal sites, conferring protection. H&E, paraffin, × 120.

cells (M cells), which have few microvilli but extend invaginations of the basolateral membrane to enclose lymphocytes and leukocytes. M cells sample microbes, ingested foreign molecules, and IgA complexes, and by interacting with immune cells sensitize populations of lymphocytes that are delivered to gut lymph nodes, thus amplifying the immune response. Activated lymphocytes are returned to the intestinal mucosa, where as plasma cells they secrete antibodies.

Enteroendocrine cells may be seen among epithelial cells but are more common in the basal region of the crypts. They have cytoplasmic granules adjacent to the basal lamina. In a similar deep location in crypts are Paneth cells, which have an apical distribution of granules thought to be capable of destroying microorganisms. These cells are absent from most of the large intestine.

LARGE INTESTINE

The large intestine comprises the colon (with cecum, from which the appendix arises), rectum, and the upper two-thirds of the anal canal. Colonic mucosa has a similar organization to that of the small bowel, except that it lacks villi.

Colon

The colon has a smooth surface when viewed macroscopically, but in histological sections the mucosa usually presents an undulating appearance, with occasional in-foldings because of local muscle contractions at postmortem and in response to chemical fixation (Fig 14.38a & b). The characteristic feature is millions of crypts of Lieberkühn or colonic glands, oriented as straight tubular glands that extend

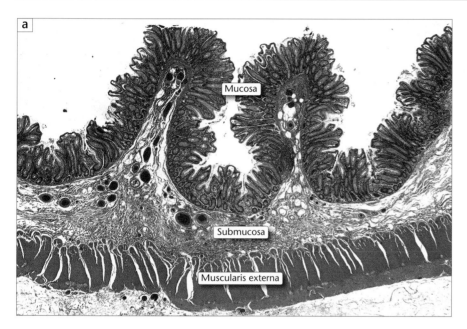

◀ Fig 14.38a Colon. The principal components of the large intestine are the mucosa, submucosa, and muscularis externa. Folds in the mucosa are not permanent, being formed by local contractions of either of the last two muscle layers. The mucosal epithelium should not be mistaken for villi, since the villi are comparatively large and arise independently, with separation between neighboring villi. H&E, paraffin, × 15.

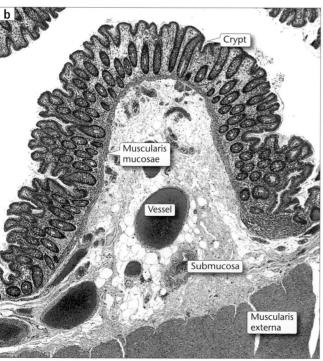

◀ Fig 14.38b Colonic mucosa. The colonic mucosa may show a highly irregular surface epithelium that, depending on the plane of section, shows invaginated crypts or their oblique profiles. The characteristic feature that sets it apart from the gastric or small intestinal mucosa is that it has no villi and its epithelial cells are mostly columnar cells and goblet cells forming simple crypts. H&E, paraffin, × 35.

down to the muscularis mucosae. Many goblet cells are noted, although they are outnumbered four to one by the absorptive enterocytes (Fig 14.39a–f).

The stem cells for the colonic epithelium reside at the very base of the crypts, giving rise to hundreds of cells that migrate apically and are shed at the surface of the crypts. Epithelial cell turnover is rapid, and most cells arising from the stem cells are replaced within a week.

Intraepithelial lymphocytes and enteroendocrine cells are abundant, but Paneth cells are rarely seen in the normal colon. Lymphoid follicles are commonly found in the mucosa and may extend into the submucosa.

The main functions of the colon are to supply mucus to the bowel contents, facilitating passage of feces, and to extract water and electrolytes, thereby dehydrating the luminal contents. The latter are stored in the colon prior to controlled elimination. A unique feature of the colon is the transformation of the smooth muscle coat of the outer muscularis externa into three distinct longitudinal strips, the teniae coli, which allow segments of the colon to contract independently. This action probably promotes fecal compaction and with general peristalsis results in the distal transport of luminal contents.

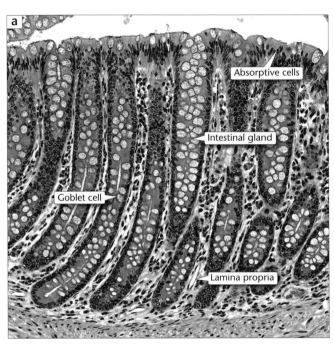

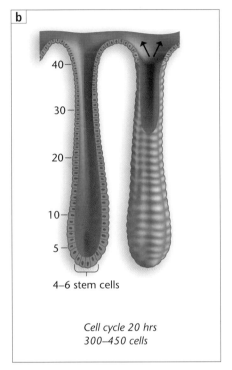

▲ **Fig 14.39a Colonic crypts.** Colonic crypts or glands with numerous goblet cells have a pale supranuclear region filled with mucous granules. On the surface, columnar absorptive cells are seen, and these cells outnumber the goblet cells in the colon. The characteristic features of colonic crypts are their alignment, which is similar to that of test tubes in a rack, and the abundance of goblet cells, together with the columnar enterocytes. In the base of the crypts, new cells arise by mitosis, and mature and migrate upward through the crypts until ultimately exfoliated from the surface. Many immunocompetent cells, notably plasma cells, occupy the lamina propria. T lymphocytes also occur there and within the mucosal epithelium. H&E, paraffin, × 120.

▲ **Fig 14.39b Diagram of cell arrangement in a colonic crypt.** The stem cells are found at the very base of the crypt, and the cell positions above this are indicated by ascending numbers. At its widest point the crypt contains about 18 cells in circumference, and, with a cell cycle duration of 20 hours, a crypt may contain more than 400 cells. The colonic epithelium undergoes continuous and rapid renewal; the average life span of a cell originating at the base of the crypt and later sloughed into the lumen is about 6 days.

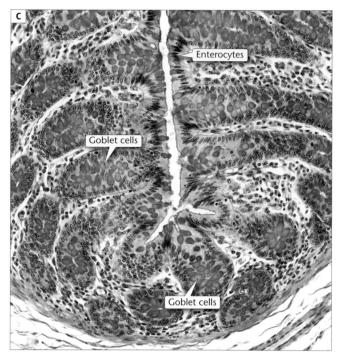

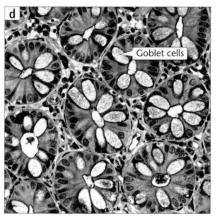

▲ Fig 14.39d Transverse section through colonic crypts, showing the radial arrangement of goblet cells and the tall intervening columnar absorptive cells. The central lumen of the gland or crypt is quite narrow and is partly filled with mucoid materials. Each gland or crypt is surrounded by the supporting lamina propria, and the fluids/electrolytes taken up by the surface epithelium of the glands are transported from the mucosa via numerous blood vessels leading to the portal system. Colonic crypts also secrete an isotonic fluid rich in potassium and bicarbonate ions, acting as a buffering agent in the lumen. H&E, paraffin, × 280.

▲ Fig 14.39c Colonic crypts and goblet cells. With special stains, the relative abundance of goblet cells and enterocytes can be demonstrated; the ratio is about 1:4. Goblet cells are intensely green owing to their high mucin content consisting of glycoproteins. The crypts contain abundant goblet cells, particularly toward the base, that often obscure the lumen. Surface epithelial cells are absorptive, taking up water and electrolytes and thus desiccating the luminal contents. Alcian blue/van Gieson's, paraffin, × 120.

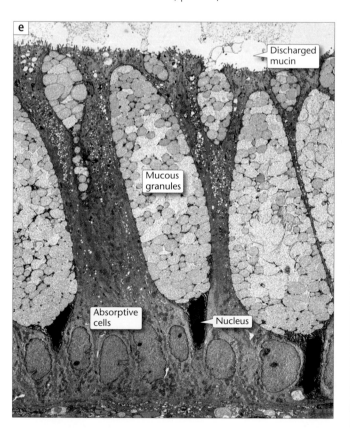

◄ Fig 14.39e Ultrastructure of colonic epithelium, showing goblet cells and absorptive columnar cells. The mucin-type proteins of goblet cells contain glycosaminoglycans, which upon release into the lumen attract water and expand in volume to form a slippery gel or mucus. The luminal contents in storage within the colon are lubricated by the mucus (about 200 mL/day) secreted from the goblet cells. For each liter of semi-fluid material entering the colon from the ileum, less than 15% remains after passing through the large intestine. The absorptive columnar cells regulate electrolyte and water content of feces but, unlike the enterocytes of the small intestine, cannot absorb glucose or amino acids in significant quantities. × 1,800.

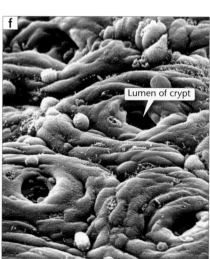

◄ Fig 14.39f Colon surface epithelium. Scanning electron micrograph of the surface epithelium of the colon, showing the circular arrangement of cells around the central lumen of the colonic crypts. × 1,000.

Appendix

The histology of the appendix is similar to that of the colon, with two main differences: the crypts of Lieberkühn are far less abundant, and the characteristic feature of the appendix is the circular arrangement of lymphoid follicles, sometimes extending into the submucosa (Fig 14.40). Because the inflamed appendix can be surgically removed with no harm, its contribution to gastrointestinal function remains uncertain.

Rectum

In the rectum the mucosa is deeper but the colonic glands contain more goblet cells than in the colon. The muscularis externa is similar to that of the colon. At the junction of the rectum and anus, the crypts of Lieberkühn are replaced with the stratified squamous surface epithelium characteristic of the anal canal (Fig 14.41a & b). The muscularis externa is thickened and forms the internal anal sphincter. In common with the stomach and small bowel, the mucosa of the colon and rectum contains many wandering lymphocytes and plasma cells, together with solitary lymphoid follicles. Scattered enteroendocrine cells are occasionally observed in the epithelium of the colonic glands.

> **Tip:** How can the differences in mucosal histology along the intestine be remembered? The **d**uodenum has **d**ual features of villi and Brunner's glands; the **j**ejunum has **j**ust villi; the **i**leum has prominent **i**mmune tissue; the **c**olon has **c**rypts; in the **a**nal canal all the foregoing are **a**bsent.

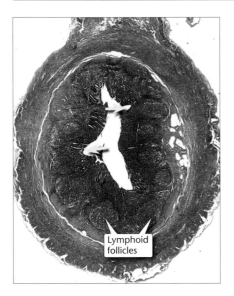

◀ **Fig 14.40 Appendix.** The vermiform (worm-like) appendix is a hollow, tubular extension of the cecum, containing prominent lymphoid follicles. Histologically the appendix resembles the colon. In young individuals the lymphoid follicles are abundant and encircle the lumen by occupying the lamina propria and submucosa; the muscularis mucosae is poorly defined. The appendiceal crypts (**arrows**) tend to be irregular in distribution and shape and are surrounded by an abundant population of plasma cells and T lymphocytes. Although considered to be an unimportant vestigial organ, the appendix probably contributes plasma cells and lymphocytes to maintain regional mucosal immune mechanisms. H&E, paraffin, × 6.

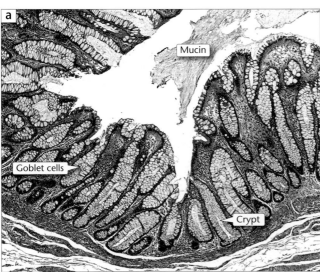

▲ **Fig 14.41a Rectoanal region.** The histology of the rectal mucosa is similar to that of the colon, but the crypts are slightly longer and goblet cells are more abundant. H&E, paraffin, × 70.

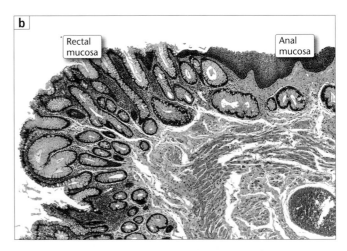

▲ **Fig 14.41b Rectoanal region.** The transition from the rectum to the anal canal occurs in the vicinity of the pectinate line. Proximally the rectal mucosa shows crypts of simple columnar epithelium, while distally the epithelium is stratified squamous. The rectoanal junction marks the endodermal origin of the hindgut and the ectodermal origin of the proctodeum or anal pit. H&E, paraffin, × 50.

ABNORMAL CONDITIONS AND CLINICAL FEATURES

Esophagus

Gastroesophageal reflux, a normal event, is a common condition in the esophagus but, if it is frequent and/or clearance of reflux material is deficient, heartburn and/or inflammation with ulceration may result. Chronic gastroesophageal reflux may change the mucosa to be similar to that of the intestine (Barrett's esophagus or metaplasia), with an increased risk of developing esophageal cancer such as adenocarcinoma, which is more common in the distal part. Alcohol and smoking are other factors involved with esophageal cancer such as squamous cell carcinoma, more common in the mid-portion. The tumour may obstruct the lumen, leading to dysphagia. The strength of the lower esophageal sphincter is the most important factor in preventing reflux.

A hiatus hernia, or sliding of the esophagus through the diaphragm, is very common and often asymptomatic. It is accompanied by heartburn and reflux and may be exacerbated when bending down.

A congenital abnormality of the esophagus in newborns is the presence of a fistula (tracheo-esophageal) and atresia (blind ending). Surgical correction is necessary.

Stomach

Gastritis may be acute and secondary to injury by aspirin, other non-steroidal anti-inflammatory drugs, ethanol, or corrosive agents. Stress is believed to induce injury, although this is controversial. Gastritis is common in very sick or intensive-care patients who develop multiple small gastric erosions and ulcers. Chronic gastritis is chiefly caused by infection with the bacterium *Helicobacter pylori*; the other major cause is autoimmune. Gastric ulcer has three main causes:

- *H. pylori* (Although it is uncertain how this bacterium causes ulcers, its involvement is shown by the prevention of recurrence after the eradication, through antibiotic treatments, of the organism.)
- Aspirin and other non-steroidal anti-inflammatory drugs
- Cancer, with carcinoma being common and epidemiologically related to *H. pylori* infection (as is gastric lymphoma) and exposure to exogenous carcinogens.

Hyperplasia of the gastric mucosa occurs in response to *H. pylori* infection, to hypersecretion of gastrin by a tumor elsewhere (usually in the pancreas: Zollinger–Ellison syndrome), or from an unknown cause. Lymphomas can occur in the stomach. *H. pylori* appears to be the cause of lymphomas of the GALT. The main regions of the stomach biopsied for histological evaluation in clinical investigations are the body and antrum, since these areas are common sites for pathological change.

Small intestine

Infections and food poisoning often cause diarrhea, resulting from viral infections of the mucosa (e.g. rotavirus) or toxins released from *Escherichia coli*, *Staphylococcus*, and cholera. Fluid and electrolytes secreted by the intestines are normally reabsorbed by the small and large intestine, but if secretion is excessive and/or absorption is decreased, diarrhea results. If untreated, nutrients from the diet fail to be adequately absorbed because of the loss of villi, leading to weight loss. Treatment with antibiotics is normally effective.

Invasion of lymphoid follicles by bacteria such as *Salmonella typhi* (typhoid fever) results in systemic illness with fever, which may be fatal. Parasites such as tapeworms, protozoa, or flukes may inhabit the bowel, but most infected individuals are asymptomatic. Celiac disease (sensitivity to gluten in cereal proteins) is associated with a flattening of the intestinal mucosa, which results in a significant loss of the mucosal surface area in the proximal small intestine, leading to malabsorption and diarrhea. The removal of dietary gluten may reduce or eliminate this reaction. Duodenal ulcer is secondary to *H. pylori* infection in more than 95% of cases. Eradication of *H. pylori* reduces recurrence of ulceration from 90% per annum to less than 2% per annum. Crohn's disease is a chronic inflammatory condition of unknown cause that affects any part of the small and large intestine in patches and commonly affects areas with the highest concentration of lymphoid follicles (terminal ileum, cecum). Fibrosis and hyperplasia of smooth muscle in the wall of the intestine may lead to obstruction of the lumen, and ulceration may be deep, causing perforation, abscess, or fistula formation. Lymphoma and carcinoma are rare, but any mass lesion can cause obstruction to the relatively small lumen of the small intestine.

Large intestine

Ulcerative colitis is a diffuse chronic inflammation, with or without epithelial ulceration, that affects only the mucosa. The inflamed mucosa may lead to bloody diarrhea, polyp formation, and anemia. Some bacterial infections, such as *Shigella*, *Campylobacter*, or *Clostridium difficile*, can cause colitis. Diverticulosis, a condition in which small parts of the mucosa are ballooned or herniated outward, is common in middle age. Hirschsprung's disease is a congenital megacolon detected in the newborn by failure to pass meconium (bowel movement), vomiting, and problems with bowel movements. It is caused by the absence of ganglia in the rectum, which becomes constricted, leading to proximal dilation of the colon and accumulation of luminal contents. Carcinoma of the large bowel is common and is the result of a combination of dietary and possible other environmental factors, together with genetic predisposition. It often arises in benign tumors (adenomas).

Appendix

Except in a few cases, the cause of appendicitis is unknown, but it is thought to be an obstructive condition followed by bacterial infection. Ulceration, gangrene, and perforation are possible consequences of untreated acute appendicitis.

Liver, gall bladder, and pancreas

The liver, gall bladder, and pancreas comprise a triumvirate of glandular organs all derived from the foregut during embryogenesis. The liver and the pancreas have both exocrine and endocrine functions, whereas the gall bladder is a sac for storage and concentration of bile. The emphasis is on the key structural features that help to identify each organ and its components, together with summaries of their major functions, many of which can be related to cell ultrastructure.

LIVER

The liver is the largest gland inside the body. It is perfused with about 1.5 liters of blood per minute, entering mainly via the portal vein and to a lesser extent from the common hepatic artery. It is often referred to as a biological factory, but with regard to the extraordinary range of hepatic functions, it is much more than a factory—rather it is a hive of industry. In addition to manufacturing products from raw materials, the liver performs other functions

analogous to those of a recycling depot, a waste-disposal unit, and a warehouse, examples of which will be discussed below.

Histologic organization

In paraffin sections, the liver is relatively easy to identify, mainly because of a rather homogeneous morphology. Basically, the liver resembles the structure of a dense sponge, in the sense that its histology is relatively simple and uniform throughout the organ; however, in a functional sense most of the substances entering the liver are significantly different when they leave the organ via the hepatic veins or the hepatic ducts of the biliary system. The gall bladder is a modified reservoir with the special function of extracting much of the water and salt in the primary bile delivered to it from the liver.

The sponge-like morphology of the liver is represented as roughly polygonal aggregations of cells that are arranged in irregular radial cords (Fig 15.1). These cords are occasionally interrupted by strands

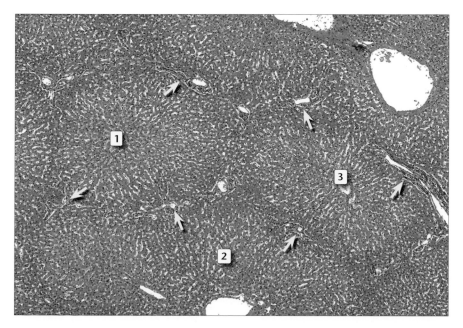

◀ **Fig 15.1 Structural organization of the liver.** Low magnification of human liver tissue, showing its sponge-like appearance. Hepatocytes and intervening spaces (vascular sinusoids) are arranged into radial patterns with indistinct margins defining three liver lobules (**1**, **2**, **3**). These borders (**arrows**) are connective tissue containing vascular, lymphatic, and biliary components with connective tissue fibers. Hematoxylin & eosin (H&E), paraffin, × 30.

of supporting tissues that contain vascular and biliary passageways. The lack of diversification of liver tissue, particularly in humans, is due to the paucity of internal supporting tissue. This is in contrast to a number of other mammalian species, particularly pigs. In pigs (and in polar bears and racoons), the liver tissue is formed into polygonal or roughly hexagonal units marked by slender profiles of supporting tissues. These units are 1–2 mm in diameter and several millimeters in length. This arrangement contributes to the traditional description of the classic liver lobule, one of three models that attempt to relate structure to function, as seen in Figure 15.2.

Liver structure models

Lobule model

The classic liver lobule is hexagonal in shape and resembles a benzene ring (six sides and six points). It consists of three recognizable components (Fig 15.3a & b):

- A central vein, seen as single holes
- Peripheral portal triads (or portal tracts) set at the angles of the polygons
- Hepatocytes (or liver cells) radiating from the central vein as anastomosing rows of cells separated by vascular sinusoids.

The classic liver lobule is usually not so readily recognizable in the human liver, and the histologic descriptions of the past that conform to this geometric model are no longer tenable. On the other hand, the lobule concept does provide some useful features that relate structure to function and emphasizes endocrine-type secretion into the blood of the central vein.

Portal lobule model

This model of hepatic functional anatomy emphasizes the exocrine role of the liver and is based on a triangle shape with central veins at the three points of the triangle. The portal tracts or triads are at the center of the triangle. They represent sites of the branches of the portal venous system (which supplies 75% of the blood that goes to the liver), the hepatic artery (25% of blood to the liver), and branches of the hepatic biliary system (which drain bile from the liver).

All these, together with small lymphatics, govern the entry of substances into the lobules and play a major role in controlling the exit of products destined for the gut (e.g. the bile).

The central vein provides a morphologic focus for the exit of all blood that enters the liver. The blood drains to hepatic veins and the inferior vena cava.

The link between the portal triads and central vein is established by the alternating columns of hepatocytes

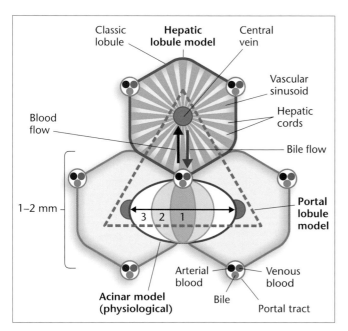

◀ **Fig 15.2 Microvascular functional units of the liver.** Diagram showing the various concepts of the histologic and functional organization of the liver. In the classic **lobule model** (blue), the central vein is at the center with portal tracts or triads in the periphery. Venous blood (blue lines) is derived from branches of the portal vein in each of the six portal triads and drains into the central vein. Arterial blood also supplies the liver tissue via hepatic arterioles within the triangular portal triads. In the **acinar model** a liver acinus (elliptical) has a central vertical axis between two portal triads, with three zones (**1**, **2**, **3**) of hepatic parenchyma of differing oxygenation and metabolic function. Several acini would make up a **portal lobule model** (broken green outline), triangular in shape and having a portal triad in its center to which bile drains.

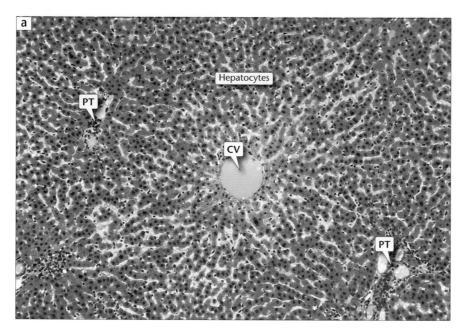

◀ **Fig 15.3a Liver lobule.** Anastomosing rows and plates of hepatocytes separated by hepatic sinusoids converge on a central vein (**CV**) located at the center of a classic lobule. The same vessel is called a terminal hepatic venule if the functional histology of the liver is considered to be based upon the hepatic acinus. Portal tracts or triads (**PT**) are the entry sites where blood from the portal vein and hepatic arteries perfuses into the sinusoids. Bile commences its exit from the liver in ducts within the portal triads. H&E, paraffin, × 60.

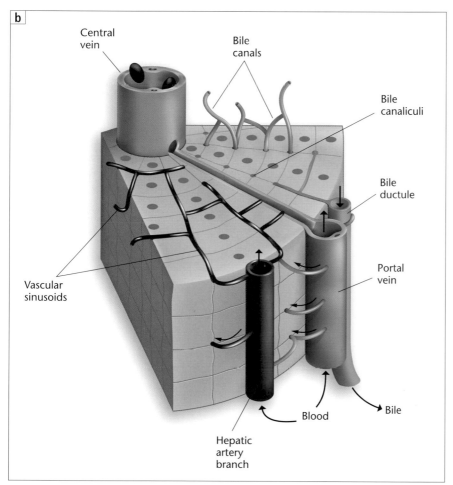

◀ **Fig 15.3b Part of a liver lobule**, with elements of a portal triad shown consisting of two blood vessels and a bile ductule. Venous and arterial blood perfuses the hepatocytes as it passes along the vascular sinusoids toward the central vein located in the center of the lobule. Bile passes in the opposite direction along the minute bile canaliculi that link to form canals, which in turn merge into ductules in each portal triad.

357

and blood sinusoids. The flow of blood is directed from the peripheral margins of the lobule to the central vein (centripetal flow). The bile is secreted into minute canals traveling between the hepatocytes; it flows in the opposite direction to bloodflow, toward the portal triads (centrifugal flow).

The "portal lobule" concept is based upon the portal triad as the central structure, with draining central or hepatic veins at the periphery, but this model has failed to gain acceptance on both metabolic and pathologic grounds.

Acinar model

Another concept of organization, the liver acinus, is based on functional considerations more than on histologic ones, and is favored by hepatologists and pathologists because it reflects numerous pathologic changes and metabolic properties of the liver (Fig 15.4). Although the acinar model is not universally accepted, it does explain the consequences of pathologic changes in terms of oxygen gradients, the distribution of drug-metabolizing enzymes, and the zones of histologic damage following ischemia and toxic insults.

The acinus is defined by an elliptical area with a short axis spanning two portal triads and a long axis defined by a line drawn between two central veins that form the outermost "poles" of the acinus. The short axis is the key feature because it contains the smallest branches of the portal venules and hepatic arterioles, both of which drain directly into the blood sinusoids. These sinusoids empty into the central veins, which

are now designated as terminal hepatic venules, since in this model they are no longer central. It should be emphasized that the acinar concept does not alter the way in which blood or bile flows in the liver.

Other models

Other interpretations of liver structure and function, based upon angioarchitecture and metabolic gradients, are the "primary lobule" or "hepatic microvascular subunits," which are six to eight wedge-shaped subdivisions of a classic hepatic lobule. While these models are helpful in explaining liver function, the organization of the liver is not readily classified into distinct histologic units. This emphasizes the complexity of its many functions.

Hepatocytes and vascular sinusoids

Liver cells form sheets, or trabeculae. These may be branched; they are usually only one cell thick and at least one surface faces a blood sinusoid (Fig 15.5). Morphologically, a sinusoid is a large capillary, which is readily seen if colored dyes are introduced into the blood vessels that supply the liver (Fig 15.6). Binucleate hepatocytes are occasionally noted. The cytoplasm of hepatocytes is eosinophilic with haematoxylin and eosin, and metachromatic with dyes such as toluidine blue. It has granularities, which are often extensive, or patchy staining representing an impressive array of organelles and inclusions commensurate with significant biochemical activity (Fig 15.7).

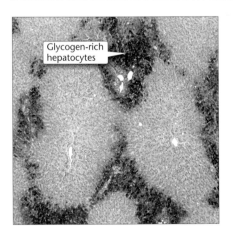

Glycogen-rich hepatocytes

◀ **Fig 15.4 Glycogen store.** Liver tissue, stained for glycogen, showing its preferential location at the periphery of the lobule. This reflects the inflow of nutrients from the gastrointestinal tract, in which the glucose component is taken up (then stored as glycogen) by peripheral hepatocytes closest to the blood vessels that emerge from the portal triads. Hepatocytes of the inner regions of the lobule lack significant glycogen deposits because of the diminished supply of glucose remaining in the blood. PAS technique, paraffin, × 25.

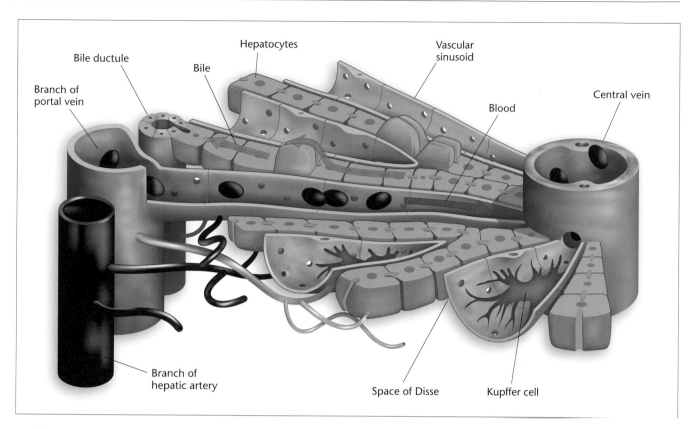

Bile ductule

Branch of portal vein

Bile

Hepatocytes

Vascular sinusoid

Blood

Central vein

Branch of hepatic artery

Space of Disse

Kupffer cell

▲ **Fig 15.5 Hepatocytes and blood sinusoids.** Hepatocytes are arranged in radial sheets or plates, very similar to the structure of a rotor fan of a jet engine. Between the cells are the vascular channels, called sinusoids because of discontinuities in the vessel endothelial walls. Blood from branches of the portal vein and common hepatic artery enters the sinusoids and is in direct contact with the hepatocytes. Kupffer cells (macrophages) reside in the sinusoids. Bile, produced by hepatocytes and secreted into a system of tiny canals between the cells, flows in the opposite direction to that of blood, and is delivered into the bile ductules in the portal triads (two vessels, one ductule), which are located at the periphery of the sheet of hepatocytes.

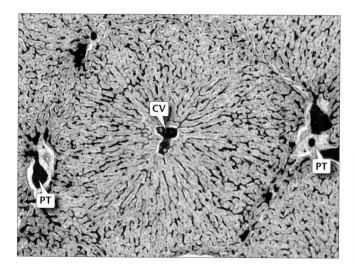

▲ **Fig 15.6 Microvascular system**. Liver tissue fixed after perfusion of a dye (red colloid) through the peripheral vascular system, demonstrating the pattern of blood flow through the portal tracts and triads (**PT**) and their relationship to hepatic sinusoids. The central vein (**CV**) region receives blood from the surrounding radially organized sinusoids, many of which are interconnected by branching. Regions close to the central vein may be poorly perfused with dye, emphasizing the acinar and microvascular concepts of zones of differing blood flow, metabolism, and oxygen gradients, and the zonal distribution of liver damage caused by toxic compounds or ischemia. Paraffin, × 50.

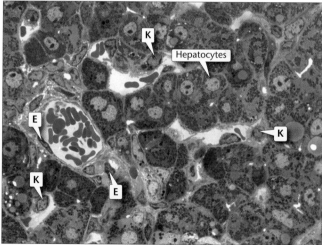

▲ **Fig 15.7 Hepatocytes and sinusoidal cells**. Thin epon resin section, showing hepatocytes, some with two nuclei and sinusoids with endothelial nuclei (**E**). Kupffer cells (**K**) are macrophages within the sinusoids anchored to the endothelium. They are phagocytic for microbes, erythrocytes, low-density lipoprotein, and immune complexes, and may produce cytokines and eicosanoids with paracrine effects on hepatocyte function. Hepatic stellate cells, or fat-storing Ito cells, within the space of Disse are modified fibroblasts that store vitamin A and can secrete collagen. This contributes to hepatic fibrogenesis in certain pathologic conditions. Toluidine blue, epon, × 420.

359

The variety and abundance of these cytoplasmic components is often employed as a model of the "typical cell" ultrastructure (Fig 15.8). It is possible to consider all of them in relation to their function, but this information is beyond the scope of this book; details can be found in the relevant texts on liver biochemistry and gastroenterology.

The chief organelles are mitochondria (> 1,000 per cell), endoplasmic reticulum of both types, Golgi apparatus, peroxisomes (500 per cell), and lysosomes (100 per cell) of all types. The chief inclusions are glycogen and lipid in varying quantities. The integrated, functional roles of these organelles and inclusions are discussed below.

Surface specializations of the hepatocyte comprise three major components:
- Desmosomes and gap junctions between adjacent cells
- Abundant short microvilli facing the vascular sinusoids
- Small, opposite-facing gutters or mini-lumens between junctional complexes, which form canals (1 μm in diameter) or bile canaliculi between adjacent cells.

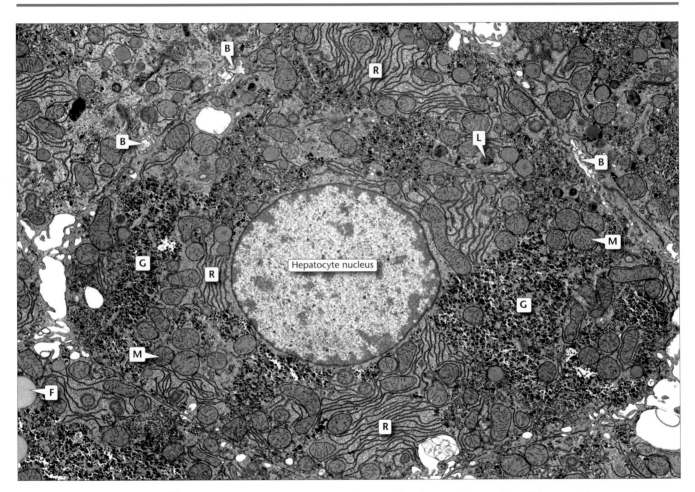

▲ **Fig 15.8 Ultrastructure of hepatocytes.** Hepatocyte, showing nucleus and cytoplasm filled with inclusions and organelles, reflecting the vast array of functions of these cells. Rough endoplasmic reticulum (**R**), glycogen (**G**), mitochondria (**M**), lysosomal bodies (**L**), and fat inclusions (**F**) are shown. The metabolic properties of hepatocytes are remarkable with regard to diversity and number (they include energy supply, nutrient utilization, biosynthesis and catabolism, waste removal, detoxification, biotransformation, immune functions, and interactions with many other organs). Equally impressive is the fact that many of these functions occur simultaneously in each cell. Note the bile canaliculi (**B**), seen as channels between hepatocytes. In three dimensions, these canaliculi are similar to conduits or grooves around the cells; they form a polygonal network in continuity with the bile ducts in the portal triads. × 7,500.

Delivery and export of substances between the blood supply and the hepatocytes is facilitated by numerous discontinuities or fenestrations of the endothelial lining of the vascular sinusoids. Between the endothelium and the adjacent hepatocyte surface is the narrow space of Disse, which is difficult to detect in paraffin sections but easily seen with electron microscopy (Fig 15.9). Within this space are the hepatocyte microvilli and delicate strands of type III collagen fibers that stain black with silver stains for "reticulin" (Fig 15.10). Hepatic stellate cells (also called lipocytes or Ito cells), which store vitamin A, are thought to produce the collagen fibers. Recent evidence suggests stellate cells are antigen-presenting cells. Lymph forms in the spaces of Disse and drains to portal triads before exiting the liver in association with blood vessels.

Macrophages known as Kupffer cells are located on the inner walls of the vascular sinusoids and represent about 10% of liver cells. Their large volume may extend across the lumen of the blood vessel, and their processes may enter the space

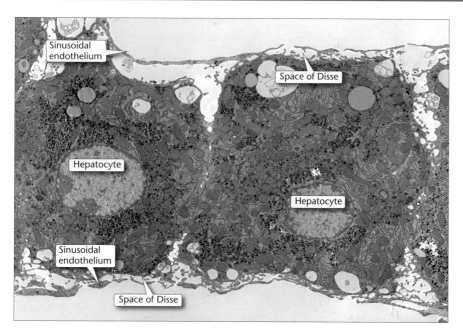

◀ **Fig 15.9 Space of Disse.** The gap between the rows of hepatocytes and the vascular sinusoids, which have no basal lamina, is called the space of Disse—a type of very loose connective tissue. The numerous fenestrations in the walls of the sinusoidal endothelium enable direct contact between blood and the hepatocytes, which is important for uptake of blood-borne products and secretion of proteins and metabolites from the hepatocytes into blood. Cells resident in the space include stellate cells and occasionally, between fenestrations, pit cells. × 3,400.

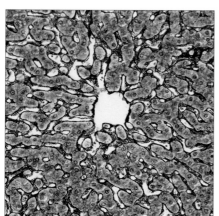

◀ **Fig 15.10 Perisinusoidal reticular fibers.** Liver tissue stained with a silver method, showing reticular fibers (type III collagen) along the hepatic sinusoids. These fibers, together with type I collagen and fibronectin, reside between the endothelium and the hepatocytes (i.e. in the space of Disse). There is no proper basement membrane. Endothelial cells are fenestrated, allowing exchange of serum proteins, metabolites, and nutrients between blood and hepatocytes but restricting direct content with blood cells, chylomicrons, and microorganisms. Gordon and Sweet's reticulin, paraffin, × 150.

of Disse (Fig 15.11a & b). These cells are long-term residents. They are derived from circulating monocytes and their function is phagocytic—they destroy particulate matter, microorganisms, and damaged red blood cells. Kupffer cells very rapidly engulf almost all bacteria or worn-out red blood cells that happen to enter the blood sinusoids. Although rare, another sinusoidal lining cell is the pit cell, or natural killer T cell, which resembles the granular lymphocyte with natural killer activity; it possibly acts against viral infection and tumor metastasis, and patrols the sinusoids to monitor the presence of antigen.

Bile ducts

As previously mentioned, bile canaliculi are formed between apposed hepatocyte surface membranes (see Figs 15.3 & 15.5). They are tiny, intercellular spaces flanked by tight junctions and form small conduits around the hepatocytes, similar in arrangement to chicken wire mesh (see Fig 15.11a & b). Through linkages they drain toward the portal triads (Fig 15.12) and reach this destination via the canals of Hering, which are lined by cuboidal cells. Ultimately these bile ducts converge and then leave the liver in the system of ducts that carries bile to the gall bladder and from there to the duodenum.

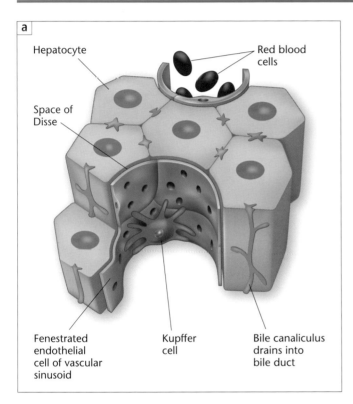

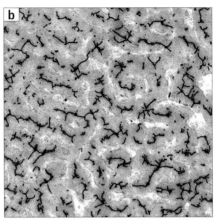

▲ **Fig 15.11b Bile canaliculi.** The tiny tunnel-like passageways between adjacent hepatocytes may be highlighted using histochemical methods specific for the metabolic properties associated with bile secretion. The canaliculi are alkaline phosphatase-positive and stain black. Note that the vascular sinusoids are unstained, the bile passageways being located centrally within plates of hepatocytes. Canaliculi drain bile away from the center of a lobule and form larger bile ductules within the portal triads. × 150. (Courtesy J Zbaeren, Inselspital, Bern, Switzerland).

▲ **Fig 15.11a Diagram of bile canaliculi.** The narrow canaliculi into which bile is secreted form a three-dimensional network of tubes that are interconnected. Osmotic pressure of the bile acids, phospholipids and other substances secreted by hepatocytes causes the flow of water into the canaliculi. Toward the periphery of a liver lobule, the bile passes into larger channels called canals of Hering, and then into the first of the bile ducts in portal triads.

Principal liver functions

Bile production

A major function of the liver with regard to digestion is the continuous production of bile, which is later concentrated and stored in the gall bladder and discharged, together with pancreatic secretions, into the duodenum. Bile contains numerous substances and, because these substances are secreted into a duct system, the biliary system constitutes an exocrine secretory mechanism. Of particular interest are bile acids (or bile salts) and bile pigment.

Bile salts are synthesized from cholesterol and act as emulsifying agents in the gut, where they facilitate the absorption of fats and are essential for absorption of fat-soluble vitamins across the gut mucosa. The bile salts are then absorbed by the terminal ileum and transported into the portal venous system. In this manner most of the bile salts are recycled back to the hepatocytes; the small fraction lost in the gut is replaced by de novo synthesis in the liver. Cholesterol and phospholipids, also present in bile, can likewise be recycled or removed via the gut.

The addition of bile pigments represents a mechanism by which the liver acts as a waste-disposal unit for the elimination of some of the breakdown products of worn-out red blood cells. Formation of bile pigments is a process that involves multiple steps. It commences with erythrocyte destruction by splenic macrophages and Kupffer cells. Briefly, part of the heme portion of the hemoglobin is converted to bilirubin, complexed to albumin, and released into the circulation and, in the case of the liver, into the vascular sinusoids. Hepatocytes take up bilirubin pigment, bind it to glucuronide, and excrete it into the biliary system, with a minor fraction released into the blood. Bile pigments are further altered in the bowel lumen and impart a characteristic color to the feces. If blood levels of bilirubin are abnormally high, jaundice—the distinctive yellowing of the skin—results.

General metabolic functions

Other substances eliminated or detoxified by the liver through the function of hepatocytes are steroid hormones and lipid-soluble drugs, which are degraded and passed to the bile. Alcohol is metabolized in the liver to acetaldehyde and acetate, with about 5% excreted unchanged in the urine, lungs, and skin. Some amino acids are broken down to ammonia, which is detoxified in the liver to form urea for elimination by the kidneys. Hepatocytes are the main cells producing plasma proteins (except immunoglobulins) such as albumin, clotting factors, the protein components of circulating lipoproteins, and the proteins that transport iron and copper.

The liver is the chief organ involved in lipid metabolism and the maintenance of lipid levels in blood. Lipids such as cholesterol, triglycerides, and phospholipids are synthesized in hepatocytes. Blood lipids are also derived from fat stores and from the diet. Some lipid is stored as fat droplets and some is directed into the bile, but much is released into blood as very low-density lipoprotein (VLDL), an important source of fatty acids for all other cells. Some fatty acids taken up by hepatocytes are converted to carbohydrates for energy.

Hepatocytes store iron, vitamin B_{12}, and folic acid, and they absorb blood glucose, which is stored as glycogen. The balance between stored glycogen and levels of blood glucose is regulated by insulin and glucagon from the pancreas. Insulin promotes glycogen synthesis; glucagon stimulates the degradation of glycogen into glucose available for release into the blood.

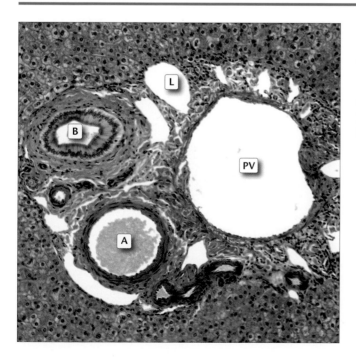

◄ **Fig 15.12 Blood and bile flow.** The portal triad is so named because it contains a portal venule (**PV**), hepatic arteriole (**A**), and a small bile duct (**B**). Often the number of hollow tubes is six or more. The vascular elements bring blood to the liver. The bile ducts receive bile from the bile canaliculi (channels between hepatocytes) with the bile flowing in the same direction as the lymph in lymphatic vessels (**L**) (i.e. in the opposite direction to that of the blood). H&E, paraffin, × 100.

GALL BLADDER

The gall bladder is a thin-walled hollow sac that performs several functions, namely:

- It acts as a reservoir for the bile produced by the liver.
- It concentrates the bile and adds a small quantity of mucus to it.
- It discharges its contents in response to the entry of fatty foods into the duodenum.

The histology of the gall bladder is simple (Fig 15.13a & b). It consists of a folded mucosa of simple columnar epithelial cells and underlying fibrovascular lamina propria; and a deeper muscularis with an external layer of supporting tissue with elastic fibers.

The outer, free surface is covered by serosa (i.e. peritoneum). The gall bladder lacks a muscularis mucosae and submucosa. Rokitansky–Aschoff sinuses are small diverticulations of the mucosa, variable in size and shape, and occasionally extending into the smooth muscle layer. The ducts of Luschka are isolated bile ducts in the subserosal connective tissue adjacent to the liver, but they do not open into the gall bladder lumen. Mucous glands of the lamina propria are found only in the neck of the gall bladder.

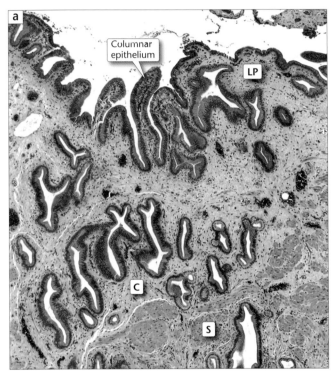

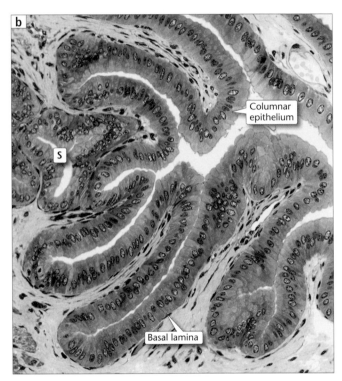

▲ **Fig 15.13a Gall bladder.** Mucosa of the gall bladder, showing folds lined by columnar epithelium with cores of lamina propria (**LP**). There is no muscularis mucosae or submucosa. Smooth muscle (**S**) is surrounded by loose connective tissue (**C**). Bile from the liver is stored and concentrated in the gall bladder. Cephalic and gastric phases of digestion stimulate initial emptying via vagal fibers to the muscle, which then contracts. Sympathetic innervation (by the celiac plexus) inhibits emptying. A strong stimulus for emptying occurs when fats and amino acids enter the duodenum; the duodenum releases the hormone cholecystokinin into the circulation, which causes muscle contraction. H&E, paraffin, × 50.

▲ **Fig 15.13b** Columnar epithelium of the gall bladder concentrates bile by absorbing electrolytes and water from the lumen that passes between the cells, across the basal lamina, and into capillaries of the lamina propria. Thus the daily production of bile by the liver (about 600 mL) is reduced in volume. There is cyclic emptying and refilling of the gall bladder, coupled to digestive and interdigestive phases. Invaginations of the surface epithelium, called Rokitansky–Aschoff sinuses (**S**), are normal; they may result from overdistension and excessive contractions of the gall bladder. H&E, acrylic resin, × 220.

About 90% of the volume of the hepatic bile is extracted within the gall bladder by absorption of sodium ions, chloride ions, and carbohydrate, followed by water. All these are transported across the epithelium into the blood vessels of the lamina propria. This activity is facilitated by a microvillus luminal surface for absorption and movement of fluids into the intercellular spaces between the epithelial cells, which expand markedly when bile is being concentrated. Bile is transported in the common bile duct.

Where it joins the pancreatic duct, the common bile duct is circumscribed by smooth muscle, the sphincter of Oddi (Fig 15.14). This is normally closed to prevent reflux of duodenal contents. When fatty substances enter the duodenum, endocrine cells of the duodenum release cholecystokinin, causing contraction of the wall of the gall bladder, relaxation of the sphincter of Oddi, and delivery of bile into the intestine.

PANCREAS

The chief structural features of the pancreas, when examined at low magnification, are its numerous lobules of acinar glands, large and small ducts located in the delicate supporting tissue septa, and the occasional circular or irregular clumps of cells that stain pink in hematoxylin and eosin sections (Fig 15.15). These pink-staining clumps of cells, collectively comprising 1–2% of the volume of the pancreas, are the islets of Langerhans—the endocrine component of the gland (see also discussion of the endocrine system, Ch 17).

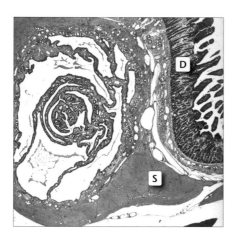

◀ **Fig 15.14 Vaterian system.** The junction of the bile duct and the pancreatic duct forms a common channel, called the ampulla of Vater, which opens into the duodenum (**D**). Surrounded by a muscular sphincter of Oddi (**S**), the epithelium shows long fronds or valvules resembling the oviduct or seminal vesicle. Sphincteric contractions regulate bile flow. Bile flow increases in response to cholecystokinin, which relaxes the sphincter. Azan, paraffin, × 20.

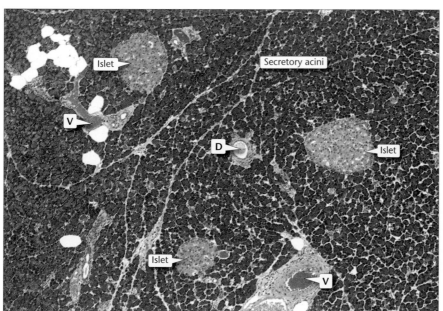

◀ **Fig 15.15 Pancreas and duct system.** The pancreas is a mixed exocrine–endocrine gland. The exocrine portion of secretory units (acini) forms the largest volume (85%); the ducts (**D**), vessels (**V**), and connective tissue make up about 12% of the volume; and the endocrine tissue—the globular islets of Langerhans—make up about 1–2%. The presence of the islets of Langerhans, variable in size but usually ovoid in shape, is one of several unique features of the pancreas that distinguish it from other similar exocrine glands, such as the lacrimal and parotid glands. H&E, paraffin, × 90.

Pancreatic acini

At higher magnification, the acinar or exocrine component is rather similar to that of the parotid gland, with basophilic cells containing apical granules clustered in groups, sometimes associated with a duct into which their enzyme-rich fluids are secreted. The unique and characteristic feature of the pancreatic acini, which differentiates the pancreas from all other exocrine glands, is the penetration of the duct cells into the central regions of the acini, which thus become intercalated and are designated as centroacinar cells (Fig 15.16a & b).

Traditionally the pancreatic acinus has been thought of as a terminal structure of the duct system, not unlike a bunch of grapes where each grape represents a cluster of exocrine cells secreting into a progressively larger and merging duct system.

However, in the human pancreas this is not the case; scanning electron microscopy and serial reconstruction studies show that acini may be tubular, with intercalated ducts emerging on opposite sides of acini, thereby forming an anastomosing and looping ductal system.

Pancreatic juice

The pancreatic juice secreted by the exocrine component contains over 20 digestive enzymes (including trypsinogens, protease, elastase, lipases, and numerous others collectively known as serine proteases), together with water and electrolytes. Approximately 1 liter of pancreatic juice is produced daily. The pancreas synthesizes and secretes more protein per gram of tissue than any other organ.

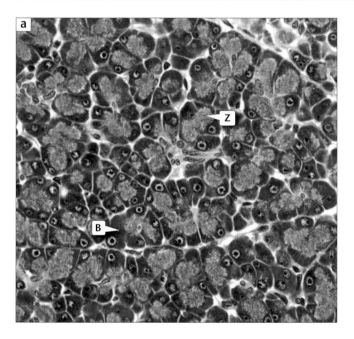

◀ **Fig 15.16a Pancreatic acini.** Acini, the enzyme-secreting units in the exocrine pancreas, are ovoid–elliptical clusters of glandular cells bordering a common luminal space. In hematoxylin and eosin sections, the basal cytoplasm (**B**) associated with the nuclei is deeply stained and shows a blue or purple color. This basophilia represents cisterns of rough endoplasmic reticulum. In the apical regions, pale-staining zymogen granules (**Z**), containing packages of inactive enzymes, face the narrow lumen. The supporting tissue is thin, composed of delicate strands of extracellular matrix and collagen. H&E, paraffin, × 250.

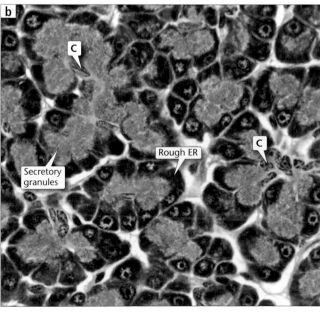

◀ **Fig 15.16b Pancreatic centroacinar cells.** Unique to the acinar complex are the centroacinar cells (**C**) which form the start of the pancreatic ducts, intercalated within the acini. Acini are not associated with myoepithelial cells commonly observed in other exocrine glands. In their absence, discharge of secretory granules from acinar cells is regulated by activation of cholecystokinin receptors on the acinar cells. H&E, paraffin, × 480.

Acinar cells are particularly basophilic owing to the enormous amount of rough endoplasmic reticulum that they contain. This endoplasmic reticulum synthesizes the enzymes, mostly in inactive form as zymogens. The zymogens are packaged and concentrated by the Golgi apparatus into condensing vacuoles. These vacuoles mature into the many zymogen granules positioned in the apex of the cell close to the lumen of the intercalated duct, into which they are discharged by exocytosis (Fig 15.17a–d).

Pancreatic juice entering the duodenum is devoid of proteolytic activity, but the duodenal mucosa synthesizes enteropeptidase, which specifically activates trypsinogen to trypsin. The latter is the trigger enzyme, and it activates all the pancreatic zymogens into enzymes essential for digestion. Secretion of alkaline fluid, rich in bicarbonate ions, originates from the duct system.

Release of pancreatic juice

Both components of pancreatic juice (zymogens and isotonic fluid) are secreted in response to a complex interaction between neural and humoral mediators, such as the sight, smell, and chewing of food together with stimulation of the secretory activities of the stomach and intestine. In the latter case, enteroendocrine cells in the duodenum release cholecystokinin and secretin into the blood; cholecystokinin stimulates the pancreas to secrete enzymes, and secretin stimulates the pancreas to secrete water and electrolytes.

Local or intrapancreatic stimulation also occurs, since a significant portion of the blood supply to the acini first passes through the islets of Langerhans, and thus the acini are exposed to blood that is rich in the hormones secreted by the islets. This arrangement is an endocrine–exocrine portal system, whereby insulin promotes the secretory activities of the acinar cells and glucagon inhibits them. Autonomic sympathetic and parasympathetic fibers are abundant in the pancreas, and ganglia within the interlobular supporting tissues and between acini are occasionally noted. Vagal stimulation induces some release of enzymes, but physiologically this is minor compared with humoral stimulation.

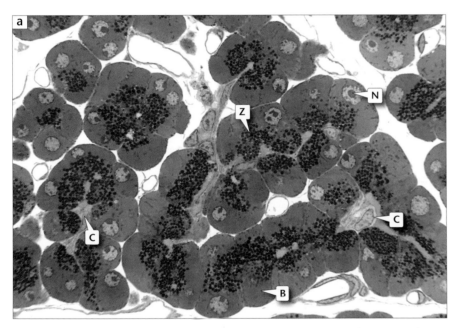

▲ **Fig 15.17a Acinar cells and secretions.** Thin epon resin section showing ovoid, elongated, and sinusoidal-type acini with centroacinar cells (**C**). Acinar cells contain nuclei (**N**) with prominent nucleoli (for ribosome production), deeply staining basal cytoplasm (**B**), indicating rough endoplasmic reticulum and protein synthesis, and many dense zymogen (**Z**) granules, which contain stored, mostly inactive digestive enzymes. Toluidine blue, araldite, × 600.

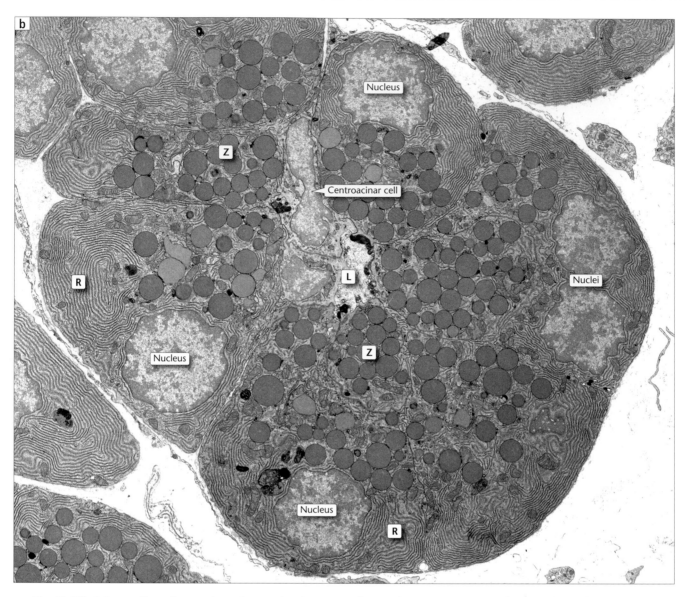

▲ **Fig 15.17b Acinar cells and secretions.** Pancreatic acinar cells have long served as model cells for studies of protein synthesis and secretion and, owing to their structural polarity, for analysis of the routes and compartmentalization of the molecules that are used in the assembly of enzymes from precursor amino acids. The nuclei show nucleoli and heterochromatin. The cytoplasm displays rough endoplasmic reticulum (**R**), and enzymes destined for the duodenum are stored in many zymogen granules (**Z**). During periods of minimal pancreatic secretion, the acinar lumen (**L**) is narrow. Large concentrations of zymogens and enzymes appear in the pancreatic duct within minutes of an appropriate stimulus, but in acinar cells synthesis of proteins from amino acids requires 1–2 hours. In order to deliver large amounts of digestive enzymes rapidly into the duodenum during food ingestion, the acinar cells store zymogen granules, the capacity of which greatly exceeds the biosynthetic abilities of the cells. × 5,000.

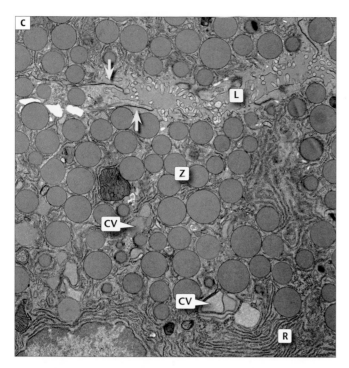

◀ **Fig 15.17c Secretory proteins pathway.** The pathway taken in the synthesis of secretory proteins involves pre-protein synthesis in the rough endoplasmic reticulum (**R**), transport through the Golgi complex, processing, sorting, and routing into condensing vacuoles (**CV**), and concentration into mature zymogen granules (**Z**), which contain about 20 different zymogens and enzymes. Zymogen granules accumulate in the apical cytoplasm, where the plasma membrane facing the lumen (**L**) shows microvilli projecting into electron-dense luminal material that contains discharged proteins following exocytosis of zymogen granules. Junctional complexes (**arrows**) provide for intercellular adhesion and seal off the acinar lumen from the intercellular space. × 6,400.

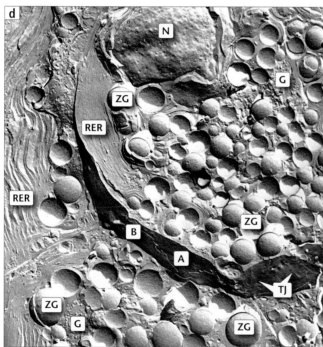

◀ **Fig 15.17d Freeze-fracture electron micrograph of a pancreatic exocrine cell.** After fixation and rapid freezing the tissue is broken along planes of fracture that often splits membranes into their inner and outer leaflets. A very thin platinum replica of the fracture surface is prepared and examined in the electron microscope. **A** and **B** = inner and outer leaflets of plasma membranes; **G** = Golgi; **N** = nucleus; **RER** = rough ER; **TJ** = tight junction; **ZG** = zymogen granules. × 5,000. (Courtesy L Orci, University Geneva; from Orci L & Perrelet A. Freeze-etch histology. Heidelberg: Springer-Verlag, 1975.)

Endocrine tissue of the pancreas

The endocrine pancreas consists of up to one million clusters or islets of hormone-secreting cells dispersed throughout the exocrine pancreas, an arrangement that facilitates local regulation of acinar cell function via an islet–acinar portal vascular system. Islets of Langerhans are complex structures with a rich vascular supply.

In H&E paraffin sections, the cells of the islets, which occur in numbers from dozens to scores in a single section, form lightly stained, compact masses with prominent capillaries (Fig 15.18a & b). Although in routine sections no evidence of cell heterogeneity is noted, the islets contain four major cell types:

- Beta cells, which secrete insulin, predominate and account for 70–80% of islet cells; they tend to occupy the core of islets.
- Alpha cells, which secrete glucagon, comprise 20–25% of islet cells, and lie mostly at the periphery.
- Delta cells are somatostatin-containing cells that make up about 5% of the islet cells and are sparsely scattered within the islet.
- Pancreatic polypeptide cells are rare, comprising only 1% of islet cells, and are found mostly at the periphery; they are also located in the exocrine pancreas.

A detailed discussion of the biology of islets of Langerhans is presented in Chapter 17.

Pancreatic hormones

Insulin plays a major role in the regulation of glucose and energy metabolism by promoting glucose uptake into cells and storage of glycogen in the liver and in skeletal muscle. Glucagon chiefly acts on the liver, where it stimulates glucose production from both glycogen breakdown and gluconeogenesis. Somatostatin suppresses insulin and glucagon release. Pancreatic polypeptide inhibits acinar exocrine secretion.

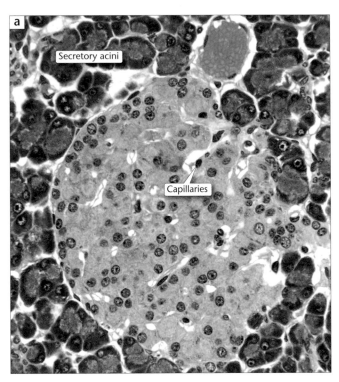

▲ **Fig 15.18a Islets of Langerhans.** Medium magnification of an islet, showing a compact mass of cells penetrated by a network of capillaries. Although islets contain four major individual cell types, these cannot readily be recognized in routine paraffin sections. During development of the pancreatic bud, islet cells and exocrine cells develop from two lineages of cells derived from endoderm. H&E, paraffin, × 220.

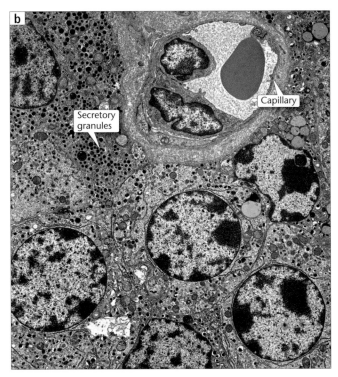

▲ **Fig 15.18b Ultrastructure of endocrine cells of an islet.** The cells contain many secretory granules, which contain hormones specific for the various types of endocrine cells. Granules such as those containing insulin or glucagon are discharged into blood vessels in response to changes in blood glucose and modulated by autonomic nerves. × 3,700.

ABNORMAL CONDITIONS AND CLINICAL FEATURES

Cirrhosis of the liver

Of all the disorders that may affect the liver, the two that are perhaps most widely recognized in the general population are cirrhosis and hepatitis. Cirrhosis is commonly believed to be an alcohol-induced liver disease, but in fact the most common cause of cirrhosis, worldwide, is chronic viral hepatitis (hepatitis C and hepatitis B virus infection). Alcohol is the next most common cause. Other causes include metabolic abnormalities, bile duct obstruction, drugs, and autoimmune disorders.

Much of the morbidity and mortality of cirrhosis is a consequence of portal hypertension (increased pressure in the portal venous system). In the cirrhotic liver, increased resistance to blood flow through the portal venous bed and sinusoids is a result of excess fibrous tissue, conversion of hepatic stellate cells to myofibroblasts, and hepatocyte hypertrophy causing sinusoidal narrowing. The collateral veins become swollen and esophageal varicosities may develop, and these may bleed. Diversion of blood from the gut past the liver may induce encephalopathy, and fluid accumulation in the peritoneal cavity (ascites).

Hepatitis

Hepatitis is characterized by inflammation, liver cell damage, and liver cell death. Hepatitis A, B, C, and D, cytomegalovirus, Epstein–Barr virus, and drugs may cause acute hepatitis. Liver function tests on serum biochemistry are abnormal, but the acute disease may be asymptomatic; alternatively it can cause severe illness and even death.

The liver usually returns to normal following resolution of the hepatitis. Chronic hepatitis can be caused by hepatitis B, C, and D infection, autoimmune hepatitis, alcohol, and a variety of drugs. Ongoing injury and abnormal regeneration of hepatocytes often leads to fibrosis and subsequent cirrhosis.

Other liver disorders

Steatosis (or fatty liver) is a common abnormality, with excess fat in the hepatocytes. It may lead to fibrosis or cirrhosis. It is associated with excessive alcohol consumption, obesity, diabetes, and some drugs.

Liver storage disease may occur if hepatocytes are deficient in those lysosomes that normally break down glycogen stored in the cell, and this may result in liver cell failure.

Cancer (or neoplasms) of the liver usually complicates cirrhosis of any cause, but it can occur in an otherwise normal liver. Treatment is unsatisfactory in most patients and, although in some instances resection may be beneficial, the prognosis is poor. Benign tumors (adenomas) are uncommon but are strongly associated with estrogen therapy. The relative risk of developing a benign adenoma is increased in users of combined estrogen–progestagen oral contraceptives but it remains an extremely rare condition.

Jaundice

Jaundice is a common presentation of liver disease. It is due either to the failure of hepatocytes to metabolize and excrete bilirubin, or to obstruction in the flow of bile from the liver (such as occurs when gall stones block the common bile duct). Jaundice, however, can also be a consequence of an increased load of bilirubin on the liver caused by, for example, excessive red cell destruction (hemolysis).

Disorders of the pancreas

Acute pancreatitis (inflammation) is characterized clinically by severe upper abdominal pain and vomiting, and it may be associated with circulatory collapse. In the affected pancreas there may be premature activation of the enzymes within the zymogen granules of the acinar cells. Autodigestion, hemorrhage, and infection may then occur. The two most common causes are gallstones in the common bile duct and alcohol.

Chronic pancreatitis has several causes and associations, but the most common is alcohol. It may manifest as chronic pain, exocrine deficiency causing fat malabsorption, or endocrine deficiency presenting as diabetes.

Neoplasms are usually adenocarcinomas and carry a poor prognosis.

Disorders of the gall bladder

Gallstones are a common disorder of the biliary system and result from excessive accumulation of cholesterol in the bile. Normally, cholesterol is made soluble in the bile by salts and lecithin, but increased cholesterol may crystallize and calcify into a stone or, if coupled with pigment, may form multiple stones. Gallstones are not harmful if confined to the gall bladder, but if they become located in the neck of the gall bladder they may obstruct the outflow and cause inflammation (cholecystitis). If they move into the bile ducts, they may cause pain, jaundice, and infection of the biliary tree (cholangitis).

Cancer of the gall bladder is uncommon; it is usually associated with gallstones and it is difficult to diagnose clinically.

Urinary system

The kidneys are glandular organs with both exocrine and endocrine properties; urine is the fluid secreted into a duct system, and renin and erythropoietin are hormones secreted into blood.

The individual's awareness of the function of the urinary system is limited mainly to the intermittent voiding of around 1–1.5 liters of urine per day. From a simplistic perspective, the function of the kidneys is to filter the blood that flows through them and to remove waste products, which are dissolved in that fraction of the filtrate excreted as urine (which is about 95% water). Collected and transported by the ureters, the accumulated urine is temporarily stored in the urinary bladder and, at various times, voided through the urethra. Put another way, a major function of the renal system is to balance the volume and composition of body water and electrolytes such that intake matches output, a function supplemented by excretion of metabolic wastes and foreign chemicals.

Together with the excretory functions served by respiration, gastrointestinal function, and sweat formation, the kidneys play a pivotal role in maintaining homeostasis; to achieve this, they perform a diverse array of functions that operate over a wide dynamic range. The net effect of this role is to compensate for diurnal variations in nutrient intake, particularly with regard to the availability of water. For example, when water intake is high, large quantities of very dilute urine are produced, with very low osmolarity; if water supply is restricted, small amounts of concentrated urine are excreted, with osmolarity greatly exceeding the osmolarity of plasma. In either case, the kidneys precisely regulate body fluid volumes and solute concentrations, and, importantly, many solutes are excreted independently of one another to ensure control of the composition of body fluids.

Major functions of the kidneys include:
- Regulation of water, electrolyte, and acid–base balance
- Regulation of body fluid osmolarity and electrolyte concentrations
- Regulation of arterial pressure
- Secretion of, and response to, hormones
- Excretion of metabolic wastes and xenobiotics.

With regard to the production of urine, the urinary system employs five processes. Four of these occur in the kidneys:

- Filtration of plasma
- Tubular reabsorption
- Tubular secretion
- Concentration.

The fifth is excretion of formed urine through the ureters, bladder, and urethra. The histologic and functional characteristics of the kidneys are heterogeneous, and a brief overview of kidney organization is appropriate to understand their basic function. Because the kidneys are so intimately involved with whole-body homeostasis (and renal failure or diseases are serious, often fatal, disorders), their physiology is accordingly complex. In this review only the major aspects are summarized; detailed discussions are available in physiology and nephrology texts.

ORGANIZATION OF THE KIDNEY

A coronal section through the human kidney reveals its association with the renal vessels and the commencement of the urinary tract, which comprises the renal pelvis and its continuation as the ureter. The substance of the kidney consists of a pale outer region—the cortex—about 1 cm in depth, and a darker inner region—the medulla—divided into 8–18 conical masses, termed renal pyramids (Fig 16.1a–c, pp 374–375). Each pyramid has its base at the corticomedullary boundary, and its apex extends toward the pelvis to form a papilla. From numerous small outlets in the papillae, urine drains into one of the expanded, cup-shaped outpouchings of the renal pelvis (i.e. the minor calyces), and then into one of the two or three larger major calyces.

Flanking each pyramid are downward extensions of cortex, called renal columns, and, together with the cap of cortex that overarches the base of each pyramid, these structures form the renal lobes, which are of anatomic more than functional significance. Renal columns provide a route whereby the renal arterial vessels subdivide and extend around each pyramid; at the corticomedullary junction, arcuate arteries diverge at right angles to supply cortical tissue, and a series of capillary networks also reaches the outer medulla. The inner medulla is supplied by long extensions of cortical arterioles, called vasa recta (histologically, large capillaries), which at various levels in the medulla form hairpin turns that contribute to ascending vasa recta, and drain into venous vessels at the corticomedullary junction. Vasa recta play an important role in maintaining a salinity gradient (discussed below).

The division of the kidney into a cortex of granular appearance and a medulla of striated appearance is mainly a reflection of the position and morphology of the individual tubules that are the functional units of the organ. How these elements perform their function of producing urine is discussed first through a description of their histology and second through a review of the principal functions.

Nephron

The nephron is the functional unit of the kidney, and is essentially a blind-ending, epithelial-lined hollow tubule that commonly originates in the renal cortex and terminates by emptying into the collecting duct system. Collecting ducts may receive distal tubules from several nephrons and the ducts join together to form openings or tiny orifices at the papillary tip of a pyramid (Fig 16.1c). In terms of histologic and functional organization, each nephron is divided into

segments that, together with a collecting duct, form a uriniferous tubule. During the development of the kidney, the nephron, strictly speaking, is that portion of the whole uriniferous tubule that arises from metanephric tissue (Fig 16.2a–c). Definitively, each nephron consists of the renal corpuscle (glomerulus and Bowman's capsule), the proximal convoluted tubule, the loop of Henle, the distal convoluted tubule, and the connecting tubule. The latter continues into the collecting duct (ending at the papilla), which is developed from the ureteric bud. Since these segments are functionally interrelated, some authorities consider a nephron to include the collecting duct.

In simple terms, the way nephrons work is that a filtrate of blood plasma is introduced into the lumen of the blind end of the tubule (the renal corpuscle) and, by a complex series of reabsorptions, secretions, and exchange of luminal contents with the supporting interstitial cells and blood vessels, urine emerges from the collecting ducts. This role necessitates many nephrons in each kidney; at times estimates have been up to 1.5 million, but based upon recent morphometric data the average is probably 600,000

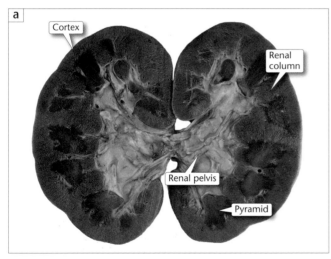

▲ **Fig 16.1a Anatomy of the kidney.** Bisected in the coronal plane, the internal morphology of the kidney reveals an outer cortex (colored brown) that borders medullary pyramids (darker brown) with their apices pointing toward the central renal pelvis. Between these structures the renal columns extend deeply to the pelvis. The renal pelvis shows a wide, funnel-shaped tube that is continuous with the ureter and in the medullary region gives tubular branches that terminate at the pyramid apices (papillae) as cup-shaped calices. Into these urine is collected when it drains from the papillae. The pelvis contains fatty tissue and neurovascular structures.

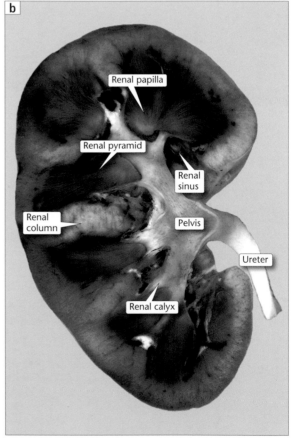

▲ **Fig 16.1b Section through the kidney,** showing the relationship between urine-forming tissues and the urine collection system. Renal pyramids are striated owing to longitudinal columns of blood vessels and tubules of the urine filtration system. Papillae point toward the calyces of the renal pelvis, which merge at the hilum to form the ureter, which exits the kidney.

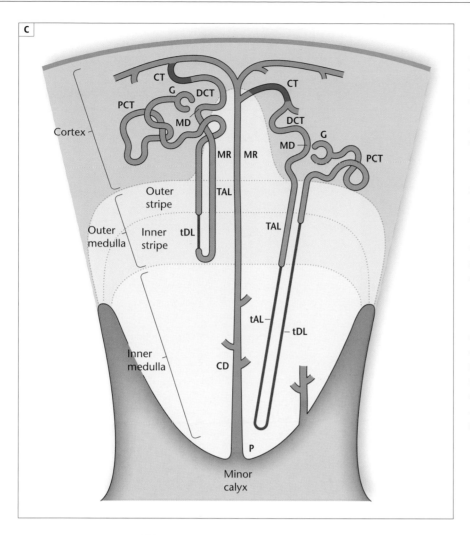

◀ Fig 16.1c Organization of a renal pyramid. In humans, the renal pyramids are conical masses of tissue within the medulla, with their tips projecting toward the minor calyx, into which urine flows. The base comprises a cap of cortical tissue, where most nephrons originate. The medulla is divided into an inner and outer zone, and the outer zone is further subdivided into inner and outer stripes. The outer stripe does not contain thin tubules, whereas the inner stripe contains the hairpin turns of short-looped nephrons and vascular bundles of capillaries (not shown) that supply the inner medulla. Commencing with the glomerulus (**G**) in the renal corpuscle, the nephron shows the following segments: proximal convoluted tubule (**PCT**); thin descending limb of Henle's loop (**tDL**); thin ascending limb of Henle's loop (**tAL**); thick ascending limb of Henle's loop (**TAL**); macula densa of thick ascending limb (**MD**); distal convoluted tubule (**DCT**); connecting tubule (**CT**); collecting duct (**CD**); papilla (**P**). The medullary rays (**MR**), actually in the cortex, contain the straight parts of the proximal and distal tubules and of the collecting ducts, all of which extend into the medulla.

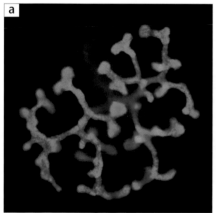

▲ Fig 16.2a Developing kidney
Fluorescence micrograph of early branching morphogenesis of a fetal kidney, showing multiple branches of the epithelial cells that have derived from the ureteric bud. As the bud grows at its tips, it induces the differentiation of the renal corpuscles and tubules (not shown). The ureteric bud becomes the collecting ducts. × 500.

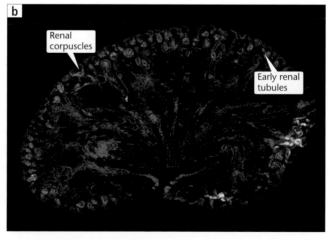

▲ Fig 16.2b Developing kidney. Fluorescence micrograph of fetal mouse kidney showing cortical distribution of developing renal corpuscles (yellow–orange) located at the distal tips of the branches of the ureteric bud. Tubules of growing collecting ducts are red. × 40. (Courtesy HT Cheng and R Kopan, Washington University, St Louis, USA.)

(range 0.3–1 million). Although mostly convoluted in the cortex, and partly straight in the medulla, nephrons are not short tubules. Depending on their location and the length of the loop of Henle, the average length of a nephron is about 4 cm; thus, the total length of all nephrons in two kidneys is perhaps 50 km. The commencement of a nephron is the renal corpuscle, described below. Renal corpuscles are located in the cortex, and nephrons can be found throughout this region, including those in

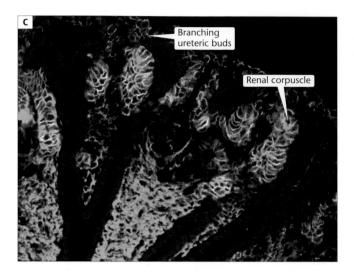

◀ **Fig 16.2c Detail of developing renal corpuscles**, showing aggregation of epithelial cells with E-cadherin (yellow). These very early cell condensates grow at the tips of the branches of the ureteric buds (cells stained red). × 400. (Courtesy R Kopan, Washington University, St Louis, USA; from Cheng HT, et al. Development 2007; 134:801–811.)

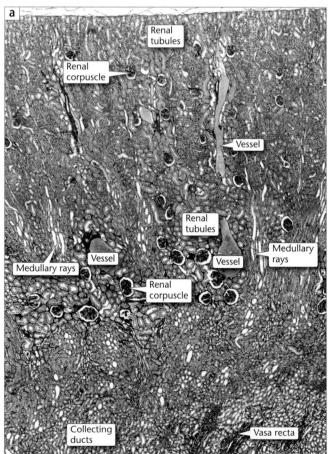

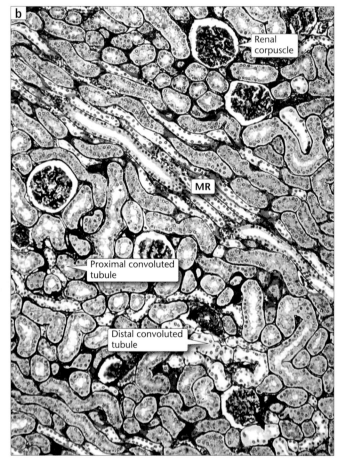

▲ **Fig 16.3a Renal cortex and medulla.** The cortex contains renal corpuscles, renal tubules, blood vessels, and medullary rays. In the medulla are many tubules of the loops of Henle and collecting ducts, sectioned in transverse, oblique, and longitudinal planes. Islands of medullary capillaries, the vasa recta, are shown. PAS, paraffin, × 20.

▲ **Fig 16.3b Renal cortex.** Scattered renal corpuscles are surrounded by tightly packed renal tubules, mostly proximal convoluted tubules and fewer distal convoluted tubules, which usually have a wider lumen, but are smaller in overall diameter. Part of a medullary ray (**MR**) is visible, and contains straight segments of proximal and distal renal tubules, and collecting ducts. All these components are supported by the interstitial tissue. Hematoxylin & eosin (H&E)/silver, paraffin, × 60.

juxtamedullary locations (Fig 16.3a & b). Two main populations of nephrons are recognized according to the length of the loop of Henle (see Fig 16.1c). Generally, nephrons that originate from superficial or midcortical regions have short loops that bend back in the outer medulla. Juxtamedullary nephrons have long loops with hairpin turns in the inner medulla. Short-looped nephrons outnumber long-looped nephrons by 7 to 1. A few nephrons have loops of Henle that do not enter the medulla.

> **Tip:** The number of nephrons (or glomeruli) formed in the fetal kidney is the maximum number made for the rest of life. Loss or dysfunction of nephrons by disease or damage is irreversible, as they are unable to regenerate.

Renal corpuscle

The renal corpuscle, on average 200 µm in diameter, is commonly known as a glomerulus, and consists of the dilated, blind-ending proximal part of a renal tubule, into which is invaginated a tuft of branched capillaries derived from an associated afferent arteriole (Fig 16.4a & b). The glomerulus proper is this tuft of capillaries; blood passes along these vessels

and emerges as an efferent arteriole that goes on to supply capillary beds and the vasa recta. The entry point of the glomerulus is known as the vascular pole of the renal corpuscle (Fig 16.5a–d).

By invaginating into the pouch-like expanded renal tubule, the glomerulus is covered by a thin, specialized layer of epithelial cells (similar to the effect of pushing a fist into a balloon). This inner or visceral layer turns back at the vascular pole and forms an outer or parietal epithelial layer in continuity with the cuboidal cells of the renal tubule. The lumen of the renal tubule, therefore, is molded to accommodate the glomerulus and forms a cup-shaped hollow space around the capillaries. This narrow cavity is called Bowman's space (or urinary or capsular space), and its visceral and parietal layers are referred to as Bowman's capsule (Fig 16.6a–c, p 379). Continuity of Bowman's space with the renal tubule lumen marks the urinary pole and is located opposite the vascular pole (Fig 16.7, p 379). Plasma that circulates through the glomerulus is filtered into Bowman's space to form a so-called ultrafiltrate, because molecules within the plasma with a radius > 4 nm or mass > 70 kDa are normally excluded from filtration. Negatively charged, large molecules are also hindered in the filtration process.

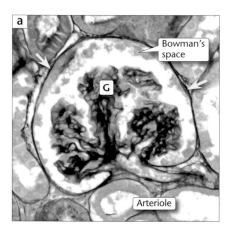

▲ **Fig 16.4a Polarity of renal corpuscles.** Afferent arteriole enters the vascular pole of a renal corpuscle and branches to form capillaries of the glomerulus (**G**). Note Bowman's space and parietal layer of Bowman's capsule (**arrows**). Silver/azure A, paraffin, × 210.

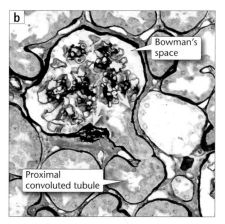

▲ **Fig 16.4b Urinary pole.** The continuity of the renal corpuscle with the proximal convoluted tubule marks the urinary pole. Note that the cuboidal epithelium of the tubule changes to squamous epithelium (**arrows**) of Bowman's capsule. H&E/silver, paraffin, × 175.

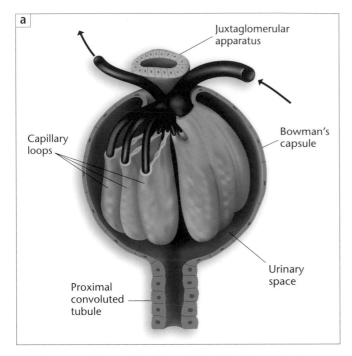

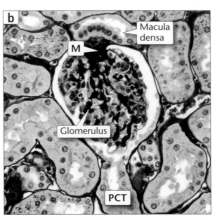

▲ **Fig 16.5b Origin of glomerulus.**
Renal corpuscle showing origin of glomerulus from the vascular pole, which contains a clump of mesangial cells (**M**) adjacent to the macula densa of the distal convoluted tubule. A decrease in Na+ or Cl− delivery through the tubule stimulates renin release from the juxtaglomerular apparatus (which may possibly involve the mesangial cells). Renin induces angiotensin II formation in blood, which (as a vasoconstrictor) may preferentially constrict efferent arterioles to adjust the glomerular filtration rate; the ultrafiltrate flows into the proximal convoluted tubule (**PCT**) at the urinary pole. H&E/silver, paraffin, × 175.

▲ **Fig 16.5a Glomerulus.** About 30 capillary loops arise from the afferent arteriole and invaginate into the sac formed by the terminal end of the proximal tubule. The outer wall of the sac is Bowman's capsule; the inner wall is applied to the capillary loops. The space in which provisional urine is formed is Bowman's space. The mesangium (modified pericytes) and macula densa (special distal tubule cells) are part of the juxtaglomerular apparatus, which contributes to control of blood flow and glomerular filtration.

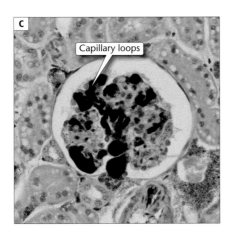

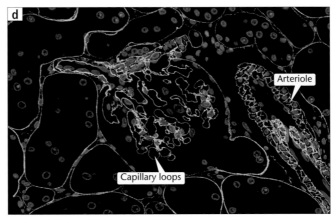

▲ **Fig 16.5c Capillary loops.**
Demonstration of the capillary loops of the glomerulus following infusion of a red dye into the arterial system. The cells between and surrounding the vessels comprise mesangial cells and podocytes. Paraffin, × 175.

▲ **Fig 16.5d Renal corpuscle.** Fluorescence micrograph of a renal corpuscle, surrounding renal tubules, and an arteriole, showing distribution of laminin—a component of basal laminae. Note the convoluted laminin of the capillary loops of the glomerulus, reflecting the large surface area of the fused basal laminae of the capillary endothelia and podocytes. Cell nuclei stained blue. Acrylic resin, × 175. (Courtesy J Zbaeren, Inselspital, Bern, Switzerland.)

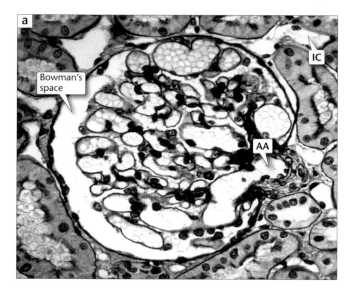

▲ **Fig 16.6a Bowman's space and glomerulus.** Glomerulus stained with the periodic acid–Schiff reaction for carbohydrates shows red-stained basal laminae of the capillary loops, which are part of the permeability barrier for filtration of plasma. Note afferent arteriole (**AA**) and interstitial capillaries (**IC**). Bowman's space is located between the parietal and visceral layers of Bowman's capsule. PAS/haematoxylin, acrylic resin, × 300.

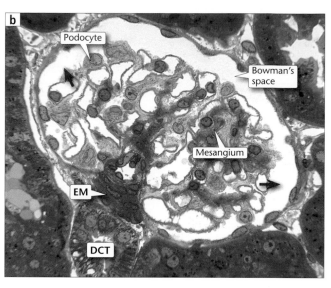

▲ **Fig 16.6b Bowman's space.** Note podocytes attached to glomerular capillaries, and the mesangial cells that provide support and are associated with extracellular matrix. Filtrate of blood plasma is filtered from the capillaries into Bowman's space in the direction of the arrows. Part of the distal convoluted tubule (**DCT**) and extraglomerular mesangium (**EM**) are indicated. Toluidine blue, araldite, × 390.

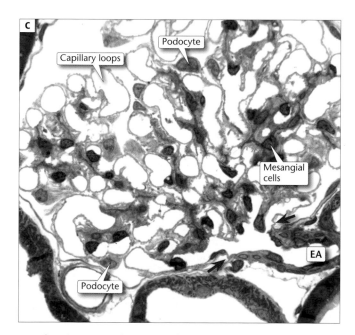

▲ **Fig 16.6c Vascular network.** The capillary loops are branched to form a vascular network that drains into the efferent arteriole (**EA**). The parietal layer of Bowman's capsule is reflected (**arrows**) to form the visceral layer, which gives rise to podocytes. Mesangial cells may modify capillary size or shape, and phagocytose matrix and foreign material trapped in the glomerulus. Toluidine blue, araldite, × 500.

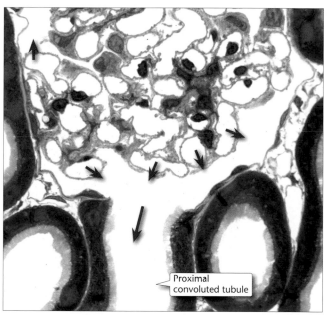

▲ **Fig 16.7 Urinary pole of the renal corpuscle**, showing the exit route (**large arrow**) of the ultrafiltrate formed as plasma is filtered across the capillaries (**small arrows**) into Bowman's space. The proximal convoluted tubule shows a brush border of microvilli, which indicates its absorptive function. The filtration rate is largely determined by capillary pressure. The composition of ultrafiltrate is very similar to that of plasma, but protein concentration is extremely low, despite glomerular capillaries being 100 times more permeable than other capillaries. Toluidine blue, araldite, × 500.

Cells of the visceral layer of Bowman's capsule, intimately associated with the capillaries, are called podocytes (Fig 16.8a–c). These are highly specialized epithelial cells with long cytoplasmic processes that wrap around the capillary loops. From their numerous branches arise very many foot processes, or pedicles, that interdigitate with foot processes from other podocytes (resembling the effect of interdigitating the fingers of each hand). Foot processes make contact with the thickened basal lamina of the capillary endothelial cells, and the narrow space between processes—the filtration slit—is bridged by a membranous slit diaphragm adjacent to the basal lamina. On the opposite aspect of the basal lamina

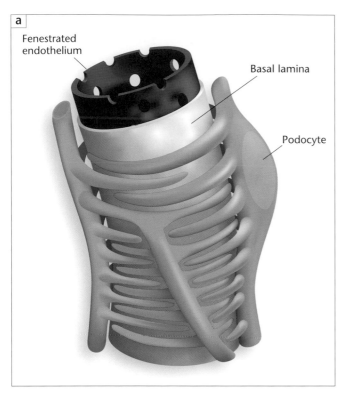

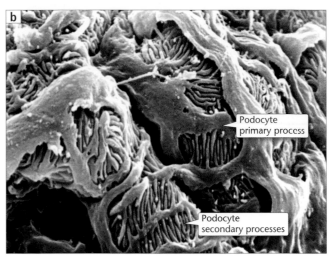

▲ **Fig 16.8b Podocytes.** Scanning electron micrograph of the external surface of the glomerulus showing how the capillaries are invisible because of the overlying podocytes. These cells have broad primary processes, from which arise many slender secondary processes that alternately interdigitate upon the underlying capillaries. × 13,000.

▲ **Fig 16.8a Podocytes.** Diagram of part of a glomerular fenestrated capillary with relatively large pores about up to 100 nm in diameter. The basal lamina is a fusion between the extracellular matrix made by the capillary and the finger-like extensions, called foot processes of podocytes, that interdigitate and embrace the vessel walls.

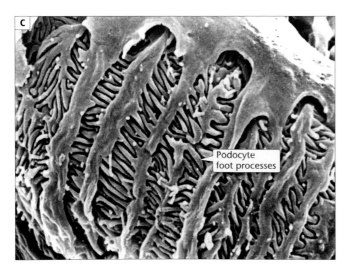

◀ **Fig 16.8c Foot processes.** Scanning electron micrograph of foot processes of podocytes. The curvature is due to the cylindrical shape of the deeper capillary to which the podocytes are applied. The slits between foot processes are the passageways through which the filtrate of blood plasma will pass and enter Bowman's space. These gaps are not open but are bridged by very small diaphragms not resolvable in this image. × 20,000.

is the thin, fenestrated endothelium of the capillaries (Fig 16.9a & b). The association of foot processes and their slit diaphragms, basal lamina (commonly called the glomerular basement membrane GBM), and fenestrated endothelium comprises the structural basis for glomerular filtration, which separates blood from the ultrafiltrate in Bowman's space. Although each component contributes to the selection filtration properties of this barrier, the podocyte slit diaphragm is believed to be the principal structure responsible for the permeability properties of the glomerulus.

The central region of the glomerulus is occupied by the mesangium, a supporting framework of connective tissue made up of mesangial cells and the extracellular matrix they secrete. These cells resemble pericytes of conventional capillaries and have contractile and phagocytic properties. Their ability to respond to vasoactive agents suggests that mesangial cells may modify glomerular blood flow or surface area (the total filtration surface area of all glomeruli in a pair of kidneys is estimated to be equivalent to a square with 50 cm sides). Immune complexes may be phagocytosed by mesangial cells and, together with increased production of mesangial matrix, may contribute to glomerular dysfunction. Extraglomerular mesangial cells (also called lacis cells, or cells of Goormaghtigh) form an outward extension from the mesangium, located in the angle between the afferent and efferent arterioles; they are a component of the juxtaglomerular apparatus (described later in this chapter).

Tip: The molecular filter of blood passing through the renal corpuscle is chiefly the slit diaphragm between podocyte foot processes, assisted by the glomerular endothelial cells and the glomerular basement membrane.

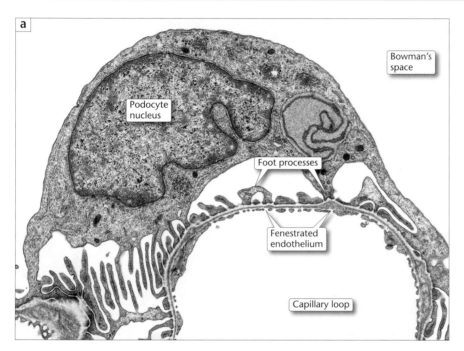

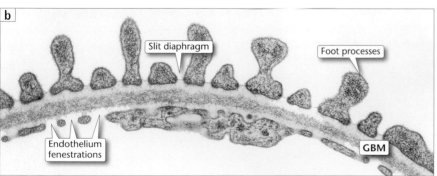

◀ **Fig 16.9a Glomerular filter.** Ultrastructure of a podocyte showing its many cytoplasmic extensions, which terminate as foot processes that attach to the basal lamina between them and the endothelium of the glomerular capillary. Gaps between the podocyte foot processes and pores in the capillary endothelium are components of the glomerular filter. × 13,000. (Courtesy H Pavenstadt, University Hospital, Freiburg, Germany, and W Kriz, University of Heidelberg, Germany.)

Fig 16.9b Ultrastructure of the glomerular filter, which consists of the porous endothelial fenestrations, the glomerular basal membrane (**GBM**), and the podocyte foot processes with interposed slit membranes. Foot processes are stabilized by actin. The slit membrane is a size-selective molecular sieve diaphragm containing podocin and a cadherin-type protein, as well as nephrin protein (a member of the immunoglobulin superfamily of adhesion molecules). The slit diaphragm may consist of two to three layers of proteins organized as molecular strands, like a zipper. Charged molecules are filtered by endothelium and the GBM; molecule mass and shape is selectively filtered by the GBM and filtration slit diaphragms. × 56,000. (Courtesy H Pavenstadt, University Hospital, Freiburg, Germany, and W Kriz, University of Heidelberg, Germany.)

Proximal tubule

Arising from Bowman's capsule, the proximal tubule is at first highly convoluted in the cortex, and becomes straight or slightly spiral as it passes through a medullary ray toward the outer medulla. Its average length is 14 mm. In histologic section, the tubules in the cortex are abundant and present circular, oblong, or U-shaped profiles characterized by a simple cuboidal epithelium with a brush border of tall microvilli (Fig 16.10a & b). After immersion fixation, the lumen is relatively narrow. Ultrastructural analysis reveals large numbers of mitochondria, and the basolateral plasma membrane is deeply folded or invaginated into the cell cytoplasm, which greatly increases the surface area compared to a non-folded membrane (similar to the apical surface area created by the microvilli). The main function of the proximal tubule, reflected in its structure, is the reabsorption of fluid and solutes that pass along it.

Loop of Henle

Passing through the corticomedullary region (Fig 16.11a & b) and entering the outer medulla, the proximal tubule shows an abrupt transition into the descending thin limb of Henle's loop, in which the lining epithelial cells are flat, with nuclei that protrude into the lumen (Fig 16.12). This appearance persists in those loops that turn back to form thin, ascending limbs. Depending on whether a nephron has a short or long loop of Henle, the thin limbs are 1–10 mm in length. Thin limbs have special permeability properties that are very important for the maintenance of a hypertonic medulla and for the urine concentrating mechanism.

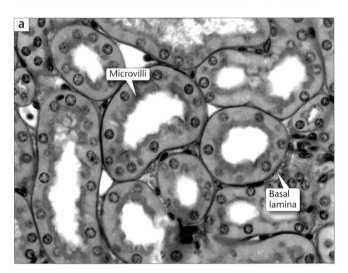

◀ **Fig 16.10a Proximal convoluted tubules**, showing carbohydrate-rich basal laminae and the microvilli. The brush border enhances reabsorption of fluid and solutes from the lumen through or between the cuboidal epithelial cells and into capillaries. These tubules also secrete organic bases and H^+ into the lumen. The brush border of microvilli enables the tubules to reabsorb about 70% of the glomerular filtrate. The membrane contains Na^+, H^+, and Cl^- antiport exchangers and enzymes that digest small amino acids. PAS/haematoxylin, paraffin, × 300.

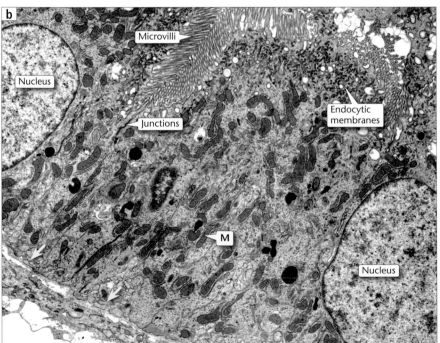

◀ **Fig 16.10b Ultrastructure of proximal convoluted tubule**, showing microvilli, intercellular junctions, mitochondria (**M**) for energy supply, and infolded basal membrane (**arrows**), which contains Na^+, K^+-adenosine triphosphatase complexes that pump Na^+ out of the cell and transport glucose and amino acids. The ionic gradient draws water from the lumen. Endocytic membranes and vacuoles reabsorb and digest proteins of low molecular weight, which (as amino acids) are returned to the peritubular capillaries. × 5,300.

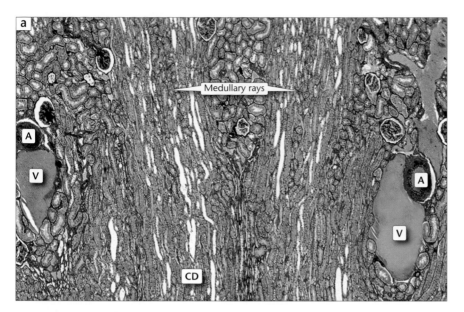

◀ Fig 16.11a Corticomedullary region. Medullary rays extend upward from the cortex into the medulla, and contain straight parts of proximal and distal tubules and collecting ducts (**CD**) with wide lumens. The arteries (**A**) and veins (**V**) are related to arcuate vessels that arise at the corticomedullary junction. Medullary rays are prominent because they provide the route by which the descending and ascending limbs of the loop of Henle reach the inner medulla. Juxtamedullary nephrons have the longest loops, but in the human kidney most cortical nephrons have relatively short loops. Methylene blue–silver, paraffin, × 35.

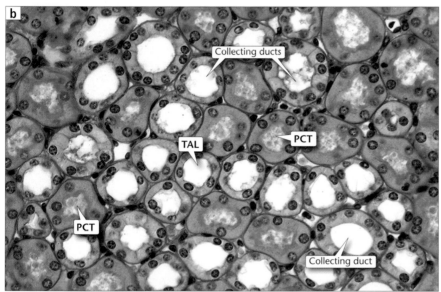

◀ Fig 16.11b Transverse section through a medullary ray, that shows collecting ducts with distinct cell outlines, straight portions (pars recta) of proximal tubules (**PCT**; note brush border), and thick ascending limbs (**TAL**) of the loop of Henle. The TAL extrudes Na^+ into the interstitium but is impermeable to water, so the osmolarity of the tubular fluid decreases as it approaches the cortex and the distal tubule. PAS/hematoxylin, paraffin, × 210.

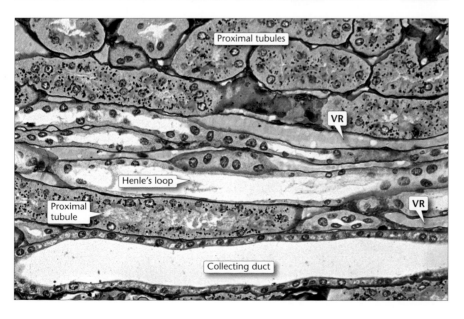

◀ Fig 16.12 Loop of Henle. The limbs of Henle's loop are recognized by association of thin-walled tubules and parallel capillaries that represent ascending and descending vasa recta (**VR**). Renal tubules, if not collapsed or shrunken, show a lumen, whereas the capillaries contain plasma and erythrocytes. By comparison, a collecting duct is a much wider part of the uriniferous tubule. Proximal tubules that belong to other nephrons are indicated. Methylene blue–silver, paraffin, × 200.

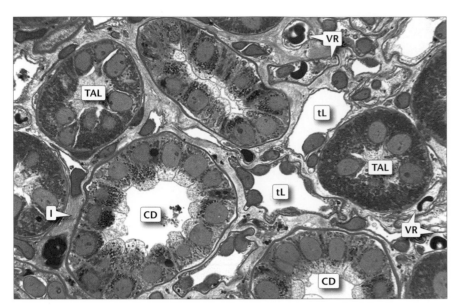

◀ **Fig 16.13 Ascending and descending limbs.** Close relationship between collecting ducts (**CD**), thick ascending limbs (**TAL**), and thin limbs (**tL**) of the loop of Henle and the peritubular capillaries, or vasa recta (**VR**). Water moves from thin limbs to interstitium (**I**) in response to the high osmolarity of the interstitial region created by Na+ movement from the TAL, the cells of which contain many mitochondria to energize the active transport of Na+ through the base of the tubule. Collecting ducts reabsorb water from lumen to interstitium in response to antidiuretic hormone. Toluidine blue, araldite, × 700.

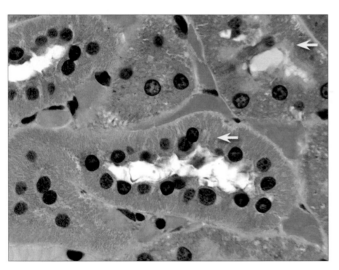

◀ **Fig 16.14 Distal convoluted tubule.** These tubules have no brush border, but their numerous mitochondria (**arrows**) provide the adenosine triphosphate necessary for active transport of NaCl reabsorbed from luminal fluid, which amounts to 5–10% of the filtered load of NaCl. This nephron segment, although relatively impermeable to water, is not homogeneous in either morphology or function, and is a transitional tubule that leads to the connecting segment or tubule. H&E, paraffin, × 490.

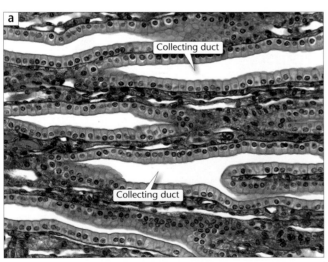

▲ **Fig 16.15a Collecting ducts.** Longitudinal section of collecting ducts, showing orderly cuboidal epithelium and prominent plasma membrane borders between cells. These ducts reabsorb water and urea and partly determine urine volume and concentration. Permeability is regulated by antidiuretic hormone, and also aldosterone. H&E/alcian blue, paraffin, × 175.

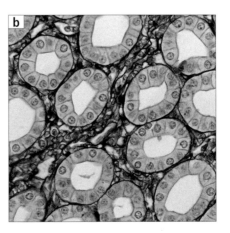

▲ **Fig 16.15b Collecting ducts.** Transverse section through the inner medulla, showing many collecting ducts with wide lumens. In the interstitium are medullary interstitial cells that support a rich vascular plexus of capillary loops and the thin limbs of the loop of Henle. Collecting ducts are permeable to water in the presence of antidiuretic hormone, which also increases urea permeability; the urea is recycled in the nephron and contributes to the high osmolarity of the inner medulla. PAS/hematoxylin, paraffin, × 230.

Distal tubule

Distal tubules are composed of three histologically distinct segments:
- Thick, ascending limb of Henle's loop
- Macula densa
- Distal convoluted tubule.

The transition from thin to thick ascending limbs (tAL to TAL) is recognized by the appearance in the latter segment of low cuboidal cells (Fig 16.13) and, at the ultrastructural level, by abundant mitochondria and invaginations of basolateral membrane. These features are associated with active transport mechanisms in which salt is reabsorbed into the interstitium, to produce a dilute tubule fluid and hypertonic interstitium. The ascending thick limb extends upward toward the cortex and returns to the parent renal corpuscle; at the contact point with the extraglomerular mesangial region, the cells are narrow and clustered side by side to form the macula densa. This structure is a type of chemoreceptor that monitors luminal Cl⁻ concentration and is involved with adjustment of the glomerular filtration rate (GFR). Beyond the macula densa is the distal convoluted tubule, characterized (compared with proximal tubules) by lower height of the cuboidal epithelium, no brush border of microvilli, and usually a wider lumen (Fig 16.14).

The combined length of the TAL and distal tubule is about 15 mm. Distal convoluted tubules are relatively impermeable to water, but reabsorb NaCl.

Connecting tubule and collecting duct

Connecting tubules represent transitional segments between distal convoluted tubules and the long collecting ducts that extend to the papillary region of the renal pyramid. Some nephrons drain directly into a single connecting tubule, whereas others join together and form arcades of this segment. Cortical collecting ducts show a cuboidal cell lining which becomes taller, to form columnar cells, as the ducts descend through the medulla (Fig 16.15a & b). Cortical ducts consist of pale-staining principal cells (which reabsorb Na⁺ and water) and darker-staining intercalated cells (proton and HCO_3^- secretion); this second cell type disappears in medullary parts of the duct. At the papilla, collecting ducts expand in diameter (to more than 100 µm) to form the ducts of Bellini, identified by tall columnar cells with lumina that open onto the surface of the papilla (Fig 16.16a & b). Urine emerging from the papilla enters the space created by the associated renal calyx (numbers of calyces form the large renal pelvis that is the

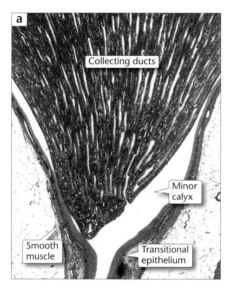

▲ **Fig 16.16a Renal papilla.** Low magnification of a papilla with apex projecting into the lumen of a minor calyx. The external wall of the calyx has smooth muscle that is continuous distally with the wall of the ureter, but proximally it extends into the medullary region. Here it meets the wall of the pyramid and encircles its base (the Ringmuskel der Papille). Coordinated peristaltic contraction of this smooth muscle exerts a rhythmic pumping action on the renal medulla, a function that promotes emptying of tubules in the papilla (first proposed in 1862 by Henle). H&E/alcian blue, paraffin, × 25.

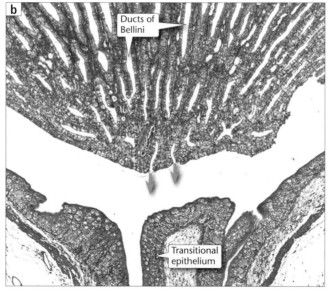

▲ **Fig 16.16b Section through the apex of a renal pyramid.** Collecting ducts terminate, with prior fusions, at a papilla to form wide ducts (of Bellini), which open, sieve-like (**arrows**), at the area cribosa. The cavity of the minor calyx is lined by transitional epithelium and conveys urine from the papilla to the renal pelvis. The papillae are thought to work as pumps through alternating pressures that are generated by peristaltic contractions of the calyces of the renal pelvic wall. H&E, paraffin, × 30.

funnel-shaped commencement of the ureter). The renal pelvis is not a rigid and motionless hollow space but, because of smooth muscle in the walls of the calyces and pelvis, it exhibits peristaltic contractions, normally at a rate of 2–3/minute in the human. In response to circulating levels of antidiuretic hormone (ADH, from the hypothalamic–posterior pituitary system), a major function of the collecting ducts is to control the reabsorption of water, which determines urine volume and concentration.

Juxtaglomerular apparatus

The juxtaglomerular apparatus consists of three components:
- Macula densa, described earlier in the text
- Juxtaglomerular cells in the wall of the afferent arteriole, which supply the glomerulus
- Extraglomerular mesangial cells in the cleft formed between afferent and efferent arterioles, also mentioned earlier.

Macula densa cells are believed to respond to NaCl concentrations in the distal tubule, and in turn regulate the release of renin from granules in the juxtaglomerular cells, which resemble myoepithelial cells. Renin is a participant in the renin–angiotensin system (RAS), the physiologic role of which is to regulate glomerular filtration and increase renal tubular reabsorption of Na$^+$ and water. The RAS controls body fluid homeostasis in response to a fall in blood pressure. At present the role of the extraglomerular mesangial cells is unclear. The juxtaglomerular apparatus may be influenced by sympathetic innervation to the afferent arteriole, causing constriction, and reduction in GFR and urine production.

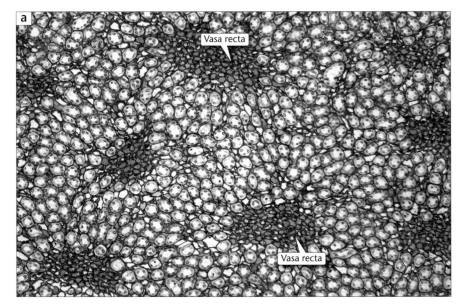

◀ **Fig 16.17a Vasa recta.** Vasa recta are columns of capillaries that are prominent in the medulla. They are comprised of descending vessels that originate from glomerular efferent arterioles that extend into the inner medulla, and return as venous or ascending vessels that drain into corticomedullary veins. In the outer medulla, the vasa recta form vascular bundles, mainly surrounded by thick and thin limbs of Henle's loop. Methylene blue/silver, paraffin, × 50.

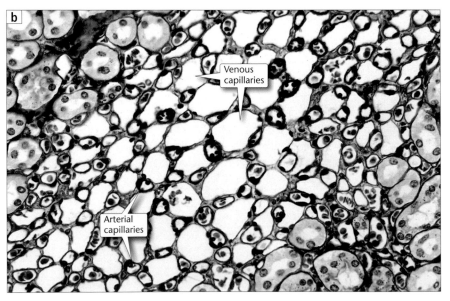

◀ **Fig 16.17b Vasa recta.** The vasa recta have a slow blood flow and operate a countercurrent exchange mechanism of water and solutes between their plasma and the interstitial fluid. These capillaries supply nutrients and remove wastes from the interstitium, but they do not wash away the solutes within the medulla that are necessary to maintain the gradient of salinity. Descending or arterial capillaries are smaller and have thicker walls than ascending or venous capillaries. Van Gieson's, paraffin, × 175.

INTERSTITIUM AND BLOOD SUPPLY

Interstitial cells (mainly fibroblast-like), and macrophages and lymphocytes, together with extracellular matrix, comprise about 10% of the cortex. This proportion increases in the medulla, in which numerous lipid-rich interstitial cells are found. In histologic sections, the medullary interstitium shows a gelatinous-type appearance, indicative of much matrix into which electrolytes and water, among other substances, accumulate as part of the exchange mechanisms that operate between the interstitium, the loops of Henle, and the collecting ducts.

The principal features of the vascular supply are described above, but it is important that blood flow through the organ must be high so that the kidney can filter blood plasma in sufficient quantities to regulate its composition, remove wastes, conserve or excrete water, and to maintain homeostasis. The kidneys receive more than 20% of cardiac blood output, most of which circulates in the cortex and only 1–2% in the medulla. The blood in the vasa recta (long, straight capillaries) in the medulla flows in opposite, parallel directions, and together the descending and ascending vessels intermingle to form vascular bundles (Fig 16.17a & b). Their close association permits a countercurrent exchange mechanism that is important for maintaining the salinity gradient within the medulla (see below, *Countercurrent concentrating system*).

MAIN PHYSIOLOGICAL FUNCTIONS

Through filtration of the blood that passes through the glomeruli, about 180 liters of filtrate per day enters the renal tubular system. Although this is an impressive feat, it represents only 20% of the plasma volume that enters the glomeruli; the larger fraction continues into the efferent arterioles. The average volume of plasma in the body is about 3 liters, and, since the filtrate is derived from plasma, it follows that this same volume of plasma is filtered and reabsorbed many times over 24 hours. With regard to electrolytes, about 1.5 kg of salt is filtered during this same period. The greater part (99%) of the filtrate is reclaimed as it passes through the segments of the nephron: by processes of tubular reabsorption, secretion, and concentration, the final urine excreted from the kidney is very different from the initial glomerular filtrate.

Filtration

Filtration of plasma across the glomerular filtration barrier depends not only on the size and charge of substances in the blood, but also on net filtration pressure, which is about 10 mmHg; that is, plasma moves out of glomerular capillaries to form an ultrafiltrate in Bowman's space. The resultant GFR is, on average, about 125 mL/min for both kidneys, and is adjusted in several ways:

- Autoregulation by the juxtaglomerular apparatus, which constricts or dilates the afferent arteriole in response to changes in blood pressure
- Constriction, by sympathetic stimulation, of the afferent arteriole in situations of shock or maximum physical activity
- Through the RAS and, in response to a fall in blood pressure, production of angiotensin II. This in turn causes vasoconstriction (especially of the efferent arteriole), increased reabsorption of water by renal tubules, and secretion of aldosterone (salt-retaining hormone) from the adrenal cortex, which enhances water and sodium reabsorption.

Reabsorption

The proximal convoluted tubule reabsorbs about 70% of the glomerular filtrate, water and urea being reabsorbed by osmosis and/or simple diffusion. Salt, glucose, and amino acids are taken up via active transport, facilitated diffusion, or antiport exchangers. Other ions pass across the epithelium by paracellular routes. The amount of water and salt reabsorbed depends upon the osmotic and pressure characteristics of the associated blood vessels, which are adjusted by the GFR, and thus proximal tubule reabsorption is matched to GFR, a mechanism termed glomerulotubular balance.

Countercurrent concentrating system

The countercurrent concentrating system comprises the medullary tissues, loops of Henle, collecting ducts, and the vasa recta, which together maintain a salinity gradient in the medullary interstitium and, with regulation by ADH, can concentrate the urine and control water loss. The concentrating mechanisms are not understood in full, but the theory is essentially correct, based upon available information. Formation of concentrated urine depends on two mechanisms, shown in Figure 16.18: the countercurrent multiplier and countercurrent exchanger.

Countercurrent multiplier

The countercurrent multiplier maintains a high salt concentration in deep medullary tissue. It is referred to as a multiplier because it enhances the salinity gradient in this region, and is described as countercurrent because it relies upon tubular fluid that flows in opposite directions—that is, down thin descending limbs (tDLs) and up tALs and TALs. In the tDL, water easily permeates into the interstitium, but not NaCl, and in approaching the salty environment of the loop more water leaves the tubule, which now contains fluid of high osmolarity. The salinity gradient in the medulla is produced by transport of Na⁺ (and Cl⁻), but not water, out of the ascending limb, and the fluid in this tubule gradually becomes more dilute (less osmolarity) as it approaches the cortex. Thus, the high osmolarity in the loop, equivalent to that in the interstitium, is in part generated by the closeness of the two limbs and their positive feedback relationship.

The collecting duct assists with the creation of elevated medullary osmolarity by its differential permeability to urea and water, controlled by ADH. Water leaves the collecting duct if ADH is present, thus concentrating the urine, but the reabsorbed water tends to dilute the medullary interstitium and so the volume reabsorbed must be kept small. This is achieved (by ADH) by significant water (but not urea) recovery in the cortical collecting duct. In the medullary duct, both water and urea can leave the tubule, and the urea, now in the deep interstitium, contributes about 40% of the osmolarity in the medulla. Urea is also recycled back into the tDL and eventually passes again into the collecting duct, which excretes variable amounts of urea according to how much water is reclaimed under the influence of ADH.

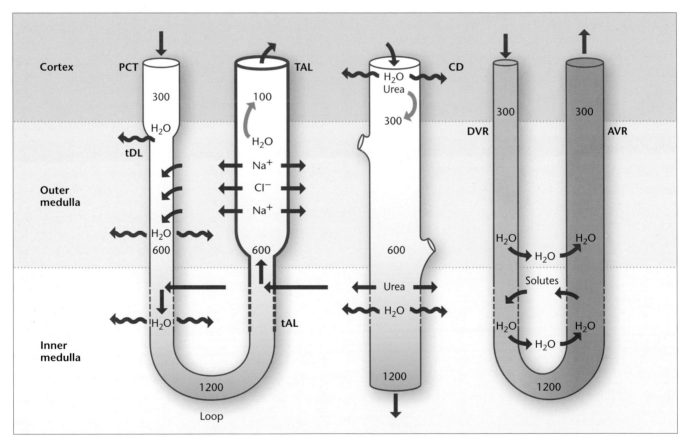

▲ **Fig 16.18 Countercurrent system.** A simplified scheme of tubular fluid and blood composition in the presence of ADH (antidiuretic hormone), in which urine becomes concentrated and hypertonic, but contains normal amounts of solutes. Key: **PCT**, proximal convoluted tubule; **tDL**, thin descending limb of loop of Henle; **Loop**, loop of Henle; **tAL**, thin ascending limb of loop of Henle; **TAL**, thick ascending limb of loop of Henle; **CD**, collecting duct; **DVR**, descending vasa recta; **AVR**, ascending vasa recta. The thickened wall of the ascending limb indicates impermeability to water, and in the vascular bundle the AVR is slightly larger in diameter. The countercurrent multiplier increases osmolarity (mOsm/L) toward the loop indicated by permeability of water and active transport of Na⁺ (Cl⁻ follows passively); the medullary interstitium has high osmolarity since solutes are trapped within it. Fluid that leaves the TAL is hypotonic to plasma. The collecting duct resorbs water and, in the medullary portion, also allows diffusion of urea into the interstitium, with recycling back into thin limbs. The vasa recta, with a sluggish blood flow, engages in countercurrent exchange of water and solutes, and thus maintains high osmolarity in the tip of the vascular loop and the interstitium.

Countercurrent exchanger

The countercurrent exchanger involves the vasa recta. As blood enters the medulla, water diffuses out and solutes diffuse in, and so blood has a higher solute concentrate than the interstitium. In the ascending vasa recta, which pass into a decreasing salty interstitium, water is regained and solutes diffuse out. The vasa recta do not wash away the solutes, which maintain medullary hypertonicity.

Main reabsorptive processes

A summary of the main reabsorptive processes and the volume and composition of selected substances in the urine is given in Figure 16.19, but note that more than 20 substances (ions, organic solutes) are measurable in urine.

> **Tip:** If the renal medulla had normal capillaries, the interstitial tissue would equilibrate with blood plasma. The high osmolarity in the medullary interstitium is maintained by the countercurrent exchange functions of the vasa recta. They ensure no net change in medullary water and solute content.

KIDNEY AS AN ENDOCRINE ORGAN
Renin–angiotensin system

The renin–angiotensin system (RAS) is a cascade of intra- and extrarenal reactions initiated by falling arterial pressure or distal tubule volume depletion. Renin is then released from juxtaglomerular cells; this enzyme circulates in blood and converts plasma angiotensinogen (mainly produced by the liver) into angiotensin I. This peptide is converted into angiotensin II (mainly in the lungs), which acts as a circulating hormone. Angiotensin II is a vasoconstrictor and regulates the GFR; it promotes water uptake by stimulating ADH release, and it enhances sodium retention by stimulating aldosterone secretion from the adrenal cortex.

Erythropoietin

Erythropoietin (EPO) is produced predominantly by the kidneys, and is a growth factor that stimulates erythrocyte production in the bone marrow. It is made by fibroblast-type cells in the peritubular interstitium of the cortex and medulla. Its rate of production is inversely proportional to the oxygen-carrying capacity of the blood. How oxygen levels are detected and then EPO produced by the kidney is not clear. Chronic renal failure is very often associated with anemia, which is treated effectively with recombinant EPO.

Vitamin D

The active form of vitamin D is a hormone produced in the kidney. When exposed to ultraviolet radiation in sunlight, the skin forms calciferol (called vitamin D_3) from cholesterol. Calciferol is converted in the liver into 25-OH-D_3, which, in the kidney, and under parathyroid hormone control, is converted into 1,25-$(OH)_2$-D_3, or calcitriol, a steroid hormone. This form of vitamin D increases calcium absorption from the intestine and increases osteoclast activity.

Nephron segmental reabsorption as percentage of the glomerular ultrafiltrate								
Segment	N^+ (%)	H_2O + antidiuretic hormone (%)	H_2O − antidiuretic hormone (%)	K^+ (%)	Glucose (%)	PO_4^{2-} (%)	Urea + antidiuretic hormone (%)	H_2O − antidiuretic hormone (%)
Proximal tubule	70	70	70	80	100	95	50	50
Loop of Henle	20	5	4	ca. 5				
Distal tubule and collecting ducts	9	24	13	ca. 5			−20	10–20
Total	99	99	87	ca. 90	100	95	30	60–70
Amount excreted per day (mmol or L)	180 mmol	1.6 L	23 L	60 mmol	0 mmol	30 mmol	200–400 mmol	

▲ **Fig 16.19** Patterns of distribution of substances during the formation of urine along the renal tubule system. (Based on data from: Lote CJ. Principles of renal physiology, 3rd edn. London: Chapman and Hall, 1994; and Greger R, Windhorst V, eds. Comprehensive human physiology. Berlin: Springer-Verlag, 1996.)

URINARY TRACT
Ureter

The ureters are simple, muscular tubes (Fig 16.20a & b), about 3–5 mm in diameter, that transport urine to the bladder by peristalsis, which is initiated in the renal calyces and transmitted to the renal pelvis and ureter. Within the smooth-muscle wall of the ureter, sympathetic and parasympathetic nerves connect with intramural neurons and fibers to modify peristalsis. The mucosal lining, usually stellate in cross section because of elastic fibers in the lamina propria, is transitional epithelium, similar to that found in the renal calyces and pelvis.

Bladder

In keeping with its role as a reservoir both for the storage of urine and expulsion of urine into the urethra, the urinary bladder is composed of a thick, smooth muscular wall, a mucosa of transitional epithelium (impermeable to urine), and a wide lamina propria that contains vessels and fibroelastic connective tissue (Fig 16.21a & b). Said to consist of three layers, the muscularis of the bladder in histologic sections shows interlacing and spiral orientations of muscle bundles. Depending on the forces applied to the mucosa in relation to filling and emptying the bladder, the cells of the transitional epithelium change their morphology from flat, squamous-type shapes into large, cylindrical shapes that bulge into the lumen (Fig 16.22a & b). Epithelial thickness is also variable, ranging from three to six or more cell strata in relation to changes in

bladder distension. Contractions of the muscularis are associated with the micturition reflex, which involves autonomic and pelvic nerves and is subject to higher voluntary control that originates in the brain.

Urethra

The urethra is a fibromuscular tube and, in the male, is associated with the prostate gland, urogenital diaphragm, and penis, and therefore respectively surrounded by glandular tissue, muscle sphincters, and erectile tissue. Initially lined by transitional epithelium, the mucous membrane gradually changes into stratified columnar (Fig 16.23) and finally stratified squamous cells in the distal part. The female urethra shows similar changes, although the epithelium (except during micturition) is crescentic and apposed. Throughout its length, the urethra is surrounded by an outer coat of skeletal and smooth muscle fibers.

DISORDERS AND CLINICAL COMMENTS
Renal failure

Renal failure is broadly defined as a fall in GFR (to 30 mL/min or less), with retention of electrolytes, nitrogenous wastes, and water, and a decrease in urine volume. The factors that cause failure are related to inadequate blood supply, intrinsic disorders of the renal vasculature or nephrons, and failure to clear urine from the excretory passages. Acute renal failure may occur in response to reduced cardiac output, hemorrhage, tissue destruction by toxic

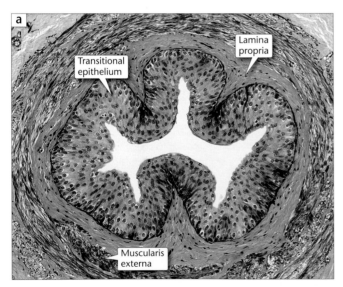

▲ **Fig 16.20a Proximal ureter.** Transverse section of proximal ureter showing typical transitional epithelium, fibroelastic lamina propria, and circular muscularis externa. Urine passes along the ureter in peristaltic waves when the lumen changes from stellate to ovoid. Masson's trichrome, paraffin, × 60.

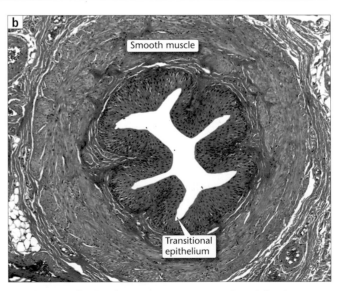

▲ **Fig 16.20b Distal ureter.** Transverse section of distal ureter with thick, smooth-muscle coats (sometimes seen in three layers) and thin lamina propria. Through autonomic nerve supply, the muscle ensures that peristaltic forces deliver urine from the ureter into the bladder. H&E, paraffin, × 40.

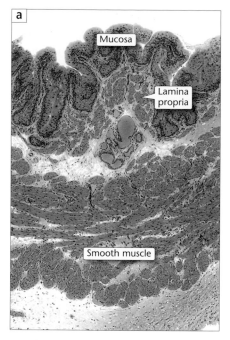

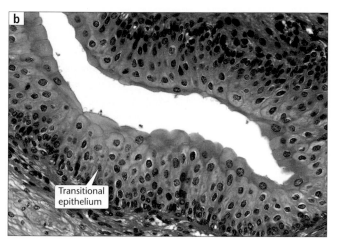

▲ **Fig 16.21b Bladder.** Transitional epithelium of the bladder is impermeable to urine; for this impermeability it depends upon a thick plasma membrane that faces the lumen, together with intercellular tight junctions. The dome-like appearance of the superficial cells is typical of relaxed bladder mucosa, which is usually four to five cell layers in depth and contains cuboidal and columnar cells. H&E, paraffin, × 150.

▲ **Fig 16.21a Bladder.** Low magnification showing non-distended, folded mucosa, and small strands of smooth muscle in the lamina propria, which is a normal finding but is not described as a muscularis mucosae. The external smooth muscle—showing three interwoven divisions—functions to allow bladder filling and contraction during the micturition reflex. H&E, acrylic resin, × 12.

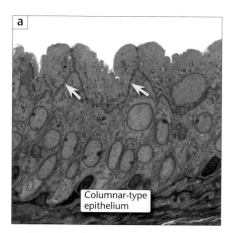

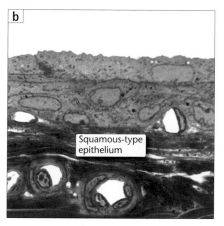

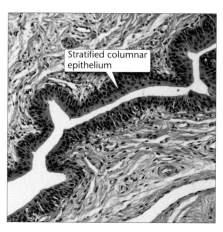

▲ **Fig 16.22a Urinary epithelium with relaxed bladder.** This shows stratification of the transitional epithelium, and the adluminal region that contains prominent intercellular junctions along the plasma membranes (**arrows**). The luminal surface membrane is scalloped and thrown into irregular folds because of the plasticity of each cell and the increase and decrease in membrane surface area that accompanies bladder filling and voiding. How membrane area is expanded is shown in Figure 16.22b. Toluidine blue, araldite, × 400.

▲ **Fig 16.22b Urinary epithelium with distended bladder.** This shows the thin epithelial layer and squamous-type cells. The surface area of the relaxed cells has increased by incorporation of disks (plaques) of membrane, which are stored in the cytoplasm and inserted into the apical plasma membrane as the mucosa is stretched by the accumulation of urine. This process is reversible and is accompanied by all cells changing shape and position within the epithelium. Toluidine blue, araldite, × 400.

▲ **Fig 16.23 Urethra.** Transverse section of penile urethra, showing a stratified columnar epithelium surrounded by the erectile tissue of the corpus spongiosum, which contains elastic, collagenous, and smooth-muscle fibers, together with vascular sinusoids. The female urethra in non-distension is folded or stellate in cross section, with a similar mucosa to that of the penile urethra, and the surrounding tissue is loose, fibrous connective tissue with a rich blood supply. H&E, paraffin, × 40.

compounds (heavy metals, carbon tetrachloride), or obstruction of the urinary tract—for example, by renal calculi (kidney stones caused by precipitation of calcium, phosphate, urate, and protein). Chronic renal failure results from a wide variety of renal diseases affecting nephrons or the vasculature, in which a gradual decline in renal function is associated with progressive and irreversible loss of functioning nephrons. Chronic renal failure is the end result of all chronic renal diseases.

Glomerular diseases

Diseases that affect the glomeruli are a major focus of attention in experimental and clinical nephrology, and a variety of factors, which include systemic diseases such as infection, may injure glomeruli. Classification of glomerular disorders may be based upon morphologic criteria, such as non-inflammatory glomerulopathies and inflammatory glomerular lesions (glomerulonephritis, GN). Alternatively, glomerular disorders may be classified as primary glomerular diseases (in which the kidney is the only or main organ affected), and secondary glomerular diseases (in which systemic disorders—microorganisms, metabolic, immune, or vascular—result in damage to the glomeruli).

Although the pathogenesis of many glomerular diseases is poorly understood, immune mechanisms underlie most cases of primary GN. Different forms of GN are characterized by light, electron, and immunofluorescence microscopy, in which various types of glomerular hypercellularity are identified (e.g. mesangial cells, endothelium, neutrophilic accumulation, thickened basal lamina, sclerosis that involves deposition of hyaline matrix). Inflammation of glomeruli in GN can lead to kidney failure by destroying nephrons, and up to 50% of patients who require dialysis or transplantation show chronic GN. Obliteration of glomeruli is the end point in all cases, and is associated with interstitial fibrosis and atrophy of many of the cortical renal tubules.

Urinary tract infection

Pyelonephritis is defined as a combined inflammation of the renal parenchyma, calyces, and pelvis. Bacterial infection results in the acute form; however, the causes of the chronic condition are less clear, but can be related to infection in combination with obstructive lesions, or to reflux from the ureter and bladder. Pyelonephritis may arise as a consequence of urinary tract infection (UTI) that involves the ureters, bladder, prostate gland, or urethra. Histologically, the affected kidney shows patchy necrosis or abscess formation that contains inflammatory cell infiltrates and purulent (pus) exudate. The renal tubules and interstitium are mainly affected.

Cystitis is an inflammation of the bladder, the common site for UTI, and is usually caused by *Escherichia coli* that enters by retrograde movement from the urethra. The mucosa may be hyperemic or show hemorrhage or pus formation and, in chronic infection, the epithelium may be lost, which results in ulceration. In most cases, appropriate antibiotic treatment is effective.

Endocrine system

Traditionally, the endocrine system is considered to consist of distinct glands or tissues that secrete organic compounds or chemical messengers called hormones into the circulatory system, where they specifically stimulate or otherwise cause a change in metabolic activity in designated target tissues or organs. In responding to the hormonal stimulus, the target cells/tissues may secrete one or more substances into the circulation, which, in turn, may regulate the synthesis and/or secretion of hormones by the endocrine gland. This system is termed feedback control and is an important part of endocrine function. In other cases, hormones may act directly on target tissues, which may not produce some form of feedback response. The endocrine system performs the role of communication and regulation, usually in response to normal physiologic changes within the body, or in response to alterations of the external environment to ensure that all components of the body's metabolism operate in a coordinated manner.

Our understanding of endocrinology, traditionally based on the study of the principal endocrine glands (hypothalamus, pituitary, thyroid, parathyroids, adrenals, pancreatic islets, pineal, gonads, and placenta), now includes many other cell types specific for particular organs (such as the gastrointestinal tract) or scattered in a variety of tissues. A hormone is a biologically active substance released into and transported in blood or lymph, and includes compounds that may act locally on cells through the extracellular fluid (paracrine regulation), or even initiate responses from the cell(s) that produced the hormone (autocrine function).

An understanding of the structure and function of endocrine tissues is relevant to the diagnosis and treatment of endocrine disorders and related disease conditions. A variety of endocrine-based disorders are commonly encountered in medical practice (e.g. thyroid and reproductive disorders, and particularly diseases such as diabetes, which is a major health problem).

PRINCIPLES OF ENDOCRINE FUNCTION
Types of hormone

There are four main types of hormone:
- *Peptide and protein hormones* vary in molecular weight and amino acid sequences; examples are hypothalamic hormones, insulin, and growth hormone. Glycoprotein hormones such as follicle-stimulating hormone (FSH) contain covalently attached sugars.
- *Steroid hormones* have a common steroid ring, and are all derived from cholesterol; examples are androgens, estrogens, and glucocorticoids.
- *Tyrosine or amine-derived hormones* include thyroid hormones and adrenomedullary hormones (epinephrine, norepinepherine). Dopamine, synthesized from tyrosine, and serotonin, from tryptophan, also belong to this group.
- *Fatty acid derivatives* (prostaglandins, leukotrienes) are a special category concerned with vascular function.

Synthesis and secretion

Peptide or protein hormones are synthesized as for other proteins, stored in cytoplasmic granules, and exocytosed when secretion is required. Most peptide hormones are synthesized as larger precursors (preprohormone), cleaved into prohormone, then stored in the form of granules and processed to form the definitive hormone.

Steroids are synthesized in mitochondria and smooth endoplasmic reticulum (ER); they are not stored, but released by diffusion.

Catecholamines (epinephrine, norepinephrine) are synthesized from tyrosine, stored in granules, and released by exocytosis. Thyroid hormones are stored extracellularly as precursors in colloid-filled cavities in the thyroid gland; the colloid enters the thyroid cells, releasing active thyroid hormones into the blood.

Transport and clearance

Most amine and peptide or protein hormones are water soluble, circulating as unbound, free hormones that are readily degraded in blood, liver, or kidneys and have plasma half-lives of minutes to hours. Steroid and thyroid hormones are lipid-soluble, being carried in blood bound to plasma proteins chiefly produced in the liver. Free hormone is a minor fraction of the total circulating hormone pool. Bound hormones tend to have long plasma half-lives (days); they enter cells slowly and are degraded slowly, and loss by renal filtration is low.

Hormone action

Hormones act on target cells by initiating characteristic biologic responses via specific receptors. Receptors for peptide or protein hormones and catecholamines are located in cell plasma membranes; receptors for steroids and thyroid hormones are usually found in the cell nucleus. When bound to membrane receptors, hormones activate second messenger molecules, which in turn initiate reactions that alter the metabolism in the cytoplasm and/or nucleus. For nuclear receptors, the hormone alters gene transcription and translation, resulting in synthesis and secretion of new proteins. In some cases, a protein hormone (e.g. FSH) stimulates the secretion of a steroid hormone (e.g. estradiol) in a target endocrine organ (e.g. the ovary). In other cases, a protein hormone (e.g. prolactin) directly stimulates new protein synthesis (e.g. milk) in target tissue (e.g. the mammary gland). Hormones producing a synergistic response are those in which the combined biologic effects of two or more hormones greatly exceed their individual actions (e.g. FSH and testosterone acting on the spermatogenic process).

Control of secretion

Feedback regulation, neural control, and factors maintaining cyclic, rhythmic, or pulsatile patterns of hormone secretion are major determinants of how and when hormones are released. Feedback control is often negative—that is, products of a stimulated target cell inhibit further hormone secretion; this is a simple first-order feedback loop. Second- or third-order feedback loops are common. Positive feedback loops amplify the secretion of the primary endocrine cells. Neural input (e.g. stress, excitement, fright, and injury) can inhibit or stimulate hormone secretion. Cyclic or pulsatile hormone secretion is common, modified by endogenous circadian rhythms (sleep–wake cycles, adrenal function) or longer cyclic patterns such as the ovarian menstrual cycle. Photoperiod or temperature may modify hormone secretion through sensory pathways connecting the central nervous system (CNS) and some endocrine glands. Much of the cyclic control of the endocrine system, responding to afferent inputs from all levels of the CNS, is governed by the hypothalamus, which regulates the pituitary gland through neural and blood vascular connections.

HYPOTHALAMUS AND PITUITARY

The hypothalamus and pituitary gland form a complex neuroendocrine circuit, the pituitary often being considered to be the "master" endocrine gland because its hormones regulate the activities of numerous other endocrine glands and tissues (Fig 17.1). However, the pituitary itself is under the command of the hypothalamus, which consists of groups of neurosecretory neurons (termed nuclei) that synthesize hormones (mostly peptides), which are transported to the pituitary gland. These hormones are blood-borne releasing hormones acting on the anterior pituitary, or other peptides reaching the posterior pituitary by transport down connecting axons. Capillary plexuses in the hypothalamus are linked to blood sinuses in the anterior pituitary by venous channels, together forming the hypothalamo-hypophyseal portal circulation.

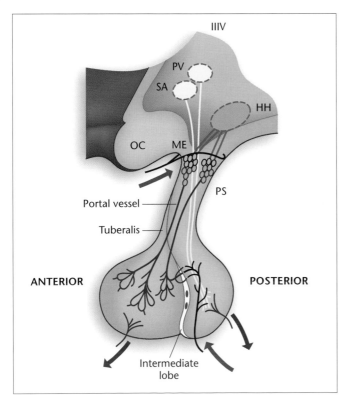

◀ **Fig 17.1 Hypothalamus and pituitary.** The median eminence (**ME**) and pituitary stalk (**PS**) contain a capillary plexus, which drains into portal vessels containing releasing factors from nerve terminals originating in the hypothalamic–hypophyseotropic area (**HH**). Portal vessels terminate in vascular sinusoids in the anterior pituitary, supplying its secretory cells. Large neurons in the paired supraoptic (**SA**) and paraventricular (**PV**) nuclei (located above the optic chiasm, **OC**, on each of the lateral walls of the third ventricle, **IIIV**) run down the pituitary stalk and terminate in the posterior pituitary. Here, they release either oxytocin or vasopressin into a capillary plexus.

The pituitary, or hypophysis, comprises two major parts; the anterior part (adenohypophysis) is derived from the developing oral cavity and contains epithelial cells, whereas the posterior portion (neurohypophysis) is part of the brain (Fig 17.2a & b). The cell types of the anterior pituitary are described according to the target tissue stimulated by the hormones they secrete. There are six main anterior pituitary hormones, all proteins, which are secreted by five different cell types (Fig 17.3). Various cell types of the anterior

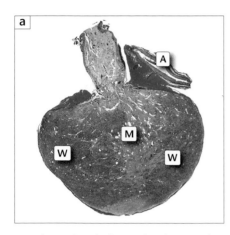

▲ **Fig 17.2a Pituitary gland.** Coronal section through the pituitary stalk and anterior pituitary of a bovine pituitary gland, enclosed by a capsule in continuity with the sellar diaphragm, through which the pituitary stalk passes. The anterior pituitary may show a central "mucoid wedge" (**M**) and two "lateral wings" (**W**) reflecting, in part, concentrations of cells with characteristic secretory granules and staining properties. Deep staining also is attributable to the rich venous blood supply. Part of the superior hypophyseal artery (**A**), which supplies the median eminence and the origin of the portal system, is shown. Mallory-Azan, paraffin, × 4.5.

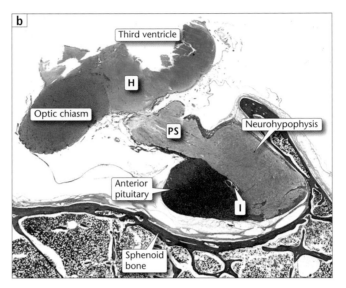

▲ **Fig 17.2b Sagittal section of primate pituitary**, showing anterior and posterior parts; the latter, the neurohypophysis, has lighter staining owing to its content of neurons derived from the hypothalamus (**H**) via the pituitary stalk (**PS**). The anterior pituitary, in contrast, contains secretory cells and the portal plexus derived from the median eminence and pituitary stalk. The intermediate lobe (**I**) shows a colloid-filled cyst, a remnant of Rathke's pouch. Note the sphenoid bone, optic chiasm, and third ventricle. Cells of the anterior pituitary synthesize and secrete hormones into efferent veins and the systemic circulation. The neurohypophysis does not produce hormones, but stores peptides (formed in the hypothalamus within nerve fibers) and releases these hormones into the circulation. It also contains glial cells, termed pituicytes. Masson's trichrome, paraffin, × 8.

Cell	% of cells	Hormone	Hypothalamic control	Target	Main action
Somatotrophs	40–50	Growth hormone (GH)	Growth hormone-releasing hormone (GHRH), somatostatin (SRIF) (inhibitory)	Bone, viscera, soft tissues	Growth promotion
Thyrotrophs	5	Thyroid-stimulating hormone (TSH)	Thyrotropin-releasing hormone (TRH), somatostatin (SRIF) (inhibitory)	Thyroid	Secretion of thyroid hormones
Corticotrophs	15–20	Adrenocorticotropin (ACTH)	Corticotropin-releasing hormone (CRH), arginine vasopressin (AVP)	Adrenal cortex	Secretion of cortisol
Lactotrophs	15–20	Prolactin (PRL)	Thytropin-releasing hormone (TRH), dopamine (inhibitory)	Mammary gland (and probably many others, e.g. Leydig cells)	Milk secretion
Gonadotrophs	10	Follicle-stimulating hormone (FSH), luteinizing hormone (LH)	Gonadotropin-releasing hormone (GnRH)	Gonads	Production of gametes, secretion of sex steroids

▲ **Fig 17.3 Anterior pituitary—histology and function.** The six major hormones produced by the anterior pituitary can be classified into two groups on a structural basis—single-chain proteins (GH, PRL, ACTH) and glycoproteins with two subunits (FSH, LH, TSH).

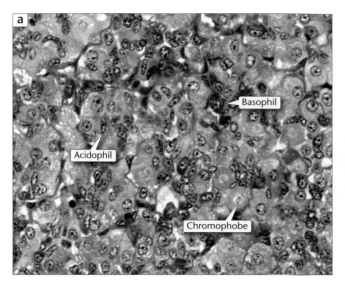

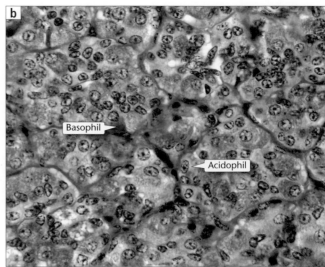

▲ **Fig 17.4a Anterior pituitary.** Arranged in clumps or cords, the secretory cells can be classified as chromophobes (poorly stained) or chromophils (well stained); the latter are subdivided into acidophils (pale pink, eosinophilic) and basophils (deep pink), reflecting granule content. This classification cannot discriminate between the five different cell types secreting six main hormones. Somatotrophs (growth hormone) and lactotrophs (prolactin) are acidophilic. Corticotrophs (adrenocorticotropic hormone), thyrotrophs (TSH), and gonadotrophs (FSH and LH) are basophilic cells. Chromophobes are thought to be quiescent chromophils. All the cells are supported by a reticular network and surrounded by vascular sinusoids, which deliver stimulatory (or inhibitory) factors from the hypothalamus or peripheral endocrine-target organs, and into which the various anterior pituitary hormones, stored in cytoplasmic granules, are discharged by exocytosis. Mallory-Azan, paraffin, × 400.

▲ **Fig 17.4b Anterior pituitary.** With the PAS–orange G stain, acidophils stain orange and basophils pink or magenta, whereas the chromophobes appear gray or lack staining. This method, although useful, still provides empirical information, and immunocytochemical techniques, although able to differentiate specific cell types, obscure structural detail. A combination of these two methods, together with electron microscopy, can provide accurate details of cell distribution, abundance, and secretory activities. PAS stains corticotrophs, thyrotrophs, and gonadotrophs owing to the glycoprotein nature of the secreted product or, in the case of corticotrophs, to the processing of the precursor glycoprotein pro-opiomelanocortin (POMC) into ACTH within secretory granules. PAS/orange G, paraffin, × 400.

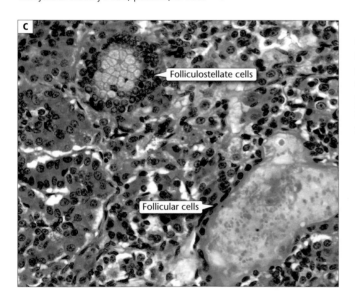

◀ **Fig 17.4c Anterior pituitary.** Follicular and folliculostellate cells are not uncommonly found in the anterior pituitary. They may surround a lumen with colloid or cellular debris and are probably damaged or dysfunctional secretory cells. Folliculostellate cells, whose function is poorly understood, occur throughout the anterior pituitary, including the intermediate lobe, where they may contribute to cysts typical of this region. Hematoxylin & eosin (H&E), paraffin, × 325.

pituitary can be identified with routine staining methods (Fig 17.4a–c), but they are best identified at the ultrastructural level using correlations between immunocytochemistry and granule morphology, the latter representing storage of the hormone (Fig 17.5a–c). The posterior pituitary (Fig 17.6a & b) consists of nerve fibers from the hypothalamus, their terminals being in close association with capillaries. Posterior pituitary hormones are peptides (Fig 17.7), which are synthesized in the hypothalamus, then bound to carrier proteins, and stored in granules in the axon terminals until discharged by exocytosis.

> **Tip:** Both divisions of the pituitary gland develop from ectoderm, but the anterior part (adenohypophysis) arises from the roof of the oral cavity, whereas the posterior part (neurohypophysis) develops from neural ectoderm (brain).

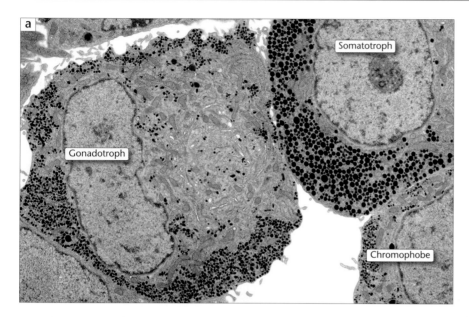

◀ **Fig 17.5a Pituitary cell types.** Ultrastructure of anterior pituitary cells, showing a gonadotroph with granules of variable size (250–450 nm) and a somatotroph with many granules, mostly 350–450 nm in diameter. Chromophobes show few, if any granules, and are probably quiescent or degranulated acidophils and basophils. × 4,200.

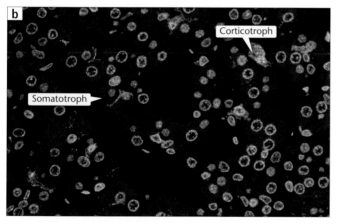

▲ **Fig 17.5b Pituitary cell types.** Immunofluorescence of rat pituitary cells, showing somatotrophs with red fluorescent secretory granules of growth hormone and corticotrophs with green fluorescent granules of adrenocorticotropic hormone. × 350. (Courtesy J Zbaeren, Inselspital, Bern, Switzerland.)

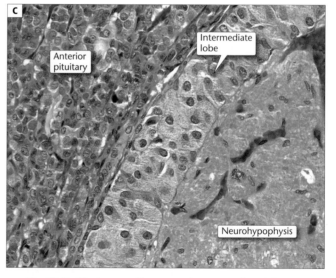

▲ **Fig 17.5c Pituitary cell types.** The intermediate lobe, part of the anterior pituitary, is a thin strip bordering on the posterior pituitary. It contains ciliated, mucous, and endocrine cells with variable immunoreactivity for pituitary hormones. Spaces or cysts with colloid may occur and may develop into Rathke's cleft cysts, occurring in about 15% of otherwise normal pituitary glands. In humans, the function, if any, of this lobe is unknown; the localization of cleavage products of pro-opiomelanocortin may not be of physiologic significance. H&E, paraffin, × 400.

THYROID

Microscopically, the two lobes of the thyroid gland are divided into lobules, each of which contains numerous follicles. These follicles, in humans numbering in the many thousands, are of variable dimension and are lined by a single epithelial layer of flattened, cuboidal, or low columnar cells. The lumen contains a protein-rich material called thyroid colloid, varying in amount according to gland function (Fig 17.8a–d). The thyroid gland synthesizes and secretes triiodothyronine (T_3) and tetraiodothyronine (thyroxine; T_4), which are formed in the follicle lumen as a component of a protein solution (the colloid) that is practically all thyroglobulin, a large-molecular-weight glycoprotein. Follicle cells produce the thyroglobulin and also concentrate iodine from the blood. Iodine is made available by dietary intake and is a trace element essential for the production of active hormone. Severe iodine deficiencies in the fetus may result in mental retardation and "cretinism." As thyroglobulin is exocytosed into the colloid, it is iodinated to form mono- and diiodotyrosines. The latter are coupled together within the thyroglobulin molecule to form T_3 (mono plus diiodo) and T_4 (diiodo plus diiodo), which may then be stored within the colloid for up to 3 months.

The thyroid secretes greater quantities of T_4 than T_3; most of the T_4 is converted in peripheral target tissues into T_3, which has far greater biologic potency. In contrast to protein hormones that act through cell membrane receptors, thyroid hormones bind to nuclear receptors and activate DNA transcription in most cells to stimulate general metabolic activity. The production and secretion of thyroid hormones are activated by thyroid-stimulating hormone (TSH) from the anterior pituitary, and thyroid hormones suppress TSH secretion by negative feedback. Secretion of TSH is also regulated by the hypothalamic releasing hormone — thyrotropin releasing hormone (TRH) — which stimulates TSH release, and by somastostatin, which is inhibitory. In the interfollicular stroma or

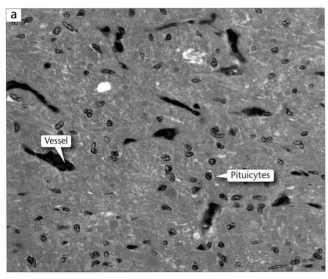

▲ **Fig 17.6a Posterior pituitary.** Also called the neurohypophysis, this tissue contains the hypothalamic peptide hormones oxytocin and vasopressin, which are stored in granules in axons and released into blood vessels. Glial cells, or pituicytes, ensheath the axons, coordinating secretion. Oxytocin and vasopressin are produced from larger precursor molecules, other cleavage products being neurophysins, which are co-secretory products (formerly thought to be carrier proteins) but have no biologic activity. Oxytocin stimulates uterine contractions during labor and causes milk expulsion from mammary gland alveoli. Vasopressin or antidiuretic hormone (ADH) mainly acts in renal tubules, reducing urine flow by increasing water absorption. H&E, paraffin, × 250.

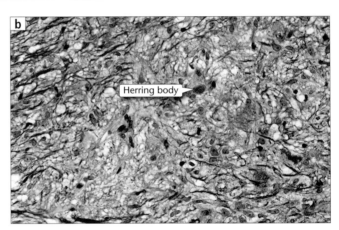

▲ **Fig 17.6b Posterior pituitary.** Distal aspect of the infundibular process connecting the median eminence to the posterior pituitary, showing many unmyelinated axons and the Herring bodies that are focal dilations of the axons containing neurosecretory granules. These granules are oxytocin and ADH. Mallory-Azan, paraffin, × 250.

Hormone	Control	Target	Main action
Vasopressin (antidiuretic hormone ADH)	Blood pressure and volume, osmotic pressure	Kidney, vascular smooth muscle	Reabsorption of water, vasoconstriction
Oxytocin	Sucking stimulus, stretch receptors	Mammary gland, uterus	Milk ejection, parturtion

▲ **Fig 17.7 Posterior pituitary hormones.** Vasopressin (ADH) and oxytocin are nonapeptides with remarkably similar molecular structure but very different physiologic actions.

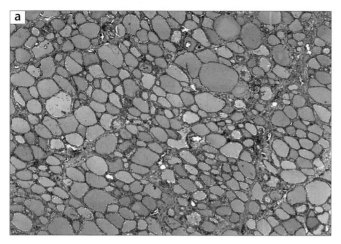

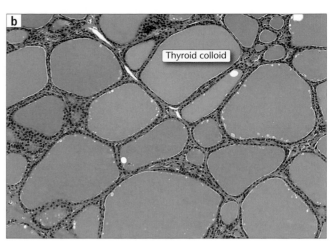

▲ **Fig 17.8a Thyroid gland.** Typical thyroid histology, showing some of the thousands of follicles, which consist of a rim of cuboidal follicular cells and a colloid-filled lumen that contains the iodinated glycoprotein thyroglobulin. Connective tissue with blood and lymphatic vessels, and autonomic nerves, surround all follicles. Thyroxine (tetraiodothyronine, T_4) and triiodothyronine (T_3) are stored within thyroglobulin, both synthesized after uptake of circulating iodine; this iodine is used by follicular cells to iodinate the thyroglobulin, which these cells also synthesize. Underactive follicles have increased amounts of colloid; overactive follicles have a reduced colloid content. H&E, paraffin, × 10.

▲ **Fig 17.8b Detail of thyroid follicles**, showing close association between the colloid and follicular cells. Gland activity is controlled by TSH from the anterior pituitary (TSH is regulated by hypothalamic TRH), which stimulates T_3 and T_4 secretion, in turn suppressing TSH by negative feedback. Thyroglobulin, in small colloid droplets, is endocytosed by follicular cells and via lysosomes, and T_3 and T_4 are separated from the thyroglobulin (which is degraded to yield recyclable iodide) and released into blood. In target cells, most of the T_4 is converted into the biologically more potent T_3. Both hormones bind to nuclear DNA and stimulate selective protein synthesis. H&E, paraffin, × 90.

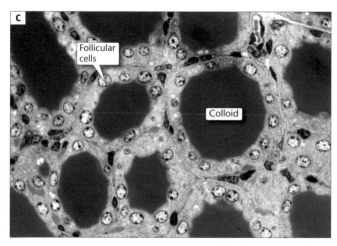

▲ **Fig 17.8c Higher magnification of thyroid follicles**, showing the lumens filled with thyroid colloid. Colloid is a gelatinous material containing thyroglobulin, a glycoprotein with 1% iodine, and comprises about half of the protein content of the thyroid gland. The granular–particulate morphology of the follicular cytoplasm represents endoplasmic reticulum, lysosomes, and colloid droplets. Toluidine blue, araldite, × 480.

follicles, are single or small groups of calcitonin-secreting cells, also known as parafollicular, "clear," or C cells (Fig 17.9). Calcitonin has a hypocalcemic effect in mammals by inhibiting bone resorption and lowering circulating calcium and phosphate; that is, it counteracts the effects of parathyroid hormone (see below). In humans the physiologic role of calcitonin is questionable, because it is parathyroid hormone that mainly controls calcium levels in extracellular fluids.

> **Tip:** Thyroid follicular cells secrete their products in opposite directions and at the same time—thyroglobulin into the colloid-filled lumen, and T_3 and T_4 into the blood.

PARATHYROID GLANDS

The parathyroid glands, normally four in number, are small (3–5 mm) ovoid structures located on the posterior surface of the thyroid (Fig 17.10). They secrete parathyroid hormone (PTH), a peptide that controls calcium and phosphate concentrations in the blood. PTH is synthesized by chief cells—small cuboidal cells with pale cytoplasm (Fig 17.11a & b). Beginning at puberty, a second, larger cell type appears, called oxyphil cells, identified by their eosinophilic cytoplasm; their function is unknown and they may represent aged chief cells no longer secreting PTH. Occasionally, water-clear cells have been described in human parathyroid glands, but

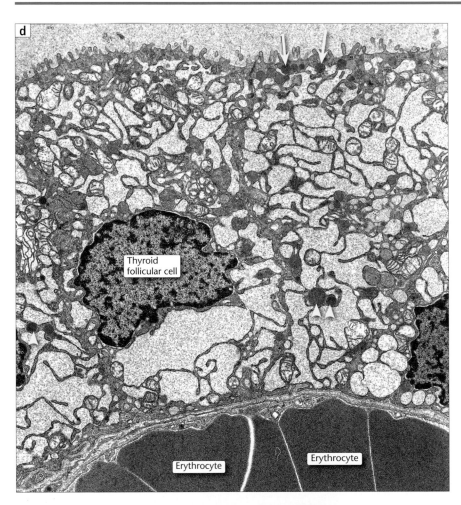

◀ **Fig 17.8d Ultrastructure of thyroid follicular cells**, with dilated rough endoplasmic reticulum (ER) containing particulate matter that represents the production of thyroglobulin protein. Lysosomes near the apical membrane accumulate iodinated thyroglobulin endocytosed from the colloid (**arrows**). Following TSH-induced proteolysis of thyroglobulin in endolysosomes (**arrowheads**), T_4 and T_3 are formed and diffuse out of the base of the cell into capillaries filled with red blood cells. × 7,500. (Courtesy P Cross, Stanford University, USA.)

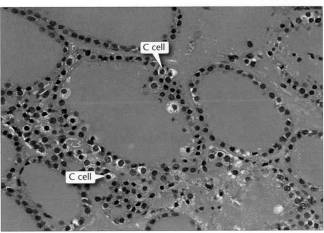

◀ **Fig 17.9 Parafollicular cells.** Also known as clear or C cells and located between follicular cells or in the connective tissue, these cells secrete the peptide calcitonin, a hypocalcemic hormone of uncertain physiologic importance in humans. Calcitonin suppresses bone resorption by inhibiting osteoclast activity, and decreases calcium and phosphate reabsorption by renal tubules. However, thyroidectomy or hypersecretion of calcitonin (in certain thyroid tumors) has little effect on calcium homeostasis in humans. C cells are of neural crest origin and cytochemically belong to the APUD (anine precursor uptake and decarboxylation) system of diffuse neuroendocrine cells. H&E, paraffin, × 300.

their function also is unknown. PTH directly increases the rate of bone resorption, thereby raising serum calcium and phosphate levels, and has direct effects on the kidneys to reduce the excretion of calcium but increase the excretion of phosphate in the urine. The net effect of PTH on bone and renal metabolism is to maintain calcium and phosphate homeostasis. In the

kidney, PTH stimulates the enzyme 1α-hydroxylase, and this results in the formation of the active form of vitamin D, which is secreted into the blood to facilitate calcium absorption in the intestine. PTH secretion is controlled by plasma calcium concentrations acting as a classic negative feedback mechanism.

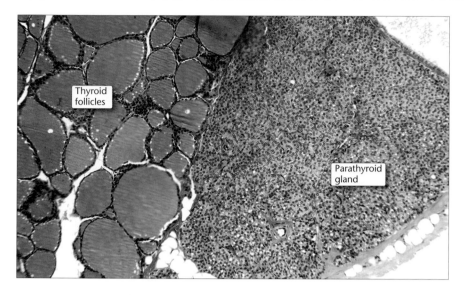

◄ Fig 17.10 Parathyroid glands. Essential for life, parathyroid glands are usually four in number (but may range from 2 to 12). They are flat, discoidal glands located behind the thyroid, about 4 × 3 × 1 mm in size. A fibrous capsule and septa divides the parenchymal cells into irregular lobules; these mostly contain aggregated, small chief cells, which secrete parathyroid hormone (PTH), and occasionally include small nodules of larger, eosinophilic oxyphil cells, thought to be non-functional chief cells. PTH strongly regulates calcium homeostasis, acting mainly on bone and the kidney. H&E, paraffin, × 90.

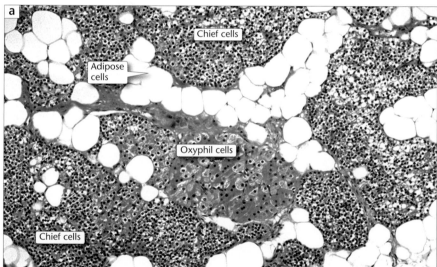

◄ Fig 17.11a Parathyroid cells. Chief cells, adipose cells, and oxyphil cells are shown. Secretion of PTH by chief cells is regulated by plasma calcium levels (i.e. increased calcium inhibits PTH secretion and hypocalcemia stimulates PTH release). PTH increases renal calcium reabsorption (but decreases phosphate reabsorption), and promotes conversion of 25-hydroxyvitamin D to 1,25-dihydroxyvitamin D. This metabolite increases calcium absorption by the gut. PTH also induces bone resorption, raising plasma calcium levels and neutralizing further PTH release. In bone, PTH removes calcium phosphate directly from bone matrix and, via intermediary factors from osteoblasts, stimulates osteoclasts to resorb mineral constituents of bone and bone matrix. H&E, paraffin, × 125.

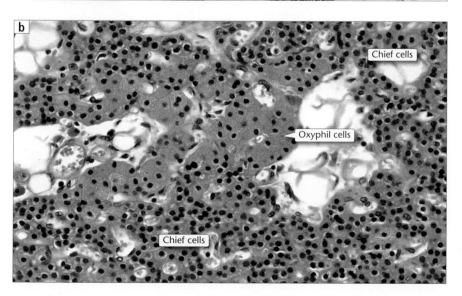

◄ Fig 17.11b Parathyroid oxyphil cells. Nodules of oxyphil cells are recognized by their large size compared with chief cells and by their eosinophilic cytoplasm, which contains mitochondria but is lacking in secretory granules typical of chief cells. Oxyphil cells arise in the parathyroid gland after puberty and occur more frequently beyond the age of 40. In hyperparathyroidism, hyperplasia of oxyphil cells or water-clear cell hyperplasia (cells with abundant rough ER) are occasionally noted. Oxyphil cells may be derived from chief cells, but their function is unknown. H&E, paraffin, × 350.

ADRENAL GLAND

In humans, each adrenal gland is composed of two endocrine components, the outer cortex and the inner medulla (Fig 17.12a–c). The adrenal cortex consists of steroidogenic cells arranged into three zones, each concerned with the production of specific hormones. Disorders of adrenocortical function may result in a range of conditions that carry significant morbidity and mortality.

Cortex

Cells of the cortex show characteristic features within each zone (Fig 17.13a–d). The superficial zone is the thin zona glomerulosa (cells in clumps), secreting the mineralocorticoid aldosterone, which acts mainly on the kidney to regulate electrolyte and fluid balance, chiefly by promoting sodium reabsorption. Adjustment of extracellular fluid volume results in changes in blood pressure, and aldosterone additionally may

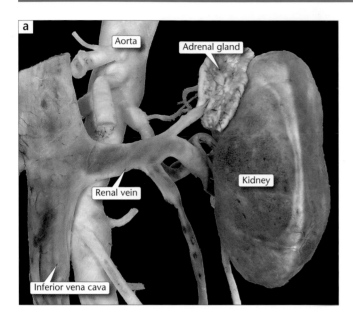

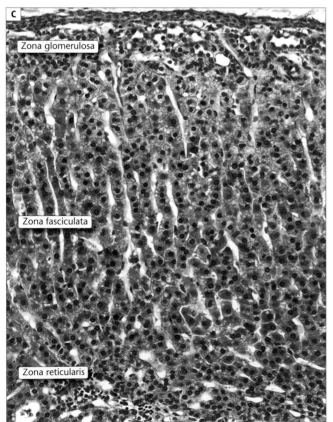

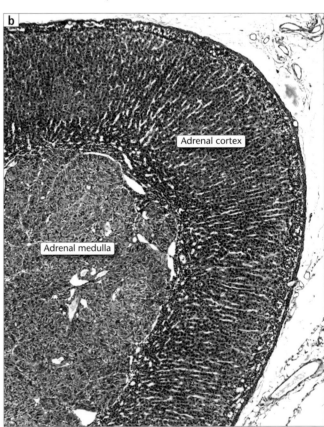

◀ **Fig 17.12a Adrenal gland.** The adrenal (suprarenal) glands sit at the superior poles of the kidney and are discoid in shape, with angular borders giving a pyramidal appearance. They are supplied by branches of the inferior phrenic, aorta, and renal arteries and drain into the vena cava or (as shown on the left) into the renal vein.

▼ **Fig 17.12b Distinct cortex and medulla of adrenal gland.** The cortex comprises up to 80% of the adrenal gland and exhibits strata of steroidogenic cells, which develop from mesoderm; the medulla develops from the neural crest and comprises postganglionic sympathetic neurons lacking axons or dendrites. These cells produce epinephrine (adrenaline) and norepinephrine (noradrenaline). H&E, paraffin, × 40.

◀ **Fig 17.12c Detail of the adrenal cortex**, showing superficial (zona glomerulosa), central (zona fasciculata), and deep (zona reticularis) zones, each of which comprises characteristic cell types involved with synthesis and secretion of a range of steroid hormones. The zones are arranged in irregular columns and nests of cells, and supplied abundantly with blood vessels. H&E, paraffin, × 130.

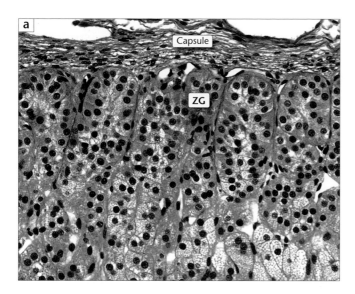

▲ **Fig 17.13a Adrenal cortex zones.** The zona glomerulosa (**ZG**) is a narrow, inconstant band of cortex deep to the adrenal gland capsule. Its cells contain some lipid, and are clustered to form hairpin-like columns bordered by fibrovascular stroma. The transition to the zona fasciculata is not sharp. The ZG synthesizes and secretes aldosterone (a potent mineralocorticoid) in response to angiotensin II or increases in potassium. Aldosterone controls blood pressure and, by increasing sodium reabsorption in renal tubules, regulates sodium balance. The renin–angiotensin system is an important regulator of aldosterone secretion. Renin (from the juxtaglomerular apparatus of the kidney) is a circulating enzyme that converts angiotensinogen (from the liver) to angiotensin I, in turn converted to angiotensin II in the lungs. H&E, paraffin, × 300.

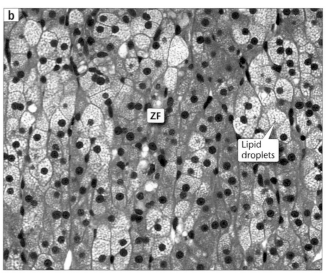

▲ **Fig 17.13b Zona fasciculata.** The zona fasciculata (**ZF**) occupies about half the depth of the adrenal cortex, and shows columns of lipid-rich cells (steroidogenic substrate) with intervening capillaries. The ZF and deeper zona reticularis are ACTH-responsive, cortisol (an important glucocorticoid) being chiefly derived from the ZF. Cortisol stimulates gluconeogenesis by the liver and decreases glucose use by tissues, thus raising blood glucose concentrations, an effect opposite to that of insulin. Cortisol also reduces protein synthesis (except in the liver), increases plasma fatty acids (used for energy), and has anti-inflammatory actions. Stress may stimulate hypothalamic CRH; the resulting ACTH secretion acts on the ZF to produce cortisol, which, via negative feedback, inhibits CRH and ACTH release. H&E, paraffin, × 300.

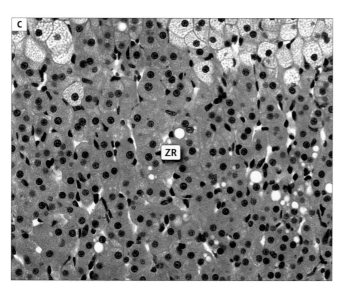

▲ **Fig 17.13c Zona reticularis.** The deepest layer of the adrenal cortex, the zona reticularis (**ZR**), shows compact cells with sparse lipid, and numerous lysosomes and lipfuscin pigment. ZR cells are in part derived from cells originating in the upper two layers. Via ACTH stimulation, the ZR produces weak androgens such as dehydroepiandrosterone (DHEA), its sulfate DHEAS, and androstenedione. Their roles are not clear, but before puberty, DHEAS secretion from the ZR is elevated, possibly contributing to the appearance of pubic and axillary hair. H&E, paraffin, × 300.

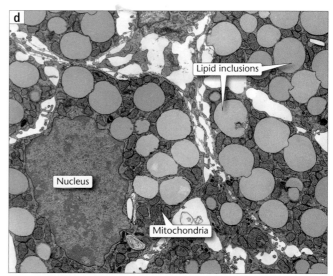

▲ **Fig 17.13d Ultrastructure of zona fasciculata cells,** showing many mitochondria and lipid inclusions typical of steroidogenic cells. Lipid inclusions provide for storage of cholesterol in the form of fatty acid esters. For steroid synthesis, cholesterol enters the mitochondria and, together with smooth endoplasmic reticulum, is converted by enzymes to a series of intermediate metabolites, leading to the production of cortisol. × 5,000.

raise blood pressure by facilitating the effects of vasoconstrictive agents on vascular smooth muscle.

The middle layer is the zona fasciculata (cells in columns), which occupies about 70% of the volume of the cortex. The cells are large, with lipid inclusions reflecting steroidogenic activities, in this case glucocorticoid production, cortisol being the dominant hormone. Cortisol is essential for life, affecting carbohydrate, protein, and fat metabolism; it exerts anti-inflammatory properties (hydrocortisone is a common therapeutic agent) and is involved with modifying the body's reaction to stress.

The inner, deepest layer is the zona reticularis (cells in an irregular network), which is characterized by small eosinophilic cells that secrete the weak androgenic steroids dehydroepiandrosterone (DHEA and its sulfate, DHEAS) and androstenedione; these are converted by peripheral tissues to active androgens and estrogens. Maturation of the zona reticularis before puberty results in increasing circulating levels of DHEA and DHEAS which promote the growth of axillary and pubic hair, a phenomenon known as the adrenarche. Secretion of glucocorticoids and androgens is regulated by adrenocorticotropic hormone (ACTH); aldosterone is controlled mainly by angiotensin II.

> **Tip:** Mnemonic for layers of the adrenal cortex—**G**o **F**ind **R**ex (zona **g**lomerulosa, **f**asciculata, **r**eticularis). Mnemonic for the secretions of the adrenal cortex—"salt, sugar, sex" for mineralocorticoids, glucocorticoids, androgens.

Medulla

The adrenal medulla contains cells of neuroectoderm origin, organized into nests and cords with a rich vascular support framework (Fig 17.14a–c). Often designated as chromaffin cells (staining with chrome salts), the cells are postganglionic sympathetic neurons (with no axons), with storage granules containing the catecholamine hormones, mainly epinephrine and norepinephrine. Their secretion, usually maximal in response to an emergency (the "fight or flight" reaction) is stimulated by sympathetic terminals from splanchnic nerves. Chromaffin cells also synthesize neurotensin, substance P, and enkephalins—opioid-type peptides that may have analgesic properties. Stimuli such as exercise, injury, anxiety, pain, cold, and hypoglycemia cause rapid discharge of catecholamines into the circulation.

ENDOCRINE PANCREAS

The islets of Langerhans produce polypeptide hormones, the most important being insulin and glucagon, both involved with the control of glucose homeostasis. Scattered through the pancreas, islets are readily identified as circular aggregations of pale-staining cells accompanied by a rich capillary supply (Fig 17.15a & b). Impairment of production of insulin or of the peripheral action thereof constitutes a heterogeneous range of ailments known as diabetes mellitus, which is a major cause of morbidity and mortality in humans. Insulin is produced by β cells

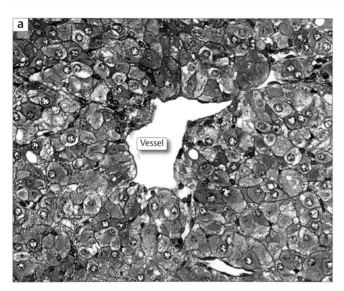

▲ **Fig 17.14a Adrenal medulla.** Adrenal medulla contains chromaffin cells (modified sympathetic postganglionic neurons), which synthesize and secrete norepinephrine and epinephrine, and shows glial-type cells, a rich vascular supply, and nerve fibers. Epinephrine is released into blood for distribution to target cells throughout the body. Exercise, anxiety, pain, and cold are among the stimuli that trigger the release of these catecholamines. Little medullary norepinephrine reaches the systemic circulation. Masson's trichrome, paraffin, × 450.

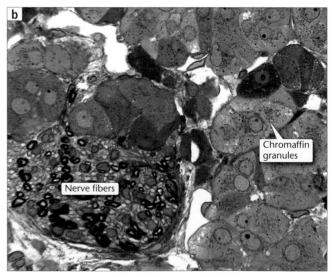

▲ **Fig 17.14b Chromaffin cell granules** contain either epinephrine or norepinephrine, the former predominating, together with proteins such as chromogranin for granule packaging. Released by exocytosis, epinephrine induces tachycardia, bronchodilation, inhibition of gut motility, and hyperglycemia. Chromaffin cells also produce opioid peptides which, in some circumstances, may act as endogenous analgesics. Sympathetic nerve fibers are indicated. Toluidine blue, araldite, × 800.

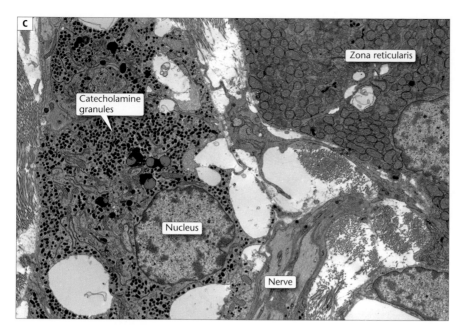

▶ **Fig 17.14c Ultrastructure of the boundary between the zona reticularis and the adrenal medulla.** A chromaffin cell is noted in proximity to an axon of a cholinergic nerve that will synapse with the cell. Hundreds of catecholamine-containing granules occupy the cytoplasm of the chromaffin cell. Upon release by exocytosis, the principal secretory product, epinephrine, quickly increases heart rate, dilates blood vessels to skeletal and cardiac muscle, and causes piloerection, papillary dilation, and other responses associated with stress or threat. × 3,800.

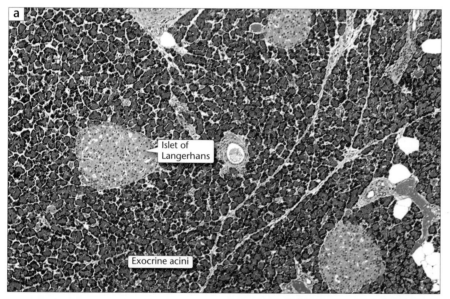

▶ **Fig 17.15a Endocrine pancreas.** The endocrine component of the pancreas, or islets of Langerhans, about 1 million in total, are compact, lightly stained cell clusters occupying 1–2% of the volume of the adult pancreas, with a rich blood supply. Four main cell types are described: β cells producing insulin make up about 70% of the cells; α cells producing glucagon, about 20% of cells; δ cells producing somastostatin, about 5–10% of cells; PP cells producing pancreatic polypeptide, about 1–2% of cells. Each of the hormones, stored in granules, is exocytosed into blood vessels. H&E, paraffin, × 100.

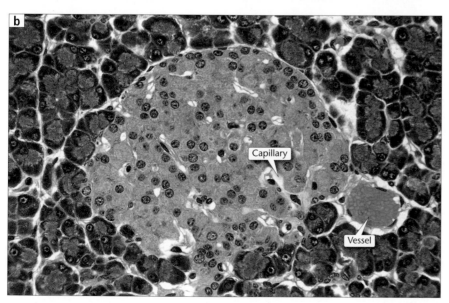

▶ **Fig 17.15b Endocrine pancreas.** Islets show a profuse vascular supply and contain abundant autonomic nerve fibers, but in H&E-stained specimens, individual endocrine cell types cannot be differentiated; this requires immunocytochemistry. The chief secretagogues of insulin and glucagon are glucose and amino acids. Insulin promotes storage of glycogen in muscle and liver, decreases lipolysis, increases fat storage in adipose tissue, and stimulates general protein synthesis. Glucagon stimulates glucose release from liver glycogen, thus raising blood glucose levels, and increases release of fatty acids (used as an energy source) from adipose tissue. H&E, paraffin, × 430.

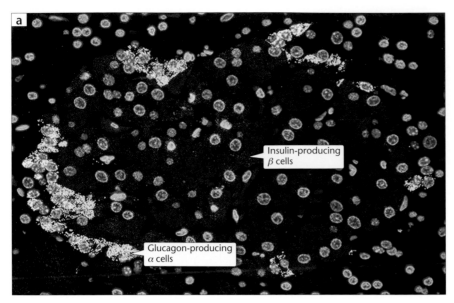

▲ **Fig 17.16a Islet cells**. Double immunofluorescence showing the abundant supply of β cells (red) in the core of an islet and α cells (yellow) at the periphery. Note the rich supply of granules in these cells, which, respectively, store insulin and glucagon. Islets have on average about 2,500 cells, most of which are β cells. Beta cells, rather than embryonic-type stem cells, are believed to be the major source of new β cells during adult life. Beta cells also produce amylin, C peptide and a host of molecules of mostly unknown physiologic relevance. × 450. (Courtesy J Zbaeren, Inselspital, Bern, Switzerland.)

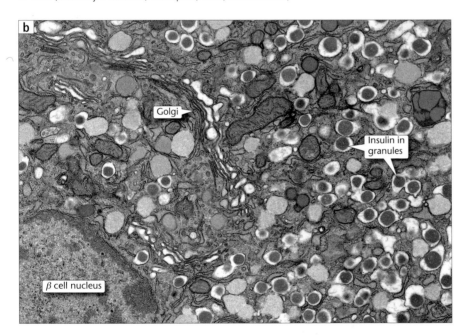

▲ **Fig 17.16b Ultrastructure of an insulin-secreting β cell**, showing many dense-core vesicles storing insulin. The structure of vesicles shows interspecies variation. Insulin synthesis begins with formation of preproinsulin, which is cleaved to proinsulin in the rough ER and in the Golgi is further modified and packaged into secretory granules containing proinsulin. The mature insulin molecule is stored in a zinc-complexed crystalline form in the dense-core vesicles that are exocytosed with release of their contents into the circulation. × 17,000.

(which account for about two-thirds of each islet cell population), glucagon is secreted by α cells, somatostatin is derived from δ cells, and pancreatic polypeptide hormone is produced by the PP cells, about 1% of the islet cells (Fig 17.16a & b). Although the islets occupy about 2% of the volume of the pancreas, they receive 10% or more of its blood supply, which facilitates their secretory responses to humoral stimuli. Islets have a portal circulation, in which blood flows from β to α to δ cells. The α and β types are extremely sensitive to fluctuations of glucose, which modulates islet hormone secretions that normally self-regulate blood glucose in a narrow physiologic range.

The entry of insulin and glucagon into pancreatic veins and the hepatic portal vein ensures that the liver is exposed to high levels of these hormones, thus regulating the availability of glucose and its storage as glycogen (Fig 17.17). Glucose is an essential energy supply for all tissues, and control of its availability is therefore crucial, especially for tissues such as the brain, retina, and germ cells of the gonads, all of which have an absolute requirement for glucose. Insulin lowers blood glucose by enhancing glucose uptake in muscle and fat tissue, and it promotes energy storage by increasing uptake of fatty acids into adipose tissue. Insulin stimulates tissue growth and regeneration by stimulating the synthesis of proteins, DNA, and RNA.

Glucagon exhibits effects on carbohydrate metabolism that are opposite to those of insulin. It raises blood glucose levels by acting on the liver to promote the breakdown of glycogen, and it stimulates glucose production from amino acids or lactate. The effects of insulin and glucagon are antagonistic; insulin is said to be a hypoglycemic hormone, whereas glucagon is a hyperglycemic hormone. Pancreatic somatostatin, from the δ cells, inhibits insulin and glucagon secretion, possibly by paracrine (i.e. local) effects within the islet. It also inhibits gastrointestinal tract motility and secretion, suppressing the rate of digestion and absorption of nutrients from the gut. Pancreatic polypeptide hormone inhibits enzyme secretion from the pancreatic exocrine glands and reduces the secretion of bile. Its physiologic role may be to conserve digestive enzymes and bile, particularly during the interdigestive period.

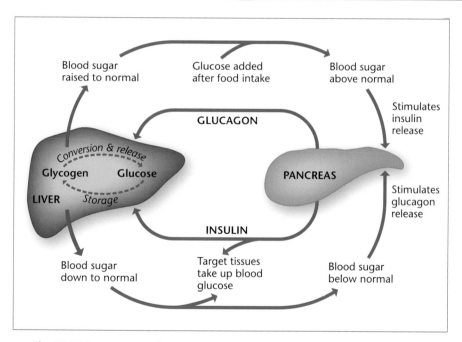

▲ **Fig 17.17 A summary of the relationship between the endocrine pancreas, the liver, and circulating blood levels of glucose.** When blood glucose levels are elevated after a meal, insulin is secreted from the pancreas and promotes glycogen formation in the liver and glucose uptake by tissues, thus lowering blood sugar levels. In turn, between meals or in fasting, low blood glucose levels stimulate release of glucagon, which promotes the release of glucose (from glycogen) from the liver. Blood sugar levels are then raised. Insulin is thus a hypoglycemic hormone and glucagon is a hyperglycemic hormone; the two hormones produce effects that oppose each other.

PINEAL GLAND

Resembling the shape of a pine cone, the pineal gland is a small organ (about 6 × 4 mm) projecting in the midline from the roof of the diencephalon. The pineal is lobulated by connective tissue with islands of parenchymal cells (Fig 17.18a & b). In lower vertebrates the pineal gland is a photoneuroendocrine transducer, converting light into neural and humoral signals. In seasonally breeding mammals such as hamsters, its main biologically active hormonal secretory product, melatonin, regulates gonadal function (through hypothalamic and pituitary hormones) in response to seasonal changes in photoperiod. Melatonin is produced from tryptophan by pinealocytes—pale, stellate-type cells that are arranged into clusters within the pineal gland, associated with neuroglial cells and supported by a stroma of connective tissue cells. In humans, circulating levels of melatonin show a circadian rhythm, being elevated at night and almost undetectable during the day. As humans are not seasonal breeders, the role, if any, of melatonin in the physiology of normal reproductive function is unclear. However, the drowsiness and disorientation accompanying rapid reversal of time zones (jet lag) can be alleviated with melatonin, suggesting a role for this hormone in regulating CNS function.

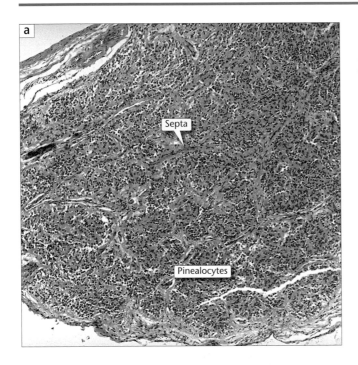

◀ **Fig 17.18a Pineal gland.** The pineal gland is a lobulated, highly cellular structure with connective tissue septa from the external pia mater, containing blood vessels and nerves entering via the pineal stalk of the third ventricle. Most of the cells are pinealocytes, which synthesize and secrete melatonin into the cerebrospinal fluid or blood; glial cells may show calcification (brain sand) with age. H&E, paraffin, × 80.

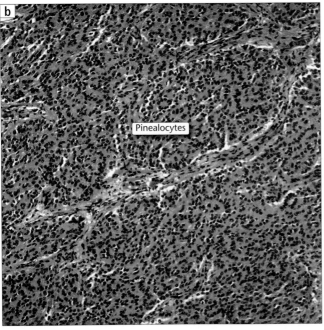

◀ **Fig 17.18b Pineal gland.** The concentrated arrangement of pinealocytes obscures their contacts with nerve fibers and capillaries. The light–dark cycle and the suprachiasmatic nucleus of the hypothalamus, via a complex pathway originating in the retina, drives melatonin synthesis. Serum melatonin is low in the day but markedly elevated at night, and may regulate the onset of sleep. Melatonin mediates the effects of photoperiod changes on reproductive function in seasonally breeding mammals. H&E, paraffin, × 125.

DISPERSED NEUROENDOCRINE SYSTEM

Hormone-secreting cells may occur as single cells or in small groups. Previous histochemical studies showed that these peptide- and amine-secreting endocrine cells shared several metabolic processes, specifically to take up amine precursors and decarboxylate them into amines, hence the acronym APUD (amine precursor uptake and decarboxylation) cells. In view of their similarities to neurons, the term paraneuron can be used to describe some neuroendocrine cells. Neuroendocrine cells show both neuronal and endocrine traits; that is, they secrete peptides or bioactive amines through neurosecretory or synaptic vesicle-like granules, which enter the blood, are released into a lumen, or act locally on adjacent cells. Hence, many of the neuroendocrine cells can produce compounds that function either as a hormone or a neuropeptide. Neuroendocrine cells exhibit a wide variety of shapes but are poorly stained in hematoxylin & eosin (H&E) histologic sections. The gut and the respiratory tract contain numerous neuroendocrine cells.

Selected examples of organs that contain neuroendocrine cells are summarized as follows:

- The *gastrointestinal tract* contains 16 or more neuroendocrine cells, producing more than 30 hormones (Fig 17.19). The *stomach* contains G cells, ECL (enterochromaffin-like) cells, and D cells (also in small bowel), which, respectively, secrete gastrin, histamine, and somatostatin. The *small bowel* contains S cells, which produce secretin, stimulating HCO_3^--rich fluid from the pancreas; CCK, or I, cells, which secrete cholecystokinin, stimulating pancreatic enzyme secretion; K cells, which secrete GIP, or glucose-dependent insulin-releasing peptide, stimulating insulin release; M cells, which secrete motilin, stimulating smooth muscle contractions; and N cells, which secrete neurotensin, regulating gastric motility.
- The *lung* contains single or aggregated neuroendocrine (NE) cells, known as neuroepithelial bodies. NE cells are chemoreceptors that secrete amine or peptides into capillaries, acting on bronchiolar smooth muscle. They may secrete peptides involved in fetal lung development.
- The *skin* shows Merkel cells in the epidermis, which store neurotransmitter peptides and release them to adjacent nerve terminals in response to pressure.

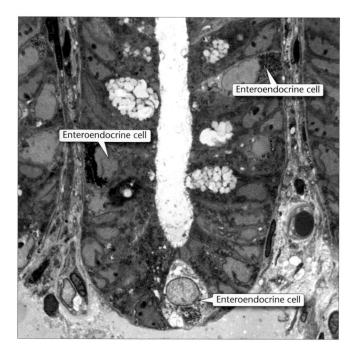

◀ **Fig 17.19 Enteroendocrine cells.** These cells shows basal secretory granules, which upon release may act locally as paracrine factors, or enter the blood, or activate afferent nerves. Gastrointestinal endocrine cells make up less than 1% of intestinal epithelial cells, but constitute the largest and most complex endocrine organ, and are represented by at least 10 different cell lineages based on peptide and amine secretory products. These cells have been called argentaffin or argyrophilic cells (silver-precipitating), or enterochromaffin cells (dichromate-staining), but these staining methods are non-specific and do not always allow detection of all enteroendocrine cells. Toluidine blue, araldite, × 900.

409

PARAGANGLIA

Paraganglia are neuroendocrine tissues that are derived from the neural crest and are widely distributed and associated with parts of the sympathetic nervous system (e.g. the adrenal medulla is the largest sympathetic "paraganglion") or with some parasympathetic nerves (e.g. the carotid body). Small sympathetic paraganglia are found in the retroperitoneum. In H&E histologic sections, paraganglia form clusters or cords of polygonal-type cells (neuroendocrine), surrounded and supported by glial cells. Chromaffin or silver stains, electron microscopy, or immunocytochemical reactions show cytoplasmic secretory granules in the neuroendocrine cells used for endocrine, paracrine, neurotransmitter, or neuromodulatory functions. These cells produce catecholamines or indolamines and several regulatory peptides, notably enkephalins. The adrenal medulla responds mainly to neuronal signals but extra-adrenal sympathetic and parasympathetic paraganglia are stimulated by chemical stimuli (e.g. hypoxemia). Sympathetic paraganglia are believed to function primarily as endocrine tissues because of their close proximity to capillaries, whereas parasympathetic paraganglia probably act on associated sensory nerve endings.

OTHER HORMONE-SECRETING TISSUES

The kidney secretes renin (an enzyme) into the blood, in which it has hormonal-like action in the renin–angiotensin system to reduce sodium and water excretion and regulate the volume of extracellular fluid. Parts of the renal tubular system secrete erythropoietin, which stimulates erythrocyte production in bone marrow. The same kidney tissues synthesize 1,25-dihydroxyvitamin D (originating from vitamin D in the diet or produced in skin), which facilitates calcium absorption by the small intestine. The placenta produces (human) chorionic gonadotropin (hCG), which maintains the function of the corpus luteum during early pregnancy. Other hormones secreted include placental lactogen (hPL), which stimulates breast development; progestagens and estrogens, which maintain the uterine lining during pregnancy and stimulate mammary gland development; and placental corticotropin-releasing hormone (CRH), which is important in the third trimester and in the onset of labor. The testis and ovary secrete a variety of hormones (Fig 17.20a & b)—chiefly sex steroids such as testosterone, and estrogens and progestagens, which are reviewed in more detail in Chapters 18 and 19.

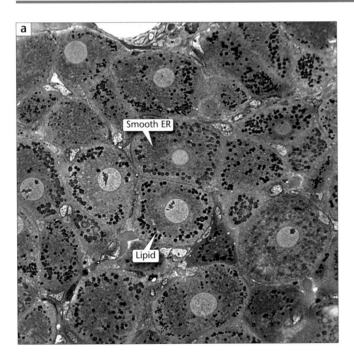

▲ **Fig 17.20a Endocrine cells of the ovarian corpus luteum.** Luteal cells of the ovarian corpus luteum are typical of endocrine cells synthesizing and secreting steroid hormones, notably progesterone and estrogen. The cytoplasm shows lipid inclusions and regions with mitochondria and smooth ER, all involved with steroidogenesis. The corpus luteum is a temporary tissue, forming from granulosa cells after ovulation, ultimately degenerating and being replaced with connective tissue to form the corpus albicans. Toluidine blue, araldite, × 550.

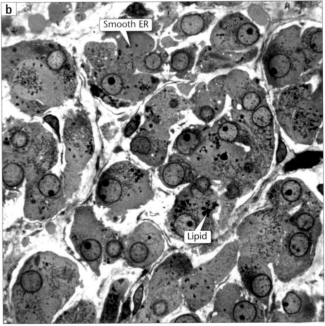

▲ **Fig 17.20b Endocrine cells of the testis.** Clusters of Leydig cells occupy the intertubular tissue of the testis and synthesize and secrete androgens, mainly testosterone, in response to stimulation by luteinizing hormone produced by the anterior pituitary. The basophilic cytoplasm contains much smooth ER, mitochondria, and granules representing lipid droplets. Formed during sexual maturation, most adult Leydig cells probably persist during adult life, although their total number tends to decline with increasing age. Androgens diffuse into the extracellular tissue and enter the seminiferous tubules and the testicular venous system. Toluidine blue, araldite, × 700.

18

Female reproductive system

The chief components of the female reproductive system that contribute to the normal physiology of reproductive function are the ovaries, uterine tubes, uterus, and, during pregnancy, the mammary glands and placenta.

In the female a single gamete, the oocyte, is usually released by the ovary in each menstrual cycle, together with considerable quantities of sex steroid hormones. The ovary also produces a variety of peptides—growth factors and regulatory peptides—which act both locally and on other tissues essential for reproduction.

The uterine tubes (oviducts, or Fallopian tubes) serve (i) to bring together an ovum and sperm, allowing fertilization to occur, and (ii) to convey the conceptus to the uterus.

Fertilization of the oocyte usually occurs in the ampulla of the uterine tube. The inner lining of the uterus provides a suitable environment for implantation of the fertilized oocyte and supports the development of the placenta and an embryo into a fetus. At the end of pregnancy, contractions of the muscular wall of the uterus during labor induce delivery of the fetus through the (now dilated) narrow canal of the cervix into the vagina (birth canal).

Expression of milk by the breasts is induced by the suckling stimulus from the newborn child, the secretory capacity of the mammary glands having been developed during pregnancy.

Coordination of the functions of these organs is largely dependent upon the activities and interactions between the brain (hypothalamic–pituitary axis) and the histologic and secretory status of the tissues in each organ. The timing of secretion and the sites of actions of the hypothalamic, pituitary, and ovarian hormones are essential to understanding the physiology of reproductive function.

The ovarian cycle relates to the episodic release of an oocyte from the ovary at ovulation. Before ovulation, ovarian secretion is characterized by estrogen dominance. After ovulation, progestins are the dominant ovarian steroids secreted by the ovary, although the primate ovary also produces estrogens in quantities in excess of or equal to the non-pregnant follicular phase (before ovulation). Cyclical release of these steroids induces physiologic and behavioral cycles that affect the whole body. In animals, this defines the estrous cycle; in humans and some primates, these changes constitute the menstrual cycle.

OVARY
Adult structure
The ovary contains an internal supporting or connective tissue called the stroma, in which the cortex is cellular, consisting of many fibroblasts together with intercellular matrix and collagen fibers. A central core, or medulla, of loose, supporting tissue shows fibroblasts, vascular elements, and nerves. In adult ovaries the outer cortex is poorly vascularized and contains many primordial follicles, each consisting of an oocyte (the female gamete or germ cell) surrounded by flattened stromal cells, termed follicular or granulosa cells.

Oocytes originate from primordial germ cells, which colonize the embryonic gonad from the yolk sac and via mitosis form oogonia in the ovary. This starts at 6 weeks' gestation. Oogenesis is the process by which oogonia develop into mature oocytes (ova) and is a special type of reductive cell division termed meiosis. Meiosis involves two successive divisions, which produce primary and then secondary oocytes, the latter containing a haploid set of chromosomes. Adult ovaries show variations in histology, which are determined by the numbers and sizes of the growing follicles that develop continuously during reproductive life (Fig 18.1a–c).

Fetal–neonatal ovary
During growth of the fetal ovary, several million oogonia are produced by mitosis, many of which commence meiosis, but not all of which complete it to yield primary oocytes. Oocytes in clusters become associated with flat, spindle-shaped stromal cells called pregranulosa cells. This association between a germ cell and somatic cells (that later become endocrine cells) comprises a follicle, which is the fundamental

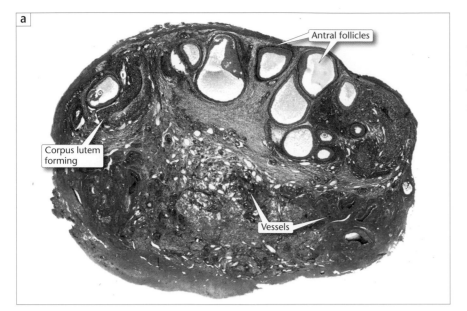

◄ Fig 18.1a Ovary morphology.
Primate ovary with a range of growing follicles, most of which show antrums (intrafollicular cavities) filled with follicular fluid. The medullary stroma of connective tissue contains many blood vessels and several corpora lutea. Masson's trichrome, paraffin, × 10.

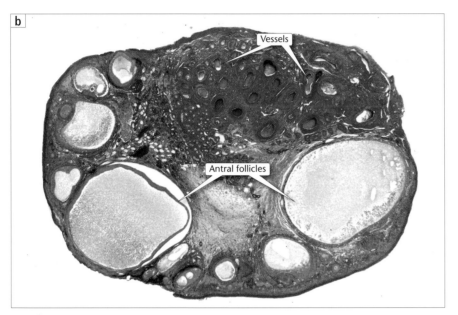

◄ Fig 18.1b Ovary morphology.
Primate ovary showing numerous antral follicles, two of which are very large, although the oocytes are not in the section plane. One or perhaps both of these follicles (the reserve stockpile of follicles) may ovulate. The central medulla is richly supplied with blood vessels, which enter the ovary from a point on the ovary termed the hilus. Masson's trichrome, paraffin, × 10.

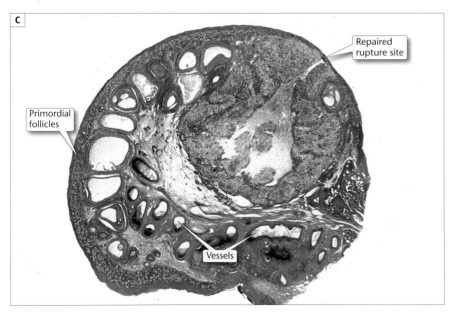

◄ Fig 18.1c Ovary morphology.
Primate ovary shortly after ovulation of an oocyte, leaving a large, forming corpus luteum. The previous rupture site of the follicle is noted. The cortex contains many small primordial follicles (the reserve stockpile of follicles) and growing follicles with antrums. In the medulla many blood vessels are noted. Masson's trichrome, paraffin, × 10.

reproductive unit in the female (Fig 18.2a–c). The oocytes do not proceed beyond prophase of meiosis and remain arrested at the diplotene stage until just before ovulation. For some follicles, this "suspension of activity" may persist for 45–50 years or more. Many follicles die in the fetal ovaries, declining to about 1 million per pair at the time of birth. In postnatal life, follicle numbers continue to decline; from 6 to 9 years of age there are about 500,000 in paired ovaries, of which there are up to 400,000 or more (variable between individuals) remaining at puberty.

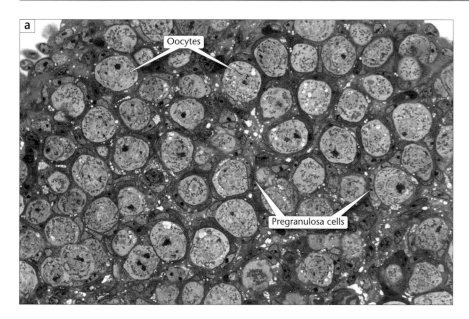

◀ Fig 18.2a Fetal ovary. Late fetal ovary packed with many clusters of oocytes. Stromal cells, termed pregranulosa cells, are being acquired around the oocytes, enclosing them. Together, these cells plus an oocyte make up a follicle. If oocytes fail to associate with pregranulosa cells they degenerate; during ovarian development, many oocytes are eliminated, probably by apoptosis. Toluidine blue, araldite, × 300.

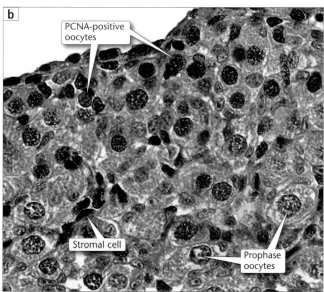

▲ Fig 18.2b Neonatal ovary. Neonatal mouse ovary, showing immunoreactivity for proliferating cell nuclear antigen (PCNA), which localizes with germ cells and stromal cells. PCNA is a marker for DNA synthesis in proliferating stromal cells, and for oocytes replicating their DNA before entering prophase I of meiosis. Some oocytes are not PCNA-positive, suggesting their progression into prophase. Labeled stromal cells multiply to become pregranulosa cells, which contribute to follicle formation. Hematoxylin, paraffin, × 250.

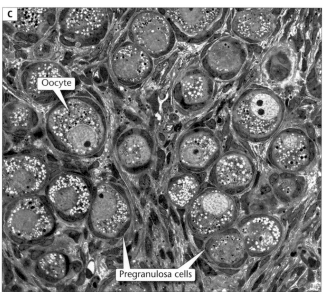

▲ Fig 18.2c Fetal sheep ovary, showing follicles comprising oocytes surrounded by squamous pregranulosa cells that are derived from the ovarian stroma. The first follicles form in the core of the fetal–neonatal ovary and later in the cortex. Collectively these early follicles become the reserve stock of follicles that are classified as primordial follicles. On a daily basis some are recruited to grow, but those that remain may survive for years until ultimately depleted. Toluidine blue, araldite, × 325.

Follicle development

After birth and up to the menopause, the human ovary contains two main classes or populations of follicles; by far the larger, in terms of numbers, is a store or pool of non-growing follicles, and the other is a continually emerging population of growing follicles that enter folliculogenesis (Fig 18.3).

The former category of follicles—the non-growing follicles—represents a reserve stockpile from which a variable number (about 15 per day in 20-year-old women to one per day in 40-year-old women) enter the growth phase. Normally only one of these follicles will ovulate; the others degenerate. The store of reserve follicles is therefore constantly depleted. The total numbers of follicles in paired ovaries between the ages of 20 and 38 has been estimated on average at 200,000 although this varies widely between individuals (range 10,000-600,000). Beyond the age of 38 years the decline in total follicle numbers is accelerated, with about 5,000 remaining by the mid-40s. The store of follicles is normally exhausted at or before about 55 years of age.

Follicle types

The classification of follicles, based chiefly on their histology and to a lesser extent on their function, can present a confusing picture, because the terminology used varies between textbooks and between authors. Investigations into the dynamics of human follicular growth and its endocrine regulation have provided new insights into the functional histology of the ovarian follicle, which at times differs from traditional descriptions. Follicles may be classified histologically into two main categories: pre-antral and antral. This classification is based on the absence or presence, respectively, of a fluid-filled cavity partly surrounding the oocyte. Pre-antral follicles may be primordial, primary, or secondary. Antral follicles are tertiary or Graafian follicles, the latter being the largest; a preovulatory follicle is a mature Graafian follicle. Entry of follicles into the growth phase and their subsequent development is called folliculogenesis. Folliculogenesis terminates with one follicle undergoing ovulation, with the remainder, at some point, showing degeneration, or atresia (Fig 18.4a & b).

Tip: Oogenesis and folliculogenesis are different processes. Oogenesis refers to the proliferation and meiotic maturation of the female germ cells; it begins after primordial germ cells colonize the primitive fetal ovary and ends with follicle atresia or when a sperm fertilizes an ovulated oocyte. Folliculogenesis refers to the growth of follicles in the ovary.

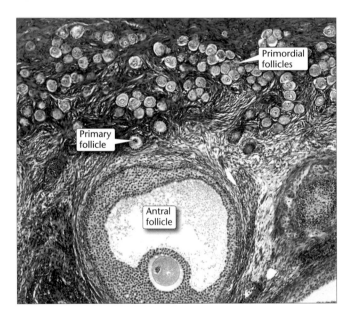

◀ **Fig 18.3 Follicle population.** Primate ovary showing the main types of follicles—primordial follicles in great numbers; slightly larger and far fewer primary follicles; and larger secondary and antral follicles. Oocytes in primordial follicles are just visible, but they grow considerably in size in association with growth of the follicle. The fluid-filled antrum of a growing follicle is shown. Masson's trichrome, paraffin, × 60.

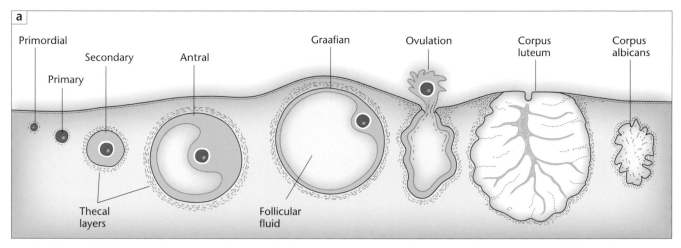

▲ Fig 18.4a Follicle types. Drawn not strictly to scale this diagram illustrates the sequence of follicle types as they grow, terminating in ovulation of the oocytes and conversion of the follicle into a corpus luteum and ultimately a corpus albicans. Growth of follicles is regulated by a complex interplay of follicle-stimulating hormone (FSH), luteinizing hormone (LH), and follicle-derived peptides and sex steroid hormones. The steroids not only stimulate follicle growth but are essential for maintenance of other tissues such as the fallopian tubes, uterus and breasts.

Stage	Process	Follicles	Cell division and follicle development	Germ cells	Chromosomes (n) DNA (c)
Embryo	Differentiation, migration, and proliferation	None	Mitosis up to 5 months	Primordial germ cells, oogonia	2n 2c
Fetus	Meiosis I begins; arrest in diplotene of prophase	Primordial follicles; 4–6 months—small pre-antral follicles; 8–9 months—antral follicles	Meiosis I	Primary oocytes	2n 4c
Newborn	Incomplete folliculogenesis	Primary, secondary, small-to-medium antral follicles	Initiation process (several months)	Primary oocytes	2n 4c
Childhood	Incomplete folliculogenesis	Antral follicles	Arrest in dictyate (up to 50 years)	Primary oocytes	2n 4c
Puberty	Complete follicular maturation	All classes	Folliculogenesis (approximately 85 days)		
Regular cycles	Complete follicular maturation; first meiotic division	Preovulatory (or Graafian) follicle	Preovulatory follicle (approximately 36 hours)	Secondary oocytes / Polar body	1n 2c
Ovulation	Meiosis II begins; arrest in metaphase	Ovulatory follicle	Meiosis II Ovulated follicle survives 6–24 hours	Polar body degenerates	1n 2c
Fertilization	Meiosis II completed; zygote formed	Corpus luteum	Zygote forms 1–2 hours after fertilization	Polar body degenerates	1n 1c plus 1n 1c from sperm = zygote

▲ Fig 18.4b Life history of follicles and germ cells in the ovary. This diagram shows the life history of germ cells from the formation of an embryonic gonad to fertilization. When primordial germ cells occupy the embryonic gonads at 5–6 weeks they are called oogonia. With mitotic proliferation and entry into meiosis I, the fetal ovaries may together contain up to 4–5 million germ cells. This number declines through atresia (dashed circles) to about 1 million at birth and to about 400,000 at puberty. Only around 400 will ovulate during the years of fertility; the remainder undergo atresia. In the adult, it may take up to nine menstrual cycles for a primordial follicle to mature into an oocyte capable of ovulation.

417

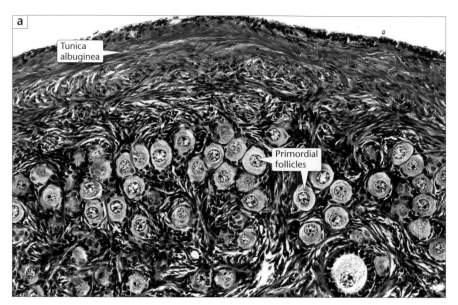

▲ **Fig 18.5a Primordial follicles.** Adult ovary with typical collections of small primordial follicles in the cortical region, which shows many stromal cells but rare blood vessels. The oocytes are arrested at diplotene of meiosis I (the so-called dictyate stage) and in humans may remain in this phase for 50 years. How this suspension of activity is maintained is not known. Note the primary follicle identified by oocytes' enlargement and a shell of cuboidal granulosa cells. Masson's trichrome, paraffin, × 130.

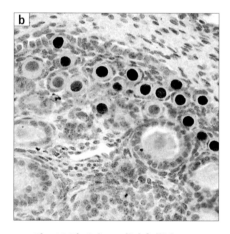

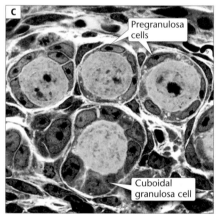

▲ **Fig 18.5b Primordial follicles.**
Immunocytochemistry for germ cell nuclear antigen (GCNA) in an early postnatal mouse ovary. Label is localized to the oocytes of primordial follicles; primary follicles are not labeled. GCNA is a marker of oocyte maturation and indicates incomplete meiotic maturation prior to arrest at diplotene. If such oocytes do not reach diplotene, they fail to form follicles and are eliminated from the follicle pool. Depending on the species, the oversupply of oocytes formed in the fetal ovary is reduced in number during fetal and postnatal life. Hematoxylin, paraffin, × 130.

▲ **Fig 18.5c Primordial follicles.** High magnification of early follicles showing several small primordial follicles with a ring of squamous-type pregranulosa cells enclosing a single oocyte. When activated and recruited into the growth phase that characterizes the commencement of folliculogenesis, the follicle is said to pass through a transition phase. During this time the oocyte has enlarged and is surrounded by granulosa cells transforming into cuboidal shapes. Toluidine blue, araldite, × 800.

Primordial follicles

Two types of follicles make up the reserve pool (Fig 18.5a–c):

- Primordial follicles, the largest proportion
- Intermediary follicles, with a mixture of squamous and cuboidal pregranulosa cells.

A proportion of follicles in the reserve store thus show maturational rather than growth changes, and, although the duration of this phase is not known with certainty, it may take several months or longer. Activation of a small number of primordial follicles each day in preparation for entering the growth phase is independent of gonadotropins and is believed to be regulated by local growth factors. The factors that recruit a dozen or so resting follicles, leaving many thousands unactivated, remains unknown.

Primary and secondary follicles

Within the reserve population, a small proportion of primordial follicles slowly transform, via the intermediary stage, into primary follicles (Fig 18.6a & b) surrounded by a single layer of cuboidal granulosa cells, a basal lamina, and the initial development from the oocyte of the glycoproteins of the zona pellucida. These glycoproteins will become an increasingly thick, clear amorphous egg coat of specialized extracellular matrix that adheres to the oocyte surface.

If leaving the non-growing pool, the primary follicle displays enlargement of the oocyte, proliferation of granulosa cells to form multiple layers, and epithelioid transformation of the surrounding stromal cells into a theca interna layer. This type of follicle is called a secondary pre-antral follicle and forms a further category of growing follicles, with an average diameter of 120 μm. At this stage the mitotic activity of granulosa and theca cells increases (Fig 18.7a & b). Blood and lymphatic capillaries form in the theca interna layer, which communicate with similar vessels in the outermost theca externa, which is composed of stromal fibroblastic cells. The follicles express receptors for pituitary gonadotropic hormones, with follicle-stimulating hormone (FSH) receptors located on granulosa cells, and luteinizing hormone (LH) receptors associated with theca interna cells.

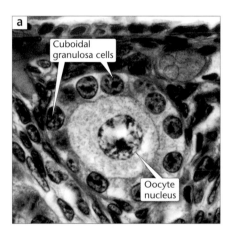

◀ **Fig 18.6a Primary follicles.** These follicles are easily identified by their single layer of cuboidal granulosa cells, which have differentiated from the earlier squamous-type pregranulosa cells. A primary follicle signals commencement of follicle growth. The transition time from primordial to primary follicle is not known with certainty, but in humans is probably many weeks. Local factors, perhaps arising from the oocytes and/or the stromal cells, probably control the entry of follicles into the long growth phase. Hematoxylin & eosin (H&E), paraffin, × 900.

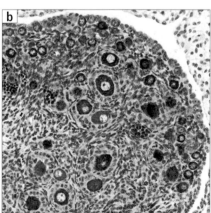

◀ **Fig 18.6b Primary follicles.** Once activated to grow, oocytes in primary follicles become metabolically active, as evidenced by the synthesis of cytoplasmic proteins. The oocytes seen here are positive for a microtubule-stabilizing protein (a Y-box protein). Significant production of mRNA and proteins in oocytes is essential not only for folliculogenesis but also for activation of the oocyte if fertilized. Immunocytochemistry for Msy2/hematoxylin, paraffin, × 75.

Although FSH and LH are crucially important factors for later stages of folliculogenesis, their precise role in the initiation of follicular growth is not known. Whereas hypophysectomy of adults does not block initiation, anencephalic fetuses lack early growing follicles, suggesting that entry into the growth phase may be complexly regulated by local or extraovarian endocrine factors, in conjunction with gonadotropins.

Antral follicles

The appearance within the follicle of an enlarging fluid-filled antrum signals the formation of a tertiary, or antral follicle (Fig 18.8a–c). Most growing follicles never reach this stage and die by a process termed atresia (Fig 18.9a & b). If the follicle is healthy, further development becomes increasingly dependent upon adequate stimulation by FSH and LH,

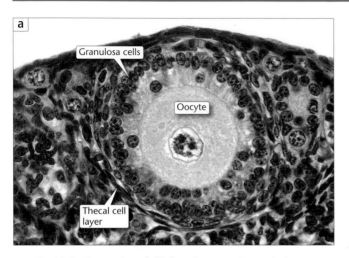

▲ **Fig 18.7a Secondary follicles.** Now growing actively, secondary follicles are identified by at least two layers of granulosa cells (also called follicle cells), which proliferate by mitosis. The oocyte's nucleus and its cytoplasm have enlarged considerably compared with those of the nearby primordial follicles. Local capillaries and peripheral stromal cells are now organized concentrically to form the thecal cell layers that are a source of androgenic hormone for the granulosa cells to convert to estrogens. H&E, paraffin, × 325.

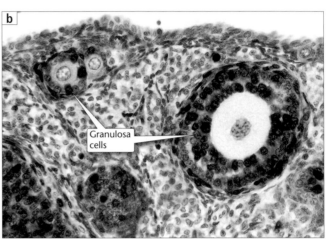

▲ **Fig 18.7b Secondary follicles.** Immunocytochemical reaction for PCNA, which identifies cells preparing for mitosis. Note the positive labeling of granulosa cells, and the stromal cells, which represent fibroblasts and wandering leukocytes. Oocytes show non-specific labeling. Proliferation and maturation of granulosa cells is regulated by factors originating from the oocytes, and the influence of FSH. Granulosa cells acquire FSH, estrogen and androgen receptors; thecal cells acquire LH receptors. Hematoxylin, paraffin, × 300.

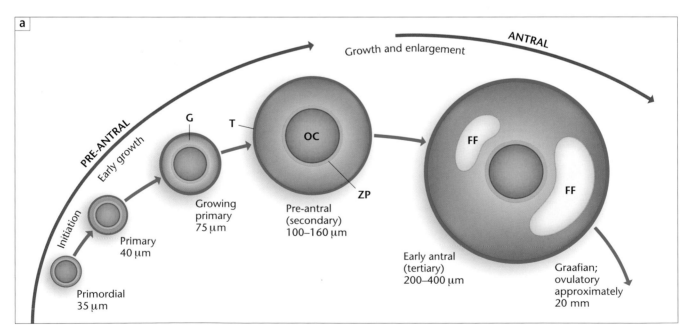

▲ **Fig 18.8a Growth of antral follicles.** Maturation and enlargement of ovarian follicles with average diameters for the various classes. The oocyte itself (**OC**) stabilizes at 80 μm in secondary follicles. Granulosa cells (**G**), zona pellucida (**ZP**), thecal layers (**T**), and antrum with follicular fluid (**FF**) are indicated. In the human ovary these phases occur very slowly over several months.

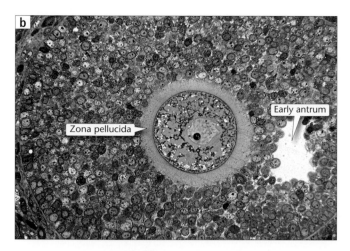

◀ **Fig 18.8b Growth of antral follicles.** Early antral follicles show development of a cavity, or antrum, containing follicular fluid. This is initially composed of proteoglycans and hyaluronan, synthesized by the granulosa cells under stimulus from follicle-stimulating hormone. The oocyte shows a nucleus with nucleolus, and a cytoplasm rich in mitochondria and granules. The zona pellucida forms a thick shell or coat surrounding the oocytes and comprises three major glycoproteins (designated as ZP proteins) synthesized by the oocyte. In ovulated oocytes, the ZP proteins induce the sperm acrosome reaction, determine the species specificity of fertilization, and prevent polyspermy. Early ZP transcripts are expressed in resting follicles well before the zona pellucida is detected by morphologic analysis. Cytoplasmic processes in the zona provide gap-junctional communication between the oocyte and granulosa cells. Toluidine blue, araldite, × 325.

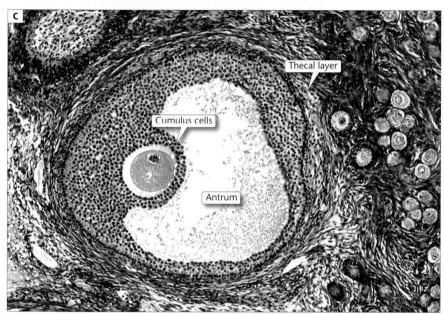

◀ **Fig 18.8c Growth of antral follicles.** Groups of growing antral follicles, dependent upon gonadotropins, are said to be recruited and will continue to grow, or undergo atresia. The antrum expands in volume from multiple cavities, and granulosa cells adjacent to the oocyte form the cumulus layer that remains with the oocyte beyond ovulation. Mural granulosa cells form the peripheral layer. The theca is richly vascularized, providing entry of substrates for the biosynthetic activities of thecal and granulosa cells, and an exit route for steroid and peptide hormones produced in the follicle. A basal lamina marks the border between the follicle and the thecal cell layer. Masson's trichrome, paraffin, × 110.

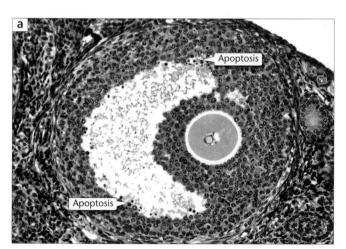

▲ **Fig 18.9a Atretic follicles.** Most follicles undergo degeneration, or atresia, and this can occur at any stage of folliculogenesis, although it is detected most frequently in antral follicles. An early indication of follicle demise in antral follicles is the appearance of apoptotic granulosa cells. Although it is not known how many apoptotic cells definitively mark the follicle in the early stage of atresia, some believe it is as few as five. H&E, paraffin, × 150.

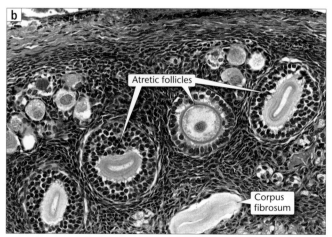

▲ **Fig 18.9b Atretic follicles.** Atretic pre-antral follicles quickly lose the oocyte, and the zona pellucida is thickened and irregular. The result is a hyalinized connective tissue mass, the corpus fibrosum, which is resorbed. The cause or causes of pre-antral atresia are not known with certainty, but probably result from lack of local growth factor/hormone support. H&E, paraffin, × 120.

particularly after the cyclic pattern of blood levels of these hormones is established at puberty. Antral follicles enlarge in diameter by way of an increase in fluid volume and proliferation of granulosa and thecal cells, although oocyte diameter stabilizes at about 80 μm. Graafian follicles are large antral follicles at the preovulatory stage and in humans are about 20 mm in diameter (Fig 18.10a & b). Primary and some early antral follicles occur in the fetal ovary during the second and third trimesters, but these all undergo atresia. Growth and then atresia of follicles also occurs in most babies and infants, and several antral follicles averaging 3 mm in diameter occasionally may be visible on ovarian ultrasound, but no medium-sized antral follicles (i.e. ones with a diameter of more than 5 mm) are seen. The restricted growth of follicles before puberty is very likely the result of lack of gonadotropin support at this time of life.

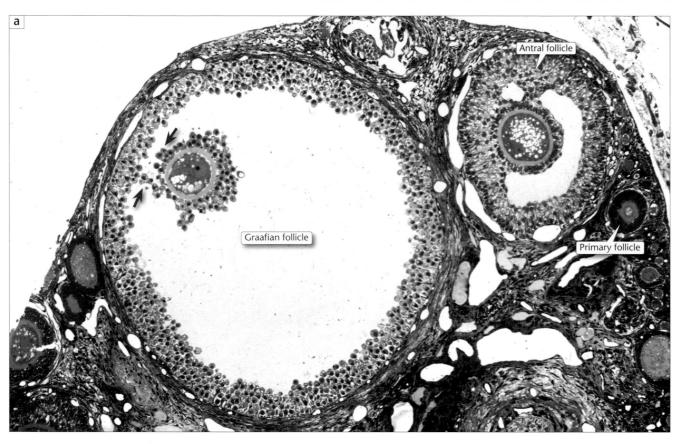

▲ **Fig 18.10a Graafian follicle.** The largest healthy follicle (5–8 mm) is selected from the cohort of recruited follicles and becomes dominant, increasing in size up to 20 mm as the preovulatory follicle. Dominance is associated with atresia of the cohort, and temporary suspension of recruitment. The cumulus mass (**arrows**), or corona radiata, will detach from the mural granulosa cells. Follicular fluid expands in volume by fluid transudate from thecal vasculature. This follicular fluid contains gonadotropins, steroids, and various peptides and protein hormones such as inhibin. Note the thinning of theca and tunica albuginea, through which the oocyte–cumulus complex will be expelled at ovulation. Toluidine blue, araldite, × 150.

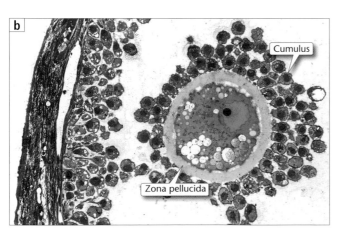

◀ **Fig 18.10b Oocyte of a mature follicle.** The cumulus–oocyte mass in ovulatory follicles shows a zona pellucida around the oocyte, surrounded by the cumulus oophorus of attendant granulosa cells. The latter produce an extracellular matrix rich in hyaluronan. The matrix assists the approach of a spermatozoon toward the oocyte during fertilization. Just before ovulation, the cumulus bridge to the follicle granulosa cells is severed, leaving the cumulus–oocyte mass suspended in follicular fluid. Toluidine blue, araldite, × 350.

That the early stages of follicle growth do not necessarily require stimulation by gonadotropins is verified by cultures of ovarian tissue in which primordial follicles can develop into early secondary follicles, suggesting regulation by local ovarian factors. In prepubertal girls, pregnant women, patients with Kallmann's syndrome, or women taking oral contraceptives, gonadotropin output is either reduced or non-cyclic, and yet some antral follicles up to 2–5 mm in diameter may occur in the ovary. These observations indicate that growth of early antral follicles requires only tonic levels of gonadotropins, and this growth is therefore referred to as tonic or basal follicular growth.

At around 12–13 years of age, onset of menstruation (the menarche) occurs, but this is not usually associated with ovulation (the release of an oocyte from a mature follicle). Regular ovulatory menstrual cycles commonly occur 6 months to several years after the menarche. In the postpubertal ovary, the primary oocyte contained within the largest Graafian follicle resumes meiosis about 24 hours before ovulation to form two cells, a similarly sized secondary oocyte and a tiny polar body (Fig 18.11a & b). The second phase of meiosis continues only for the large secondary oocyte, and again development is arrested, this time at metaphase II; the oocyte completes its division into a mature oocyte and another small polar body only if fertilized by a sperm. Polar bodies degenerate. Primary follicles may take up to 90 days (>3 menstrual cycles) or longer to reach ovulation, with all but one destined to undergo atresia. On average, only about 400 follicles ovulate during the reproductive years (approximately 13 ovulations each year for about 30 years or more).

Why is it that so many more follicles commence growth between puberty and menopause but all of these are destined to die? The answer lies in the fact that the ovary, and specifically the follicles, must produce appropriate quantities of sex steroids and protein hormones for fertility and maintenance of secondary sex characteristics. As follicles grow, they produce more of these hormones and therefore an adequate number of hormone-producing follicles is essential. To maintain these healthy follicle numbers when many others are simultaneously lost through atresia, the ovary recruits a group each day from the reserve stock of primordial follicles to begin growth. This guarantees a supply of the hormones that are necessary for fertility.

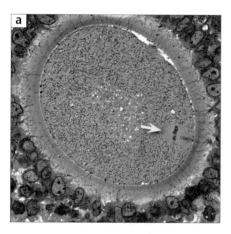

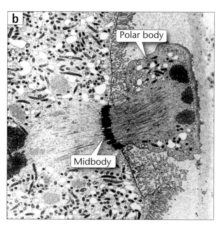

▲ **Fig 18.11a Meiotic maturation.** Coincident with the midcycle surge of gonadotropins, the oocyte, arrested in dictyate, resumes meiosis I several hours before ovulation. The nucleus disappears (by germinal vesicle breakdown), and condensed chromosomes and spindles (**arrow**) are located adjacent to the plasma membrane. Cell division is unequal, producing a tiny daughter cell (a polar body) and a large secondary oocyte. The secondary oocyte proceeds into meiosis II but again is arrested, at metaphase II, until the oocyte is fertilized. This triggers completion of meiosis with formation of a second polar body. Toluidine blue, araldite, × 550.

▲ **Fig 18.11b Ultrastructure of polar body extrusion** during meiosis I in an oocyte of an ovulatory follicle. Note the chromosomes linked at the future cleavage furrow by a midbody. Polar bodies degenerate in the zona pellucida, or in the perivitelline space if the oocyte is ovulated. Arrest of the oocyte in metaphase of meiosis II is possibly regulated by the protein kinase product of the c-mos proto-oncogene, Mos. This is thought to inhibit the degradation of spindle microtubules necessary for sister chromatid separation. Arrest of meiosis may occur to prevent inappropriate DNA replication before fertilization. (Courtesy H Moore, Sheffield University, UK, and D Taggart, University of Adelaide, Australia.) × 2,500.

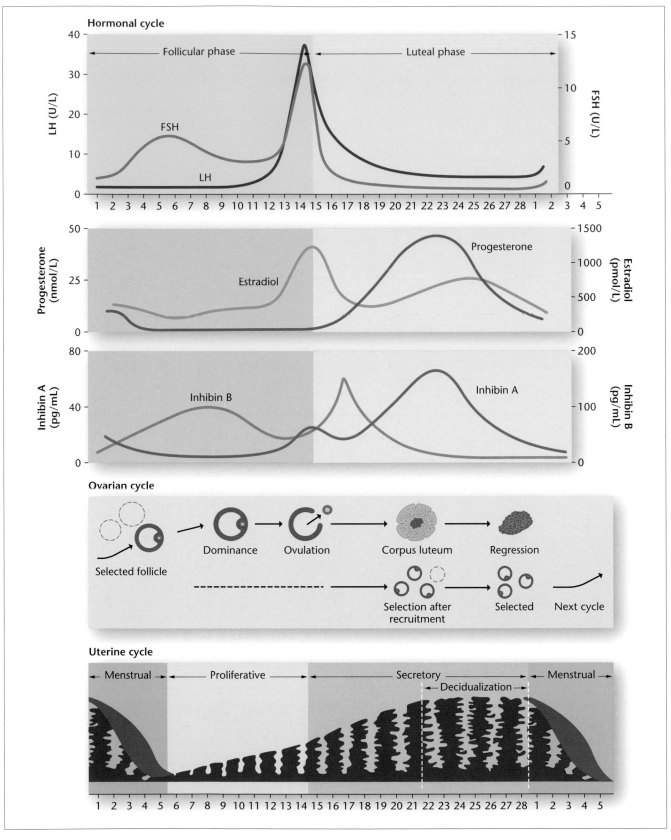

▲ **Fig 18.12 The human menstrual cycle.** The diagram shows changes in plasma concentrations of hormones, development of follicles and corpus luteum, and changes in the endometrium during the menstrual cycle. In the **hormonal cycle** (top three graphs), inhibin B is probably secreted by antral follicles in response to FSH; it possibly limits the duration of the midcycle rise in FSH. Inhibin A is secreted by the corpus luteum and its decline, together with falling steroid levels, contributes to the rise in FSH in the follicular phase. In the **ovarian cycle**, only follicles selected to provide one dominant follicle are indicated. This phase lasts 20–25 days. In the **uterine cycle**, the stratum basalis is not shed at menses and provides for regeneration of the mucosa. (Hormone profiles adapted from Groome NP, et al. J Clin Endocrinol Metab 1996; 81:1401–05.)

Follicle growth versus atresia

The hormonal control of follicle growth during the menstrual cycle is driven by the regular discharge of pulses of gonadotropin-releasing hormone from specific nuclei of the hypothalamus; this in turn stimulates secretion of FSH and LH from the anterior pituitary (Fig 18.12). Luteinizing hormone stimulates the theca interna to produce androgen, which is then converted to estrogens by aromatase enzyme in the adjacent granulosa cells under specific FSH stimulus (Fig 18.13). The peptide hormones inhibins and activins produced by granulosa cells of follicles respectively inhibit and activate FSH secretion by the pituitary. In addition these peptides have intraovarian effects on androgen and estrogen production. Thus by their actions on the pituitary and the ovary, inhibins and activins modulate the functions of the granulosa cells during follicle growth.

In humans, the maturation of growing follicles is regulated by a balance between their survival and atresia. In young adult women, two or three antral follicles (each about 2–5 mm in diameter) are recruited for development (chiefly by FSH) during the second half of the menstrual cycle preceding the next cycle in which ovulation will occur (i.e. some 20 days before ovulation). From this group of growing antral follicles stimulated by FSH, the most advanced follicle destined to become the ovulatory follicle is said to be "selected." It produces estrogen and inhibins (peptides), which circulate in peripheral blood, thereby restraining or suppressing FSH to levels that are insufficient to support further development of the other follicles. Essentially the other follicles are starved of their supply of FSH and then undergo atresia. The now "dominant" antral follicle (with a continuously enlarging diameter of more than 10 mm) survives in this environment of reduced FSH because it acquires increased responsiveness to gonadotropins, assisted by local regulatory factors that amplify the actions of FSH and LH. The high secretion of estrogen by the dominant follicle now exerts positive feedback at the pituitary level. This initiates a sharp surge in gonadotropin release, which induces ovulation by rupture of the mature follicle.

> **Tip:** All healthy ovaries in humans, from babies to adult women, contain growing follicles. The prepubertal ovary is not "quiescent" or non-functional, but it fails to produce mature follicles because appropriate hormone stimulation is lacking until puberty.

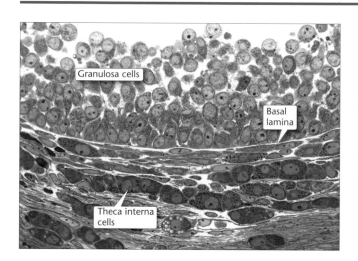

◀ **Fig 18.13 Theca interna.** The ovary secretes progestins, androgens, estrogens, and protein hormones, notably inhibins. Steroid production and regulation in follicles is compartmentalized in the theca interna and granulosa cells. LH stimulates theca cell production of aromatizable androgens (androstenedione, testosterone), which cross the basal lamina for conversion by aromatase enzyme into estrogens in granulosa cells, initially under stimulus from FSH but later also by stimulus from LH in large antral follicles. The output of hormones by large follicles contributes to control of the menstrual cycle, timing of ovulation, and fertility. Toluidine blue, araldite, × 550.

Corpus luteum

Following ovulation the follicle is retained within the ovary and is easily recognized due to its large size and unique morphology (Fig 18.14a–c). Granulosa and theca interna cells of the ruptured follicle show histologic and functional transformation into the respective granulosa and theca lutein cells of the corpus luteum, and the entire mass of this tissue becomes richly vascularized via growth of blood vessels through its supporting connective tissue. In response to stimulation by LH, the corpus luteum secretes progesterone, estrogens, and inhibin, together with

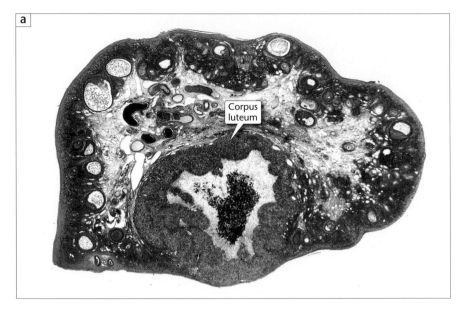

◀ **Fig 18.14a Corpus luteum.** Primate ovary postovulation, showing the fate of the ovulatory follicle that is retained by the ovary and converted into endocrine tissue termed the corpus luteum. As ovulation requires rupture of the follicle to expel the oocytes–cumulus mass, vascular disruption and invasion of new vessels gives coagulated blood and fibrin accumulation in the resealed antral cavity of the corpus luteum. Note the folding of the luteal wall as it compacts to replace the core with connective tissue and blood vessels. Masson's trichrome, paraffin, × 12.

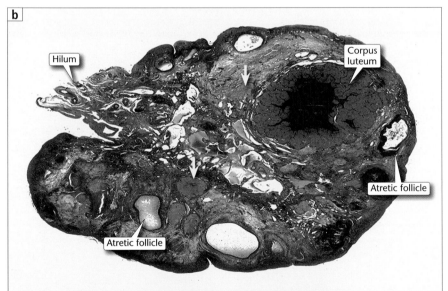

◀ **Fig 18.14b Corpus luteum.** Human ovary at late luteal phase of menstrual cycle (age 39 years), showing a compacting corpus luteum with a central fibrin blood clot, which indicates that ovulation has occurred recently. Large antral follicles are noted, some of which are atretic, with fibrous clotting. Primary follicles are uncommon. The medulla contains blood vessels entering and exiting via the hilum, and fibrous aggregations (**arrows**) represent residual atretic follicles and corpora albicantes. Masson's trichrome, paraffin, × 4.

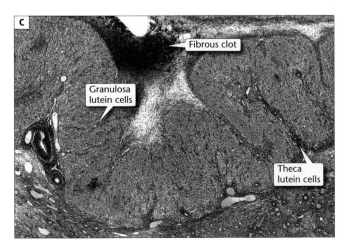

◀ **Fig 18.14c Corpus luteum.** Following oocyte release, granulosa cells in the follicle wall differentiate (luteinize) into granulosa luteal cells through specific stimulus from luteinizing hormone. They acquire variable quantities of lipid and steroidogenic and protein synthetic capacity. Theca cells also luteinize and reside in small numbers at the periphery of masses of luteal cells or granulosa luteal cells; at times these are called paraluteal cells. The fibrotic clot in the center (formerly the antrum) diminishes as the corpus luteum compacts itself and acquires a rich blood supply. Masson's trichrome, paraffin, × 40.

relaxin. Luteal cells show typical features of steroid-secreting cells with smooth endoplasmic reticulum and lipid inclusions (Fig 18.15a & b). The corpus luteum is pink in color owing to its rich blood supply; it is yellow when mature and in regression.

Progesterone prepares the uterine mucosa for the implantation of a fertilized oocyte, but in non-pregnant conditions the corpus luteum regresses and degenerates (a process termed luteolysis) within 2 weeks of ovulation. At that time it becomes fibrosed or pigmented owing to hemoglobin degradation (corpus nigricans); it is then hyalinized into opalescent, whitish connective tissue called the corpus albicans (Fig 18.16a & b). Ultimately it is

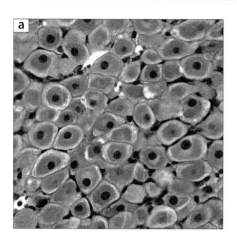

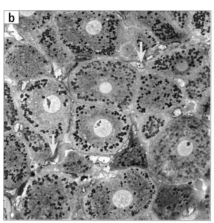

▲ **Fig 18.15a Luteal cells.** Large granulosa luteal cells predominate in the corpus luteum. They exhibit a central nucleus, a cytoplasm that shows eosinophilic staining (because of the mitochondria and lysosomes), and peripheral regions with less staining (indicating smooth endoplasmic reticulum)—i.e. they contain organelles for steroidogenesis. The thin extracellular areas contain fibroblasts and many capillaries. Serum luteinizing hormone maintains luteal function. Luteal cell secretion of progesterone continues the maturation of the endometrium initiated before ovulation and brought about by estrogen secretion from the ovarian follicles. H&E, paraffin, × 160.

▲ **Fig 18.15b Luteal cells**, showing cytoplasm with lipid and smooth endoplasmic reticulum. Endothelial cells and fibroblasts (**arrows**) are more numerous than luteal cells. Most luteal cells secrete progesterone, but theca luteal cells produce androgen substrate, which is aromatized to estrogens by granulosa luteal cells. The corpus luteum is pivotal to the control of the menstrual cycle; it secretes androgens, growth factors, and particularly inhibin A, progesterone, and estrogen, which exert negative feedback regulation of pituitary secretion of follicle-stimulating hormone, thereby inhibiting follicular development. Toluidine blue, araldite, × 400.

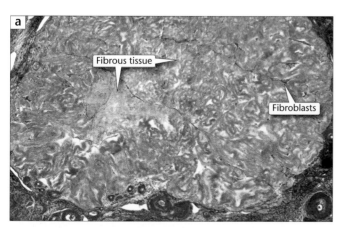

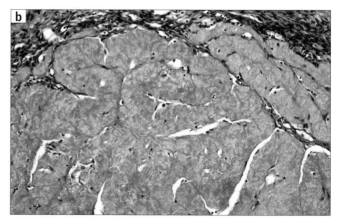

▲ **Fig 18.16a Corpus albicans.** Luteolysis is accompanied by fibroblastic invasion. These fibroblasts synthesize collagen and extracellular matrix, which produces a whitish, hyaline appearance. The resulting corpus albicans is a well-circumscribed structure with convoluted borders. Persisting in one or more subsequent menstrual cycles, older corpora albicantes contract in size and are usually resorbed, although typically their demise is prolonged in postmenopausal women. Masson's trichrome, paraffin, × 60.

▲ **Fig 18.16b Detail of a corpus albicans**, showing that all the regressing luteal cells have been removed via the phagocytic activities of macrophages that accompany the conversion of the highly cellular corpus luteum into a mass of connective tissue. The scattered nuclei in the corpus albicans are fibroblasts and capillary endothelial cells. H&E, paraffin, × 150.

resorbed into the stroma. The number of corpora lutea or corpus albicans is a reliable indication of prior ovulations.

Luteolysis effectively terminates the ovarian–menstrual cycle; the declining progesterone, estrogen, and inhibin levels allow resumption of the follicular phase of development in response to increasing FSH levels and high-frequency, low-pulse amplitude of LH secretions. Proof that the ovary regulates the timing of the menstrual cycle is shown by the fact that, in monkeys, ovaries transplanted into castrated males exhibit normal monthly ovulatory cycles.

If implantation occurs, the developing placenta secretes human chorionic gonadotropin, which prevents luteal regression, or luteolysis, by supporting the function of luteal cells and extending the phase of progesterone secretion. The corpus luteum of the menstrual cycle is said to be "rescued" during early pregnancy, and it survives for up to 5–6 weeks until the placenta assumes the dominant role of secreting progesterone and estrogen, the so-called luteal–placental shift. In humans, the corpus luteum may persist throughout pregnancy, but its low activity is not essential for fetal survival.

UTERINE TUBES

Extending between the ovary and the uterus, the uterine tube is a muscular tube that is narrow medially but wider and funnel-shaped adjacent to the ovary (Fig 18.17a–c). The distal mucosa is branched and folded, and it exhibits a columnar epithelium with ciliated and secretory cells. The ciliated cells are believed to assist transfer of the oocyte from the ovary to the uterine tube. The secretory cells are responsible for nutrient supplies to oocyte, zygote, and the conceptus, the main nutrients being pyruvate, glucose, amino acids, and proteins.

Secretory activity is cyclical and maximal at the midpoint of the menstrual cycle. After coitus, living sperm may pass along the tube within several hours, possibly assisted by peristaltic-type contractions of the smooth muscle, fluid flow, and sperm motility. The passage of the zygote, or conceptus, through the

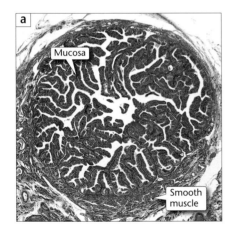

◀ **Fig 18.17a Ampullary region of the uterine tube**, showing the myosalpinx of two layers of smooth muscle for tubal contraction, and the endosalpinx, or mucosa, which forms many complex folds. The mucosa secretes fluid to create a luminal environment suitable for fertilization. Ciliated mucosal cells, abundant in the ampulla, encourage oocyte transport along the uterine tube; this is assisted by contractions of the outer wall. Ciliogenesis is cyclic and estrogen-dependent. H&E, paraffin, × 20.

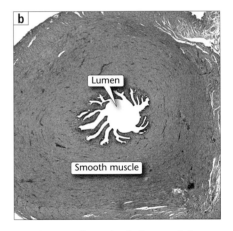

▲ **Fig 18.17b At the isthmus of the uterine tube**, the smooth muscle, now in three layers, predominates, and the lumen is narrow with a few short, longitudinal folds of mucosa. Ciliated mucosal cells are few, with secretory cells dominating. The secretory cells respond to cyclic changes in estrogen levels; this response is marked by apocrine secretion of granules. H&E, paraffin, × 20.

uterine tube is much slower (it takes about 3 days) and is thought to be the result of ciliary activity of the mucosa.

> **Tip:** Progesterone is a natural steroid produced by the ovary and, in addition to other actions, may be said to be an antiestrogenic hormone. Progestins and progestogens are natural or synthetic agents that mimic in full or in part the biologic actions of progesterone.

UTERUS

Myometrium

The wall of the uterus is thick (1–1.5 cm) and contains three indistinct layers of smooth muscle, together with collagen and elastic fibers. These layers of smooth muscle are called the myometrium (Fig 18.18).

The myometrium undergoes considerable hypertrophy and hyperplasia during pregnancy, in preparation for the contractile forces required to expel the fetus during labor.

Endometrium

An inner glandular mucosa, the endometrium (variably 0.5–5 mm in depth) consists of tubular glands extending down from the surface into connective tissue called the stroma. The deeper zone of the endometrium, termed the stratum basalis, is a reserve tissue that regenerates the upper two-thirds (the stratum functionalis), which is subject to cyclic growth, degeneration, and loss of tissues in concert with the pattern of ovarian activity. The breakdown of the functionalis produces the clinical presentation of the menstrual cycle.

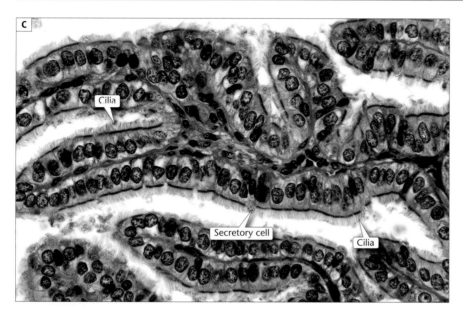

◀ **Fig 18.17c Oviduct mucosa** is a simple columnar epithelium with ciliated cells and secretory cells. Secretory cells are filled with numerous granules and their glycoproteins and proteins are released via exocytosis; other granules appear to release mucus-type products via apocrine secretion, particularly in non-human primate oviducts. These secretions are believed to regulate sperm and cumulus–oocyte transport and possibly prevent ectopic implantation. Intraepithelial lymphocytes may populate the epithelium. Masson's trichrome, paraffin, × 450.

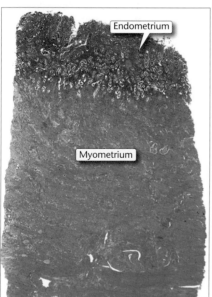

◀ **Fig 18.18 Uterus.** The human uterus is somewhat pear-shaped. It has a very thick smooth-muscular wall with connective tissue and abundant blood vessels, which is called the myometrium (the inner two-thirds are shown here). Toward the cervix, smooth muscle is replaced with fibrous tissue. A narrow central cavity is lined by a glandular mucosa called the endometrium. The myometrium is dense and capable of considerable enlargement during pregnancy. In contrast the endometrium is soft and easily disrupted, for example during various surgical procedures. H&E, paraffin, × 8.

The endometrium and the menstrual cycle

Proliferative phase

The cyclic changes in the histology of the endometrium are regulated by ovarian steroids. Briefly, estrogen from the ovaries during the follicular phase of the ovarian cycle acts on the endometrium in the proliferative phase of the menstrual cycle to stimulate growth and height of the tubular glands within the mucosa (Fig 18.19a–c).

Secretory phase

With the emergence of the corpus luteum in the luteal phase of the ovarian cycle, progesterone stimulates

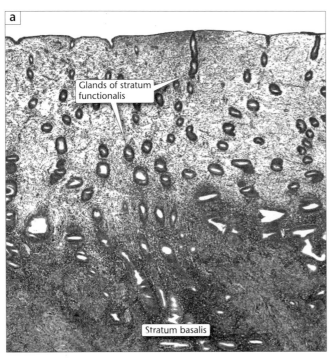

▲ **Fig 18.19a Early proliferative endometrium.** Responding to estrogen levels secreted by the ovary, the glands, stroma, and vessels proliferate synchronously, thereby contributing to increasing thickness of the stratum functionalis. The glands are short, narrow, and straight, and begin to increase in length. The surface columnar epithelium is flat and is not convoluted. H&E, paraffin, × 20.

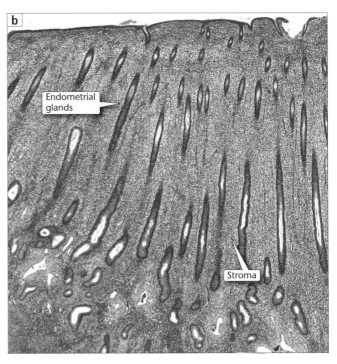

▲ **Fig 18.19b Mid-proliferative endometrium.** At this stage the endometrium has grown in thickness and its glands are very long and narrow, with some early signs of convolutions. The stroma is very cellular, containing mesenchymal-type cells and extracellular matrix. Estrogen induces development of all elements of the endometrium. H&E, paraffin, × 20.

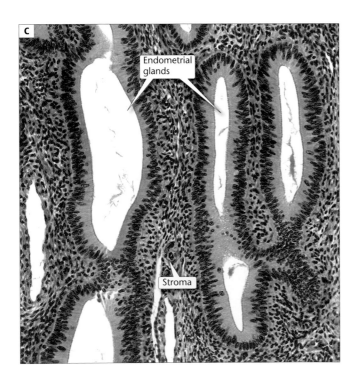

◀ **Fig 18.19c Endometrial glands** have pseudostratified columnar epithelia containing numerous mitotic cells with some ciliated cells. The first wave of stromal cell proliferation, stimulated by estrogen, is evident by the dense aggregation of these cells between the glands. Later in the menstrual cycle, stromal cells enlarge to become decidual cells in readiness for implantation. H&E, acrylic resin, × 200.

further glandular maturation. This involves secretion of glycogen by the glandular cells, together with extensive coiling and lengthening of the rich vascular supply to the mucosa. This is the secretory phase of the menstrual cycle (Fig 18.20a–e).

In the latter part of the secretory phase, beginning around day 21 of the menstrual cycle, the superficial stroma of the endometrium undergoes spontaneous decidualization. The stromal cells proliferate into cuboidal decidual cells and leukocytes are abundant. If there is no implanting conceptus, menstruation is inevitable.

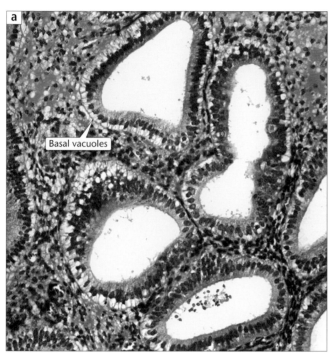

▲ **Fig 18.20a Early secretory endometrium.** The earliest histologic evidence of ovulation based upon uterine morphology is the basal vacuolization and glycogen content of the glandular epithelial cells. Several days later, vacuoles shift to a supranuclear location. The stromal cells become spindle-shaped, with more cytoplasm. Early secretory endometrium is stimulated by periovulatory estrogen, which induces estrogen and progesterone receptors within this tissue. Later, progesterone becomes the principal hormonal stimulus for the secretory endometrium. H&E, paraffin, × 200.

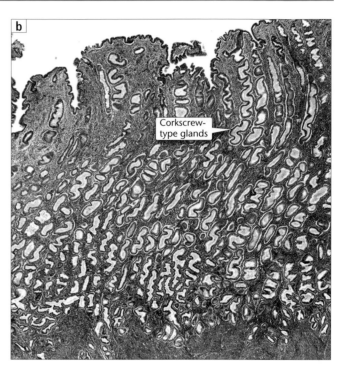

▲ **Fig 18.20b Mid-secretory endometrium.** The glands are now coiled resembling corkscrew shapes and are primed to become secretory due to stimulation by progesterone. The eosinophilic matter in the glands is their secretory product. H&E, paraffin, × 20.

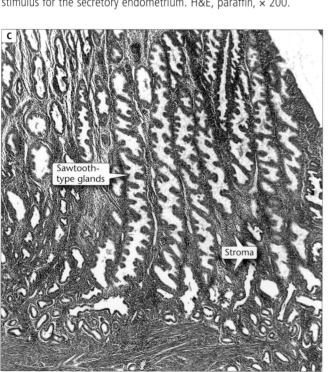

◀ **Fig 18.20c Late secretory endometrium**, showing characteristic sawtooth appearance of the glandular mucosa. Stromal cells are again very abundant, and characteristically predecidual cells are noted in the stroma around the arterioles. These cells become decidual cells, which control leukocyte infiltration, contribute to the formation of the placenta, and secrete prolactin; they also possibly play an immunomodulatory role. H&E, paraffin, × 20.

431

Menstrual phase

The menstrual phase is precipitated by luteolysis of the corpus luteum, withdrawal of hormonal support, and changes in the vascular supply of the endometrium, which deprive the endometrial glands of blood for varying intervals. The majority of the endometrium breaks down into the products of menses: non-clotted blood, dead or degenerating tissues, and some fluid, on average about 50 mL in volume (Fig 18.21). The deepest layer of the endometrium, the stratum basalis, remains and serves as a reserve tissue for endometrial growth and vascularization in the next cycle.

Cervix

The cervix is the inferior part of the uterus, extending into the vagina as a short cylinder with a narrow, slit-like lumen. It consists mostly of connective tissue overlaid with a glandular mucus-secreting epithelium inside the cervical canal. Squamous epithelium covers the external os seen inside the vagina (Fig 18.22a & b). A transformation zone exists where these epithelial linings meet, and is an important and common site of dysplasia that may become malignant.

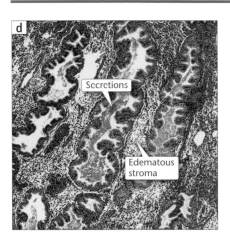

◀ **Fig 18.20d Secretory endometrium**, showing glandular coiling with luminal secretions of glucose and specific glycoproteins. Other endometrial proteins include transferrins, cytokines, growth factors, prostaglandins, and globulins. The stroma is edematous, owing to a hormone-driven increase in blood flow and loosening of the extracellular matrix. The stratum basalis remains relatively unchanged. H&E, paraffin, × 100.

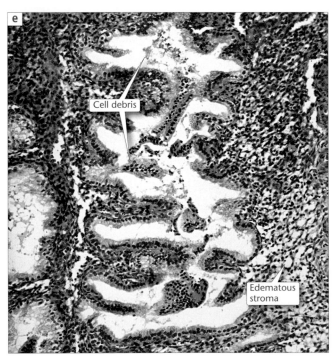

◀ **Fig 18.20e Detail of endometrial glands in the late secretory stage**, showing exfoliated cells, cell fragments, and vacuolization in their lumens. This feature, along with the edematous stroma and abundant blood vessels, is characteristic of a premenstrual condition, in which the upper or functional layer of the endometrium is soon to be shed at menstruation. H&E, paraffin, × 180.

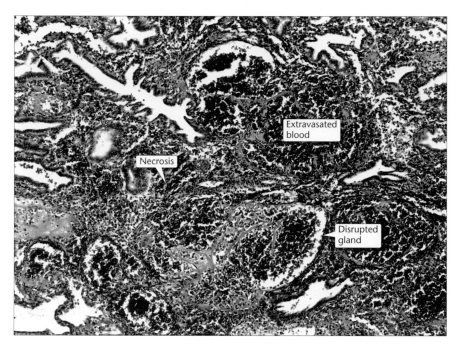

▲ **Fig 18.21 Menstruation.** Menstruation is inevitable unless there is an implanting embryo. Withdrawal of progesterone is followed by prostaglandin release, rupture of the vasculature, leukocytic infiltration, and ischemic necrosis, with subsequent sloughing of the functionalis. Bleeding is controlled by (i) local vasoconstrictors (endothelin), (ii) fibrinolysis to prevent clotting within the tissue (under stimulus of prostacyclin and nitric oxide), and (iii) repair of blood vessels (under stimulus of cytokines and angiogenic growth factors) in preparation for the next cycle. H&E, paraffin, × 180.

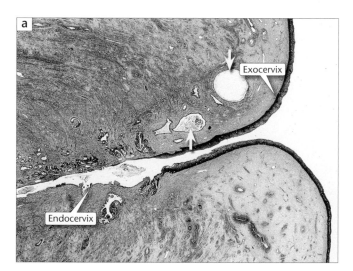

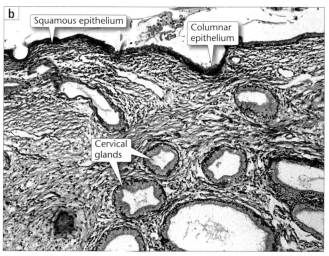

▲ **Fig 18.22a Cervix.** The mostly fibrous neck of the uterus, the cervix consists of the exocervix, with stratified squamous epithelium, which abruptly changes to the endocervix, with mucin-secreting columnar epithelium. The location of a squamocolumnar junction (**arrows**) within the endocervical canal is typically a postmenopausal feature. This transformation zone is the site where the majority of neoplasms arise. A Nabothian follicle is shown. Masson's trichrome, paraffin, × 12.

▲ **Fig 18.22b Cervix.** The transition from squamous to columnar epithelium is shown (**arrow**), together with clefts or invaginations of surface epithelium lined by mucous-type cells. Mucus secretion regulates the entry of sperm into the uterus, initiates sperm capacitation, and protects the uterus from microorganisms in the vagina. H&E, paraffin, × 60.

433

VAGINA

Extending between the cervix and the external genitalia, the vagina is a hollow tube comprising an outer adventitia of connective tissue, a middle component of fibromuscular tissues, and a mucosa of stratified squamous epithelium (Fig 18.23a & b). It lacks glands, but receives fluid secreted by the cervical glands and an exudate of fluid from the deeper blood vessels of the lamina propria, which itself contains many elastic fibers. The mucosa is thrown into transverse folds, or rugae, and, although not cornified, the epithelial cells at midcycle show an abundance of glycogen correlating with estrogen stimulation.

PLACENTA

The placenta is a temporary storage, vascular exchange, and endocrine organ that comprises fetal and maternal parts (Fig 18.24a & b). The fetal part of the placenta, the villous chorion, is

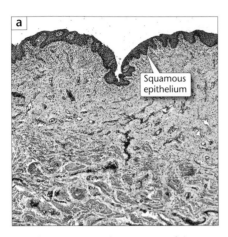

▲ **Fig 18.23a Vagina.** Mucosa of the vagina, showing non-keratinized squamous epithelium, with extensive vascular supply in the lamina propria. Deep to this are bundles of smooth muscle. The epithelial cells are rich in glycogen and hormone-responsive, being maximally abundant at ovulation, but they atrophy without hormone stimulation (e.g. before puberty and after menopause). Bacteria (lactobacilli) are abundant and utilize glycogen as a substrate for lactic acid production, maintaining a low pH environment in the vagina. H&E, paraffin, × 30.

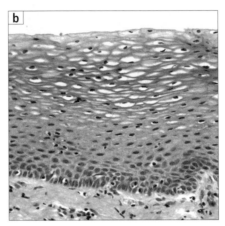

▲ **Fig 18.23b Vaginal mucosa** consisting of nonkeratinized stratified squamous epithelium that is continuously shed during the menstrual cycle; unlike non-human primates, the cells do not vary in phenotype with the cycle. H&E, paraffin, × 100.

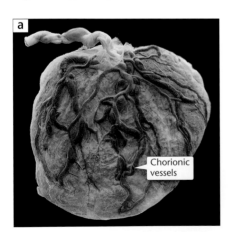

▲ **Fig 18.24a Placenta.** Museum specimen, showing the fetal surface with branches of the umbilical vessels. The smooth appearance is due to the adherent amniotic membrane.

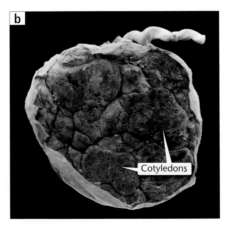

▲ **Fig 18.24b Placenta.** Reverse aspect showing the maternal surface with numerous lobes, which consist of cotyledons separated by septa of the decidua basalis derived from the uterus. Internally, each lobe or cotyledon has two or more villous stems that branch into vascularized villi.

attached to the decidua basalis of the endometrium by the trophoblastic cell layer. Each villus is highly branched and tree-shaped, and surrounded by the intervillous space into which maternal blood flows from the endometrial vessels as funnel-shaped spurts (Fig 18.25a–c). Vessels within the villi, communicating with the fetus, are separated from the intervillous space by the double-layered trophoblast (syncytiotrophoblast and cytotrophoblast) on the surface of the villi. This is known as the placental membrane or barrier. Villi are continuously flushed with maternal blood, which carries O_2 and nutritional requirements for the fetus, and removes CO_2 and wastes from the fetus.

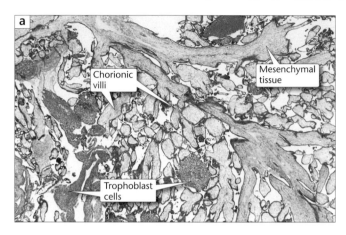

◀ **Fig 18.25a Early human placental tissue,** showing branching chorionic villi that extend into mostly empty spaces, representing the intervillous spaces or lacunae that in life would be filled with maternal blood. Villous cores have mesenchymal tissue, but the absence of capillaries classifies the villi as the secondary type. Primary villi are solid extensions of cytotrophoblast cells. H&E, paraffin, × 15.

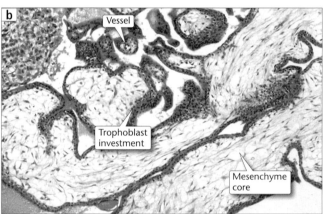

◀ **Fig 18.25b Placental tissue: detail of secondary villi,** showing central mesenchyme covered with outer syncytiotrophoblast and inner cytotrophoblast cells. Growth of trophoblast to form new branches of villi is noted. When blood vessels develop within the villi, they are classed as tertiary villi. Empty spaces in vivo are filled with blood derived from the maternal circulation. H&E, paraffin, × 60.

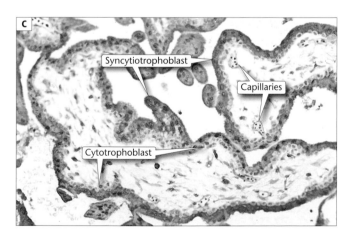

◀ **Fig 18.25c Placental tissue.** Immunocytochemical demonstration of the location of human chorionic gonadotropin to the syncytiotrophoblast layer covering the surface of branching villi. Note the early appearance of villous capillaries, which indicates the formation of tertiary villi. Human chorionic gonadotropin is secreted in association with the developing implanting blastocyst and by the placenta, increasing to peak levels at 9–12 weeks of pregnancy and then at lower but stable levels thereafter. Hematoxylin, paraffin, × 60.

MAMMARY GLAND

Mammogenesis is hormone-dependent. At puberty, breast development is stimulated chiefly by estrogens, which cause the lactiferous duct system to grow. After the establishment of menstrual cycles, estrogen, progesterone, and adrenal corticosteroids induce breast enlargement, with progesterone inducing additional growth of ducts and primitive lubulo-alveolar glands. The mammary gland is divided into lobes supported by dense connective tissue and fat (Fig 18.26).

Alveolar-type glands occur in lobules within each lobe, and their growth in pregnancy is maximal in the first trimester. This growth involves increased branchings of the ducts and increased alveolar numbers (Fig 18.27a–c). The nature of the hormonal stimuli for this growth is not entirely clear, although estrogen, progesterone, and prolactin are required.

Milk produced by the breasts originates from secretory alveolar glands and ducts that converge as excretory ducts at the tip of the nipple (Fig 18.28a & b).

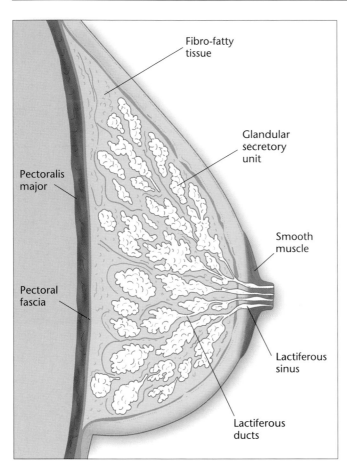

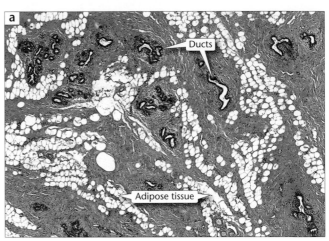

▲ **Fig 18.27a Breast tissue.** Low magnification of inactive breast tissue (non-pregnant, non-lactating), showing that the glandular structures make up the minor component of the tissue. Much of the breast in this condition comprises fatty and connective tissues. In adults, cyclic changes occur during the menstrual cycle; in the luteal phase, there is more cell proliferation and associated increase in breast size. H&E, paraffin, × 20.

▲ **Fig 18.26 Mammary gland.** Sagittal section through the mature breast, showing its division into lobular units consisting of secretory acini or alveoli. These are grouped around small and major ducts, which lead to lactiferous sinuses that empty into the nipple. The breast can be considered as a modified sweat gland that is hormonally dependent. As a derivative of ectoderm, the breast is located superficially to the fascia that invests the pectoralis major.

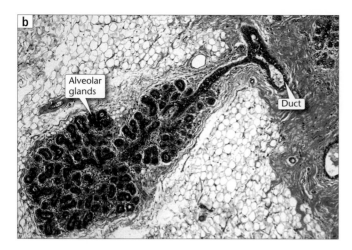

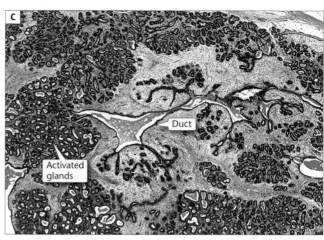

▲ **Fig 18.27b Breast tissue.** Higher magnification of a tubuloalveolar glandular unit in the breast that is connected to a small duct merging with part of an intralobular duct. The quantity of surrounding fibro-fatty tissue is characteristic of the inactive breast. Myoepithelial cells enclose alveolar glands. Alveolar cells show histologic changes during the menstrual cycle; they are small and eosinophilic in the follicular phase, and larger and vacuolated in the luteal phase. Estrogen is a stimulus for duct growth, whereas progesterone facilitates ductal branching and gland development throughout the reproductive years. If there is no pregnancy, the growth of glands and their ducts will be restrained. H&E, paraffin, × 40.

▲ **Fig 18.27c Breast tissue.** During pregnancy, estrogen and progesterone greatly stimulate the glandular system and fibro-fatty tissue is sparse, as seen here. The formerly simple glands now show extensive proliferation and branching, their ducts leading to large intra- and interlobular duct systems that ultimately lead to the ducts entering the lactiferous sinuses. Alveolar secretion begins during the second trimester of pregnancy, and the secretory products within the glands and the ducts are visible by the third trimester. H&E, paraffin, × 30.

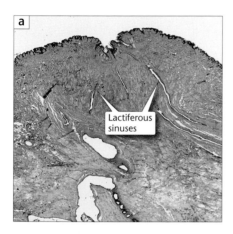

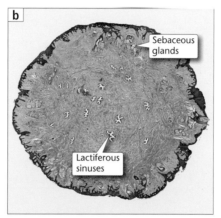

▲ **Fig 18.28a Nipple.** Low magnification of a vertical section through the nipple of inactive breast, showing the convergence of several narrow lactiferous sinuses, which will empty through the nipple. Note the presence of some deeper, dilated duct structures, but the absence of glandular tissues. H&E, paraffin, × 5.

▲ **Fig 18.28b Nipple.** The nipple in cross section contains 20 or more lactiferous sinuses, or ducts, which open onto the surface. Suckling stimulates areolar nerves connected via the spinal cord to the posterior pituitary, releasing oxytocin into the bloodstream. Oxytocin causes contraction of the myoepithelial cells of the alveoli, which produce more milk via simultaneous stimulation with prolactin, also present in the blood. Sebaceous glands deep to the epidermis are indicated. H&E, paraffin, × 10.

Lactation

Lactogenesis refers to glandular cell secretion of lactose, casein, fats, and (soon after parturition) antibodies that convey passive immunity to the newborn (Fig 18.29a & b). Approximately 0.5–1 liter of milk per day may be expressed.

The suckling stimulus sends nerve impulses to the paraventricular and supraoptic nuclei of the hypothalamus and, by way of a complex series of actions on the pituitary, prolactin and oxytocin are released—prolactin from the anterior pituitary, and oxytocin from the posterior pituitary. These hormones stimulate milk ejection from the alveolar glands. Suckling at both breasts when feeding twins causes a greater release of prolactin than the stimulation of just one breast.

Breastfeeding in women delays resumption of ovarian cyclicity and menstruation for several months or even up to 3 years or more postpartum, depending on the duration and frequency of suckling. Lactational amenorrhea is thus nature's method of contraception, relying on the suckling stimulus and prolactin to inhibit ovulation at the hypothalamic–pituitary site. This occurs chiefly by suppression of the normal pulsatile secretion of LH.

ABNORMAL CONDITIONS AND CLINICAL FEATURES

Disorders of the ovary

The ovary may develop cysts. These are usually derived from follicles but are rarely associated with serious clinical conditions. Polycystic ovaries (Stein–Leventhal syndrome) contain numerous cysts, 10 or more, each 2–8 mm in diameter. There are no corpora lutea. Polycystic ovary syndrome is associated with infertility owing to chronic anovulation. This is often due to excessive androgen production by theca cells.

Tumors of the ovary most commonly arise from epithelial components (more than 60% of primary ovarian cancers; most malignant ovarian cancers come from the surface) or the germ cells (25% of primary ovarian cancers). From the germ cells a teratoma may form; this tumor develops tissues representing two or three of the embryonic germ cell layers (i.e. ectoderm, mesoderm, and endoderm). Many teratomas therefore contain skin, hair, cartilage, bone, and respiratory epithelium, but few show malignant transformation.

One example of the failure of follicular development is Turner's syndrome, in which the chromosome constitution is 45,X. Turner's syndrome occurs in about one in 5,000 live female births. This condition is analogous to accelerated ovarian aging, since all follicles degenerate in childhood, resulting in streak ovaries. Consequently, individuals with Turner's syndrome do not undergo puberty and do not menstruate.

Disorders of the uterine tube

Inflammation of this tissue is termed salpingitis. It causes fusions or adhesions of the mucosa and thus partial or complete blockage. This is often caused

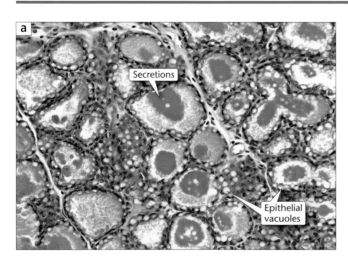

▲ **Fig 18.29a Lactation.** Active breast, showing alveolar lumens filled with milk secretion, which contains lactose, fats, proteins including immunoglobulins, amino acids, minerals, and vitamins. Note the many vacuoles in the epithelial cells, representing lipid droplets released by an apocrine secretory process. Proteins (e.g. caseins) and carbohydrate (e.g. lactose) are co-released as secretory granules via exocytosis. Each alveolus is surrounded by thin myoepithelial cells. H&E, paraffin, × 150.

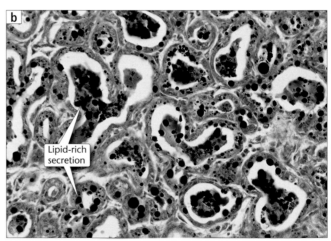

▲ **Fig 18.29b Lactation.** Secretory alveoli stained with osmium to show the location and quantity of lipid-rich secretory products in the gland lumens and cells. Note that this secretion has lipid droplets (black) and brown-stained materials representing other secretory products, some of which are small fragments of the cells released by an apocrine secretory mechanism. Initiation of milk production, as opposed to milk ejection, is chiefly regulated by prolactin from the pituitary gland. Osmium tetroxide, frozen section, × 150.

by microorganisms such as *Chlamydia trachomatis* and *Neisseria gonorrhoeae*, which is why sexually transmitted diseases commonly cause infertility in women. Ectopic pregnancy, or extrauterine implantation of an embryo, commonly occurs in blocked or dysfunctional uterine tubes.

Disorders of the uterus

Hyperplasia of the endometrium may occur in response to excessive estrogen production. Hyperplastic endometrium can go on to become cystic or to show adenomatous transformation or malignancy. A common reason for this is the chronic anovulation of polycystic ovary syndrome, but it can also be due to a persistent dominant follicle or a hormone-producing ovarian tumor.

Endometriosis is a condition in which glands and connective tissue stroma arise outside the uterus. These may be associated, for example, with the ovaries or the attachments of the uterus. Endometriosis is often associated with severe period pain (dysmenorrhea), infertility, or both. It is possibly caused by abnormal cellular differentiation of the peritoneal lining or by retrograde menstruation. Dyspareunia (painful intercourse) may also be a symptom of endometriosis.

Benign smooth muscle tumors (leiomyomas) are common in the myometrium and may attain a diameter of 30 cm. Abnormal epithelial transformation of the squamous–columnar junction of the uterine cervix is an important cause of cancer mortality; in most cases it can be successfully treated by early detection with the Papanicolaou cervical cytology or smear test.

Hormonal contraceptives are associated with a decrease in the incidence of pelvic inflammatory disease as well as uterine and ovarian cancer. After the menopause, hormone replacement therapy, using daily estrogen administration sometimes with progesterone, is effective in suppressing hot flushes, headache, depression, and osteoporosis.

Disorders of the breast

Mastitis is common in postpartum lactation and at weaning. The breasts are tender and lumpy because of duct obstruction. Mastitis is usually caused by an acute bacterial infection, and it is alleviated by increased milk expression or by antibiotics.

Gynecomastia of the male breast is quite common at puberty. It involves increases in the supporting tissues and is often idiopathic, but in adult men it may be associated with elevated estrogen from drug ingestion, tumors of the testis or adrenals, and various endocrine syndromes.

Carcinoma of the breast is a common malignancy, occurring in 1 in 13 women. It often involves the glandular elements and/or the ducts, where islands of epithelial cells often present as non-invasive carcinoma in situ or, with malignant transformation, into invasive carcinoma. Local excision or partial radical mastectomy are usual treatments, followed by radiotherapy and drug treatments that block/destroy estrogen receptors or decrease blood estrogen levels. The antiestrogen strategies are used in cases of hormone-receptor-positive tumors, which make up two-thirds of breast cancers.

Multiple pregnancies

Twins occur spontaneously in about 1% of births. When two oocytes are released and fertilized, dizygotic twins result. Dizygotic twins can be of the same sex or of different sexes, and make up around 70% of all twins. Monozygotic twins (identical twins, who are always of the same sex) result from one fertilized oocyte. The division into twins usually begins in the blastocyst stage at about 7 days, when the inner cell mass divides to produce two early embryos.

439

Male reproductive system

The main functions of the male reproductive system are to manufacture spermatozoa, to deliver these as semen into the female reproductive tract, and to produce male sex steroid hormones, known as androgens. The organs contributing to these functions are:

- The testes
- A duct system that conveys sperm produced in the testis to the urethra
- Accessory glands that supply fluid components to the semen, the latter being discharged as the ejaculate through the penile urethra.

The tissue components of the male reproductive system are hormone-dependent; testosterone—the main androgen produced by the testis—is an essential hormone for sperm production and also for the normal functional integrity of the ducts and accessory glands. Testosterone and its biologically active metabolites (such as dihydrotestosterone) are important in every phase of life (e.g. fetal sexual development, puberty, male phenotype, and behavior). Testicular function is regulated by the anterior pituitary hormones, luteinizing hormone (LH), and follicle-stimulating hormone (FSH), synthesized and secreted under hypothalamic control of gonadotropin-releasing hormone (GnRH). Communication between the testis and the hypothalamo-pituitary system occurs via steroid and protein hormones of testicular origin.

Structure–function relationships of the male reproductive organs can be summarized as follows:

- **Testes:** Seminiferous tubules produce spermatozoa; intertubular Leydig cells synthesize and secrete testosterone.
- **Ducts:** Efferent ductules absorb testicular fluid and convey sperm to the epididymis; the epididymis accumulates, matures, and temporarily stores sperm; the vas deferens delivers sperm to the prostatic urethra.
- **Accessory glands**: Seminal vesicles secrete the bulk of the seminal fluid, contributing fructose (the energy source for sperm) and coagulating proteins to semen; the prostate gland supplies zinc (bactericidal), proteolytic enzymes (liquefaction of

the ejaculate), and prostaglandins (contractions of female tract) to semen; bulbourethral glands secrete alkaline lubricant for the distal urethra.

TESTIS

The testes produce sperm by the process of spermatogenesis, and they synthesize and secrete androgens from biochemical reactions, referred to as steroidogenesis. Spermatogenesis and steroidogenesis occur in separate histologic compartments in the testis—the seminiferous tubules and the intertubular tissue respectively. These compartments are functionally and physiologically interactive. The normal adult human testis ranges in volume from 12–20 mL and is enclosed by a thick, fibrous capsule, the tunica albuginea, which posteriorly extends inward, forming the mediastinum testis. Here the connective tissue contains many interconnected channels, the hollow spaces providing passageways for exit of sperm from the seminiferous tubules to the epididymis. The tunica vasculosa, deep to the tunica albuginea, extends septa into the testis, thus dividing the organ into 250–300 pyramidal lobules, each of which contains one to three seminiferous tubules (Fig 19.1a & b). The mediastinum is also the focal point for blood vessels supplying the testis through the lobular septa or from peripheral locations through the capsule. During the years of postnatal growth, testis volume (median for paired testes) is 1 cm³ up to 1 year, 3 cm³ at ages 5–10 years and 23 cm³ at 14–18 years. Beyond this age, paired testis volume may reach 40 cm³.

Seminiferous tubules

Each seminiferous tubule is a convoluted loop; both ends empty through straight tubuli recti into the rete testis, the epithelium-lined channels of the mediastinum. The rete is continuous with the efferent ducts, transporting sperm to the epididymis (Fig 19.1).

A normal human ejaculate may contain 100 million or more sperm; therefore, the two testes together may

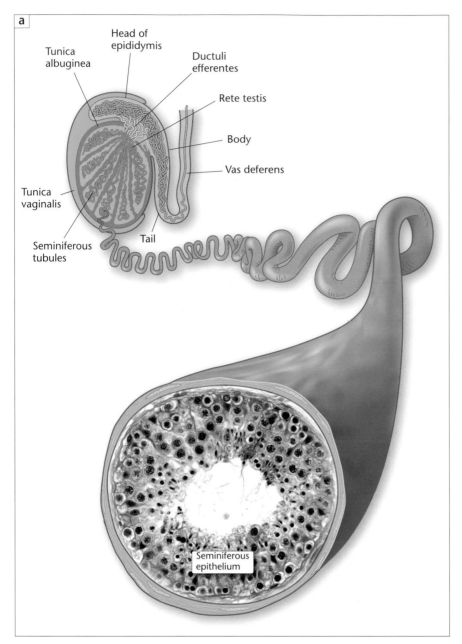

a

Head of
epididymis

Tunica
albuginea

Ductuli
efferentes

Rete testis

Body

Vas deferens

Tunica
vaginalis

Tail

Seminiferous
tubules

Seminiferous
epithelium

◄ **Fig 19.1a Testis and excretory ducts.** The testis is surrounded by a tough, fibrous capsule called the tunica albuginea, with an inner layer called the tunica vasculosa. Septa form many lobules, each containing one to several convoluted loops of seminiferous tubules; the ends of these empty into channels called the rete testis, which is a mass of connective tissue within the mediastinum testis. Sperm pass through the ductuli efferentes to the head of the epididymis, at the top of a single, coiled tube that also forms the body and tail of the epididymis. From the latter, the vas deferens passes through the spermatic cord and inguinal canal, and then joins the seminal vesicle duct to form the ejaculatory duct in the prostate gland. The seminiferous epithelium contains germ cells, spermatogonia, spermatocytes, and spermatids all supported by Sertoli cells. The seminiferous tubule, shown in cross section, is bounded by several layers of peritubular tissue.

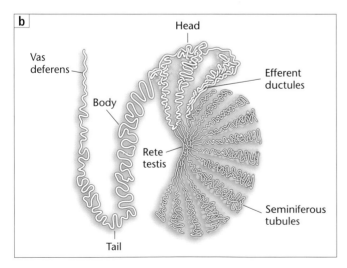

b

Head

Vas
deferens

Body

Efferent
ductules

Rete
testis

Seminiferous
tubules

Tail

◄ **Fig 19.1b Tubules of the testis and epididymis.** Loops of highly convoluted seminiferous tubules—from one to three per lobule—join as single, straight tubules to open into an anastomotic series of ducts termed the rete testis. From these, at the posterior pole of the testis, passageways of the extratesticular rete drain into the strongly coiled efferent ductules that enter and make up a significant part of the head of the epididymis. The epididymis is a single duct, again convoluted, that distally continues as the ductus (vas) deferens.

produce around 1,000 new sperm every second. How this is achieved is well known from a histologic aspect, although details of the hormonal regulation of this remarkable and complex process remain unknown. Seminiferous tubules are 150–200 μm in diameter, 30–80 cm in length, and with about 500 tubules per testis their total length in two testes is up to 500 m.

Owing to their convolutions, tubules present as circular, elliptical, and irregular shapes in histologic sections, supported by intertubular connective tissue with clusters of Leydig cells. The tubules are lined internally by a complex stratified epithelium—the seminiferous epithelium (Fig 19.2), which consists of various types of male germ cells (or spermatogenic cells) and a single type of supporting cell, the Sertoli cell. The seminiferous epithelium is traditionally considered to be the exocrine component of the testis, because it produces (immotile) spermatozoa that leave the testis by ducts. It is also an endocrine tissue, however; the Sertoli cells synthesize and secrete several

hormones with peripheral and/or local intratesticular actions (inhibin/activin, estrogen).

Peritubular tissue

Human seminiferous tubules are bordered by a lamina propria (or tunica propria), 3–5 μm in width, which contains a basal lamina, collagen, and several layers of myofibroblasts or peritubular cells (Fig 19.3). Human myoid cells contain filaments of actin and vimentin. The peritubular tissue, providing structural support, may show peristaltic contraction–relaxation in response to local vasoactive agents such as nitric oxide and vasopressin (to modulate sperm transport), and it possesses androgen receptors. Stimulation of these receptors may be involved with secretion of paracrine factors that act on the seminiferous epithelium, although details of this are not well defined. Mesenchymal cells are also found in the peritubular tissue and have been shown to be capable of differentiating into Leydig cells.

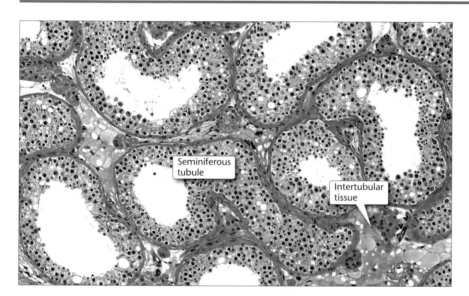

◀ **Fig 19.2 Testicular parenchyma.** Human testis showing convoluted seminiferous tubules, about 250 m in total length per testis, and the intertubular connective tissue containing islands of Leydig cells, which produce testosterone. Tubules are bordered by a thick layer of peritubular tissue. Hematoxylin & eosin (H&E), paraffin, × 100.

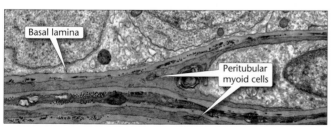

◀ **Fig 19.3 Peritubular tissue.** Surrounding each tubule are several layers of myofibroblasts, collagen, and extracellular matrix. In addition to support for the tubules, peritubular cells have contractile function; they secrete various peptides, possibly influencing the function of Sertoli cells and spermatogonia via paracrine action. In some species the peritubular tissue partly restricts the entry of macromolecules into the tubules from the intertubular tissue. × 10,000.

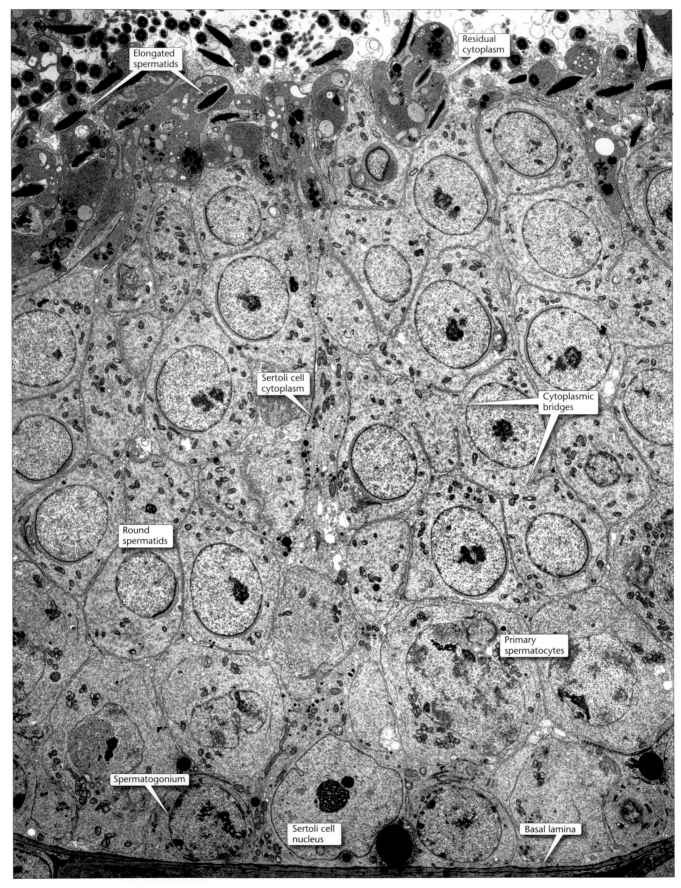

▲ **Fig 19.4 Seminiferous epithelium.** Ultrastructure of mouse seminiferous epithelium, showing the basal location of a Sertoli cell nucleus and several spermatogonia. Sertoli cells provide the structural framework for all the germ cells, which are supported by Sertoli cell cytoplasmic extensions from the base to the luminal aspect of the epithelium. Arranged in strata are the primary spermatocytes and the round and elongated spermatids. Note the intercellular cytoplasmic bridges linking round spermatids. Associated with the sperm heads are irregular masses of excess spermatid cytoplasm that are discarded during sperm maturation and subsequently phagocytosed and digested by the Sertoli cells. × 2,700.

Seminiferous epithelium

Germ cells of the seminiferous epithelium are arranged as strata of variable depth; from base to lumen, these cells are spermatogonia, spermatocytes, and round and elongate spermatids (Fig 19.4). The seminiferous epithelium itself represents on average 40% of the volume of the testis. All germ cells are supported, physically and functionally, by the columnar Sertoli cells, identified somewhat inconspicuously by basally located, irregular nuclei often with a nucleolus. Sertoli cell cytoplasm extends from the basal lamina to the tubular lumen, with thin lateral processes filling the interstices between the germ cells.

Spermatogenesis is the process of cell proliferation and maturation by which the early diploid germ cells, the spermatogonia, are transformed over a time period of about 70 days into haploid spermatozoa (Fig 19.5). Not all germ cells survive during spermatogenesis, and, depending on the species, significant attrition (up to 50% or more) of germ cells by apoptosis can occur at any phase of their development.

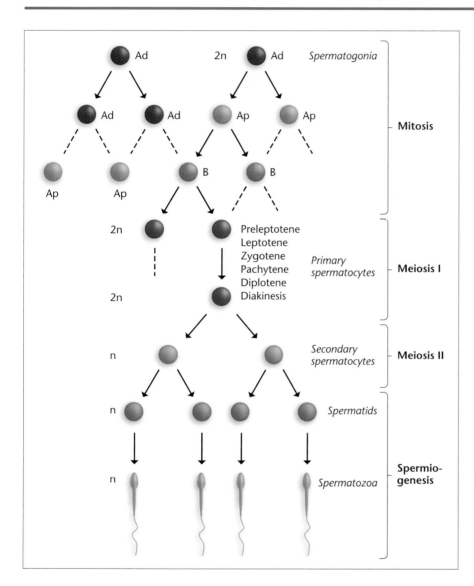

◀ **Fig 19.5 Germ cells of human spermatogenesis.** Maintenance of spermatogenesis is secured by proliferation and renewal of spermatogonial stem cells, meiotic maturation of spermatocytes into spermatids, and differentiation of the latter into spermatozoa, the whole process lasting 10 weeks. Dark and pale type A spermatogonia (Ad, Ap) are stem cells. Ad spermatogonia are reserve cells, dividing if the epithelium is damaged or dysfunctional. Ap spermatogonia may self-renew or divide to produce type B spermatogonia, which proliferate at defined intervals; the division yields primary spermatocytes, which enter meiosis. Homologous chromosomes pair in meiosis I and align, forming synapses at pachytene, when genetic material is exchanged between paternal and maternal homologs. Primary spermatocytes have diploid chromosome number, but DNA synthesis at preleptotene results in each chromosome having two chromatids (DNA content is twice the diploid content). Secondary spermatocytes (from meiosis I division) contain a haploid chromosome number, each composed of two chromatids. Division at meiosis II produces spermatids (haploid DNA and chromosomal content), which transform into spermatozoa —a process termed spermiogenesis. As spermatogonia do not separate at mitosis (incomplete cytokinesis), they, and all their derivative germ cells, are interconnected by cytoplasmic bridges, so forming families, or clones, of germ cells, and remain connected until spermatozoa are released (spermiation). Not every germ cell survives during spermatogenesis. In the human testis, one third or more of the germ cells degenerate by apoptosis; compared with other primates and other mammals, human spermatogenesis is relatively inefficient.

445

Spermatogenesis

Spermatogenesis is the process by which germ-line stem cells self-renew and supply differentiating spermatogonia, which constantly add to the population of germ cells. It can be subdivided into three consecutive sequences, which are visible histologically:

1. **Mitotic divisions** of spermatogonia, in humans classified into type A dark (Ad, self-renewing stem cells), type A pale (Ap, produced by Ad spermatogonia), and type B (produced by type Ap)
2. **Meiotic maturation** of spermatocytes—classified as primary (produced by mitosis of type B spermatogonia)—which pass through meiotic division I, becoming secondary spermatocytes, which in turn complete meiotic division II to yield round spermatids
3. **Differentiation** with no further cell division of spermatids into spermatozoa, a process called spermiogenesis.

A convenient way to illustrate these steps of germ cell proliferation and maturation is to track their development in postnatal testes (Fig 19.6a–c).

Spermatogonia

Spermatogonia are the founder cells for spermatogenesis and reside on the basal lamina of the seminiferous tubule (Fig 19.7a–e). Depending on the species, spermatogonia may be classified on the basis of their nuclear morphology and for many species,

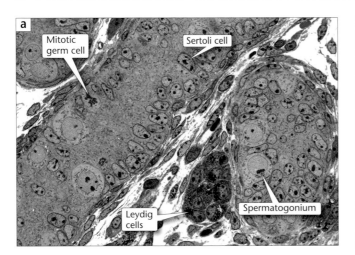

▲ **Fig 19.6a Neonatal testis** with seminiferous cords (before lumen formation), which contain many immature Sertoli cells and several large spermatogonia, one which is in mitosis. Intertubular tissue shows mesenchymal cells and a cluster of Leydig cells. Toluidine blue, araldite, × 525.

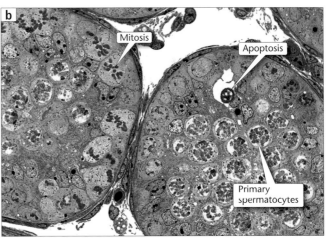

▲ **Fig 19.6b Immature prepubertal testis** during the period when spermatogenesis is initiated. Intense mitotic activity is seen among the basally located spermatogonia. Germ cells occupying the core of the cords are early primary spermatocytes with thick, condensed patterns of chromatin. Not every germ cell survives, as indicated by apoptosis. Toluidine blue, araldite, × 525.

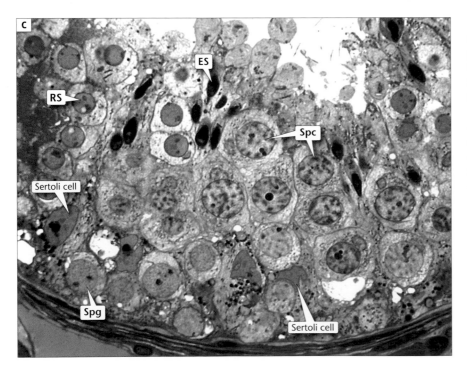

◀ **Fig 19.6c Adult seminiferous epithelium**, showing the full range of germ cell types of normal spermatogenesis. Cell types are Sertoli cells, spermatogonium (**Spg**), primary spermatocytes (**Spc**), round (**RS**) and elongating spermatids (**ES**). The long duration of germ cell development in human spermatogenesis means that the elongating spermatids are about 8 weeks older than the spermatogonia in the same segment of the epithelium. Toluidine blue, araldite, × 900.

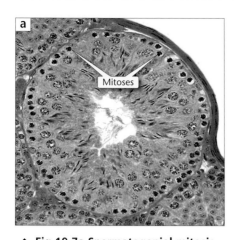

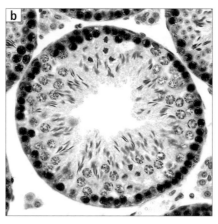

▲ Fig 19.7a Spermatogonial mitosis.
Seminiferous epithelium of rat testis at
stage XII of the spermatogenic cycle,
showing many mitoses of spermatogonia.
Dividing in synchrony is reflective of the
intrinsic and rhythmic coordination of germ
cell development that is a hallmark of
spermatogenesis. This activity is a complex
interplay of hormone stimulation and
paracrine signaling orchestrated by the
Sertoli cells. H&E, paraffin, × 140.

▲ Fig 19.7b Spermatogonia mitosis.
Similar stage of spermatogenesis (stage
XIV) after immunolabeling with proliferating
cell nuclear antigen (PCNA), showing
type A spermatogonia at or preparing to
enter the S-phase of the mitotic cycle. All
cells not in this phase are unlabeled. PCNA
immunocytochemistry/hematoxylin, paraffin,
× 140.

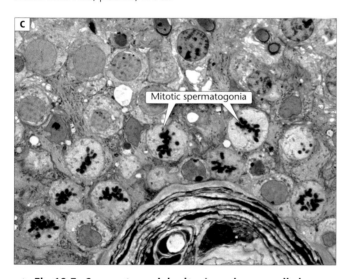

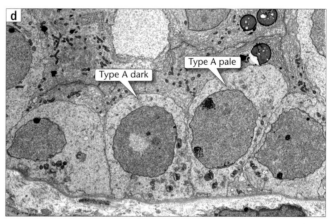

▲ Fig 19.7d Ultrastructure of human spermatogonia.
Type A dark spermatogonium is recognized by a nuclear vacuole.
It is the stem cell for spermatogenesis and, like the type A pale
spermatogonium, is in contact with the basal lamina. Spermatogonia
are believed to occupy niches in the epithelium, sites favorable
for signaling from Sertoli cells and for regulation of their survival,
proliferation, and differentiation. Spermatogonia are non-randomly
distributed around the periphery of the seminiferous tubule,
presumably for spatial arrangement of the many germ cells that
ultimately arise from them. × 2,400.

▲ Fig 19.7c Spermatogonial mitosis and germ cell clones.
Mitotic divisions of human spermatogonia (probably type B)
marked by chromosome condensations with no nucleus. These cells
apparently do not contact the basal lamina (the section is in an
oblique plane through the epithelium). The progeny of these divisions
will be preleptotene primary spermatocytes, which synthesize DNA,
each chromosome then being composed of a pair of chromatids.
Toluidine blue, araldite, × 800.

**◀ Fig 19.7e Ultrastructure of a pair of type B
spermatogonia** joined by an intercellular bridge, the result of
incomplete cytokinesis of the type Ap spermatogonium that divided
to produce them. The spermatocytes, and ultimately spermatids
that arise from these conjoined cells, will remain interconnected,
forming a clone of germ cells that passes through the process of
spermatogenesis. Cytoplasmic bridges may provide intercellular
signaling and exchange of metabolites to assist with the coordinated
development of germ cells. × 4,000.

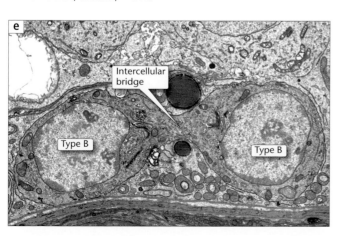

including humans, are designated as type A and B, with type A being subdivided into the dark and pale types. Type A has homogenous nuclear chromatin, whereas for type B the chromatin is clumped around the nuclear membrane. Stem cell spermatogonia are believed to occupy a stem cell niche that regulates their proliferation. The niche is maintained by local growth factors originating from Sertoli cells and intertubular tissue.

Spermatocytes

Spermatocytes (Fig 19.8a–d) are the germ cells that undergo meiosis, an extended process (3 weeks in the human male) of cell maturation involving two cell divisions. In the first division, termed meiosis I, the chromosomes of the primary spermatocytes appear as a pair of chromatids that by alignment of homologous chromosomes (maternal and paternal chromosomes) form bivalent pairs. Exchange of chromosome segments by chromosomes crossing over occurs in meiosis I in primary spermatocytes, which will divide into secondary spermatocytes containing bivalent pairs with half (the haploid) number of chromosomes. In meiosis II, which occurs in less than a day, the second meiotic division of the secondary spermatocytes results

in the chromatids of each chromosome separating to daughter cells, similar to what happens in the process of mitosis. The daughter cells, called spermatids, have the haploid chromosome number and half the DNA content of somatic cells.

Spermatids

Transformation of spermatids to spermatozoa is termed spermiogenesis (Fig 19.9a–i), in which there is no further cell division; instead there is a remarkable metamorphosis of a conventional cell into a complex, highly organized and elongated spermatozoon. A spermatozoon has a compacted nucleus, little cytoplasm and a long tail, or flagellum. Mature spermatids are released from the uppermost tips of the Sertoli cell cytoplasm and enter the fluid-filled environment of the seminiferous tubule lumen. Within the lumen of the tubules, spermatozoa are transported toward the rete testis and exit the testis to enter the initial ducts of the epididymis.

> **Tip:** Sperm produced in the testis are immotile and not capable of natural fertilization. These properties are acquired by passage through the epididymis.

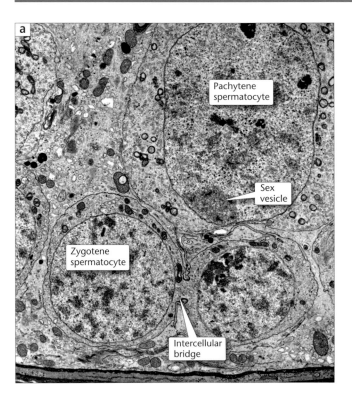

◄ **Fig 19.8a Ultrastructure of primary spermatocytes.** Zygotene spermatocytes are joined by an intercellular bridge. The chromosomes, each comprising two chromatids, give distinctive clumps or thickened masses in the nucleus, which represents the commencement of pairing of homologous chromosomes. Pairing, referred to as synapsis, thus forms bivalents consisting of two chromosomes and a total of four chromatids. As a result of considerable increase in cell size, the pachytene spermatocyte is the largest of the round germ cells. Although the bivalents are extensively aligned at pachytene they appear diffuse in the thin sections required for electron microscopy. It is within this phase, lasting for days, that certain lengths of the paired chromosomes exchange DNA, a process called crossing over or genetic recombination. The sex vesicle contains the X and Y chromosomes that also pair, but cross over only at one small region at the end of the chromosome. × 3,400.

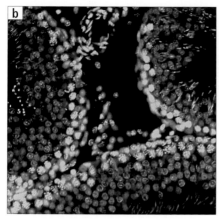

▲ **Fig 19.8b Primary spermatocytes.**
The high content of chromatin in primary spermatocytes is demonstrated with diamidinophenylindole (DAPI), which is a fluorescent probe for DNA. The most intensely labeled germ cells are the peripheral spermatogonia and the larger spermatocytes, many showing strands of chromatin. DAPI fluorescence, paraffin, × 150.

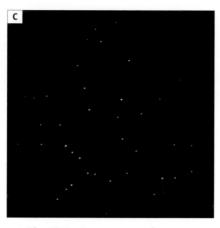

▲ **Fig 19.8c Synaptonemal complexes.** Fluorescence preparation of a human spermatocyte stained with antibodies to show lengths of synaptonemal complex axes (red) and foci representing crossing-over sites of bivalents (green). These sites are proteins that are about 90 nm in diameter. × 2,000. (Courtesy W Baarends, Erasmus University, Rotterdam, The Netherlands.)

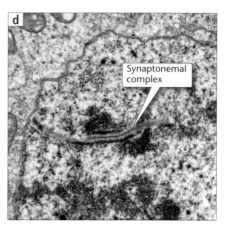

▲ **Fig 19.8d Ultrastructure of a synaptonemal complex** in a pachytene primary spermatocyte. Resembling a zipper shape, the complex has two lateral fibrils and a central element. Portions of the paired chromosomes are associated with the synaptonemal complex, and loops of their DNA will be aligned on opposite sides and available for crossing over. Synaptonemal complexes are assembled during leptotene and zygotene of prophase I. × 13,000.

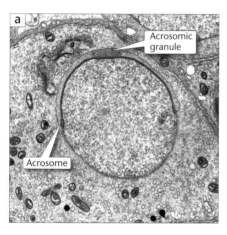

▲ **Fig 19.9a Round spermatid.** A cap-phase round spermatid, showing how the Golgi apparatus has contributed to the formation of the acrosome, with the cranial pole marked by the acrosomic granule. When fully formed, the acrosome contains glycoproteins and lysosomal enzymes for penetration of the zona pellucida of the oocyte. × 6,000.

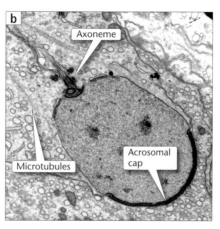

▲ **Fig 19.9b Elongating spermatid.** A spermatid that is beginning to elongate shows a more mature acrosomal cap and remodeling of nuclear shape, with condensation of chromatin. The developing flagellum, or axoneme, is anchored to the caudal aspect of the nucleus via a modified pair of centrioles. Tracks of microtubules are oriented caudally in association with the elongation of spermatid cytoplasm. × 7,400.

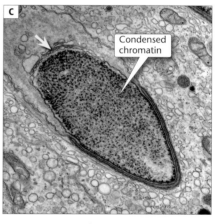

▲ **Fig 19.9c Late cap-phase spermatid,** showing DNA condensation, in which nuclear histones are replaced by protamines, allowing close aggregation of chromatin fibers. Nuclear compaction produces folds of excess or redundant nuclear membrane (**arrow**), which, with most of the cytoplasm, will be detached from the mature spermatid at spermiation. × 9,500.

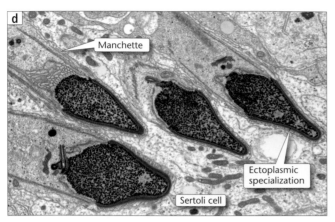

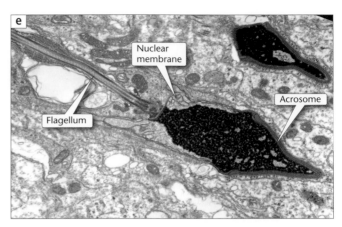

▲ **Fig 19.9d Acrosome-phase spermatids**, showing transformation of the nucleus into a pyriform shape, together with significant compaction of chromatin. The acrosomes now cover much of the leading edges of the nuclei. The trailing cytoplasm is dense and bordered by the manchette, a cylinder of microtubules serving to organize the caudal displacement of cytoplasm and its organelles. Spermatids are embedded in crypts of Sertoli cell cytoplasm and stabilized with specialized spermatid–Sertoli cell junctional complexes, termed ectoplasmic specializations. × 5,000.

▲ **Fig 19.9e Early maturation-phase spermatid**, showing further nuclear remodeling, with a prominent acrosome. Compaction of the nucleus results in folds of redundant nuclear membrane. The flagellum is attached to the nucleus via a connecting piece surrounding the centriole. × 8,000.

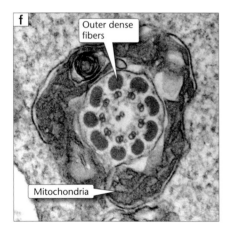

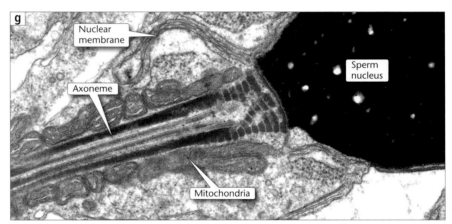

▲ **Fig 19.9f Flagellum.** Cross section through the flagellum, showing the central axoneme, which comprises a 9 + 2 arrangement of microtubules and nine outer dense fibers that serve to stiffen the tail—they run longitudinally and eventually taper and disappear at the end of the tail. Mitochondria form a sheath in the middle piece of the tail and provide the energy source for flagellar motility. × 60,000.

▲ **Fig 19.9g Spermatid.** Detail of neck and flagellum, showing the continuity between the cross-striated columns of the connecting piece and the outer dense fibers of the axoneme. Mitochondria surround the middle piece of the tail. The tail is articulated with the nucleus via the implantation fossa. × 31,000.

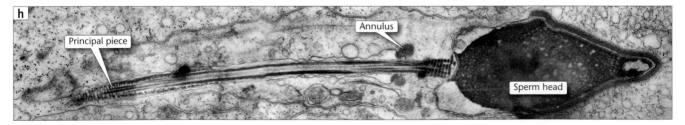

▲ **Fig 19.9h Longitudinal section through a late-elongating spermatid.** Note the annular material that will displace caudally; it will be followed by organization of the mitochondria into a sheath around the flagellum to form the middle piece. A glancing section of the developing principal piece shows rib-type structures linking not nine outer dense fibers but just two longitudinal columns, collectively called the fibrous sheath. × 14,000.

Coordination of germ cell development

Spermatogenesis is a coordinated process initiated by the entry of early primary spermatocytes (from mitosis of type B spermatogonia) into meiosis. Each seminiferous tubule displays particular collections of germ cells and stages of germ cell development, representing but one moment in the prolonged sequence of spermatogenesis. Put another way, the histologic features of any part of the seminiferous epithelium containing multiple layers and types of germ cells is a freeze-frame image of a dynamic epithelium that in vivo is slowly but continuously changing in morphology. In most mammals, longitudinal segments of the seminiferous epithelium show the same developmental stage of spermatogenesis (Fig 19.10a & b), followed

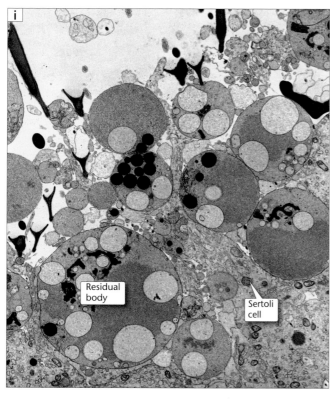

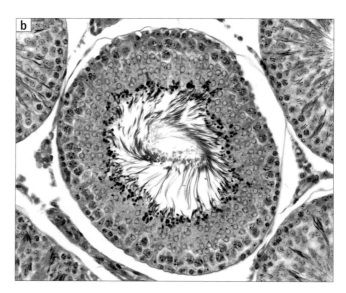

◀ **Fig 19.9i Mature spermatids.** As mature spermatids are released from the Sertoli cells, their previously discarded cytoplasm is packaged into spherical "residual bodies." These contain lipid, vesicles, organelle remnants, and ribosomes. Residual bodies are retained by the Sertoli cells, which eliminate them by phagocytosis and digestion. × 3,400.

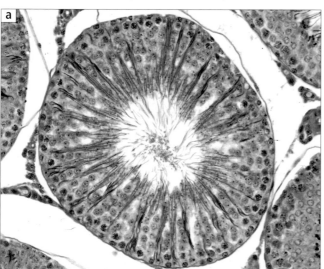

▲ **Fig 19.10a Germ cell coordination.** Cross section of rat seminiferous tubule at stage V of the spermatogenic cycle. The entire seminiferous epithelium shows uniform radial coordination of germ cell development. H&E, paraffin, × 180.

▲ **Fig 19.10b Germ cell coordination.** If the tubule in Fig 19.10a had been examined about 4 days later it would have looked like the tubule in this image, which is at stage VIII. The seminiferous epithelium retains its synchrony of spermatogenesis and the elongated spermatids have matured fully and are being released into the tubule lumen. For most mammals the stages of spermatogenesis are arranged serially along the tubules, subject to sites where the sequence is occasionally reversed. H&E, paraffin, × 180.

sequentially by slightly more advanced (or earlier) stages along the length of the tubule. These defined histologic stages are designated by Roman numerals (I–XIV for rats; I–XII for guinea pigs; I–VIII for rams, stallions and bulls; I–XII for monkeys, and I–VI for humans); a complete, uninterrupted sequence of these stages constitutes what is termed the wave of spermatogenesis. The series of histologic changes occurring in a given epithelial area, between two successive appearances of the same stage, is defined as the cycle of the seminiferous epithelium, or the spermatogenic cycle. In humans, one cycle is about 16 ± 1 days. As spermatogenesis takes at least 70 days, each germ cell passes through the cycle four times before its final release as a spermatozoon. By observing over time the locations, associations and morphological development of specially labeled germ cells, the seminiferous epithelium in the human has six defined stages all visible in histologic sections (Fig 19.11).

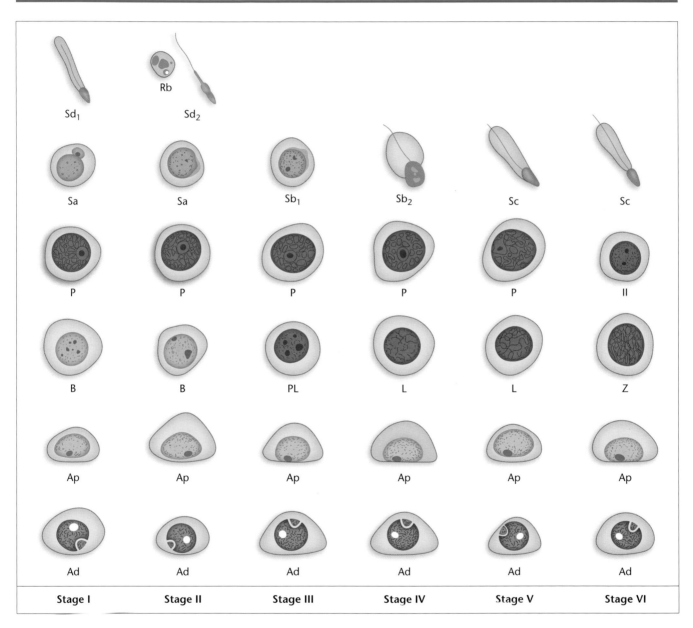

▲ **Fig 19.11 Human spermatogenic stages.** The six histologic stages of the human cycle of the seminiferous epithelium are shown, based upon visible germ cell associations (stages I–VI) and tracing their development with time. In this "road map" of spermatogenesis, the starting point is the spermatogonium at the left of the bottom row. Development proceeds from left to right along each row, moving upward from the bottom row. Mature spermatids are finally released at stage II. Germ cells pass through the stages nearly 4½ times; this requires about 70 days in humans. **Ad, Ap, B** = spermatogonial types; **PL, L, Z, P** = preleptotene, leptotene, zygotene, pachytene primary spermatocytes; **II** = secondary spermatocytes; **Sa, Sb, Sc, Sd** = phases of spermiogenesis; **Rb** = residual body.

The arrangement of stages in humans and several primate species is somewhat irregular, if not random. In cross section, a tubule may show two to four different stages, unlike in other species where only one stage is seen in transverse sections (Fig 19.12). In some cases, this seemingly chaotic pattern in humans is organized as a series of helices along the tubule (Fig 19.13).

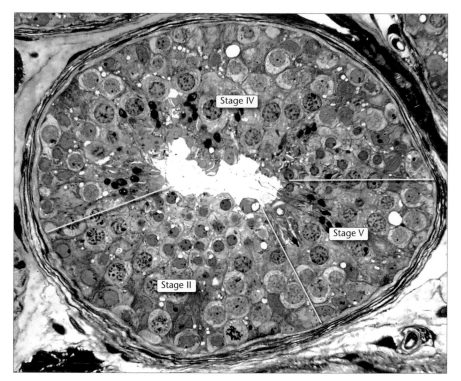

◀ **Fig 19.12 Multi-staged human seminiferous tubules.** Cross section of a human seminiferous tubule, illustrating several stages within the seminiferous epithelium. Similar histology is seen in other primates (chimp, baboon, macaque, marmoset). How multi-staged tubules maintain coordination of spermatogenesis is unknown, but is probably related to local/paracrine signaling by the Sertoli cells and precise activation of spermatogonial stem cell proliferation. The families or clones of germ cells derived from the germ-line stem cells occupy distinct subregions around the circumference of the tubules. Specific clusters of germ cell types may be adjacent to one another but in age can be significantly younger or older. Toluidine blue, araldite, × 400.

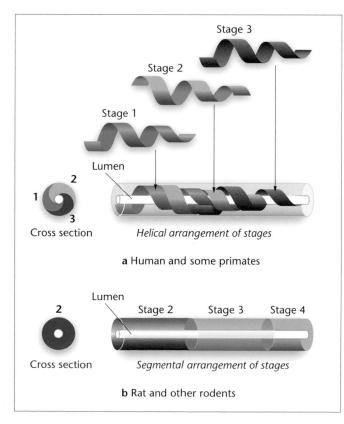

◀ **Fig 19.13 Organization of germ cell stages.** Diagrammatic representation of the arrangement of stages of spermatogenesis. In humans and some primate species (**a**), there are random patterns or gyrating spirals along the tubule. Two to three stages are seen in a transverse histologic section. For most non-primate mammalian species (**b**), the stages have an orderly sequence, occasionally reversed for several stages then reverting to the original order. For both models, stages of germ cell development are coordinated, in part or largely by interaction with the Sertoli cells. In comparison to single-stage tubules (many rodents), the occurrence of multi-stage tubules is not correlated with efficiency of spermatogenesis, but points to an evolutionary trend associated with New World monkeys, great apes, and humans.

Germ cell tumors

A common precursor of testicular germ cell tumors is the carcinoma in situ (CIS) cell. CIS cells are large cells in the seminiferous tubules and in advanced cases replace all other germ cell types (Fig 19.14a & b). It is thought that CIS cells arise in utero when gonocytes undergo malignant transformation. The pathogenesis is uncertain but may be due to hormonal disturbances and possibly to "endocrine disruptors" such as natural and synthetic estrogens and antiandrogens. Such agents may be found in plastics and some pesticides, but the link between such disruptors and reproductive disorders remains hypothetical.

Sertoli cells

The association between Sertoli cells and germ cells is analogous to trees in an orchard, with the germ cells resembling spheres that are located on the earth around the tree trunks and supported by the branches as they rise up through the four or five layers representing the seminiferous epithelium (Fig 19.15a–c). Sertoli cells occupy as much as 25% of the volume of the seminiferous epithelium. At its base each Sertoli cell is in contact with five or six other Sertoli cells, and each may support up to 50 germ cells throughout the depth of the seminiferous epithelium. To support the main body of the cytoplasm, the Sertoli cells

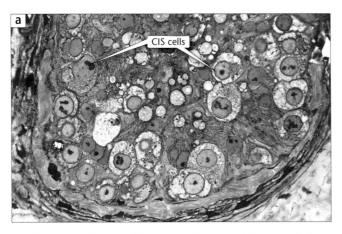

▲ **Fig 19.14a Germ cell tumors.** Human seminiferous tubule with carcinoma in situ (CIS), identified by large cells with vacuolated cytoplasm containing glycogen and positive reactivity for placenta-like alkaline phosphatase of unknown significance. There are no normal germ cells. Gene expression studies of CIS cells showing a similarity of CIS cells to embryonic stem cells suggest that CIS originates in utero from fetal gonocytes. Most testicular germ cell tumors originate from CIS cells. Toluidine blue, araldite, × 500.

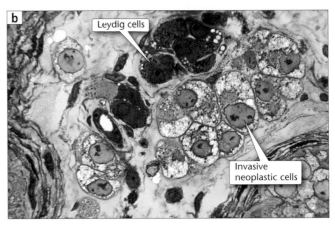

▲ **Fig 19.14b Germ cell tumors.** CIS cells in the intertubular tissue of the testis. Because they are extratubular, these cells may pose a risk for metastatic spread within the lymphatic vessels to sites beyond the testis. In cases of testis cancer with CIS there is a 50% risk of developing invasive growth within 5 years and 70% risk within 7 years. The management of unilateral CIS is by orchidectomy, or by localized radiotherapy in bilateral cases. Toluidine blue, araldite, × 500.

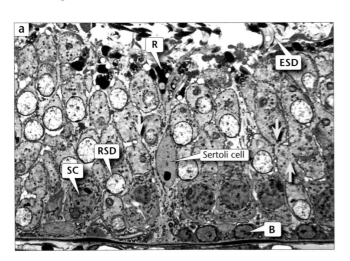

◀ **Fig 19.15a Sertoli cells.** Rat seminiferous epithelium, showing Sertoli cell nuclei and columnar cytoplasm extending from the base to the luminal aspect of the epithelium, partly or completely surrounding the germ cells. This arrangement provides physical and functional support for spermatogenesis. Note type B spermatogonia (**B**), pachytene primary spermatocytes (**SC**), and round and elongated spermatids (**RSD**, **ESD**), the latter discarding their excess cytoplasm as residual bodies (**R**), which in a later stage are phagocytosed by Sertoli cells. Cytoplasmic bridges (**arrows**) occur between spermatocytes and between spermatids. Toluidine blue, araldite, × 620.

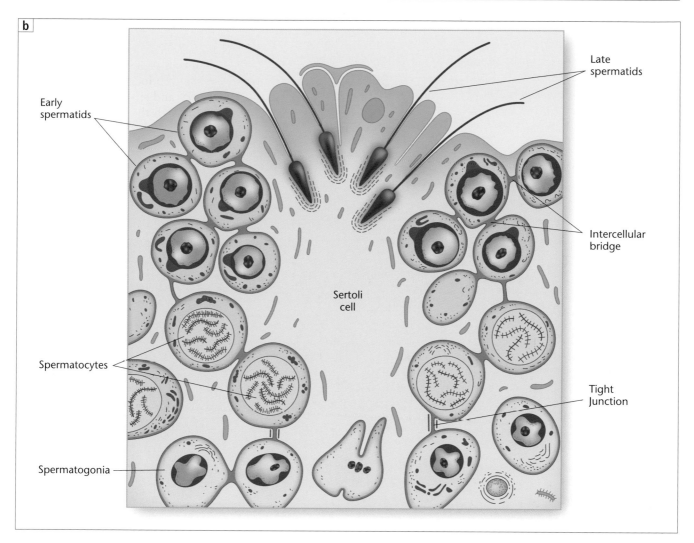

b

Early spermatids

Late spermatids

Intercellular bridge

Sertoli cell

Spermatocytes

Tight Junction

Spermatogonia

▲ **Fig 19.15b Sertoli cell.** The Sertoli cell divides the epithelium into basal and adluminal compartments by means of special tight junctions of the blood–testis barrier. Spermatogonia (and early spermatocytes, not shown) are in the basal compartment. More mature spermatocytes and round and elongating spermatids are in the adluminal compartment. All germ cells are supported by Sertoli cell cytoplasm. Testosterone binds to androgen receptors in Sertoli cells and peritubular myoid cells, initiating biochemical reactions (largely unknown but probably cyclic, in concert with the stages of spermatogenesis)

that stimulate germ cell development. FSH is of major importance in the prepubertal testis (to stimulate Sertoli cell proliferation as the testis grows in size) and possibly is required for quantitative spermatogenesis in the adult. FSH binds to the basal Sertoli cell plasma membrane and stimulates numerous metabolic functions (e.g. cyclic AMP, androgen binding protein, and inhibin production; fluid secretion) and is probably involved with spermatogonial development. Testosterone is essential for spermatogenesis; FSH (in adults) augments the stimulatory actions of testosterone.

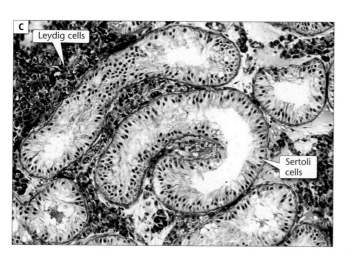

c

Leydig cells

Sertoli cells

◀ **Fig 19.15c Sertoli cells.** In the absence of germ cells the tubules are filled only with Sertoli cells. This appearance may be found in various conditions including cryptorchidism, idiopathic infertility, hypopituitarism, or certain congenital conditions (e.g. Kleinfelter syndrome). Masson's trichrome, paraffin, × 80.

contain an impressive cytoskeleton of microtubules (Fig 19.16). Microtubules no doubt are involved with intracellular transport and distribution of organelles and macromolecules that show cyclic variations in synchrony with the spermatogenic cycle. These changes are also required to modify the shape of the Sertoli cells as the ever-changing germ cells proliferate and are repositioned during their development.

Blood–testis barrier

In addition to supporting the germ cells and engineering their release into the tubule lumen (spermiation), the lateral plasma membranes of adjacent Sertoli cells near their base form specialized tight junctions, termed the blood–testis barrier, segregating the epithelium into anatomic and physiologic compartments (Fig 19.17a–c). The basal compartment contains germ cells up to early primary spermatocytes; the adluminal compartment contains all other germ cells. The latter environment is thus a unique physiologic milieu that favors the development of male gametes and probably maintains an immunologically privileged site within the seminiferous tubules.

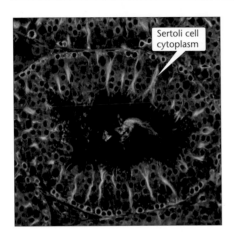

▲ **Fig 19.16 Sertoli cell cytoskeleton.** Mouse testis immunostained for tubulin, a protein found in cytoplasmic microtubules. The radial arrangement of slender green fluorescent columns represents the body of the Sertoli cells, which extend through the seminiferous epithelium. The Sertoli cell cytoskeleton provides the necessary structural framework that supports the multiple layers of germ cells. Immunofluoresence, paraffin, × 150.

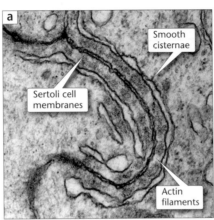

▲ **Fig 19.17a Ultrastructure of the inter-Sertoli cell junction,** a cell surface specialization that restricts entry of macromolecules into the deeper aspects of the seminiferous epithelium. It is often called the "blood–testis" barrier and comprises fusions of the apposed Sertoli cell plasma membranes, bundles of actin filaments, and smooth membrane cisternae. × 40,000.

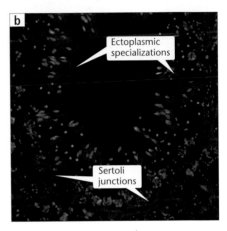

▲ **Fig 19.17b Inter-Sertoli cell junction.** Immunofluorescence preparation of a seminiferous tubule, showing the location of espin, stained red. Espin is an actin-bundling protein of the Sertoli cell junctions, also known as ectoplasmic specializations. Espin is also noted near elongating spermatids, where it is part of the ectoplasmic specializations between spermatid nuclei and Sertoli cells. These interfaces provide adhesion between the cells, which is lost as spermatids are released at spermiation. DNA in cell nuclei is stained blue with DAPI. Immunofluorescence, paraffin, × 150.

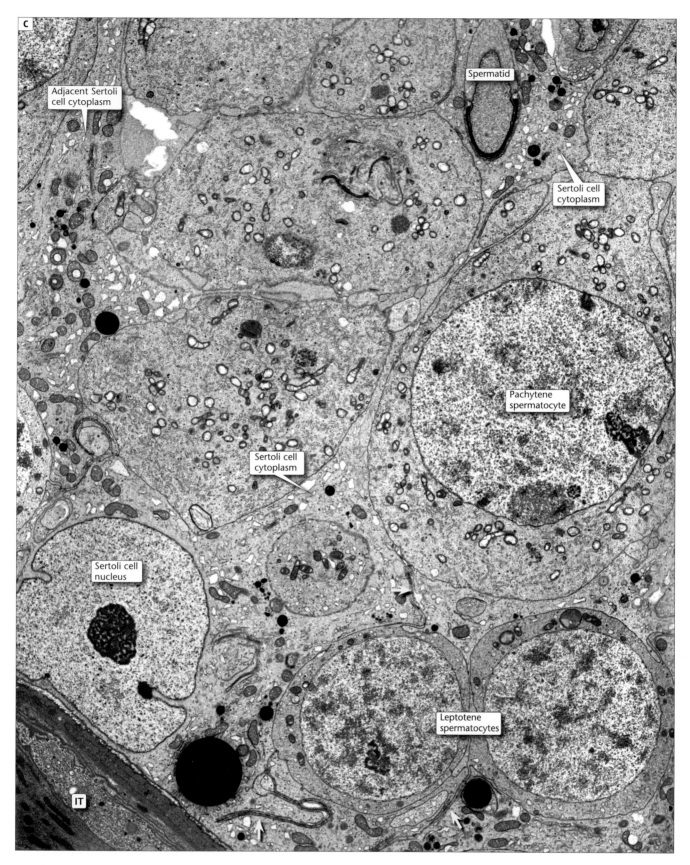

▲ Fig 19.17c Sertoli cell ultrastructure. Electron micrograph showing a Sertoli cell nucleus whose cytoplasm extends to surround leptotene and pachytene primary spermatocytes and an elongating spermatid. Sertoli cell cytoplasm contains all the common organelles, but lipid inclusions are often abundant, representing the product of germ cell phagocytosis and the ingestion of spermatid residual cytoplasm after spermiation. Note inter-Sertoli cell junctional complexes (**arrows**) located below and above the leptotene spermatocytes. These junctions selectively restrict the entry of macromolecules into the epithelium from the intertubular tissue (**IT**) and constitute the blood–testis barrier. × 4,700.

457

Physiology

The functions of Sertoli cells are many and varied, and include fluid production, synthesis and secretion of numerous proteins and enzymes, metabolic conversions, phagocytosis of degenerating germ cells (which is significant in the human testis), and production of known and putative growth factors. Sertoli cells are also the target of an increasing number of substances with hormone-like actions both external to and within the testis. The principal role of the Sertoli cells is to support spermatogenesis in response to hormonal regulation by FSH and testosterone (see below).

> **Tip:** Sertoli cells proliferate in the postnatal, prepubertal testis to establish a stable non-growing cell population from puberty and into adult life. Because the germ cells depend upon the Sertoli cells for their development, the numbers of Sertoli cells per testis may be one determinant of sperm output and fertility.

Intertubular tissue

Loose connective tissue surrounds the seminiferous tubules and contains blood vessels, occasional nerves and lymphocytes, and an ill-defined lymphatic system. Leydig cells in the adult human testis form clusters in the intertubular tissue, often associated with macrophages (Fig 19.18a & b). Depending on the species, the proportion of intertubular tissue in the adult testis that is occupied by Leydig cells is commonly 10%–20%, but can be much higher—up to 60%, for example, in the boar, zebra, and some marsupials. Human fetal Leydig cells are especially abundant at 14–18 weeks' gestation, but at the time of birth have declined in number. In postnatal and prepubertal testes, mature or adult-type Leydig cells appear in the intertubular tissue. At the ultrastructural level, Leydig cells show an abundant content of smooth endoplasmic reticulum that is associated with steroidogenesis (Fig 19.19).Through receptors on their plasma membrane, Leydig cells are stimulated by LH (from the anterior pituitary) to synthesize and secrete large quantities of testosterone and lesser amounts of other androgens. Testosterone diffuses into the nearby seminiferous tubules, where it is required for spermatogenesis, and also enters the systemic circulation for peripheral distribution to its numerous target organs. Polygonal or needle-type crystals of Reinke are seen in Leydig cells (Fig 19.20a–c). These contain proteins, but their function is unknown. They also occur in the chimpanzee and in a species of rat, *Rattus fuscipes*.

Hormonal regulation of the testis

The maintenance of quantitatively normal spermatogenesis in the adult testis is dependent on appropriate stimulation of the testis by FSH and LH, both of which, as already mentioned, are secreted by the anterior pituitary gland in response to hypothalamic gonadotropin-releasing hormone (GnRH) and modified by various regulatory factors, including feedback from the testis. FSH binds to and acts specifically on the Sertoli cells; LH stimulates secretion of testosterone

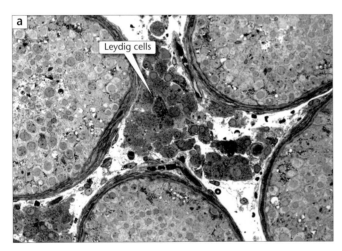

▲ **Fig 19.18a Leydig cells.** Intertubular tissue of the human testis with clusters of Leydig cells that are steroidogenically very active. These cells respond to LH stimulation by secreting androgens that diffuse into the nearby seminiferous tubules. Other structures in the intertubular tissue include blood vessels, lymphatics, macrophages, and connective tissue cells. Toluidine blue/basic fuchsin, araldite, × 180.

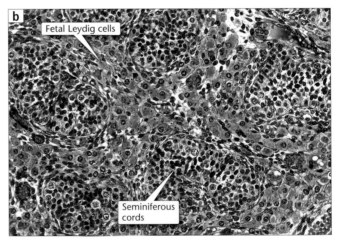

▲ **Fig 19.18b Leydig cells.** Human fetal testis at 19 weeks' gestation, showing a high proportion of Leydig cells between the seminiferous cords. The Leydig cell cytoplasm is intensely eosinophilic because of the abundance of smooth endoplasmic reticulum required for androgen production. Proliferation of fetal Leydig cells is regulated by placental chorionic gonadotrophin and pituitary LH. As the source of androgens during fetal life, the Leydig cells support testis development and androgen-dependent organ differentiation. H&E, paraffin, × 170. (Tissue courtesy R Anderson, College of Medicine, University of Edinburgh, Scotland.)

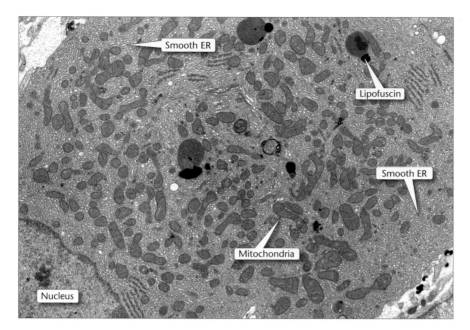

◀ Fig 19.19 Human Leydig cell structure. **Fig 19.19 Human Leydig cell structure.** As steroidogenic cells, Leydig cells have cytoplasm that contains a rich supply of tubular smooth endoplasmic reticulum (ER), together with many mitochondria, both of which are mandatory for the synthesis of testosterone. In Leydig cells, testosterone is synthesized from cholesterol. In mitochondria, cholesterol is converted to pregnenolone, a rate-limiting step stimulated by LH acting via specific plasma membrane receptors. The large surface area of smooth ER contains enzymes necessary for further conversion to progesterone, and then to androstenedione or (predominantly) androstenediol, and finally to testosterone. Steroids are produced continuously, with testosterone by far the main product, ensuring high local concentrations within the testis. × 8,000.

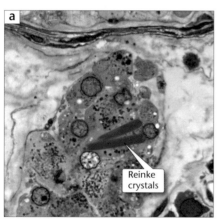

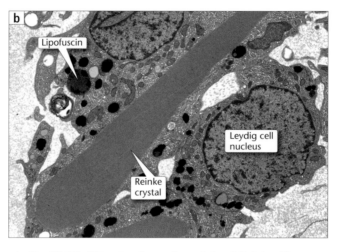

▲ **Fig 19.20a Reinke crystals.** Human testis showing a cluster of Leydig cells with spherical nuclei and cytoplasm containing rod-shaped Reinke crystals. Cytoplasmic granules represent lipid and lipofuscin inclusions. Toluidine blue, araldite, × 600.

▲ **Fig 19.20b Ultrastructure of crystals of Reinke.** These are polygonal, rod, or needle-shaped inclusions composed of protein subunits in an hexagonal array. Their function is unknown but they occur in Leydig cells of the chimp and a species of wild rat, and increase in abundance with age and in response to withdrawal of LH. Lipofuscin pigment granules, derived from lysosomes, also increase with age. The remaining cytoplasm contains mitochondria and smooth ER for steroidogenesis (testosterone production). × 4,000.

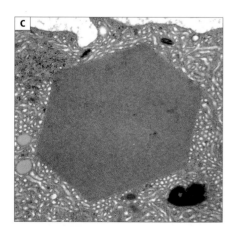

◀ **Fig 19.20c Reinke crystals.** At high magnification, Reinke crystals display an orderly pattern of hexagonal lattice-like subunits, with the surface exposed directly to the cytoplasm. Subunits are thought to assemble from aggregations of paracrystalline inclusions. Reinke crystals increase with advancing age but their function remains obscure. × 12,000.

by the Leydig cells. Testosterone is an absolute requirement for spermatogenesis, for which, acting via receptors located in peritubular cells and Sertoli cells, it stimulates germ cell development by mechanisms that remain unknown. The role of FSH in adult men is uncertain, although the available evidence suggests that both FSH and testosterone acting synergistically are necessary for quantitatively normal sperm production.

A key role of the Sertoli cell in stimulating and coordinating spermatogenesis is emphasized by the finding that germ cells do not possess receptors for FSH or testosterone. Although Sertoli cells of the fetal testis have no androgen receptors, androgens support fetal Sertoli cell proliferation perhaps via indirect effects involving androgen receptors on peritubular myoid cells. In postnatal testes, knockout of the androgen receptor specifically in Sertoli cells results in severe disruption of spermatogenesis from puberty onwards. Thus functional androgen receptors in Sertoli cells are an absolute requirement for maintenance of normal spermatogenesis.

The duration of spermatogenesis and the cycle (in days) is fixed, but is variable between different species. If rat germ cells are transplanted into mouse testes, they maintain their normal rate of development, suggesting that mouse Sertoli cells can support rat spermatogenesis, but the latter is independently programmed with regard to the duration of germ cell maturation.

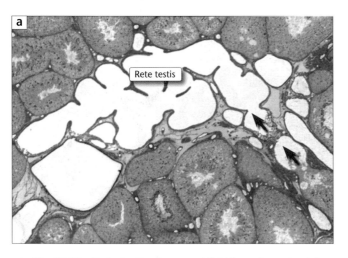

▲ **Fig 19.21a Rete testis.** Sperm and fluid from the ends of the seminiferous tubules empty into (**arrows**) channels with epithelial lining, which form the rete testis within the connective tissue of the mediastinum testis. The rete testis connects with the extratesticular efferent ducts leading to the head of the epididymis. Toluidine blue, araldite, × 30.

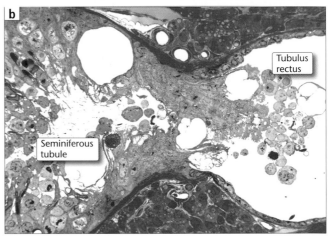

▲ **Fig 19.21b Rete testis.** Termination of a seminiferous tubule is marked by its narrowing with a plug of modified Sertoli cells, some germ cells, and a slender channel. This arrangement may prevent reflux of luminal contents of the tubulus rectus. Toluidine blue, araldite, × 200.

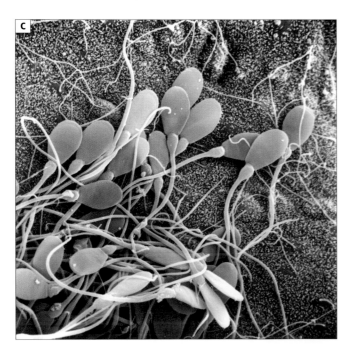

◀ **Fig 19.21c Rete testis viewed by scanning electron microscopy**, showing mature sperm passing along the surface of channels that form the most extensive part of the rete testis. The epithelial lining consists of squamous or cuboidal cells with microvillous projections. In the subepithelium, myoid cells probably provide a contractile mechanism for raising intrarete pressure, forcing rete testis fluid into the efferent ducts and epididymis. × 2,000.

DUCTS OF THE TESTIS

Spermatozoa pass through the rete testis (Fig 19.21a–c), leaving the testis to enter a duct system composed of the efferent ducts, epididymis, vas deferens, and the ejaculatory duct terminating in the prostatic urethra. Each segment has characteristic histologic features and serves different functions.

Efferent ducts and epididymis

The efferent ducts, up to 12 in number in humans, are coiled, forming several coni vasculosi, which amalgamate to form the start of the epididymis.

The histology of the efferent ducts is distinctive, showing a pseudostratified columnar epithelium that is stellate in cross section (Fig 19.22). This is the only part of the duct system in which the epithelium is ciliated. Functions include absorption of most of the fluid arriving from the rete testis and peristaltic contraction, which assists fluid flow toward the epididymis. About 5 m in length, the epididymis is a highly coiled tube, consisting of caput, corpus, and caudal segments (Fig 19.23). In histologic sections, many tubular profiles are noted, indicating the high degree of convolution of this single tube. The epididymal tube is ensheathed by smooth muscle cells

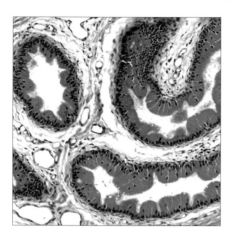

◀ **Fig 19.22 Efferent ducts.** About 12 efferent ducts connect the rete testis to the single-coiled tubule of the head of the epididymis. Each coiled efferent duct forms a conus vasculosus (a conical lobule); these lobules join, in the head of the epididymis, to form the ductus epididymidis. The efferent ducts show a scalloped outline with ciliated and non-ciliated cells; the former reabsorb more than 90% of rete testis fluid by endocytosis, water and active salt transport, and endocytic uptake of proteins. Sperm move through the ducts, probably by ciliary action and contraction of myoid cells. H&E, paraffin, × 80.

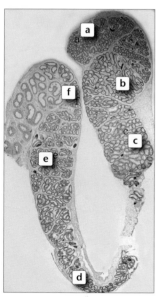

◀ **Fig 19.23 Epididymis.** Epididymis of the rat showing many profiles through this highly coiled tube. The tissue is an immunocytochemical stain for RNase, thought to be involved with sperm maturation. In the head region, the epithelium absorbs fluid, and in transit through the epididymis sperm acquire progressive motility and fertilizing capacity. The luminal fluid microenvironment is androgen-dependent and regulates sperm maturation and survival. **a** = initial segment; **b**, **c** = caput; **d**, **e** = corpus; **f** = cauda region. Immunocytochemistry, paraffin, × 4. (Courtesy Y-L Zhang, Shanghai Institute for Biological Sciences, China.)

and lined internally by a pseudostratified columnar epithelium with stereocilia (Fig 19.24a–c). Fluid (containing spermatozoa) entering the epididymis is also absorbed in the caput region, but the main functions of the organ are sperm transport (average transit time about a week), sperm maturation, and sperm storage (of limited capacity). In their passage through the epididymis, sperm acquire increasing capacity for successful fertilization; this maturation process, including the development of motility, is fully accomplished in the body (corpus or middle) of the epididymis.

Vas deferens and ejaculatory duct

Emerging from the cauda epididymis, the vas deferens is a tube with a thick layer of smooth muscle and an inner epithelium of pseudostratified columnar cells with tall stereocilia (Fig 19.25). Autonomic innervation of the vas deferens causes contractions and the transport of the luminal contents toward the ejaculatory ducts, a function that is considerably enhanced before ejaculation. Arising from the confluence of the duct of the seminal vesicle and the terminal (ampullary) region of the vas, the ejaculatory ducts with a thin muscle coat pierce the prostate gland, emptying into the prostatic urethra. During ejaculation the ducts dilate to permit the passage of sperm (from the vas deferens) and the secretions from the seminal vesicle.

Accessory glands

Secretions of the seminal vesicles, prostate gland, and bulbourethral glands contribute most of the ejaculate. The proper functioning of each of these organs is required to produce an optimum composition and quantity of fluid in the ejaculate. Biochemical analysis of fresh semen samples is one method used to assess prostate and seminal vesicle function.

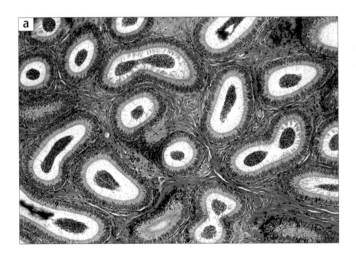

◀ **Fig 19.24a Epididymal epithelium.** Section through the epididymis, showing many individual cut profiles of a single tubule. The tall columnar epithelium faces a wide lumen, which contains fluid and sperm. Between the sectioned tubules is connective tissue, which supports a thin, peritubular layer of contractile myoid cells that assist with sperm transport via peristalsis. H&E, paraffin, × 30.

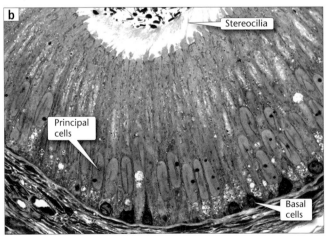

◀ **Fig 19.24b Epididymal epithelium.** Pseudostratified columnar epithelium of the epididymis showing stereocilia, and basal and tall principal cells. The peritubular myoid layer contracts intrinsically in the proximal organ but is responsive to autonomic regulation in the tail, where any stored sperm are expelled into the vas deferens during ejaculation. The many proteins secreted by the epididymal cells (more than 200 have been described) no doubt contribute to sperm maturation (the mechanisms remain largely unknown), assisted by tight junctions of the blood–epididymal barrier, and immunosuppressive factors that reduce autoimmune reactions against sperm. Toluidine blue, araldite, × 500.

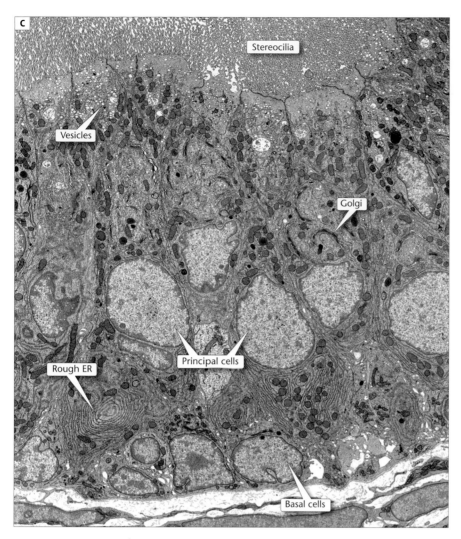

◀ **Fig 19.24c Ultrastructure of the epididymis**, illustrating basal cells and principal cells with stereocilia, which are long microvilli involved in the exchange of molecules between the cells and the lumen. Principal cells are polarized with rough ER basally, and Golgi with endocytic vesicles in the apical cytoplasm. In addition to protein secretion, the epididymal epithelium absorbs ions and water and is believed to create a current along the lumen supporting sperm transport. The epididymis is an androgen-dependent organ, and its mucosal cells are stimulated by dihydrotestosterone, a metabolite of testosterone. × 3,300.

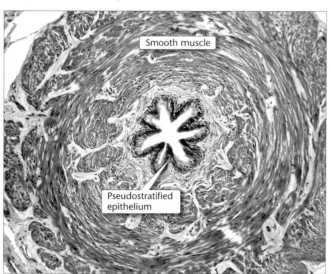

◀ **Fig 19.25 Vas deferens.** Vas (ductus) deferens is a hollow tube with a thick, trilaminar smooth muscle coat and an inner epithelium or mucosa, often stellate in cross section. The epithelium is pseudostratified columnar with stereocilia. Via sympathetic innervation, contractions force sperm along the vas during ejaculation, but at other times the vas slowly transports sperm to the ampulla and beyond, thus providing a limited storage capacity. After vasectomy, sperm are phagocytosed by the vas and to a lesser extent, the epididymal epithelium. H&E, paraffin, × 30.

Seminal vesicles

These androgen-dependent paired vesicles are elongated, convoluted sacs consisting of a dilated, coiled tube, with the inner pseudostratified columnar epithelium lining a complex array of folds, ridges, and branchings of the lamina propria (Fig 19.26a & b). Smooth muscle is noted in the main subcapsular wall and around the internal convolutions. The secretory product is a yellowish, viscous fluid containing proteins (which coagulate after ejaculation), fructose, and prostaglandins, all in high concentration.

Prostate

The prostate gland is about the size of a walnut and is a composite of glandular and non-glandular stromal components within a common capsule, the latter extending fibromuscular septa into the parenchyma of the gland (Fig 19.27a & b). The prostate gland consists of the following zones:
- Peripheral zone (70% of glandular mass), related to the distal prostatic urethra
- Central zone (20% of glandular mass), associated with the ejaculatory ducts
- Transitional zone (5%–10% of glandular mass), associated with the proximal prostatic urethra.

Groups of glandular elements—mucosal, submucosal, and main prostatic glands (which predominate)—are arranged concentrically around the prostatic urethra. The main glands consist of tubuloalveolar elements (with simple or pseudostratified epithelium) that resemble branched channels with alveoli or saccules and blind endings.

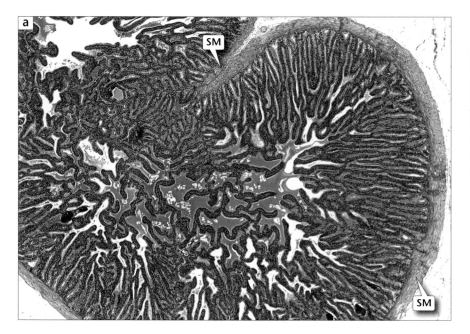

◀ **Fig 19.26a Seminal vesicles.** The paired seminal vesicles are androgen-dependent, tubulosaccular glands with internal folds of connective tissue that form branches, ridges, and crests lined by a secretory epithelium. Saccules are associated with smooth muscle (**SM**), their sympathetic innervation causing, at ejaculation, discharge of luminal contents into the main duct, confluent with the terminal vas deferens. H&E, paraffin, × 30.

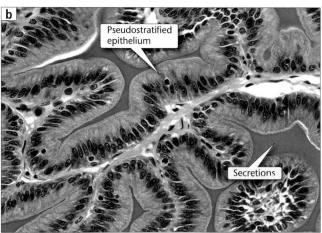

◀ **Fig 19.26b Seminal vesicle epithelium.** Epithelium of the seminal vesicle is pseudostratified columnar with basal cells—the former secretory, the latter probably stem cells. The secreted proteins are released via granule exocytosis and include semenogelin and fibronectin, which provides the structural component of the ejaculated seminal plasma or coagulum, a semi-solid gel. H&E, paraffin, × 280.

Prostatic secretion is a watery liquid that contributes about one-third of the ejaculate volume and contains zinc, citric acid, prostaglandins, and proteolytic enzymes. The prostate gland is an androgen-dependent organ, and the conversion of testosterone into dihydrotestosterone in the prostate stimulates its growth, possibly leading to the development of androgen-dependent tumors.

Bulbourethral glands

Also known as Cowper's glands, these tubular and alveolar-type glands, within the urogenital diaphragm, empty their mucous secretions into the associated urethra. This clear secretory product, which usually appears before ejaculation, is thought to provide lubrication of the distal urethra.

Penis

The erectile tissues of the penis—the corpora cavernosa and the corpus spongiosum (which encircles the urethra)—are masses of labyrinthine trabeculae of fibromuscular tissues, ramified by vascular or cavernous spaces that become filled with blood during

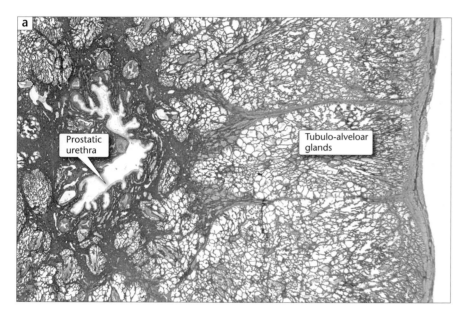

◀ **Fig 19.27a Prostate gland.** The main prostatic glands are tubuloalveolar in shape, surrounded by fibromuscular tissue, which forms lobules that are often indistinct. Prostatic secretion is colorless and appears before seminal vesicle secretions during ejaculation. It is rich in zinc, citric acid, acid phosphatase, fibrolysin, prostate-specific antigen (PSA), and other proteases involved with liquefaction of semen. Van Gieson's, paraffin, × 10.

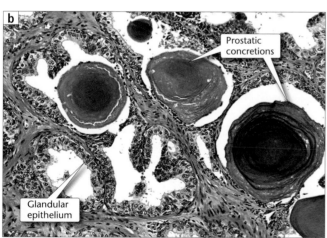

◀ **Fig 19.27b Prostate gland.** Prostatic glands show a heterogeneous epithelium secreting proteins under androgen regulation. Testosterone, dihydrotestosterone, progesterone, and estrogen are implicated in benign prostate hyperplasia and adenocarcinoma, both abnormalities afflicting many men with increasing age. Measurement of serum PSA in used in early detection of prostate cancer and evaluation of its progression. With increasing age, prostatic concretions may arise in the glands, forming ovoid, concentrically lamellated bodies containing proteins, nucleic acids, cholesterol, and calcium phosphate, which may calcify. Concretions are thought to be mixtures of prostatic secretions and debris from degenerated epithelial cells. H&E, paraffin, × 80.

erection (Fig 19.28a & b). Far greater quantities of blood, maintained at high pressure during erection, fill the cavernosa compared to the spongiosum. The latter, containing a venous plexus, also fills with blood, but as the spongiosum contains more connective tissue it remains less turgid, allowing semen to pass along the urethra. The epithelium of the penile urethra is stratified columnar, changing into non-keratinized stratified squamous epithelium near its termination. Invaginations along its length form urethral glands (of Littré), which secrete mucoid substances thought to protect the epithelium against urine.

ABNORMAL CONDITIONS AND CLINICAL FEATURES

Testis

Disturbances of fertility may arise from a large range of disorders, examples of which are intrinsic disorders of the testis, hypothalamic–pituitary disturbances, disorders of the seminal ducts or accessory glands, various diseases, genetic causes, occupational or environmental influences, or disorders of androgen target organs. The following comments are restricted to histopathologic changes of the testis. Clinical evaluation of the male partner, in cases of suspected infertility (i.e. failure of pregnancy in a couple during 1 year of regular, unprotected intercourse) in whom andrologic factors have been excluded, will involve a semen analysis and other investigations. Normally the ejaculate is ≥2 mL in volume, sperm concentration is ≥20 million/mL, total sperm count is ≥40 million, motility is ≥50%, and morphology is ≥30% with normal form. Oligozoospermia is defined as <20 million sperm/mL; azoospermia is defined as no spermatozoa appearing in the ejaculate. Taken together, and with regard to spermatogenesis, subnormal seminal parameters are frequently found in patients with idiopathic infertility (unexplained infertility; i.e. the cause is unknown and therapy is empirical and often ineffective).

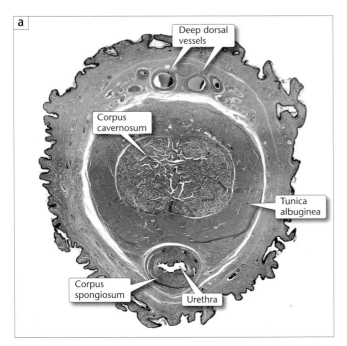

▲ **Fig 19.28a Penis structure: body.** Cross section through the body of the penis, showing the erectile tissues of two central corpora cavernosa fused in the midline, and surrounded by a thick tunica albuginea, which also encompasses the erectile tissue of the single corpus spongiosum. The urethra passes through the latter. Deep to the skin are fascial layers including the deep and dorsal arteries and veins. H&E, paraffin, × 4.

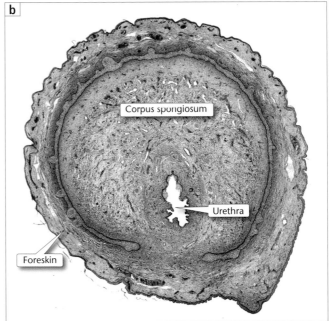

▲ **Fig 19.28b Penis structure: glans.** Cross section through the glans penis, showing the expanded corpus spongiosum erectile tissue transmitting the distal penile urethra, seen as a sagittal slit. The erectile tissue comprises dense connective tissue and many blood vessels with smooth muscle in their walls. The prepuce, or foreskin, displays an inner and outer epithelium; it covers the glans and is attached at its neck. H&E, paraffin, × 6.

Maldescent of the testis, or cryptorchidism, usually unilateral, may occur in 0.5% of adult men and in 2%–3% of human newborn males. Spontaneous descent into the scrotum usually occurs within several months from birth. Elevated temperature of the cryptorchid testis is incompatible with spermatogenesis and, if untreated, results in spermatogenic arrest or almost complete absence of germ cells with peritubular thickening. Sertoli cells and Leydig cells remain, the latter continuing the secretion of androgens. Cryptorchid testes are associated with increased risk of testicular tumor malignancy. Orchitis occurs in a minority of patients who suffer mumps (paramyxovirus) after puberty and results in impaired spermatogenesis of variable severity, occasionally leading to tubule degenerations or, at times, infertility. Childhood vaccination against the virus may prevent orchitis developing as a complication of infection.

Absence of germ cells—aplasia, or Sertoli-cell-only syndrome (SCO)—can occur in focal tubules or in all tubules, but the Leydig cells are present and androgenic parameters often are normal. Germ cell aplasia may be congenital or acquired (drugs, viral infections, irradiation, cryptorchidism). Partial or complete spermatogenic arrest may result from many different causes such as genetic defects in germ cell maturation, systemic diseases, radiotherapy, or chemotherapy. Klinefelter syndrome (47,XXY) is associated with infertility, small testis volume or hypogonadism (2 mL), hyalinized seminiferous tubules, absence of spermatogenesis and reduced numbers of Leydig cells, and low serum testosterone levels. Testicular tumors are rare (about 2–5 per 100,000 males) and most arise from germ cells, with a high degree of malignancy. The cause of such neoplasms remains largely unknown (although there is increased risk associated with cryptorchidism), and frequently they present as a swelling or lump in the testis. Seminomas (proliferating gonocytes) and non-seminomas (embryonic cells) can arise from neoplastic gonocytes representing a precancerous stage (carcinoma in situ, CIS); the latter resemble large spermatogonia with abundant glycogen and, when present, are often within small seminiferous tubules with impaired spermatogenesis. Current treatment strategies (surgery, chemotherapy, and radiotherapy), if instituted in the early stages, are very successful in effecting high cure rates.

Seminal ducts

Infections of the epididymis, vas deferens, seminal vesicles, or urethra by microorganisms, particularly bacteria, may result in obstructive azoospermia, pain, swelling, and/or general malaise. Non-specific urethritis (NSU) is a relatively common infection and is often caused by *Chlamydia*. Treatment with antibiotics is usually successful, but in some cases microsurgical reconstruction of the obstructed portion of the tract may be required (vasoepididymostomy, vasovasostomy).

Prostate

Enlargement of the prostate gland is an almost inevitable consequence of old age, occurring in 80% of men by the eighth decade of life. Benign prostatic hyperplasia (BPH) arises from the transitional zone and is androgen dependent and possibly also estrogen responsive. Symptoms include urinary obstruction and bladder irritation. Transurethral prostatectomy, when indicated, is highly effective in removing the hyperplastic tissue. Alternatively, treatment with 5a-reductase inhibitor may be effective in suppressing tissue overgrowth. Prostate carcinoma is the second most common cause of cancer-related deaths in men in their 60s and older and, although the causes(s) are unknown, genetic, hormonal, and environmental factors are all implicated in its pathogenesis. Most of these carcinomas arise from the glands of the peripheral zone and if untreated metastasize to local organs, lymph nodes and elsewhere, particularly to bone. Assay of blood levels of PSA (prostate-specific antigen) produced by normal and abnormal prostatic epithelial cells is often elevated in prostatic disorders and is one of a range of diagnostic tests used to assess and differentiate between prostate hyperplasia, prostatitis, and carcinoma. Treatment of the latter varies—surgery, radiotherapy, or hormonal therapy are currently used, the latter to counteract or block the androgen-dependent growth of advanced tumors.

Special senses

The sensory components of the nervous system provide for the detection, transmission, and analysis of information derived from inside and outside the body. Many aspects of sensory information relating to the tissues and organs in the body are not consciously registered by the central nervous system (i.e. the cerebral cortex, cerebellar cortex, and brain stem). The conscious perception of stimuli originating from the external environment gives rise to sensations which, to varying degrees, are integrated together, thereby allowing interpretation of the outside world and reaction to it.

TASTE BUDS

The sensation of taste plays an important role in the selection of food and liquids, and operates in conjunction with the sense of smell, thermoreception, and mechanoreception to determine the density and texture of the food or liquid. Taste buds are small, intraepithelial specializations, each one shaped like a barrel, that occur chiefly in the tongue, with a few in the epiglottis, soft palate, and pharynx.

Structure

In humans, there are several thousand taste buds, each about 50 μm in diameter. They act as chemoreceptors and contain several cell types—tall, slender taste receptor cells (TRC); accompanying supporting cells; and small basal cells (Fig 20.1a & b). Taste buds are not permanent structures and have a lifetime of about 14 days. New taste buds are formed in response to innervation of the lingual epithelium, which is thought to stimulate development of the basal cells into taste and supporting cells; the supporting cells are possibly a stage in the cycle of taste-cell differentiation. Taste buds are commonly found on the sides of the vallate papillae of the tongue, and also on the smaller but more numerous fungiform papillae that are scattered over the anterior two-thirds of the tongue. They are absent from the filiform papillae.

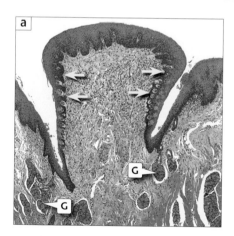

▲ **Fig 20.1a Taste buds.** A circumvallate papilla of tongue is shown, with taste buds (**arrows**) in the lateral walls. Serous glands (**G**) of von Ebner empty into furrows, or clefts. The secretions of these glands wash the surface epithelium clear of particulate matter, enabling continuous stimulation of the taste buds. Hematoxylin & eosin (H&E), paraffin, × 40.

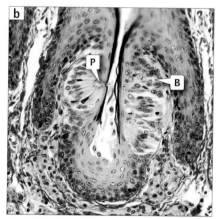

▲ **Fig 20.1b Taste buds.** Taste buds open into apical pores (**P**), where microvilli from receptor cells extend into the overlying mucus layer and detect taste stimuli. Dark cells provide a supporting function and may represent stages in the development of taste cells, since taste cells are replaced every 10–14 days. Basal cells (**B**) are the stem cells for this process. Van Gieson's, paraffin, × 250.

Function of taste buds

Serous secretions delivered to the surface epithelium from exocrine glands intrinsic to the tongue assist with washing the taste buds, allowing detection and solubilization of molecules that excite the taste receptors. The receptor taste capabilities are traditionally grouped into four main categories— sweet, sour, salty, and bitter. A fifth type of taste, umami (savory), is elicited by certain amino acids such as monosodium glutamate.

These taste stimuli are detected by entry into the apical taste-bud pore, where receptors are found on microvillous extensions of the taste cells. The receptors depolarize the taste cells (which do not possess axons), and the resulting action potentials release neurotransmitters, which stimulate afferent nerve terminals in the taste bud, passing signals to several cranial nerves and then to the cerebral cortex. A single afferent nerve can carry more than one type of signal, depending on the type of chemical stimulus; therefore, for example, one taste bud can be excited by several or all four primary taste stimuli.

In the past it was believed that particular tastes could be mapped to discrete regions of the tongue; sweet taste (from organic compounds) and salty taste (from ionized salts) are mainly detected on the tip and anterolateral aspects, sour taste (from acids) on the lateral margins of the tongue, and bitter taste (mostly from organic substances) mainly on the posterior surface of the tongue. This concept has been shown not to be accurate, because responsiveness to all five taste modalities is present in all areas of the tongue. TRCs aggregated in taste buds are tuned to respond to single tastes and are innervated by individually tuned nerve fibers. Each taste quality is perceived by the activities of non-overlapping receptors and fibers.

OLFACTORY MUCOSA

The olfactory mucosa is a ciliated, pseudostratified columnar epithelium in the roof of the nasal cavity, lying close to the cribriform plate of bone (Fig 20.2a & b). Afferent nerves pass from the olfactory epithelium

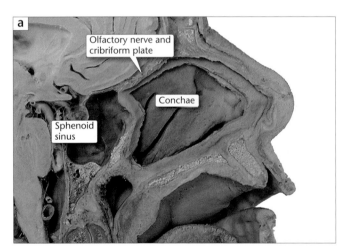

▲ **Fig 20.2a Olfactory mucosa.** Sagittal section of nasal cavity, showing the conchae covered with respiratory mucosa. The superior concha is the location of the olfactory mucosa that contains the olfactory receptors supplied by branches of the olfactory nerve passing through perforations in the cribriform plate of the ethmoid bone to the olfactory bulb.

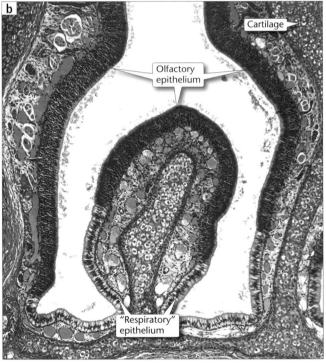

▲ **Fig 20.2b Olfactory mucosa.** Section through a developing concha in a fetal mouse nasal cavity, showing the mucosa with pale-staining segments of respiratory-type epithelium, and abrupt transition points to the olfactory epithelium with tall dense-staining columnar epithelium. The curved shelves of cartilage will, with further development, become plates of bone. Conchae serve to increase the surface area of contact between inspired air and the mucosa, which has a rich neurovascular supply. H&E/alcian blue, paraffin, × 50.

470

through the cribriform plate and then to the olfactory bulb. The olfactory mucosa has a total area of about 5 cm².

Cells of the olfactory mucosa

The olfactory area can be differentiated from the large area of respiratory-type epithelium lining the nasal cavity by two criteria:

- The epithelium is tall (50 µm) and lacks mucous cells.
- Serous glands (the glands of Bowman) and bundles of unmyelinated axons are noted in the lamina propria (Fig 20.3).

The olfactory epithelium consists of three types of cells:

- Basal cells
- Tall supporting cells, whose apices extend microvilli into the seromucous layer that covers the epithelium
- Olfactory sensory cells, which are slender bipolar neurons that expand apically and extend between 5 and 20 non-motile cilia in between the microvilli.

Hence the olfactory epithelium is a neuroepithelium and its neurons are the only nerve cells that continually degenerate but are regenerated from the basal cells.

Olfactory receptors

Membrane receptors in the cilia detect odorants, and among the millions of sensory cells (the neurons) each receptor detects a subset of the 10,000 or so different detectable odors. When odorant molecules bind to receptors, cell depolarization and action potentials are triggered. There are about 350 intact or functional odorant receptor genes. Many more are mutated and non-functional. Axons of neurons expressing the same receptor project to the same glomerulus (synaptic units) in the olfactory bulb.

Depending on the method of classification, the number of primary odors ranges from six to several dozen. The repertoire of distinct receptor populations for odorants in humans is possibly about 30, since there are about this number of specific anosmias (inability to detect a particular odorant).

How is the odorant response terminated? One mechanism may be the increasing airflow that is produced by sniffing, supplemented by watery dilution at the lumenal surface through the serous secretions delivered by Bowman's glands, which serve to remove remnants of odoriferous molecules. Perhaps the most effective mechanism is provided by the supporting cells, which contain enzymes that inactivate odorants via hydroxylation and glucuronidation.

Tip: The olfactory sensory neurons are the only part of the nervous system directly exposed to the external environment and are continuously replaced over a period of 4–8 weeks throughout life. This property has generated interest in their potential as stem cells for repair of damaged or degenerative neural tissues.

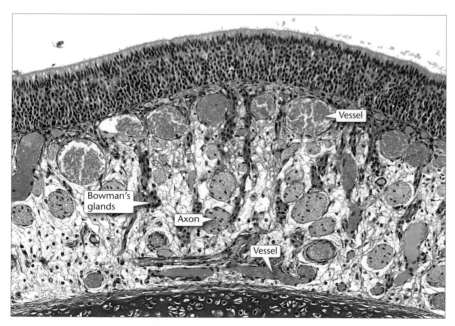

▲ **Fig 20.3 Olfactory epithelium.** The characteristic features are the tall, pseudostratified columnar epithelium with a ciliated surface but no mucous cells. Serous glands of Bowman are seen. Fascicles of axons are derived from the olfactory cells (bipolar neurons) within the epithelium. Numerous blood vessels in the lamina propria contribute to the warming of inspired air and, when expanded, cause swelling of the mucous membranes. H&E/alcian blue, paraffin, × 125.

THE EAR

Anatomically the ear is subdivided into external, middle, and inner regions. The inner comprises the organ of hearing and the organs that detect linear and rotatory accelerations. Detailed information about the structure and function of all the components contributing to the sense of hearing and equilibrium can be found in texts of anatomy, physiology, and neuroscience. The main topic of the discussion here is the functional histology of the cochlea, which, as the organ of hearing, is clinically important in relation to deafness.

External and middle ear

Sound waves travel through the external auditory meatus into the external auditory canal, and from there to the outer surface of the tympanic membrane (eardrum). The surfaces of all these structures are lined by epidermis. Sebaceous and ceruminous glands (similar to sweat glands) secrete sebum and a yellowish waxy substance into the canal. This restricts the entry of foreign materials.

The energy of sound waves causes vibration of the tympanic membrane, which is coupled to the cochlea of the inner ear by a chain of three small bones called ossicles (the malleus, incus, and stapes), and so causes oscillations of the fluids inside the cochlea.

The ossicles extend across the middle ear, or tympanic cavity, which is itself in communication with the mastoid air cells of the temporal bone and the eustachian tube (internal auditory canal). The eustachian tube opens into the nasopharynx and allows equalization of atmospheric air pressure between the middle ear and the external auditory meatus.

Inner ear

The cavity known as the inner ear is made up of:
- The sensory apparatus for hearing, the cochlea (containing the organ of Corti)
- The system of membranous sacs and tubes that detects changes in equilibrium (the vestibular apparatus).

Both sensory organs are encased in dense bone in order to protect and insulate the delicate vibrations of the fluids that they enclose. The cochlea is a spiral canal lying inside bone; the vestibular apparatus (utricle, saccule, and semicircular canals) is also located in bone, but its canals, ampullae, and sacs are membranous ducts or tubes lying close to the surrounding osseous labyrinth, although they are suspended in perilymph—a fluid similar to extracellular fluid. All of the membranous labyrinth contains endolymph fluid. Hair cells occur in the inner epithelial linings of the cochlea and vestibular apparatus.

The hair cells

In the otolithic organs—the utricle and saccule—linear accelerations (such as occur when riding in an elevator) are detected by bending of columnar hair cells, which then become depolarized and send action potentials destined for the cerebellum and the oculomotor system. The stereocilia of hair cells are embedded in a gelatinous mass of calcium carbonate crystals (otoliths), which, when deflected, set up the sensory stimulus to the hair cells. A similar mechanism operates in the ampullae of the semicircular canals, which respond to angular accelerations. The hair cells protrude into a gelatinous septum, the cupula, which extends like a diaphragm across the ampulla (Fig 20.4a–c). Displacement of the surrounding endolymph deflects the cupula, and the hair cells generate afferent impulses.

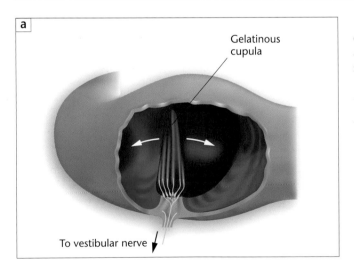

a

Gelatinous cupula

To vestibular nerve

◄ **Fig 20.4a Semicircular canal.** Representation of the inner ear, showing the ampullary part of a semicircular canal and the ampullary crest oriented transversely across the canal. The crest has supporting and sensory cells, the latter extending hair bundles (cilia) into the tall cupula, which is a gelatinous mass suspended in the ampulla. With head rotation in the plane of the canal, the rotating canal causes movement of endolymph in the opposite direction. This force bends the deformable cupula and also the specialized stereocilia, resulting in stimulation of the vestibular nerve.

The cochlea

The cochlea is similar in appearance to a snail's shell. Its tube has about 2.5 turns, which spiral around a core, or modiolus, of spongy bone that contains the spiral ganglion where nerve fibers from the sensory (auditory) hair cells arrive (Fig 20.5). The nerve stimuli ultimately pass to the auditory cortex.

Although hair cells in the cochlea are basically mechanoreceptors sensitive to extremely delicate vibrations or displacement of the lymph-filled canals

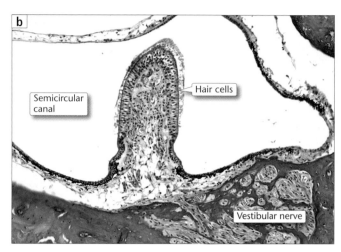

▲ **Fig 20.4b Ampullary region of a semicircular canal**, where part of the semicircular duct has been dislodged during specimen preparation. The canals contain endolymph, into which the ampullary crest extends with a core of connective tissue that supplies its surface with branches of the vestibular nerve. Remnants of stereocilia protrude from the surface sensory hair cells into the gelatinous cupula, which is not visible, having been dissolved during preparation. When endolymph is moved in response to head movements, the cupula is bowed, thus bending the hair cells, which either excite or suppress neurotransmitter release onto the sensory nerve fibers. This mechanism provides awareness of angular accelerations as distinct from simple motion. H&E, paraffin, × 100.

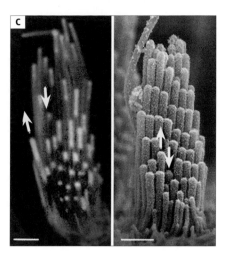

▲ **Fig 20.4c Vestibular hair cells.** *Left:* Actin-green fluorescent protein-transfected hair cells, showing longer and shorter stereocilia (**arrows**). This reflects turnover of actin cores as part of the dynamic shaping of functional architecture of the stereocilia bundle (bar = 2 μm). *Right:* Stereocilia packed in characteristic rows forming hair bundles, which, when deformed by bending, transmit mechanical energy to the hair cells to which they attach. **Arrows** show slight differences in stereocilia lengths (bar = 1 μm). (Courtesy B Kachar; from Rzadzinska AK et al. J Cell Biol 2004; 164:887–97.)

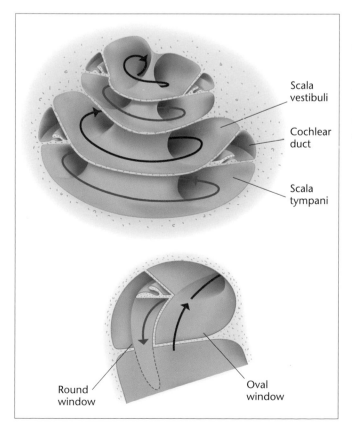

◀ **Fig 20.5 Cochlea.** Representation of the cochlea consisting of a central axis of bone, the modiolus, that contains branches of the auditory nerve and spiral ganglion. Spiraling around the axis are canals with the sensory receptor for hearing—the organ of Corti—located in the cochlear duct, also known as the scala media. Transmitted through the oval window, sound waves generate oscillations in the cochlear fluid ascending in the scala vestibuli toward the apex and descending in the scala tympani to the cochlear window. High frequencies are detected in basal spiral canals and low frequencies in the upper canals.

within the cochlea, the histology is very complex. In general terms, the spiral turns of the cochlear tube contain three longitudinal compartments—two outer canals (filled with perilymph) that meet in continuity at the end, or core, of the spiral (the helicotrema), and a central cochlear compartment or duct filled with endolymph. Each compartment is kept separate by a membrane that, in sections, gives the impression of multiple sacs inside each turn of the spiral (Fig 20.6). At the tympanic cavity, the outer canals are closed by the stapes at the oval window and by a membrane at the round window. The piston-like action of the stapes displaces the lymph contents of the cochlea's three internal compartments, which causes one of the membrane partitions, the basilar membrane (Reissner's membrane), to move up and down. On this membrane are found the hair cells of the organ of Corti, which are stimulated by the shearing motion between the hairs (stereocilia) and an overlying, hanging-roof-type structure called the

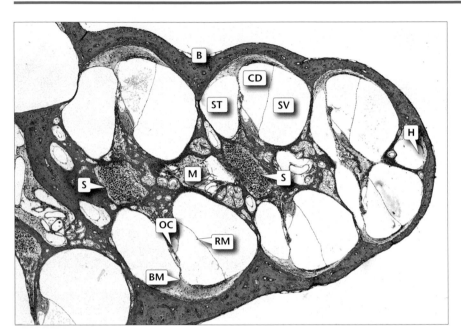

▲ **Fig 20.6 Cochlear sacs.** Spiral turns of the cochlear tube form lymph-filled sacs in section, surrounded by compact bone (**B**) with a central core of spongy bone, the modiolus (**M**). Each part of the turn shows three compartments: the cochlear duct (**CD**) with endolymph, the scala vestibuli (**SV**), and the scala tympani (**ST**) with perilymph, the latter two in continuity at the helicotrema (**H**). Reissner's membrane (**RM**, or the vestibular membrane) and the basilar membrane (**BM**) provide the partitions. Detection of sound occurs in the organ of Corti (**OC**), which sends nerve signals to the spiral ganglia (**S**). The spiral ganglia are connected to the cochlear nerve, which transmits to the brain. H&E, paraffin, × 25.

tectorial membrane (Fig 20.7a & b). There are four rows of hair cells; three rows of about 20,000 outer hair cells and a single row of about 3,500 inner hair cells. Inner hair cells are the primary source of sound transduction. Individual stereocilia are interconnected by delicate filaments at the ends of stereocilia, which are called tip links and are rich in cadherin protein

(Fig 20.8). When the stereocilia are bent, the tip links (which are probably like stiff cables) open mechanically gated ion channels that depolarize the stereocilia. This activates neurotransmitters at the base of the hair cells, which in turn stimulates the auditory nerve. Outer hair cells are thought to amplify local movement of the basilar/tectorial membranes.

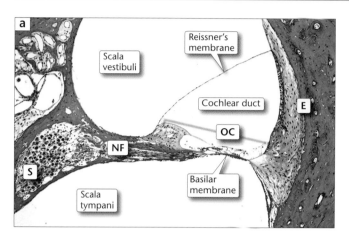

▲ **Fig 20.7a Cochlea and organ of Corti.** Section through one turn of the cochlea, with Reissner's membrane and the basilar membrane defining the scala vestibuli, cochlear duct, and scala tympani. The epithelium of the stria vascularis (**E**) secretes endolymph into the cochlear duct and is unusual for having intraepithelial blood vessels. Sound energy is transmitted through the scala vestibuli, which presses against the cochlear duct and moves it into the scala vestibuli; the sound energy is then dissipated by the scala vestibuli, causing an up-and-down displacement of the basilar membrane. The organ of Corti (**OC**) responds to this movement and sends nerve impulses to the spiral ganglia (**S**) via cochlear nerve fibers (**NF**). H&E, paraffin, × 70.

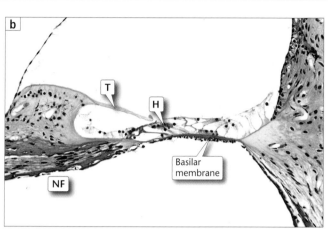

▲ **Fig 20.7b Organ of Corti.** The up-and-down displacement or vibration of the basilar membrane of the organ of Corti causes shearing of the stereocilia of the hair cells (**H**) against the fibrous, overarching tectorial membrane (**T**). In a process called mechanoelectrical transduction, deflection of the stereocilia initiates nerve impulses transmitted by the cochlear nerve fibers (**NF**) that innervate the organ of Corti. The threshold of hearing is equated to an extremely small deflection of a hair bundle (about ± 0.003°)—analogous to one finger-breadth's displacement of the pinnacle of the Eiffel Tower. H&E, paraffin, × 150.

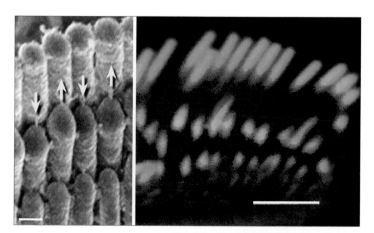

▲ **Fig 20.8 Organ of Corti hair cells.** *Left:* Stereocilia of packed rows of the hair bundle, showing tip links connecting individual stereocilia (bar = 250 µm). *Right:* Actin-green fluorescent protein-transfected hair cells, showing variability in shape and length of stereocilia tips that may reflect recovery from injury (bar = 2 µm). (Courtesy B Kachar; from Rzadzinska AK et al. J Cell Biol 2004; 164:887–97.

THE EYE

The ability of the eye to convert light signals into nerve impulses that are processed and sorted by the retina and the visual cortex of the brain is a phenomenon that is often taken for granted. On the other hand, defects in vision—less than perfect eyesight regardless of age—are common and are not considered to be trivial. A basic knowledge of the microstructure of the eye, using suitably prepared specimens, shows that the eye is similar to a photographic camera. The capture, focusing, and analysis of the enormous amount of information in a visual image begin in the eye, all on a miniature scale (Fig 20.9a & b).

The components of the eye with functional

histologic importance may be summarized as follows:

- *Eyelids and lacrimal glands* provide physical protection and lubrication of the anterior, exposed ocular surface.
- The *corneoscleral coat* is the outermost of three layers forming the globe of the eye, with the anterior portion forming the transparent cornea.
- The *uveal tract* forms the middle layer of the eyeball, composed anteriorly of the iris and ciliary body and extending posteriorly to the vascularized choroid.
- The *lens* is a biconvex, elastic structure, anterior to which is a chamber of aqueous humor, and posterior to which is the vitreous body occupying the inner cavity of the eye.

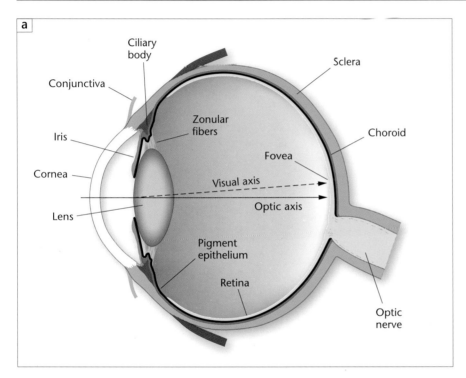

◀ **Fig 20.9a Vertical section through the eye.** The optic axis passes through the middle of the lens to reach the retina between the optic disc (optic nerve) and the fovea, a pit-like depression in the retina. The eye is directed toward a fixation point on the visual target. Light from the fixation point passes along the visual axis to the fovea, which has the highest visual resolution of any part of the retina.

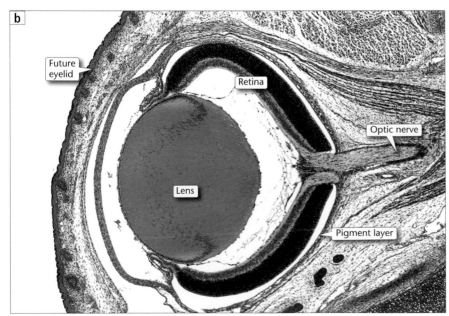

◀ **Fig 20.9b Anatomy of the eye.** Fetal eye showing relatively large lens, with rows of lens fiber nuclei forming a bow-shaped arrangement. The eyelids are fused and close over the deeper cornea. The intraretinal space between the neural retina and the pigment epithelium will disappear as these layers fuse. H&E/alcian blue, paraffin, × 50.

- The *retina* forms the innermost layer and consists of nerve cells in multiple layers, supporting cells, a photoreceptor layer, and a pigmented epithelium.
- The *optic nerve* is a tract of the central nervous system that receives fibers from the retina and supplies vascular elements to the superficial strata of the retina.

Eyelids and associated structures

The eyelids (Fig 20.10a & b) are lined externally by skin and internally by the conjunctival epithelium, a thin mucous membrane that moistens the ocular surface. Skeletal muscle fibers and sweat glands are present in the subcutaneous tissue, reinforced posteriorly by the tarsus, a plate of dense connective tissue that confers rigidity and conformation with the eyeball.

Modified sebaceous glands contribute to an oily film over the tears. The tears themselves are produced by the lacrimal gland, which is located in the upper lateral margin of the orbit (Fig 20.11). The tear film is about 40 μm deep (the oily film, about 0.1 μm deep) and contains immunoglobulin A, lysozyme, and anti-inflammatory proteins.

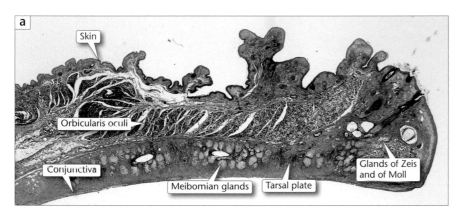

▲ **Fig 20.10a Eyelid.** The curvature corresponds to that of the eyeball. The upper margin is epidermis and the lower margin is the conjunctiva. Fibers of the palpebral part of orbicularis oculi muscle serve to close the eyelid. Sebaceous (Meibomian) glands are embedded in tough connective tissue, called the tarsal plate. In the vicinity of eyelashes are ducts/glands of Zeis (sebaceous) and Moll (apocrine). Masson's trichrome, paraffin, × 15.

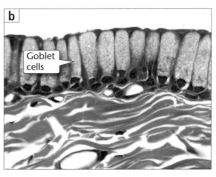

▲ **Fig 20.10b Inner eyelid.** The conjunctiva is a mucous membrane lining the inner eyelids and extends to the cornea. Its goblet cells may be numerous, and they provide mucin to the tear film for normal vision. The conjunctiva's blood supply delivers antibody, complement, and leukocytes to counter infection and remove cellular debris. H&E, paraffin, × 380.

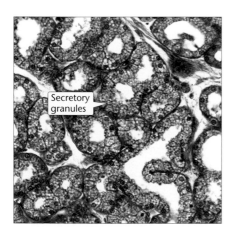

◀ **Fig 20.11 Lacrimal gland.** The lacrimal gland is tubuloacinar with prominent mucous-type secretory granules, which, when released, form the tears. The tear film has a moistening function and supplies the major refractive interface of the eye. Immunoglobulins (chiefly immunoglobulin A), lysozyme, lactoferrin, and other substances in tears combat infection and participate in inflammatory reactions at the ocular surface. Masson's trichrome, paraffin, × 200.

Cornea and sclera

The cornea makes up about one-sixth of the corneoscleral envelope (Fig 20.12a). It is shaped like a watch glass and is the most transparent tissue in the body. It is the primary refractive component of the eye, contributing about 43 diopters—more than the lens, which contributes 17–25 diopters, depending on its accommodation or focusing power. The diopter is the

measure of refractive strength, 1 D = 1 m^{-1},with light passing through a 1 D lens being focused at 1 m.

The outer surface of the cornea is a shallow, stratified squamous epithelium resting on Bowman's membrane, a lamina of collagen. The corneal stroma, about 1 mm thick, is a hydrated, multilayered arrangement of precisely oriented strata of collagen fibers, each bundle running obliquely or perpendicularly

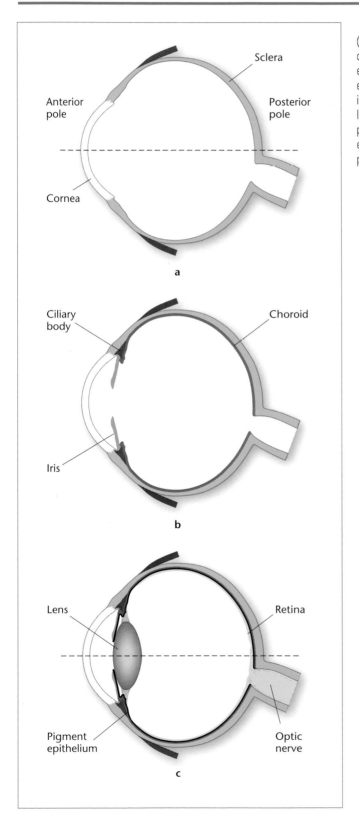

◀ **Fig 20.12 Layers of the eye.** The corneoscleral envelope (**a**) consists of the transparent cornea and the tough, inelastic sclera of the globe. It confines intraocular pressure and preserves the eye's dimensions. The uvea (**b**) is the middle vascular tunic of the eyeball. It consists of the vascular choroid, ciliary body, and iris; it is the source of intraocular fluid and nourishes the outer, avascular layers of the retina. Innermost is the retina (**c**), which terminates posterior to the ciliary body, but its outermost or underlying pigment epithelium continues into the ciliary process; there is a similar pigment layer in the iris.

to the others, thereby reducing interference of light rays and giving the cornea its transparent properties (Fig 20.13a & b). The inner surface is bounded by Descemet's membrane (again made up of collagen fibers—collagen type VIII) and an endothelium. Since the cornea is avascular but metabolically active, the endothelium supplies it with oxygen and nutrients from the adjoining aqueous humor, and acts as a barrier against edema by moving ions and water out of the stroma.

The sclera is a robust coat of collagen, fibroblasts, and some elastic fibers. It extends from the cornea to the optic nerve. It protects the eye from trauma, maintains intraocular pressure, and provides attachment for extraocular muscles. As the outermost coat of the eye, the sclera defines the size of the eyeball. In neonates its diameter is 10–17 mm and in adults 22–23 mm.

Uveal tract

The uvea forms the middle coat of the eyeball (Fig 20.12b). It consists of three parts:
- The choroid
- The ciliary processes
- The iris.

Choroid and ciliary processes

The highly vascularized choroid lies on the inner aspect of the sclera and ends anteriorly, beyond the terminal margin of the retina at the ciliary processes, which are the second components of the uvea (Fig 20.14).

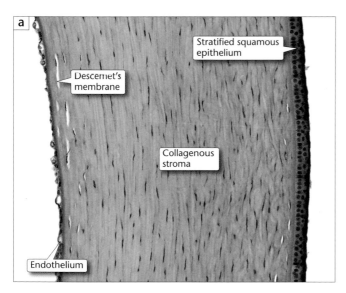

◀ **Fig 20.13a Cornea.** Anteriorly the cornea is limited by a stratified squamous epithelium with endothelium posteriorly. In between is the avascular stroma of some 200–300 parallel lamellae of collagen, which are often oriented at right angles. The anterior curvature and smooth surface of the interface between the tear film and the air provide 70% of the refractive power of the eye. Branches from the trigeminal nerve give a rich nerve supply to the cornea, providing warning of injury from foreign bodies. H&E, paraffin, × 120.

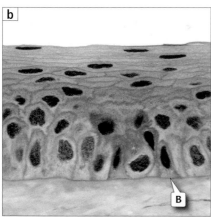

▲ **Fig 20.13b Cornea.** Anterior stratified squamous epithelium of the cornea contains glycogen for energy supply (the cornea is avascular) and rests on a thick basal lamina (**B**) called Bowman's layer. Repair after injury is achieved by centripetal sliding of cells, and new cells form in the epithelium by limited cell division and migration from the periphery of the cornea to the center. H&E, paraffin, × 350.

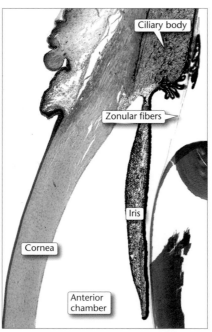

◀ **Fig 20.14 Anterior eye.** The sclera extends to form the cornea, behind which is the anterior chamber. The vascular tunic of the eyeball (the uveal tract) consists of the ciliary body with smooth muscle, which regulates the curvature of the lens via its attachment through the zonular fibers. Pigmented epithelial cells of the ciliary processes extend to the iris to give a characteristic color. The smooth muscle of the iris controls its length to adjust the diameter of its central aperture, the pupil. H&E, acrylic resin, × 12.

The choroid supplies the retina—which it underlies—with essential nutrients, and it contains fibroblasts, leukocytes, and scattered melanocytes. At the level of the outer margin of the lens, the choroid is modified to contribute to the core of the ciliary processes (Fig 20.15a–c), which are irregular finger-like processes covered by a double epithelial layer derived from the ora serrata, the serrated anterior extension of the retina. The superficial ciliary cells are not pigmented, but the cells of the inner layer next to the core of connective tissue are highly pigmented.

Aqueous humor is secreted by the ciliary epithelium and flows into the anterior and posterior chambers of the eye between the cornea and lens. Both of these structures receive nutrient supply from the aqueous humor, which has a total volume of about 250 μL. This fluid is normally drained constantly by the canal of Schlemm (from where it passes into veins) at the

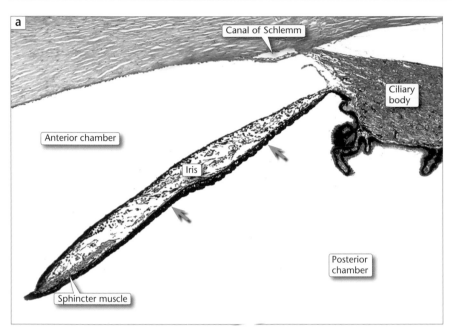

▲ **Fig 20.15a Ciliary apparatus and iris.** The iris extends from the ciliary body and defines the anterior and posterior chambers, both filled with aqueous humor produced by the ciliary epithelium and drained by the canal of Schlemm. The stroma of the iris is vascularized connective tissue. Melanocytes occur in this tissue and in abundance along the posterior margin (**arrows**). Dilator muscle in the stroma (myoepithelial cells) opens the pupil via sympathetic innervation (in response to low light, pain, or fear); sphincter muscle constricts the pupil via parasympathetic innervation (in response to bright light or to improve depth of focus and visual acuity). H&E, paraffin, × 20.

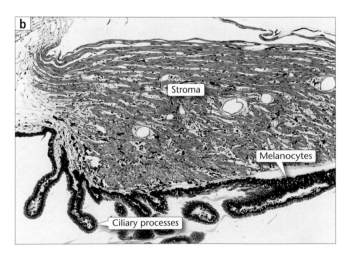

◀ **Fig 20.15b Iris.** Root of the iris showing vascularized stroma, which contains connective tissue and contractile myoepithelial cells together with melanocytes. Anteriorly the iris has no epithelial margin but a layer of fibroblast-like cells. Posteriorly, and continuous with the ciliary processes, there is a double epithelial layer—a deeper layer of melanocytes derived from the retinal pigment epithelium, and a more superficial layer of non-pigment cells derived from the continuation of the sensory retina. Ciliary processes attach zonular fibers to the lens capsule to provide support and allow modification of its shape (and hence the accommodating power) of the lens. H&E, paraffin, × 80.

iridocorneal angle. Failure of adequate drainage raises intraocular pressure, and this may damage the retina and optic nerve.

Lateral to the ciliary processes is the smooth muscle of the ciliary body. The body and its processes extend very fine, elastic-type zonular fibers to the lens, to which they provide support. Changes in refraction, and hence focus on distant or near objects, are made possible by alteration of the shape of the lens, termed accommodation. For distant vision, the circular muscles of the ciliary body relax (sympathetic innervation), stretching the zonular fibers taut and causing the lens to flatten. For near vision, the muscles constrict via parasympathetic supply and the zonular fibers relax, allowing increased curvature of the lens.

The iris

The iris, the third component of the uveal tract, is a thin diaphragm of tissue arising from the ciliary body and resting gently on the lens. The part of the iris in contact with the lens contains melanocytes, which give a blue color if few in number and a brown color if abundant (Fig 20.16). The central opening is the pupil, which is made smaller by the operation of sphincter pupillae muscles near the pupillary margin. The dilator pupillae muscles are located in the remaining iris stroma, together with a well-vascularized loose connective tissue.

The lens

The lens is the second most transparent tissue in the body—only the cornea is more transparent. The slight yellow color of the lens absorbs UV light. It is elastic and consists of an extracellular capsule with a simple cuboidal epithelium anteriorly. Toward the equator of the lens, these epithelial cells proliferate and then withdraw from the cell cycle. By switching their pattern of gene expression, these cells greatly elongate (hence the term lens fibers), losing their nuclei but retaining a very high concentration of

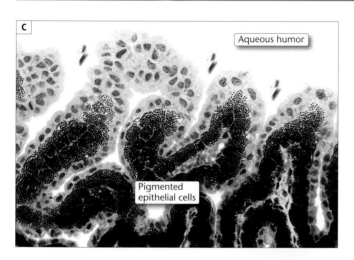

◀ **Fig 20.15c Detail of ciliary processes**, which are radial folds of the ciliary body, showing non-pigmented epithelial cells and a deeper pigmented epithelial layer. The valleys between processes (**arrows**) provide attachment for lens zonular fibers. Aqueous humor production by the ciliary epithelium occurs via ultrafiltration of fluid from fenestrated blood vessels, thus allowing large proteins to enter the stroma. These proteins do not enter the aqueous humor because they are restricted by the blood–aqueous barrier that is located at tight junctions connecting the apical poles of the ciliary epithelium. H&E, paraffin, × 400.

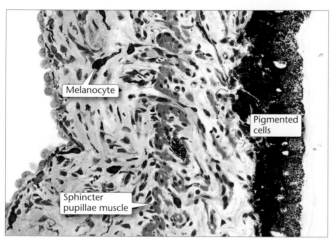

◀ **Fig 20.16 Detail of the iris**, showing the anterior border of fibroblasts and the posterior border of pigmented epithelial cells. The stroma contains loose connective tissue, with part of the sphincter pupillae muscle visible. Melanocytes occur in the stroma and near the anterior border, their numbers (excluding the pigment epithelium) determining the color of the iris. In the brown iris, melanocytes are abundant; in the blue iris, they are less abundant and as a result light of shorter wavelengths in the blue region of the spectrum is reflected. At birth the irises are blue or gray as there are only a few melanocytes present; the adult coloration is established at around 4 months of age. H&E, paraffin, × 150.

proteins, which are termed crystallins (Fig 20.17a & b). New fibers become arranged like layered shells on top of one another, and are produced throughout life, the older fibers being located at the center or nucleus of the lens. Thus the lens contains embryonic, fetal, and postnatal cells and retains every cell it has formed throughout its life.

The fibers are six-sided prisms, numbering about 2,000, and are interdigitated by ball-and-socket and tongue-and-groove membrane specializations (Fig

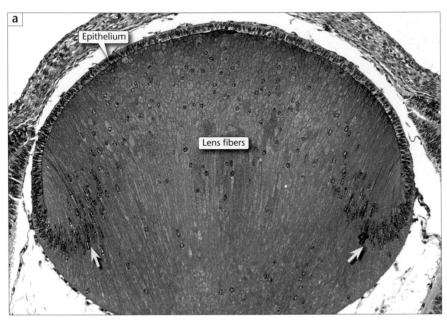

▲ **Fig 20.17a Lens.** Developing lens in the fetus, showing an anterior border of epithelial cells that migrate into the central regions, as indicated by the distribution of their nuclei, which form the lens fiber nuclear bows (**arrows**). Note the crescent-shaped shells, or lamellae, of lens fibers in the interior of the lens. H&E, paraffin, × 140.

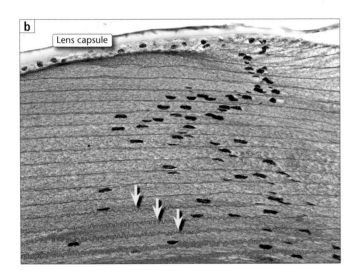

◀ **Fig 20.17b Beneath the lens capsule**, surface epithelial cells divide and greatly elongate and flatten to form a C-shaped curve as more cells are produced in the superficial region. The older cells lose their nuclei, and the so-called fibers become stacked on top of one another to form concentric layers that extend around the curve of the lens from the anterior to the posterior pole. Young lens fibers still interlock via ball-and-socket and tongue-and-groove membrane specializations (**arrows**). These structures maintain fiber order and hence transparency, and they allow limited fiber sliding and flexing during lens accommodation. H&E, paraffin, × 400.

20.18a & b). Fibers run anteroposteriorly, their ends meeting one another at Y- or star-shaped suture lines.

Tip: To focus an image, the shape of the lens is changed by the action of the ciliary muscle, which alters the curvature of the lens. A flatter lens focuses on distant objects; a rounder lens focuses on close objects. Accommodation is the ability of the lens to increase its focal power and is commonly reduced with age.

The retina

The retina packages an enormous complexity within a small region. It is histologically and embryologically a part of the central nervous system (CNS). Photoreceptor cells must be small so as to allow packing together to maximize resolution, and the retina must be thin so as to allow light to reach the rods and cones. The retina is a thin layer of neural tissue lining the inner eye. In histologic section it is

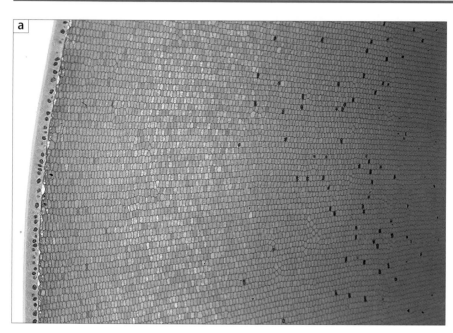

▲ **Fig 20.18a Lens fibers.** Arranged in stacked columns, the lens fibers are elongated epithelial cells that with maturation lose their nuclei and organelles and synthesize crystallin protein. Lens fibers are ribbon-type cells that form a highly packed mass, enclosed on anterior surface of the lens tissue by a germinal cell layer. The adult lens may have 2,000 lens fibers, and throughout life new lens cells arise from the lateral margins of the anterior lens epithelium. H&E, acrylic resin, × 180.

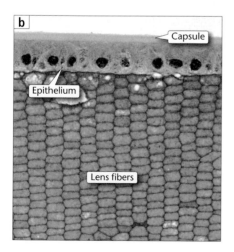

◀ **Fig 20.18b Lens fiber cells seen end-on**, showing their hexagonal shape and orderly arrangement. The cytoplasm contains more protein than is found in cytoplasm in any other cell (crystallins make up 35% of the wet weight). Fibers have gap junctions, which assist in lens metabolism; the lens derives nutrient supply for metabolism from the aqueous humor through the capsule and anterior epithelium. The lens retains all the fibers it produces; this process continues throughout life. H&E, acrylic resin, × 500.

483

highly stratified, and it is described as having 10 layers, which consist of neurons or cell bodies, synapses, one principal type of glial cell, the photoreceptive rods and cones, and an outermost postmitotic pigmented epithelium (Fig 20.19a–c). With the exception of the fovea, light must pass through nine layers of tissue to reach the photoreceptor apparatus of the rods and cones.

Because there are probably more than 50 different functional elements in the retina, a comprehensive understanding of the functional histology of this tissue is chiefly of interest to the ophthalmologist, optometrist, and neuroscientist. For students of general histology, only the major features need be discussed.

Before reaching the retina, light passes from the lens through the vitreous body, a hydrated gel-like

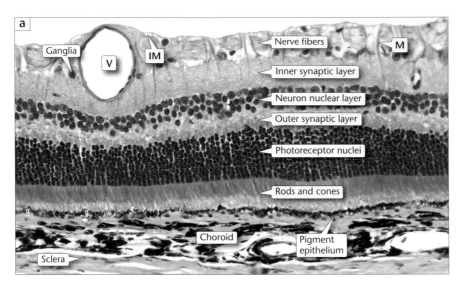

◀ **Fig 20.19a Retina.** The major features noted are the sclera, the pigmented, vascularized choroid, pigment epithelium, photoreceptor segments of rods and cones and their nuclei, an outer synaptic layer, a neuron nuclear layer, an inner synaptic layer, slender glial (Müller) cell processes (**M**), ganglion cells, and an afferent nerve fiber layer. A retinal vessel (**V**) is noted; it derives from the vessels accompanying the nerve fiber layer. The inner "limiting membrane" (**IM**) is the basal lamina for Müller cells, and above it is the vitreous humor through which light passes into the retina. H&E, paraffin, × 375.

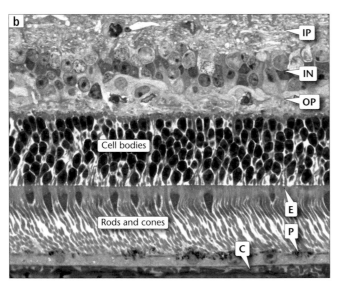

◀ **Fig 20.19b Retina section.** Thin epon resin section of retina resting on the choroid (**C**). The layers noted are the pigment epithelium (**P**), which absorbs excess scattered photons, phagocytoses the tips of rod and cone segments, and recycles retinal back to the photoreceptors; the photoreceptor layer of rod (monochrome) and cone (color) segments, which contains visual pigments; the external "limiting membrane" (**E**), which is, in actuality, an assembly of tight junctions; the outer nuclear layer of rod and cone cell bodies; the outer plexiform (synaptic) layer (**OP**) of dendrites, which is concerned with processing signals from static images; the inner nuclear layer (**IN**) of cell bodies of amacrine, bipolar, horizontal, and interplexiform neurons; the inner plexiform (synaptic) layer (**IP**) of dendrites, which deals with information received from moving images. Above these (not shown) is the ganglion cell layer, where electrical stimuli are processed into action potentials, and the optic nerve fiber layer, which passes to the optic nerve. Toluidine blue, araldite, × 625.

substance, 4–5 mL in volume and similar to egg white. The vitreous body is adherent to the lens capsule, the ora serrata, and to the optic disc posteriorly. It is mostly aqueous and is suspended in hyaluronan, together with fine collagen fibrils, which are produced by cells called hyalocytes.

In the living eye the retina is purplish-red, owing to the visual pigment (visual purple, or rhodopsin) present in the rod photoreceptors. Beneath or external to the photoreceptors is the pigment epithelium—a brown layer continued forward as the pigmented layer of the ciliary epithelium. The central retina, located

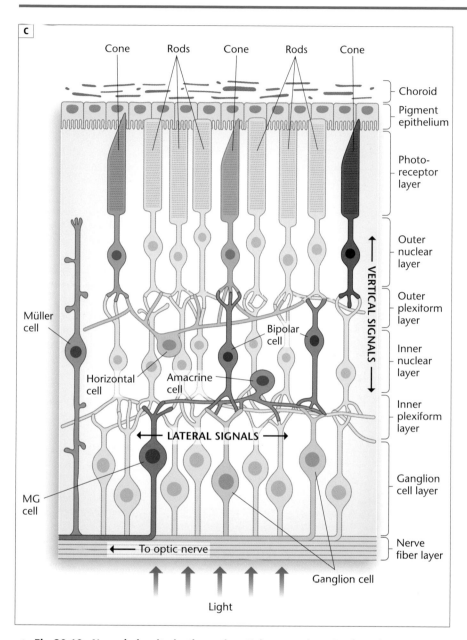

▲ **Fig 20.19c Neural circuits in the retina.** Light enters the retina from the vitreous body and passes through the neural layer before reaching the outer pigmented layer. Starting from the top of the diagram the *neuroepithelial* layer has the rods and cones and their nuclei; the *middle/ganglionic* layer has bipolar neurons (horizontal, bipolar, amacrine cells); the *ganglionic layer* of the optic nerve has multipolar neurons, with axons extending as unmyelinated fibers to the papilla of the optic nerve. The melanopsin ganglion (**MG**) cell is a newly discovered photosensitive neuron that detects blue light and may be involved with detecting dawn and dusk to contribute to body circadian rhythm. Müller cells extend through much of the retina and act as glial cells.

temporal to the optic disc, is about 5 mm in diameter and thinner at its center, where it forms the fovea (about 2 mm in diameter) with a concave indentation (0.35 mm in diameter) called the foveola. Here the retina contains only cones, providing maximum acuity of vision (Fig 20.20). The peripheral retina increases the field of vision and has far more rods than cones; in the human eye there are 100–120 million rods and 5–6 million cones.

Following the detection of light by the photoreceptor cells (see below), how are the excitation signals processed by the retina? The remaining strata of neurons perform this function. They are organized into three cellular (nuclear) layers, separated by two synaptic (plexiform) layers. Synapses between the neurons are made in the two synaptic layers before the visual information leaves the eye. The outer plexiform layer carries out spatial (static) analysis of visual input; the inner plexiform layer is concerned more with temporal (moving) aspects of light stimuli. All this information is processed by the ganglion cell layer on the superficial aspect of the retina, from where it passes to the outermost fiber layer of the optic nerve. Of the structurally different types of ganglion cells, 80% are called X type (processing detail and color), Y type (motion), W type (unknown function), and a recently described MG type that remarkably detects light directly. Blood vessels in the ganglion cell layer are accompanied by astrocytes (Fig 20.21), which support blood vessel growth and are abundant around the optic disc but sparse elsewhere.

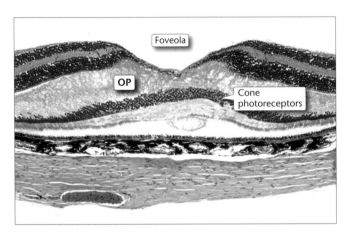

◀ **Fig 20.20 Fovea.** At the center of the fovea the retina is avascular and thinned at the foveola, which is filled with cone photoreceptors, and with cells of the overlying outer plexiform layer (OP). It represents about 1° of the visual field but provides maximum acuity (resolving power); in humans this is achieved at 4–5 years of age. In addition to the 35,000 cones in the region, there are a few blue-absorbing cones, thus the light-adapted eye is maximally sensitive to yellow light. Individual foveolar cones have one-to-one connections to the brain via a bipolar cell and a ganglion cell, giving high-resolution information, in color, which in the macaque monkey is recorded in area V4 of the visual cortex. In the peripheral retina, many rods and cones together contribute signals from the visual field; this information is pooled and resolution is coarser. H&E, paraffin, × 75.

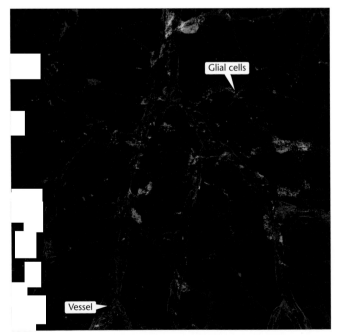

◀ **Fig 20.21 Retinal astrocytes.** Retinal glial cells stained with glial fibrillary acidic protein (red) with nuclei in green. Blood vessels are blue. Astrocytes are found in the nerve fiber and ganglion cell layers and are abundant around the optic disc, but absent from the fovea. They contact blood vessels and axons, but not ganglion cell bodies. Astrocytes emerge from the developing optic nerve, spread along the retina, and stimulate retinal angiogenesis. Immunofluoresence, × 650. (Courtesy T Chan-Ling, Department of Anatomy, University of Sydney, Australia.)

Function of the photoreceptors

Rods are receptive in dim light, whereas cones function in bright light and are responsible for color vision. The outer segments of rods have many free-floating membranous discs, and cones have many membrane folds stacked like coins (Fig 20.22). Both rods and cones contain visual pigment molecules (retinal, derived from vitamin A, bound to a protein called opsin, which varies in structure in different pigments). All rods absorb maximally in blue–green light, whereas individual cones absorb blue, or green, or red–yellow light (Fig 20.23). Red- and green-sensitive cone pigment genes are located on the X-chromosome (i.e. they are sex-linked).

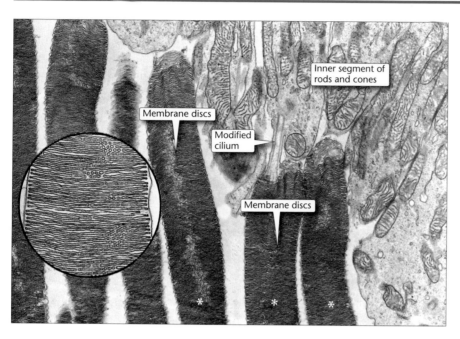

▲ **Fig 20.22 Rod photoreceptors**. Ultrastructure of rod photoreceptors with the inner segment above, and outer segments below showing many membrane discs. These are separate from the plasma membrane; they are synthesized in inner segments and assembled in outer segments, where they are replaced as the outermost discs are phagocytosed by the pigment epithelium. Disc membranes contain the photoreceptor rhodopsin molecules, consisting of retinal and opsin. Retinal may absorb from 1 to 1,000 photons, which suppress the innate electrical or so-called dark current. In turn, opsin is altered and activates transducin protein, which initiates a membrane hyperpolarization response and a signal is passed to retinal neurons. Cones do not produce new discs and have three types of opsins with maximum absorbance in the blue–violet, green–yellow, and yellow–red parts of the light spectrum. × 12,000. (From Porter KR & Bonneville MA. Fine structure of cells and tissues. Philadelphia: Lea & Febiger, 1973.)

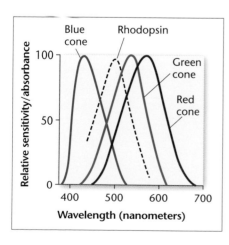

◀ **Fig 20.23 Photopigments**. Light absorbance spectra of the three cone photopigments and rhodopsin in humans. The curves overlap. Rhodopsin is the pigment found in rods and is also called visual purple because it has this color after blue and green light has been absorbed. Rods absorb widely across the visible spectrum, but detect grayscale only. Color perception by cones depends on the ratios of stimulation from different wavelengths.

When photons are absorbed by the visual pigment, they induce transformations in the pigment molecule, causing excitation of the rod or cone and separation of the retinal pigment molecule from the opsin pigment molecule, a process called bleaching. Retinal pigment molecule is reduced to vitamin A, which is recycled and changed back to retinal in the pigment epithelium. Vitamin A is also made available to the eye from the blood. New membranous discs are produced in the rods, and they migrate toward the tips of the cells, where they are phagocytosed by the pigment epithelium. Melanin granules in the pigment epithelium absorb excess light, and this reduces reflection and interference (Fig 20.24). The structure and function of the pigment epithelium declines with age, with an increasing burden of phagocytosis.

The retina is sensitive to light of a remarkable range of intensity—across about 10^{12} units; that is, from the faintest stars on dark nights (eighth magnitude, or 0.0005 lux) to the intensity of the sun (1,600 million lux). Rods and cones provide for variations in spectral sensitivity. In the dark, the eye is maximally sensitive to green; in the light the eye is maximally sensitive to yellow. So, as the sun sets, yellow flowers in the garden lose their prominence but the blue ones seem brighter, and eventually they all lose their color.

The rods have the greatest light sensitivity (faint stars are brighter about 20° lateral to the central field of vision, which coincides with the maximum density of rods in a corresponding histologic view of the retina). Color perception is associated with the cones, whose maximum density is in the central fovcola (Fig 20.25).

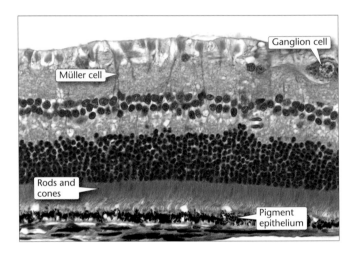

◀ **Fig 20.24 Pigment epithelium.** The basal retinal pigment epithelium is shown, containing a mixture of dark-staining melanin granules and lysosomes. The former minimize any reflection of back-scattered light from the choroid and sclera. Lysosomes degrade the tips of the outer segments of rods and cones through microvillous processes that extend from the pigment epithelium in between the outer segments. Large ganglion cells are noted in the inner retina. Their axons form the inner nerve fibers that become the optic nerve. The slender processes are those of the tall columnar Müller cells (these cells provide nutritive and organizational support), which are accompanied by capillaries from the retinal vessels within the inner nerve fiber layer. H&E, paraffin, × 375.

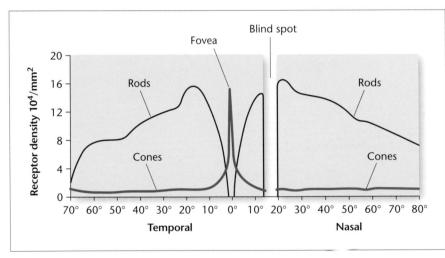

◀ **Fig 20.25 Distribution of photoreceptors.** A plot of cone and rod density as a function of position relative to the fovea, the region of the retina with the highest visual resolution. Note the absence of rods at the fovea but a high concentration of cones to give maximum acuity. No cones or rods are found at the blind spot, where nerve fibers enter the optic nerve.

The optic disc, or blind spot (Fig 20.26a & b), is the site where about 1 million axons from the fiber layer of the retinal nerve leave the eye through the sclera. Vascular supply to the inner retina, up to and including the inner nuclear layer, is provided by the central retinal artery and vein located within the optic nerve and disc.

CLINICAL NOTES ON THE SPECIAL SENSES

Taste

Taste buds are more sensitive to bitter flavors (one part in millions) than to other flavors, thus possibly constituting a protective mechanism against bitter-tasting toxic substances such as alkaloids, nicotine, and strychnine. Congestion of the mucous membranes of the head, as caused by, for example, the common cold, reduces the sense of taste.

Olfaction

Anosmia, the partial or complete inability to smell, may be caused by trauma to the head or by any tumor that impinges on the olfactory nerves. The sensation of smell is associated with behavioral responses (e.g. babies find the nipple by smell), and olfactory sensations may modify reproductive behavior in some mammals (e.g. to encourage mating, to promote the marking-out of territories, or to induce estrus or ovulation). The edema of the nasal mucous membranes associated with a cold often inhibits the sense of smell owing to excessive production of mucus.

Hearing and vestibular system

Deafness may arise from a range of disorders, including ear infection, physical damage, and nervous conditions. Conduction deafness is a consequence of blockage of the auditory canal, damage or perforation of the tympanic membrane, or otitis media (bacterium-induced middle-ear inflammation). Damage to the auditory nerve pathway or to the sensory hair cells in the cochlea contributes to sensorineural (nerve) deafness. Frequently this condition occurs in response to chronic exposure to excessively loud noise.

Disturbances of the vestibular organs or their nerve supply may cause vertigo (spinning sensation) or motion sickness and can be either intrinsic or induced. Cyclical movements of the body coupled with uncoordinated or unfamiliar visual sensations result in motion sickness. Astronauts may experience this, because although the utricle and saccule are non-functional in zero gravity, angular accelerations are detected by the semicircular canals. Ménière's disease is caused by excessive production of endolymph, which causes distortion of the membranous labyrinth with vertigo, loss of hearing, and tinnitus.

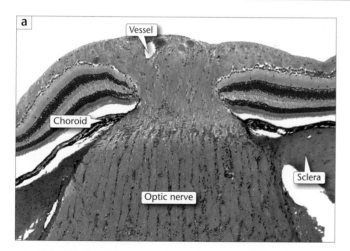

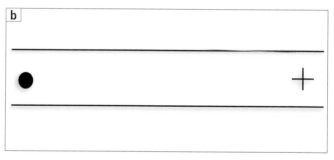

▲ **Fig 20.26b Blind spot.** Demonstration of the blind spot, where the optic disc lacks photoreceptors. Close the left eye and hold the page about 12 inches (30 cm) away. Fix your gaze on the spot and move the page closer; the cross will disappear. Repeat, closing the right eye, but fixing your gaze on the cross; the spot will disappear.

▲ **Fig 20.26a Optic nerve.** The optic nerve is formed from about one million axons from the inner nerve fiber layer, which is located on the superficial or inner aspect of the retina. Retinal blood vessels accompany the optic nerve and supply the inner layer of the retina; the outer layers are supplied by diffusion of nutrients from the choroid vessels. Vascular proteins from the choroid and sclera cannot reach the retina via the optic nerve because of tight junctions between glial cells and pigment epithelial cells (the blood–brain barrier at the optic disc). The ratio of photoreceptors to single nerve fibers in the optic nerve is 125:1, and this is thought to limit the quantity of information required for analysis by the brain. It also produces a blind spot, devoid of photoreceptors, which is sufficiently small not to interfere with vision. H&E, paraffin, × 50.

Vision

Conjunctivitis (inflammation of the conjunctiva) is a common disorder often caused by atmospheric pollutants, pollens, or microorganisms (e.g. trachoma) and resulting in redness of the eye and pain. Chemicals or ultraviolet light (e.g. from oxyacetylene welding lights or arc furnaces) may cause severe conjunctivitis, with damage to the cornea (keratitis); bacteria and viruses may also cause inflammation of the iris.

The eyes of newborn babies appear blue or slate-gray, since the formation of melanocytes in the iris is not completed until about 3–4 months after birth. If the concentration of pigment is high, the eyes appear almost black or brown; if low, the eyes may show various colors of green, blue, or gray.

If the aqueous humor in the anterior and posterior chambers does not drain normally, the raised intraocular pressure may restrict the supply of blood to the retina, resulting in neuron damage and impaired vision, a condition known as glaucoma. Treatment is effected using drugs that inhibit fluid production or increase its drainage, or by laser surgery to promote its outflow.

Disorders of image formation are common, and include astigmatism (irregular corneal curvature), in which refraction is not radially symmetrical; myopia (near-sightedness), in which focusing occurs in front of the retina; and hyperopia (far-sightedness), in which focusing occurs behind the retina. The focal plane varies in relation to the shape of the elastic lens or the shape of the eyeball. With age, the ability of the lens to change shape to accommodate for objects at infinity or at close range may be compromised, a condition termed presbyopia. In this case, the lens becomes more rigid because its capsule becomes less elastic and more lens fibers are produced.

In cataracts, a common cause of blindness, the lens becomes opaque as a result of aggregation of crystallin proteins or of edematous changes. The condition is associated with old age and may require surgical implantation of an artificial lens.

In blindness associated with diabetes (diabetic retinopathy), the capillaries and arterioles of the retina become sclerotic, and microaneurysms and hemorrhage occur. The resulting scar tissue impairs retinal function. Laser coagulation of affected vessels suppresses neovascularization and hemorrhage.

Night blindness, or poor vision in dim light, occurs if rod function is disrupted; the main cause is vitamin A deficiency in the diet.

Color blindness is usually genetically based. It affects more males than females. In red/green color blindness, which is due to a deficiency or absence of red- or green-sensitive cones, red and green are perceived as the same color.

Appendix: stains

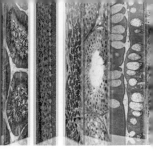

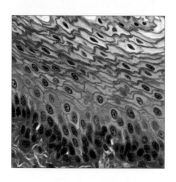

◀ Hematoxylin and eosin. Hematoxylin stains nuclei deep blue-purple due to their content of DNA, RNA, and ribosomes. Rough endoplasmic reticulum stains similarly. Eosin stains the cytoplasm pink-magenta. Extracellular materials such as connective tissues stain in varying shades of pink to red.

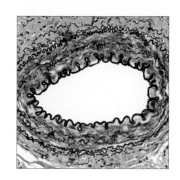

◀ Gomori's aldehyde fuchsin/Masson's trichrome. Elastin fibers stain purple with aldehyde fuchsin. Used as a counterstain, the trichrome stains cell nuclei red; extracellular matrix and collagen stain green.

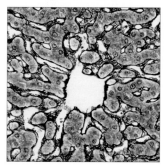

◀ Gordon and Sweet's silver method. This is an ammoniacal silver stain for reticular fibers, followed by gold chloride to give a dense black color. Counterstaining with neutral red stains cell nuclei and cytoplasm yellow.

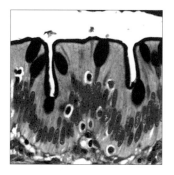

◀ Periodic acid – Schiff/ hematoxylin. The PAS reaction stains mucins/ glycoproteins a deep magenta, seen here for goblet cells, their apical brush border, and the basal lamina. Nuclei stain blue with hematoxylin as a counterstain.

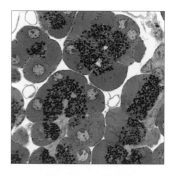

◀ Toluidine blue. A metachromatic dye, toluidine blue dissolved in sodium borate (borax) is the preferred stain for 1 μm epon/araldite sections. Tissue components show various color shifts other than that of the dye (e.g. blue-violet, and for lipids, shades of green).

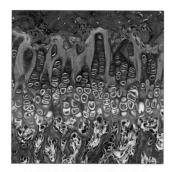

◀ Alcian blue/hematoxylin and eosin. Alcian blue stains glycosaminoglycans (such as in cartilage) shades of blue to bluish green. It is especially useful for demonstrating cartilage in endochondral ossification. Hematoxylin-eosin is used for counterstaining.

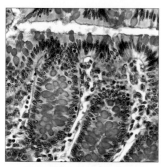

◀ Alcian blue/van Gieson's. Alcian blue normally stains mucins/glycoproteins a blue color, but the picric acid in van Gieson's shifts the color to green, and addition of indigo carmine stains nuclei red-brown, with cytoplasm stained yellow-orange.

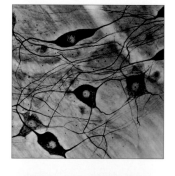

◀ Bielschowsky's silver. This is an ammoniacal silver nitrate stain to demonstrate nerve cells and their processes. Background tissue, in this case smooth muscle, is stained yellow to brown.

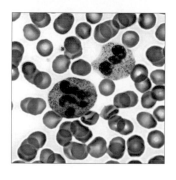

◀ Romanowsky stains. These have been modified as May–Grunwald–Giemsa, and Wright's stains for blood/bone marrow using azure B and eosin. *Azure B:* nuclei, neutrophil granules, ribosome-rich cytoplasm are blue; basophil granules are violet. *Eosin:* erythrocytes, eosinophil granules, platelets, ribosome-rich cytoplasm are red. In combination these give purple colors.

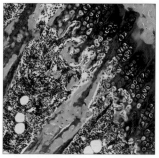

◀ Masson's trichrome. In combination with Gomori's aldehyde fuchsin, this method produces three primary colors in various shades. Cartilage stains blue-violet; osteoid is magenta; bone and collagen are blue-green. Cell cytoplasm, muscle, and most blood cells are red.

Index

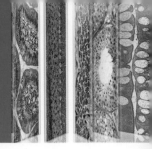

A

A bands, muscle, 138, 144, 146, 147
    cardiac muscle, 150, 151, 152
    ultrastructure, 144
aberrance of tissues, 65
ABO blood group, 93
absorption
    epithelial cell polarity and, 97
    gastrointestinal tract, 323, 324, 344–5
    Golgi apparatus role, 26–7
    water, in kidney, 382, 384, 385, 387, 388, 389
accessory sex glands (male), 441, 462, 464–5
accommodation, vision, 481, 482, 483
acetylcholine, 172, 173
    antibodies, 159
    gastrointestinal tract, 172, 328
    skeletal muscle, 146, 148
    in vesicles in axons, 146, 148, 172, 173
acetylcholinesterase, 173
achondroplasia, 256
acid hydrolases, 29
acid–base balance, 105
acidophils, 396, 397
acinar cells see pancreas, acinar (exocrine) cells
acinar glands, 111, 113
acini (acinus), 100, 101, 358
    liver, 356, 358
    lung, 297–8, 303
    pancreatic see pancreas
    salivary glands, 308, 309, 310
    tongue, 307
acne, 215, 220
acrosomal cap, 449
acrosome, formation, 449
acrosome-phase spermatids, 450
acrosome reaction, sperm, 421
acrosomic granule, 449
ACTH see adrenocorticotropic hormone (ACTH)
actin, monomers, 40
actin filaments, 9, 35, 40, 41
    assembly/growth, 40
    cardiac muscle, 150, 152
    contractile ring, in mitosis, 40, 51, 54
    drugs affecting, 40
    microvilli, 42, 43
    positioning and stabilizing, 147
    skeletal muscle, 140, 144, 146, 147
    sliding along myosin filaments, 40, 137, 147, 158
    smooth muscle, 154
    terminal web and villi, 42, 43
actinin, 147
action potential
    heart, 191
    muscle, 146, 148, 152, 153, 174
    nerve, 163, 170, 171–2
    special senses, 470, 471, 472

active transport, 114
activins, 425
acute lymphoblastic leukemia (ALL), 93
acute myeloid leukemia (AML), 93
adaptive immune system
    see immune system
adenocarcinoma, lung/bronchial, 304
adenohypophysis see pituitary gland, anterior
adenoids (enlarged pharyngeal tonsil), 318, 322
adenosine triphosphate (ATP) see ATP
ADH see antidiuretic hormone (ADH; vasopressin)
adherens junction (zonula adherens), 40, 45, 46–7, 103–4
    cardiac muscle, 46, 47, 153
adhesion proteins, in desmosomes, 47
"adhesion zippers", 103
adhesive glycoproteins, 126
adipocytes see adipose cells (adipocytes)
adipokines, 129
adiponectin, 129
adipose cells (adipocytes), 2, 33, 68, 118, 119, 128, 129
    brown/white, 33, 128, 129
    development, 129
    functions, 33, 119, 128, 129
    parathyroid gland, 401
    yellow bone marrow, 77, 78
adipose tissue, 68, 128–9, 138, 219
    benign tumors, 136
    breast, 436
    brown/white, 33, 128, 129
    functions, 119, 128, 129
adrenal gland, 402–4
    blood supply, 402
    congenital hyperplasia, 412
    cortex, 402–4
        disorders, 402, 411–12
        hormones secreted, 402, 403, 404, 411
        zones, 402, 403
    development/origin, 402
    failure, 411
    medulla, 402, 404, 410
        chromaffin cells, 404, 405
        disorders, 412
        zona reticularis, boundary, 405
adrenalin (epinephrine), 393, 404, 405
adrenarche, 404
adrenocorticotropic hormone (ACTH), 395, 403, 404
    excess/reduced levels, 411
adult respiratory distress syndrome, 303
adventitia, gastrointestinal tract, 323
aerobic respiration, 27, 28

afferent (sensory) nerves, 161
agenesis, tissues/organs, 114
agglutinins, 93
aggrecan, 125, 126, 134, 252, 255
aging, cellular, 31
agranulocytes see lymphocyte(s); macrophage
airways, 293, 295, 300, 303
    acinar, 297, 298
    trachea, 290, 291
    "transitional", 297, 298
    see also bronchi; bronchioles; trachea
albinism, 220
Alcian blue staining, 491
alcohol, 363, 371
aldosterone (salt-retaining hormone), 387, 389, 403
    actions, 402, 404
alimentary canal see gastrointestinal tract
allergic reactions, 90, 91, 261, 285
alpha cells, pancreatic, 370, 405, 406, 407
alveolar bone, 311, 312, 313
alveolar capillaries, 299, 300, 302
alveolar cells, 299, 300
    types I/II, 299, 300, 301, 302
alveolar cysts, 100
alveolar ducts, 297, 298
alveolar glands, breast, 436, 437
alveolar pressure, 298, 299
alveolar sacs, 297, 298
alveoli (alveolus), 294, 297–8
    dimensions, 299
    elastic fibers, 299
    epithelium, 300
    gas exchange and, 298, 299–302
    interstitium, 299
    macrophage in, 300, 302
    numbers and surface area, 299, 303
    structure/function summary, 302
    ultrastructure, 301
alveolus (tooth socket), 312
Alzheimer's disease, 187
amacrine cells, 484, 485
ameloblasts, 318
    development of, 314, 316, 317
    enamel development, 312, 314, 316
amelogenesis, 314, 317–18
amenorrhea, lactational, 438
amines, biogenic, 172, 296, 347
amino sugars, sulfated, 126
amnion, 63
amoeboid movement, 40
ampulla/ampullary region
    semicircular canals, 472, 473
    uterine tubes, 413, 428
    vas deferens, 462
ampulla of Vater, 365
ampullary crest, 472
amylin, 406
β-amyloid plaques, 187

amyotrophic lateral sclerosis, 187
anaerobic metabolism, 145
anal canal, 324, 352
anaphase, 50–1, 52
anaphylaxis, 285
anastomoses, arteriovenous, 201, 213
anchoring junctions see adherens junction (zonula adherens)
androgen(s), 247, 441
    excess production, 412
    receptors, 443, 455, 460
    secretion by Leydig cells, 410, 441, 458
    secretion by ovary, 425, 427
    see also testosterone
anemia, 92
anergy, 264
aneurysm, 205
angina pectoris, 159
angiogenesis, 202
angiotensin I, 387, 389, 403
angiotensin II, 387, 389, 403
angiotensinogen, 389, 403
annulus, late-elongating spermatid, 450
annulus fibrosus, 255
anosmia, 489
anovulation, 438, 439
anterior chamber of eye, 476, 479, 480
anterograde transport, 22, 24–5
antibodies (immunoglobulins), 257, 258, 263, 264, 265
    class switching, 266, 278
    classes and functions, 264
    diversity generation, 264, 278
        VDJ gene segments, 264, 266
    formation/secretion, 17, 18, 262, 263, 265, 266, 268
        in intestine, 284
    structure, 264
    see also specific immunoglobulins
antidiuretic hormone (ADH; vasopressin), 384, 386, 387, 388, 389
    actions/functions, 398
    excessive, 411
antigen(s), 258, 259, 263
    B cell activation, 263, 265, 266
    endogenous, MHC class I and, 268
    exogenous, MHC class II and, 269
    processing and presentation, 267–8, 269, 270
    T cell binding/activation, 263, 266, 268, 269
antigen-presenting cells (APCs), 257, 267
    dendritic cells, 84, 266, 269, 270
    Langerhans cells, 211
    monocytes/macrophage, 91, 119, 260, 261

antimitotic drugs, 37
antral follicles *see* ovarian follicles
aorta, 192, 193
apatite crystals, 234
aphthous stomatitis, 321
aplasia, tissue/organ, 114
apo-eccrine glands, 214
apocrine glands, 213, 214, 215
    eyelid, 477
    secretory coils, 214
apocrine secretion, 114, 214
apoptosis (programmed cell death),
    32, 58–9
    control/initiation, 58, 59
    defective, 59
    early/late, ultrastructure, 59
    granulosa cells, 421
    male germ cells, 445, 446
    nerve cells in Alzheimer's
        disease, 187
apoptotic bodies, 59
apoptotic cells, 29, 59
appendicitis, acute, 283, 354
appendix, 283, 352, 354
APUD cells, 290, 347, 400, 409
aqueous humor, 476, 480, 481, 490
arachnoid mater, 180
arcuate arteries, 373, 383
areolar nerves, breast, 437
areolar tissue *see* connective
    (supportive) tissue, loose
argentaffin (argyrophilic cells), 409
arginine vasopressin (AVP)
    see antidiuretic hormone
    (ADH; vasopressin)
argyrophilic cells, 409
arrector pili muscle, 216, 218
arteries, 193–6
    anastomoses with veins, 201
    characteristic features, 190
    constriction/dilation, 196
    dimensions, 192
    disorders, 205
    elastic, 192, 193–4
    elastic fibers in, 124, 193
    hardening (arteriosclerosis), 205
    inadequate (loss of) elasticity,
        125, 205
    muscular (medium-sized), 192,
        194, 204
    in transition, 194, 195
    role/functions, 196
    smooth muscle, 155, 193, 194
    vasa vasorum, 194, 201
    vein comparison, 204
    wall layers, 193
arterioles, 190, 194
    anastomoses, 201
    blood pressure in, 194, 195
    constricted, 194, 195
    dimensions, 192
    elastic fibers, 124
    functions, 194, 195
    muscular artery transition to,
        194, 195
    terminal, 196, 201
    ultrastructure, 195
arteriosclerosis, 205
arteriovenous anastomoses, 201,
    213
arthritis/arthrosis, 256
articular cartilage, 224, 250–3
    calcified, 252, 253
    loss in osteoarthritis, 256
    thickness, 135, 252, 253
    tidemark, 252, 253
    see also hyaline cartilage
ascites, 371
asters (astral microtubules), 39
asthma, 261, 296, 303
    allergic, 285
astigmatism, 490

astrocytes, 167–8
    fibrous type, 167
    processes, 180
    protoplasmic type, 167, 168
    retina, 486
    "territory", in hippocampus,
        168
    velate, 185
atherosclerosis (atheromata), 160,
    205
ATP, 27, 28, 44, 149
    skeletal muscle contraction,
        145, 147
ATPase, skeletal muscle, 149
atrioventricular bundle of His, 153,
    191
atrioventricular node, 153, 191
atrium, heart, 191
atrophy, 114
    cell/epithelial, 114
    muscle, 147, 159, 187
    renal, 392
    vaginal mucosa, 434
auditory nerve damage, 489
auditory system, 472–5
Auerbach's (myenteric) plexus, 163,
    173, 177, 325, 327–8
    myenteric ganglia, 163, 328
Aurora B, 54
auto-immune disease, 259
autocrine regulation, 393
autonomic ganglia, 176, 177
autonomic innervation, vas deferens,
    462
autonomic nervous system (ANS),
    161
autophagic lysosomes, 31–2
autophagy, 31–2
autoregulation
    of blood flow, 196
    of filtration, 387
AVP (arginine vasopressin)
    see antidiuretic hormone
    (ADH; vasopressin)
axillae, apo-eccrine glands, 214
axon(s), 74, 163, 164, 165–6
    acetylcholine vesicles, 146, 148,
        172
    bulb, 172
    diameters, 174
    dorsal root ganglia, 177
    hillock, 163, 164, 166
    length, 165–6
    motor end-plate, 146, 148
    myelinated, appearance, 174,
        175
    myelination, 170
        in CNS by oligodendrocytes,
            168, 170, 171
        gaps, nodes of Ranvier, 170
        in PNS by Schwann cells,
            169, 170, 171
    staining, 161, 174, 175
    synapses, 172
    terminals (boutons), 173
    transport within, 38, 42
    ultrastructure, 166, 169
    varicosities, 173
axonal transport, antero/retrograde,
    166
axoneme, 44, 99, 449
axoplasmic flow, 186
azoospermia, 466

B

B lymphocytes, 80, 92, 258, 263–6
    activation, 264–6, 270, 279
    affinity maturation, 266, 278,
        279
    defective/self-reactive, deletion,
        264, 271
    development, 84, 263, 278

B lymphocytes *continued*
    bone marrow, 263, 264,
        271
    differentiation and proliferation,
        264–5
    functions, 263–4
    in lymph nodes, 276, 277, 278,
        279
    maturation, 264, 278
        germinal centers
            see germinal centers
    memory cells, 264
    migration/circulation, 263, 276,
        277
    naïve/unprimed, 264, 279
    in palatine tonsils, 319
    proliferation in Peyer's patches,
        348
    receptors (BCRs), 263, 264
    specificity, 264, 278, 279
    in spleen, 282, 283
    surface immunoglobulins, 264
    T cell interactions, 265
    see also antibodies; plasma cells
bacteria
    crescentin, 42
    intracellular killing of, 260
    neutrophil killing of, 89
    oral cavity, 2, 321
    "organelle" in, 11
band cells (stab cells), 82, 83
Barrett's esophagus, 353
basal bodies, 42, 43, 44, 99
basal cell(s), 107
    epididymis, 462, 463
    taste buds, 469
    trachea, 290, 291
basal cell carcinoma, skin, 220
basal ganglia (basal nuclei), 180,
    182
    disorders, 182
basal lamina, 97, 99, 102, 107, 127
    alveolar cells, 299, 300, 301
    arteries, 194
    cornea, 479
    dento-enamel junction, 317
    of endothelium (in heart), 190
    primary and antral follicles,
        419, 421, 425
    renal corpuscle, 378, 379, 380
    respiratory epithelium, 290,
        291, 299
    seminiferous tubules, 443, 444,
        446
    ultrastructure, 99, 127
    see also basement membrane
basement membrane, 71, 99, 127
    capillaries, 197
    functions/location/structure,
        127
    in kidney, 99, 127
    reticular lamina, 127
    villi, in jejunum, 343
    see also basal lamina
basic multicellular unit (BMU), 233,
    236, 250
basilar membrane, cochlea, 474
basket cells, cerebellum, 184
basolateral domains, epithelium, 97
    specializations, 99
basophil(s), 82, 90–1, 261, 263
    activated, 90–1
    anterior pituitary, 396, 397
    properties, 86
    ultrastructure, 91, 261
basophilia, pancreatic acinar cells,
    366, 367
Bcl-2 protein family, 59
Bellini, ducts of, 385
benign prostatic hyperplasia, 465,
    467
Bergmann glial cells, 185

beta cells, pancreatic, 370, 404,
    405, 406
    destruction, autoantibodies, 412
    ultrastructure, 406
Betz cells, 182
bicarbonate, 87, 105, 236, 351
    secretion, 334, 339, 367
Bielschowsky's silver stain, 491
bilaminar embryonic disc, 61, 63, 64
bile
    circulation, 363, 364
    composition, 363
    concentration, by gall bladder,
        364, 365
    flow, 365
        in liver, 357, 358, 359, 363
        obstruction, 371
    formation by hepatocytes, 359,
        363, 364
    secretion, 358, 359
    storage, 364
    volume, 364
bile canaliculi, 356, 357, 360, 362,
    363
bile ducts, intrahepatic, 362, 363
bile ductules, 357, 359
bile pigments, 363
bile salts, 363
bilirubin, 87, 220, 363, 371
biofilm, 321
biogenic amines, 172, 296, 347
bipolar neurons, 484, 485
bladder, 391
    distended or relaxed, 391
    smooth muscle, 390, 391
    transitional epithelium, 390,
        391
blast cells, 80
blastocoel, 62
blastocyst, 61, 62, 63
blastomeres, 61, 62
bleaching (retinal separation from
    opsin), 488
bleeding, menstrual, 431, 432, 433
blind spot (optic disc), 476, 488,
    489
blindness, 490
blood, 67, 71, 77–93, 85–92
    analysis, 77
    as connective tissue, 117, 136
    disorders, 92–3
    formed elements, 86–92
    functions, 85
    oxygen-carrying capacity, 389
    pumped by heart in lifetime,
        190
    resistance to flow, arterioles,
        194, 195
    volume, 77, 85, 189
blood cell(s)
    development/lineages, 80, 81
    progenitors, 79
    see also erythrocyte(s);
        leukocyte(s)
blood cell analyzers, 93
blood donors, "universal", 93
blood films, 77, 86, 93
blood flow
    capillaries, 196, 201
    cerebral, 183, 196
    glomerular, 387
    in liver, 358
    velocity, 192
blood groups, 93
blood pressure, 404
    in arterioles, 194, 195
    blood vessel changes, 196
    elevated, 205
blood tests, 77
blood transfusions, 93
blood vessels, 192–202
    anastomoses, 201

blood vessels *continued*
blood–tissue exchange, 192
collagen, 123, 125
in dermis, 213
diameters, 192, 194
in epithelial tissue supporting
tissue, 102
innervation, 201
microvasculature, scheme, 196
pressure and flow, 192, 196
repair of wall, 202
villus core, in jejunum, 342
wall elasticity, 123, 125, 193–4
wall thicknesses, 192
walls, blood supply to, 201
see also arteries; arterioles;
capillaries; veins; venules
blood–air barrier, 299–302
blood–aqueous barrier, 481
blood–brain barrier, 167, 198
at optic disc, 489
blood–testis barrier, 455, 456, 457
blood–tissue exchange, 192
BMP signaling pathway, 102
bone, 67, 136, 223, 232, 240
adult, 223–33
architecture, 224, 225, 232
basic structure, 223
composition, 223, 225
morphology, 232, 233
basic multicellular unit (BMU),
233, 236, 250
blood supply, 250
calcium homeostasis and PTH,
237, 401
canaliculi, 227, 234, 235
cancellous (spongy/trabecular),
136, 223, 224, 230–1, 232,
245
compression fracture, 230
growth/development, 248–9
osteoclast action, 236
resorption/replacement, 250
strength, 230, 231
structure, 230–1
"cartilage", 239
cartilage interface, 252
cartilage relationship, 223
cells, 136, 233–8
osteoprogenitor, 233
see also osteoblasts;
osteoclasts; osteocytes
cement line, 226
collagen, 223, 224, 227, 228,
233
collar, 241
compact (cortical/dense), 223,
224, 226, 227–8
osteoclast action, 236
see also osteon (Haversian
system)
components, 223, 225
dense (compact), 136
as dense connective tissue, 72
development and growth, 223,
238–49, 246
appositional, 240, 249
cancellous bone, 248–9
criteria affecting, 238
disorders, 256
endochondral
see endochondral
ossification
endocrine control, 247
epiphyseal growth plate,
243, 244–8
estrogen receptors and, 248
intramembranous
ossification, 238,
239–40
length/width increase,
242–4

bone *continued*
long bones, 238, 242–4
onset, in embryo/fetus, 239
during puberty, 247
signaling pathways, 246–7
time frame, 244
velocity and growth spurts,
247
see also ossification
diaphysis, 242
disorders, 255–6
endosteum, 231, 233, 236
epiphyses, 224, 242, 243
erosion/demineralization, 236
fetal *see* fetus
formation, 223, 233–4, 238,
246
cartilage role, 238, 239
secondary, 240
time required, 234
see also ossification
fractures *see* fracture(s)
Haversian canals, 225,
226, 228, 229, 232,
235, 240
Haversian system *see* osteon
(Haversian system)
lacuna, 227, 232, 234, 235,
236, 250
lamellae/layers, 223, 225, 227
circumferential, 225,
232, 251
collagen orientation, 227
concentric, 227, 232
interstitial, 228, 232
parallel, 230
lamellar, 227–31, 236
formation, 234, 240
see also bone, cancellous;
bone, compact
lengthening, 242–4, 248
long
development/growth, 238,
242–4
fetus, 239, 242, 244
fractures, 228
shaft, 223, 227
see also bone, development
and growth
matrix degradation by
lysosomes, 236, 237
mature, 223
"membrane", 238–9
mesenchymal cells, 233, 239
metabolic disorders, 256
metaphysis, 224, 243, 246
mineral density decline, 256
mineralization, 223, 234, 238
nonlamellar, 227
as organ, 223
ossification centers
see ossification
osteoid *see* osteoid
osteons *see* osteon (Haversian
system)
osteophytes, 256
parallel-fibered (bundle), 223
periosteum, 231, 232, 233,
242
primary spongiosa, 240, 242
regeneration/repair, 223
remodeling, 240, 249–50, 251
cancellous bone and, 230
closing cone, 250
osteoblasts role, 233
osteon replacement, 228
rapid, 227
reversal zone, 250
resorption
canals, 249–50
control/coordination, 237–8
osteoclasts role, 236, 237

bone *continued*
parathyroid hormone effect,
401
suppressed by calcitonin,
400
surface excavation,
appearance, 237
resorption cavity, 236
skeletal muscle attachment, 140
spicules, 240, 246
spurs, 256
staining, 491
trabeculae, 136, 223, 224, 230
development, 240, 249
vascular (Haversian) canals,
225, 226, 228, 229, 232,
235, 250
Volkmann's canals, 226, 228,
232
woven (immature), 223, 227,
228, 233–4
development, 239–40, 245
remodeling, 249–50
bone-lining (osteoprogenitor) cells,
233
bone marrow, 71, 77–85, 271
adults, neonates and infants, 77
anemia, 92
B cell development, 263, 264,
271
as connective tissue, 77, 117,
136
erythropoiesis, 80, 82
functions, 77
gelatinous, degeneration, 77
hemopoiesis, 79, 80
histology, 80, 82–5
lymphocytopoiesis, 84
mast cells, 83
mesenchymal cells of, 233
microenvironments (niches),
271
monocytopoiesis, 83
morphology, 77, 78
neoplasms, 92–3
origin, 79
red (hemopoietically active),
77, 78, 136, 271
reticular fibers, 136
reticulocytes, 82
sampling, 80
staining, 491
transplantation, 93, 285
vascular sinusoids, 77, 78, 79,
271
yellow (inactive), 77, 78, 136
bone marrow smears, 77, 80
bone morphogenetic protein (BMP),
102
Bowman's capsule, 377, 378, 380
Bowman's glands, 471
Bowman's membrane, cornea, 478,
479
Bowman's space, 377, 378, 379,
387
brachial plexus, 162
brain, 17, 178–87
architecture, 178
capillaries in, 198
energy requirements, 183
repair, astrocyte role, 167
volume, 180
weights, 178
see also cerebral cortex; gray
matter; white matter; *other*
specific structures
"brainbow" transgenic mouse, 168,
182
brainstem, 183
breast, 436–8
alveolar glands, 436, 437
carcinoma, 439

breast *continued*
development, 436
disorders, 439
lactation, 436, 438
male, 439
menstrual cycle changes, 436
breast milk, 158, 436, 438
breastfeeding, 413, 438
bronchi, 292, 294–6
squamous metaplasia, 115
bronchial arteries, 300
bronchial secretions, 295, 296
bronchial tree, 293, 297
branching morphogenesis, 293,
294, 297
bronchiectasis, 44
bronchioles, 294, 295, 296
in asthma/emphysema, 303
blockage/closure, 296
cartilage lacking, 295
respiratory, 294, 296, 297, 298
terminal, 297, 298
bronchitis, 296, 303
bronchopulmonary segments, 293,
294, 295
brown adipose tissue, 33, 128, 129
Brunner's glands, 111, 113, 339
brush border (of microvilli), 42,
106, 344
proximal convoluted tubules,
379, 382, 383
small intestine, 337, 344
ultrastructure, 344
brush cells, tracheal, 290, 291, 292
buccal cavity, 305
bulbourethral (Cowper's) glands,
441, 465
bundle branches, 153
bundle of His, 153, 191
burns, 115, 221

C

C cells (parafollicular), 399–400
C peptide, 406
cadherin proteins, 46, 47, 103, 376
Cajal, cells of, 328
Cajal bodies, 13
calciferol, 389
calcification, 239
calcitonin, 400
calcitonin-secreting (C) cells,
399–400
calcitriol, 389
calcium (ions)
in cardiac ischemia, 159
homeostasis, 235, 236, 401
release/flux, muscle
contraction, 152, 159
cardiac muscle, 152
in rigor mortis, 159
skeletal muscle, 146, 148
smooth muscle, 155, 158,
195
tidemark of enthesis, 135
uptake/storage/release, smooth
ER role, 21
calcium-binding proteins, 234
calcium-induced calcium release,
152
calcium phosphate, 135, 223, 234
calculus, dental, 322
callus, 255
calmodulin, 158
calyces, renal, 374, 385
canal of Hering, 362
canal of Schlemm, 480
canaliculi
bile, 356, 357, 360, 362, 363
bone, 227, 234, 235
parietal cells, 334
cancer, 42
gall bladder, 371

cancer *continued*
  gastric, 353
  intermediate filament subtypes, 42
  liver, 371
  lung, 304
  ovary, 438
  p53 mutations, 59
  skin, 220
  testis, 454
  see also carcinoma
candidiasis, oral, 321
capillaries, 196–8
  alveolar, 299, 300, 302
  basement membrane, 197
  blood flow, 196, 201
  in brain, 198
  characteristic features, 190
  continuous, 196, 197
  dermis, 213
  dimensions, 192
  endothelium of, 197, 201, 203, 302
  fenestrated, 196, 197
  functions, 197
  glomerular *see* glomerular capillaries
  junctional, 196
  lymphatic *see* lymphatic capillaries
  network, 196–7, 213
  non-fenestrated, 196, 197
  pericytes, 197, 198
  permeability of wall, 198
  sinusoidal (discontinuous), 196, 197, 198
  tight junctions, 196, 198
  types, 196, 197, 198
  ultrastructure, 197
capillary plexus
  alveoli, 213
  dermis, 213
  hypothalamus, 394
capillary–tissue exchange, 197
capsules, of organs, 131
carbohydrate, metabolism, 21
carbon dioxide, 87, 300
carbonic acid, 236
carcinoma
  basal cell, 220
  breast, 439
  intestinal, 353, 354
  lung/bronchial, 304
  squamous cell, 220, 321
carcinoma in situ, testis, 454, 467
cardia, of stomach, 330, 332
cardiac failure, 204–5
cardiac ischemia, 159–60
cardiac muscle, 73, 137, 150–3, 192
  abnormalities, 159–60
  action potentials, 152, 153, 191
  A bands, I bands, and Z lines, 150, 151, 152
  cell junctions, 46, 47, 153
  characteristics, 137
  contraction, and calcium flow, 152–3
  "dyad", 152
  growth and development, 158
  injury, 158
  intercalated discs, 150, 151, 153
  mitochondria, 28, 150, 151
  myofibrils, 150
  myofilaments, 152
  nuclei, 150
  sarcomere, 150, 152–3
  sarcoplasm, 150
  sarcoplasmic reticulum, 152
  transverse tubule system, 152
  ultrastructure, 151

cardiac myocytes, 73, 137, 150–2, 158, 191
  see also cardiac muscle
cardiomyopathy, 159
cardiovascular system, 189–202
  characteristic features, 190
  functions, 189
  lymph system comparison, 189
  see also blood vessels; heart
carotene, 210
cartilage, 72, 133–5
  articular *see* articular cartilage
  bone formation, 238
  bone relationship/interface, 223, 252
  calcified, 244, 246, 249, 252, 253
  collagen type II, 123
  costal and respiratory, 133
  elastic *see* elastic cartilage
  epiphyseal, 242, 243
  formation, bone formation, 240, 245
  hyaline *see* hyaline cartilage
  mineralized, 135
  resting zone, in epiphyseal growth plate, 244, 245, 246
  staining, 491
  types, 133
  see also chondroblasts; chondrocytes; fibrocartilage
cartilage canals, 243
cartilage cells, 2, 133
cartilage matrix protein, 125
caspases, 59
cataracts, 490
catecholamines, 404
  epinephrine, 393, 404, 405
  excess, 412
  receptors, 394
  storage granules, 404, 405
  synthesis, 393, 404, 410
  see also norepinephrine
β-catenin proteins, 96
cathepsin K, 236
cauda equina, 162, 186
caudate nucleus, 178
caveolae, 29–30
caveoli, smooth muscle, 157, 158
"caveosomes", 30
CD markers, T lymphocytes, 266–7
CD3, 267
CD28, 267
CD34, 80, 83
celiac disease, 353
cell(s), 1–48
  adhesion, intermediate filaments role, 42
  boundary, 67
  compartments and packaging, 6–9
  complexity, 4–6
  cytoplasm *see* cytoplasm, cell death, 58–9
    see also apoptosis (programmed cell death)
  digestive processes, 28–32
  division *see* meiosis; mitosis
  fate of digested material, 31–2
  internal structures, 11–28
  membrane density/surface area, 6, 8
  mobility, actin microfilaments role, 40
  non-cellular components *vs*, 67
  order *vs* chaos (entropy), 5
  organization, 10–48
  polarity *see* epithelium
  proliferation, 48–58
    control, 48–9

cell(s) *continued*
  shape, cytoskeleton role, 36
  sizes/dimensions, 1
  structural features, 67–8
  suicide (planned depletion) *see* apoptosis
  surface, interactions with environment, 42–5
  surface specializations, 4
  two-dimensional micrographs, 4, 34
  volume, 8, 9
  see also specific cell types
cell cycle, 49–54
  checkpoints, 54, 55
  duration, 49
  G_0, G_1, G_2 phases, 49
  interphase (resting), 49
  M phase, 49–54
    see also mitosis
  S phase, 49, 100, 447
cell fate, definition, 67
cell junctions, 45–8
  adhesive (adhering), 45, 46–7, 103–4
  desmosomes *see* desmosomes epithelial cells, 71, 97, 99, 102–4
  functions, 46, 47, 48, 103, 104
  gap/communicating *see* gap junctions (nexus)
  intermediate *see* adherens junction (zonula adherens)
  tight *see* tight junctions (zonula occludens)
  types, 45, 103–4
cell-mediated immunity, 258
cell membrane *see* plasma membrane
cell-to-cell transport, gap junction role, 104
cell–cell adhesion, 103
cellular antennae, 42
cement line (tidemark), 135, 252, 253
cementoblasts, 312
cementocytes, 312
cementum, 312, 313
central nervous system (CNS), 161, 167, 178–87
  disorders, 187
  hormone secretion control, 394
  see also brain; spinal cord
central tolerance, 274
central vein, liver, 356, 357, 359
centrifugal flow, bile, in liver, 358
centrioles, 39
  modified (basal bodies), 42, 43, 44, 99
centripetal flow, blood, in liver, 358
centroacinar cells, 366, 367, 368
centroblasts, 278, 279
centrocytes, 278, 279
centromeres, 16
centrosomes, 35, 37, 39
cerebellar cortex, 182, 183
  astrocytes, 185
  dendrites, 164, 165, 184, 185
  granular layer, 183, 184
  layers, 183, 184, 185
  molecular layer, 183, 184
    ultrastructure, 185
  Purkinje cells, 164, 165, 184, 185
  Purkinje layer, 184, 185
  surface area, 183
cerebellum, 178, 182–5
  efferent/afferent pathways, 182, 184, 185
  folia, 178, 183
  functions, 184
  gray matter, 178, 182, 183, 184

cerebellum *continued*
  hemispheres, 182
  white matter, 182, 183, 184
cerebral blood flow, 183, 196
cerebral cortex, 178, 180–2
  evolutionary aspects, 181, 182
  gray matter, 178, 179
  interneurons, 182
  laminar organization, 181, 182
  layers (I-VI layers/organization), 180, 181, 182
  neuron loss, 187
  pyramidal neurons, 163, 164
  somatosensory cortex, 181
  stem cells, 182
  synaptic density, 182
  ultrastructure, 180
  white matter, 180
cerebral cortex neurons, 165
cerebral edema, 180
cerebral hemispheres, 178, 180
cerebrospinal fluid (CSF), 168, 186, 187
cerebrum, 162, 180–2
ceruminous glands, ear, 472
cervical dysplasia, 432
cervical ganglia, 176
cervix, uterine, 432, 433
  disorders, 432, 439
CFU-GEMM, 84
chaperones, molecular, 21
chemoreceptors, taste buds as, 469
chemotherapy, effect on microtubules, 37
chest pain, 159
chiasmata, meiosis, 57
chief cells, 335
  granules, and ultrastructure, 335
  parathyroid glands, 400, 401
  stomach, 331, 332, 333, 334, 335
chloride
  reabsorption from saliva, 310
  renal transport, 384, 386, 388
chloride channel, 334
cholangitis, 371
cholecystitis, 371
cholecystokinin (CCK), 339, 364, 365, 366
  cells secreting, 409
  pancreatic juice release, 367
cholesterol, 28, 363
  excess accumulation, gallstones, 371
  steroid hormone synthesis, 393, 403, 459
chondroblasts, 118, 119, 133
  formation, endochondral ossification, 241
chondrocytes, 4, 72, 119, 133, 134
  clusters (isogenous groups), 133
  ECM secretion, 133
  elastic cartilage, 134, 320
  epiphyseal growth plate, 243, 244, 245
  fibrocartilage, 135
  hyaline cartilage, 133, 134, 252
  hypertrophied, 247, 248, 249
    endochondral ossification, 241, 242, 246, 247
  islands, 119
  lacuna, 134
  proliferation, 241
chondroitin sulfate, 126, 134
chondron, 134
chordae tendinae, 150
chorion, 63
chorionic gonadotropin, human (hCG), 63, 410, 428
chorionic villi, 434–5
choroid, 478, 479–81, 484

choroid plexus, 186, 187
chromaffin cells, 404, 405
chromatids, 49, 50
chromatin, 13–17
  compacted/condensed, 14
    in apoptosis, 59
    in spermatids, 450
  non-dividing cells, 14, 16
  packaging/arrangement, 14, 16
chromatin fiber, 15
chromogranin, 336
chromophils, 396, 397
chromophobes, 396, 397
chromosome 5, 16
chromosome 19, 16
chromosomes, 13–17
  condensed, 51
  crossing-over see genetic
    recombination
  DNA length in, 16
  hierarchical organization, 15
  interphase, 14
  looped domains, 15
  normal metaphase, 14
  number, 49, 57
  polytene (Drosophila), 14
  replication, 13, 14, 49, 50
  segregation to poles in mitosis,
    53
  ultrastructure, 16
chronic fatigue syndrome, 159
chronic lymphoblastic leukemia
  (CLL), 93
chronic myeloid leukemia (CML),
  93
chylomicrons, 345
chyme, 330, 334, 335, 339
cilia, 43–4, 99, 107
  movement, 43–4
  nasal passages, 287
  olfactory receptors, 471
  primary, 43
  tracheal epithelium, 107, 290,
    291, 292
    immotile (Kartagener's
      syndrome), 44, 303
  ultrastructure, 44, 99, 291, 292
ciliary body, 34, 476, 478, 480, 481
ciliary muscle, 480, 481, 483
ciliary processes, 478, 479, 480–1
ciliated epithelium see epithelium
circadian rhythm, 408
circulation
  bile, 363, 364
  lymph, 276, 277, 303
  lymphocytes, 263, 276, 277
  pulmonary, 189, 299, 300
  systemic, 189
circulatory system, 189–205
  disorders, 204–5
cirrhosis of liver, 205, 371
cisternae, 17, 18, 22
cisternal maturational model, 24
Clara cells, 296, 297
clathrin, 30
clathrin-coated vesicles, 24, 27,
  29, 30
climbing fibers, cerebellum, 185
clonal selection theory, 258, 259,
  262, 263
closing cone, bone remodeling, 250
Clostridium tetani, 159
CNS see central nervous system
  (CNS)
coagulation, blood, 88
coagulation factors, 85
cochlea, 472, 473–5
  hair cells see hair cells
cochlear duct, 473, 474, 475
cochlear fluid, 473
cochlear nerve fibers, 475
cochlear sacs, 474

cochlear tube, 474
codons, start, 18
colchicine, 37, 100
cold spots, 219
collagen, 4
  bone, 223, 224, 227, 228, 233,
    234
    orientation in lamellae, 227
  bundles, 122, 130
    annulus fibrosus, 255
    dermis, 131, 212
    osteons, 228
    submucosa of gut, 131, 326
  content of body, 123
  cornea, 479
  in dense connective tissue, 72,
    131, 132
  fibers, 117, 121, 127
    abnormalities, 136
    disruption/rupture, 123
    in mesentery, 130
    Sharpey's, 231, 232, 312,
      313
    submucosa of gut, 131, 326
    synthesis/formation, 121,
      122
  fibrils, 121, 122, 223
  fibromas producing, 136
  heart wall, 190, 191
  intervertebral disk, 255
  in loose connective tissue, 72,
    129, 130
  precursor α-chain, 122
  properties, 122
  sheet-and-wave forms, 131
  structure, 121, 122
  synthesis, 118, 121, 122
  tendons, 132
  type I, 121, 122, 123, 125
    bone, 223, 225, 242
  type II, 122, 123, 125, 134
  type III, 122, 123, 125, 129
    space of Disse, 361
  type IV, 122, 123, 125
  type VIII, 125, 479
  type X, 125
  types, 123
collecting duct see kidney
colloid, 399
  thyroid, 398, 399
colon, 349–51
  crypts, 112, 349, 350, 351
  epithelium, 71, 324, 349, 350,
    351
    ultrastructure, 351
  fluid absorption, 323, 350
  mucosa, 349, 350
  muscularis externa, 326
colonic glands, 349, 350, 351
colony-forming units (CFUs), 80
colony-stimulating factors (CSFs),
  80, 237
color blindness, 487, 490
color vision, 487, 488
comedones, 220
common bile duct, 365
common cold, 489
common hepatic artery, 359
communicating junctions see gap
  junctions
complement, 260
conchae, 287, 288, 470
conduction deafness, 489
cones (retina), 484, 485, 487, 488
  color perception, 487, 488
  fovea, 486
  function/mechanism of action,
    487–9
confocal fluorescence microscopy,
  4
congenital adrenal hyperplasia
  (CAH), 412

congestive cardiac failure, 205
coni vasculosi (conus vasculosus),
  461
conjunctiva, 477
conjunctivitis, 490
connective (supportive) tissue, 4, 69,
  71–2, 117–36
  bone marrow as, 77, 117, 136
  cartilage, 133–5
  cell types, 118–21, 126
    migratory/transient/resident,
      119
    proliferation, 119
    see also adipose cells
      (adipocytes);
      chondroblasts;
      fibroblasts; myoblasts;
      osteoblasts
  classification, 128–36
  composition, 117, 118
  dense, 72, 130–3, 230
    irregular, 131
    regular, 132, 133
    see also bone
  disorders, 136
  disrupted, repair, 136
  functions, 117
  heart, 192
  loose, 72, 128–30
    dermis papillary region, 212
    endomysium, 143
    lamina propria of GI tract,
      325
    villus core (jejunum), 342
  matrix see collagen;
    extracellular matrix (ECM)
  mucous, 130
  specialized, 71, 136
    see also blood; bone
      marrow
  trachea, 290, 291
  types and embryonic origins, 75,
    118
  volume and complexity, 117
  see also cartilage
connexin proteins, 48, 153
connexons, 48
contraceptives, hormonal, 439
conus vasculosus, 461
cooling, sweat evaporation, 213
COPI/COPII-coated vesicles, 24
corkscrew-type glands,
  endometrial, 431
cornea, 476, 478–9
  endothelium, 479
  epithelium, 102, 115, 478, 479
  inflammation, 490
  stroma, 478, 479
corneoscleral envelope/coat, 476,
  478
cornu ammonis area (CA1), 182
corona radiata, 422
coronary artery occlusion, 205
coronary blood flow,
  autoregulation, 196
corpora cavernosa, 465, 466
corpus albicans, 417, 427–8
corpus callosum, 178
corpus fibrosum, 421
corpus luteum, 417, 426–8
  formation, 414
  granulosa luteal cells, 410, 426,
    427
  lipid inclusions in cells, 33
  menstrual cycle control, 427
  regression/degeneration
    (luteolysis), 427, 428, 432
  "rescued", 428
  theca luteal cells, 426, 427
corpus nigricans, 427
corpus spongiosum, 465, 466
Corti, organ of see organ of Corti

corticotrophs, 395, 396, 397
corticotropin-releasing hormone
  (CRH), 403, 410, 411
cortisol, 403, 404
  deficiency/disorders affecting,
    411, 412
  excess, 411
  synthesis, 403, 412
costameres, 150
cotranslational import/targeting
  of proteins, 19, 20–1
countercurrent concentrating
  system, 386, 387–9
countercurrent exchanger, 389
countercurrent multiplier, 388–9
Cowper's (bulbourethral) glands,
  441, 465
cranial nerves, 161
craniosacral innervation, 327
crescentin, 42
cretinism, 398, 411
cristae, mitochondrial, 27, 28
Crohn's disease, 353
croup, 303
cryoelectron tomography, 4, 6
cryptdins, 346
cryptorchidism, 455, 467
crypts of Lieberkühn, 102, 112
  appendix, 352
  cell cycle and turnover, 340–2,
    350
    proliferative cell detection,
      341
  cell types, 340, 344–7
  epithelial cells/enterocytes, 340,
    344
  large intestine, 349, 350, 351
  rectum, 352
  small intestine, 337, 338
    duodenum, 339
    jejunum, 340–3
  stem cells, 340–2
  structure, 340
crypt–villus axis, 340, 344–7
crypt–villus junction, 340, 346
crystallins, 482, 483, 490
crystalloid bodies, eosinophils, 34
crystalloid inclusions, 34
crystals, cytoplasmic inclusions, 34
crystals of Reinke, 458, 459
cumulus cells, 421
cumulus layer, 421
cumulus mass, 422
cumulus–oocyte mass, 422, 426
cupula, 472, 473
Cushing's disease, 411
Cushing's syndrome, 411
cuticle
  hair, 217
  nail, 218
cyclin-dependent protein kinases
  (Cdks), 54, 55
cyst(s)
  alveolar, 100
  ovarian, 438
  Rathke's cleft, 397
cyst-type structures, epithelia
  forming, 100, 101
cystic fibrosis, 303
cystitis, 392
cytochalasin, 40
cytokines, 261
cytokinesis (cytoplasmic division),
  40, 49, 50, 51, 52
  incomplete, spermatogenesis,
    445, 447
  ultrastructure of cell after, 54
cytoplasm, cell, 1, 2, 3, 5, 9, 67
  components, 3, 9
  inclusions see inclusions, cell
  protein sorting in, 19–21
cytoplasmic blebbing, 214

cytoplasmic bridges, between spermatogonia, 444, 447, 448
cytoplasmic streaming, 40
cytoskeleton, cell, 3, 34–42
 components, 3, 35, 36
 pore size, 37
 Sertoli cells, 456
 stability/rigidity, 34, 36
 three-dimensional meshwork, 37
 transport mechanisms using, 38–9
cytosol see cytoplasm, cell
cytotoxic agents, 285
cytotoxic T cells see T lymphocytes, cytotoxic
cytotrophoblast, 63, 435

D
D cells, 335, 409
deafness, 489
decidua basalis, 434, 435
decidualization, 424, 431
decorin, 121, 125
defense mechanisms, 257–8
 see also immune system
defensins, 346
dehydroepiandrosterone (DHEA), 403, 404
delta cells, pancreatic, 370, 405, 407
demyelinating diseases, 187
demyelination, 168
dendrites, 74, 163, 164, 165
 apical/basal, 164
 cerebellar cortex, 164, 165, 184, 185
 cerebral cortex, 164, 165, 179
 Purkinje cells, 172
 pyramidal neurons, 164, 165
 staining, 161
 ultrastructure, 165
dendritic cells, 80, 84, 269–70
 antigen presentation, 84, 266, 270
 class II MHC proteins, 268–9
 development, 80, 81, 84, 269
 follicular, 270, 276, 278, 279
 functions, 270
 Langerhans, 211, 269
 lymph node, 269
 migratory, 269
 plasmacytoid, 269
 small intestinal mucosa, 337
dendritic spines, 172, 185
dendritic-type cells, 211
dense bodies, smooth muscle, 157
dense fibers, flagellum of sperm, 450
dental caries, 312, 322
dental lamina, 315
dental papilla, 316, 318
dental plaque, 322
dentate gyrus, 182
dentin, 311, 312, 313, 317
 decalcification, 322
 formation/secretion (pre-dentin), 312, 316, 318
 incremental deposition (imbrication lines), 313
 mineralization, 316–17, 318
dentinal tubules, 311, 312, 313, 317
dento-enamel junction, 316–17, 318
depolarization
 heart, 191
 motor end-plates, 148, 174
 nerve, 171–2
 olfactory receptors, 471
 taste receptor cells, 470
dermal papillae, 207, 212
dermal ridges, 207
dermatitis, 220
dermatomes, 218

dermis, 208, 212–20
 blood vessels/supply, 213
 collagen bundles, 131, 212
 dense irregular connective tissue, 131
 elastic fibers, 212
 papillary, 212, 218, 219
 regenerative capacity, 213
 reticular, 212
Descemet's membrane, 479
desmin, 42, 147, 150
desmosomes, 45, 47, 103–4
 cardiac muscle, 153
 epidermis, 99, 209
 functions, 99, 104
 hepatocytes, 360
 intermediate filaments association, 41, 42, 47, 209
 stratum spinosum, 209
 ultrastructure, 47
diabetes insipidus, 411
diabetes mellitus, 404, 412
 retinopathy, 490
diakinesis, 57
diamidinophenylindole (DAPI), 449
diapedesis, 199, 202
diaphysis, 242
diarrhea, 345, 353
diastole, 193
dictyate stage, 418
digestive enzymes, 335, 366
digestive processes, 364
 by cells, 28–32
digestive tract see gastrointestinal tract
digital deconvolution microscopy, 4
dihydrotestosterone, 463
dimensions, used in histology/cell biology, 1
diopters, 478
diphtheria, 304
diplotene, 57, 415
Disse, space of, 124, 359, 361
diverticulosis, 353
DNA
 junk, 16
 length in chromosomes, 16
 linker, 14
 mitochondria, 27
 mutations, 27, 220
 packaging, in chromatin, 16
 sequencing, 16, 17
DNA vaccines, 285
dopamine, 393
dopamine-secreting neurons, loss, 187
dorsal root ganglia, 164, 176, 177, 186
 sensory fibers, 176, 177, 187
Drosophila, 14, 102, 239
Duchenne's muscular dystrophy, 159
ducts see specific ducts
ducts of Bellini, 385
ductuli efferentes see efferent ducts, testis
ductus (vas) deferens see vas deferens
ductus epididymidis, 461
duodenum, 71, 339
 ampulla of Vater opening, 365
 Brunner's glands, 111, 113, 339
 submucosa, 330, 339
 ulcer, 353
dura mater, 180
dwarfism (achondroplasia), 256, 411
dyes, basic, 17
dynein, 38, 39, 44, 51
dysmenorrhea, 439
dyspareunia, 439
dysplasia, epithelium, 115

dystrophin, 147, 151
 in brain, 159
 defects, 147, 159

E
E-cadherin, 376
ear, 472–5
 disorders, 490
 external, 472
 inner, 45, 472–5
  cochlea, 472, 473–5
  see also hair cells
 middle, 472
eccrine glands, 213–14
 ducts and secretory unit, 213
eccrine (merocrine) secretion, 114, 214
ectoderm, 64, 65, 95
 neural, 65
 somatic, 65
 tissues derived from, 64, 65, 66
ectopia, 65
ectopic pregnancy, 439
ectoplasmic specializations, 450, 456
eczema, 220
edema, 205
efferent ducts, testis, 441, 442, 461–2
 sperm transport, 441, 442
efferent (motor) nerves, 161
 see also motor neuron(s)
Ehlers–Danlos syndrome, 136
ejaculate, volume, 466
ejaculatory duct, 462
elastic arteries, 193–4
 dimensions, 192
elastic cartilage, 133, 134
 epiglottis, 134, 320
 external ear, 134
 larynx, 289
elastic fibers, 123–5
 alveoli (alveolus), 299
 arteries, 124, 193
 arterioles, 124
 bronchi and bronchioles, 296
 dermis, 212
 dysfunctional states, 125
 epiglottis, 320
 ligaments, 123
 mesentery, 123, 130
 synthesis, 123, 124, 125
elastic lamellae, 124
 arteries, 193, 194
 veins, 199
elastic lamina
 external, of arteries, 193, 194, 195, 200
 internal see internal elastic lamina (IEL)
elastin, 4, 123–5, 193
 disorders, 136
 staining, 491
electrolytes, filtered by kidney, 387
electron microscopy (EM), 4, 6, 34
embolism, pulmonary, 303
embolus, 205
embryo
 cells of, 61, 62
 cleavage stages, 61, 62
 development, 61, 62
 early
  cell types/characteristics, 62
  potential for development, 61
 rat, 76
embryogenesis, 61
 bilaminar disc formation, 61, 63, 64
 bone marrow, 79
 bones, 239
 epithelial cells, 95

embryogenesis continued
 germ layers, 61–7
 kidney, 374, 375, 376
 skeletal muscle, 141–2, 158
 vertebral column, 254
 see also fetus
embryonic disc, bilaminar, 61, 63, 64
embryonic germ layers, 61, 62
embryonic stem cells (ES), 61, 64
emphysema, 125, 303
enamel, 312
 development, 312, 314, 317–18
 inner/outer epithelia, 315, 316
enamel knot, 314, 315
enamel organ, 314, 315
enamel prisms, 312, 318
endocardium, 190, 191
endocervix, 433
endochondral ossification, 238, 240–4
 cartilage model, 241
 first sign, 241–2
 length/width increase, 242–4
 long bone, 242
endocrine cells, 111, 410
 see also specific endocrine organs
"endocrine disruptors", 454
endocrine glands, "master", 394
endocrine secretion, 114, 393–4
endocrine system, 393–412
 control of secretion, 393, 394
 disorders, 411–12
 principles, 393–4
 transport and clearance, 393
 see also hormones; specific organs
endocytic membrane, proximal convoluted tubule, 382
endocytic vesicles, 28
endocytosis, 10, 26, 27, 29, 98
 clathrin-mediated, 29, 30
 fluid phase, 30
 mechanisms, 29–30
 receptor-mediated, 27, 30
 types, 29
endoderm, 64, 95
 primitive, 61
 tissues derived from, 65, 66
endolymph, 472, 473, 474
 excess, in Ménière's disease, 489
endolysosomes, thyroid follicle, 400
endometrial glands, 430, 431, 432
endometriosis, 439
endometrium, 429, 430
 disorders, 439
 early proliferative, 430
 early secretory, 431
 glands, 430, 431, 432
 hyperplasia, 439
 late secretory, 431, 432
 menstrual cycle, 430–1
 mid-proliferative, 430
 mid-secretory, 431
 stroma, 429, 431, 432
endomitosis, 85
endomysium
 cardiac muscle, 150
 skeletal muscle, 138, 139, 140, 143
endoneurium, 170, 175, 176
endoplasmic reticulum (ER)
 collagen synthesis, 122
 as dynamic organelle, 21
 ribosomes, 17, 18, 96
 rough, 17–21
  chief cells, 335
  epididymis, 463
  hepatocytes, 5, 360
  Nissl bodies, 165

endoplasmic reticulum (ER) *continued*
    pancreatic acinar cells, 367, 368
    plasma cells, 265
    protein synthesis/sorting, 18–21
    purpose/functions, 18, 21
    as "quality check" for proteins, 21
    thyroid follicular cells, 400
    ultrastructure, 17, 18
    smooth, 5, 21
      functions, 21
      Leydig cells, 458, 459
      ultrastructure, 21
      whorled, 21
endosalpinx, 428
endosomes, 23, 27, 28–30, 31, 107
    functions, 28–9
endosteal cells, 231, 233
endosteum, 231, 233, 236
endothelial cells, 35, 201–2
    fenestrated, 87, 197, 381
      capillaries, 86, 196, 197, 198
      glomerular capillaries, 380, 381
      liver, vascular sinusoids, 361, 362
    gaps, lymphatic capillaries, 203
    nitric oxide release, 196, 201
    progenitor cells, 202
    proliferation, 202
    tight junctions between, 201
    ultrastructure, 201
endothelin, 201, 433
endothelium, 104, 201–2, 204
    arteries, 194, 195
    arterioles, 195
    capillaries, 197, 198, 201, 302
    corneal, 479
    functions, 104, 201
    glomerular capillaries, 380, 381
    heart valves, 192
    leukocyte adherence, 199, 201, 202
    lymph capillaries, 202, 203
    transendothelial transport, 197
energy, production, mitochondria, 27
enkephalins, 404
entactin, 127
enteric glia, 171
enteric nerves, 173
enteric nervous system (ENS), 161, 177, 327–9
    axon varicosities, 173
    see also Auerbach's (myenteric) plexus
enterochromaffin cells, 325, 409
enterochromaffin-like (ECL) cells, 409
enterocytes
    function (diagrammatic), 345
    large intestine, 350
    M cells, 102, 283, 348–9, 409
    small intestine, 337, 338
      jejunum, 340, 343, 344–5, 346
enteroendocrine cells, 324, 325, 409
    "closed"/"open" types, 346–7
    colon, 350
    small intestine, 346–7, 409
      duodenum, 339
      ileum, 348
      jejunum, 343, 346–7
    stomach, 409
      corpus, 332, 333, 334, 335
      pyloric region, 336
    ultrastructure, 335, 347
enteropeptidase, 367

enthesis, 135
entropy, 5
eosin, 491
eosinophil(s), 82, 90, 261
    development, 82, 83
    granules, 34, 83, 90, 261
    inflammatory reactions, 90
    lamina propria, 284
    properties, 86
    ultrastructure, 90, 261
eosinophilic series, 82, 83
ependymal cells, 168, 169, 186, 187
epiblast, 61, 64
epicardium, 190, 191
epidermis, 207, 208–12
    cell transit time, 210
    cells, 208, 210–12
      see also keratinocytes
    desmosomes, 209
    functions, 208, 209, 210
    spinous (prickle) cells, 209
    stem cells, 209
    stratum corneum, 208, 210
    stratum germinativum (basal layer), 208–9
    stratum granulosum, 208, 209, 210
    stratum lucidum, 210
    stratum spinosum, 208, 209, 211
epididymis, 441, 442, 461–2
    androgen-dependence, 463
    basal cells, 462, 463
    caput, corpus and caudal segments, 461, 462
    disorders/infections, 467
    fetal, mesenchymal cells, 120
    functions, 461
    head, 442
    principal cells, 462, 463
    protein secretion, 462
    pseudostratified columnar epithelium, 107, 461, 462, 463
    ultrastructure, 463
epigenetic, definition, 67
epiglottis, 134, 289, 320–1
epiglottitis, 322
epimysium, 140
epinephrine, 393, 404, 405
epineurium, 174
epiphyseal cartilage, 242, 243
epiphyseal growth plate, 224, 243, 244–8, 251
    endocrine regulation, 247
    fast-/slow-growing bone, 245
    function, 245
    growth during puberty, 247
    layers, 244, 246, 247
    resting zone, 244, 245, 246
    signaling pathway, 247
epiphyses, 224, 242, 243
epithelial cell(s), 2, 71, 95
    adhesion and communication, 102–6
    apical surface, 97, 98, 102
    atrophic, 114
    basal surface, 97
    characteristics and functions, 95
    ciliated, 42, 43–4, 99
    columnar, 68, 70, 96, 112
      bronchioles, 295, 296
      small/large intestine, 324, 337, 349
      see also epithelium, simple columnar
    decrease/increase in size, 114
    diversity, 95–102
    isolated/growth in culture, polarity loss, 97
    junctions between, 71, 97, 99, 102–4

epithelial cell(s) *continued*
    lateral surface, 97
    membrane domains/surfaces, 97–8
    non-linear layers, 96
    polarity, 96–100
    proliferative capacity, 100, 102
    shape changes and pattern, 96–9, 100
    single/multilayered sheets, 96
    skin *see* keratinocytes
    squamous, 68
    stem cells, 100, 102
    surface specializations, 98–9
    thymic, 272, 273, 275
    tubes derived from, 100, 101, 102
    see also epithelium
epithelial cell–mesenchymal interactions, 102, 120
epithelioid cells, 111
epithelium, 69, 71, 95–115
    abnormal/pathology, 100, 114–15
    architecture, 95–6
    atrophy, 114
    of blood vessels *see* endothelium
    building blocks (tubules, cysts) of, 100–2
    cell junctions, 71, 97, 99, 102–4
    ciliated, 42, 43–4, 99
      pseudostratified, 107, 115, 289, 290, 291
    connective tissue associated (mesenchyme), 102
    cyst-type structures, 100, 101, 102
    development and homeostasis, 95–6
      abnormal/defective, 114
    diversity, 95–102
    dysplasia, 115
    follicle-associated, 348
    functions, 95
    gingival, 313
    glands derived from, 100, 110–14
      see also glands
    hyperplasia, 114, 115
    hypertrophy, 114
    hypoplasia, 114
    inner enamel (IEE), 315, 316
    intestinal, 42, 43
      colon *see* colon, epithelium
      self-renewal, 100, 102
      small intestine, 10, 337, 338
    labile (steady-state renewable), 100
    mesenchyme interactions, 102, 120
    metaplasia, 115
    neoplasia, 115
    olfactory, 288, 470, 471
    origins and diversity, 75, 95
    outer enamel (OEE), 315, 316
    permanent (non-renewable), 100
    polarity, 96–100
    proliferative capacity, 100, 102
    pseudostratified, 107–8
      ciliated, 107, 115, 289
      goblet cells, 107, 108
    pseudostratified ciliated columnar, 107, 290, 291, 470, 471
      see also epithelium, respiratory-type
    pseudostratified columnar, 107, 287, 288, 320, 430
      efferent ducts, testis, 461
      epididymis, 107, 461, 462, 463

epithelium *continued*
    respiratory tract, 107, 287, 288
    seminal vesicles, 107, 464
    with stereocilia, 107, 461, 462, 463
    vas deferens, 463
    regenerative medicine and, 115
    respiratory-type, 41, 290, 291, 470
      bronchi, 294, 295
      distribution, 287
      epiglottis, 320
      olfactory epithelium *vs*, 471
      tracheal, 107, 290, 291, 293
      upper respiratory tract, 287, 288
    seminal vesicle, 107, 464
    seminiferous *see* seminiferous epithelium
    simple, 104–6
      polarity, 97
    simple columnar, 68, 96, 105, 106, 112
      bronchioles, 295, 296
      gall bladder, 364
      gastrointestinal tract, 324
      goblet cells with, 106
      microvilli with, 106
      small intestine, 337
      stomach, 333
    simple cuboidal, 104–5
      absorptive/secretory functions, 105
      lens capsule, 481
      respiratory bronchioles, 296, 297
    simple squamous, 104
    squamous, 68, 104
      cervix, 432, 433
    stable (conditionally renewable), 100
    stratified, 108–9
    stratified columnar, 109
      urethra, 390, 391
    stratified cuboidal, 109
    stratified squamous, 108, 109
      cornea, 478, 479
      epiglottis, 320
      esophagus/anal canal, 324
      keratinized, 109, 208, 306
      non-keratinized, 108, 109, 329, 434
      palatine tonsils, 319
      soft palate (oral aspect), 320
      tongue, 305, 306
    surface specializations, 98–9
    tracheal, 107, 290, 291, 293
    transitional, 110
      bladder, 390, 391
      proximal ureter, 390
      renal pyramid apex, 385
      urethra, 390
    tubules derived from, 100, 101, 102
    types, 75, 104–10
epitopes, 263
erectile tissue, 466
erythema migrans (geographic tongue), 321
erythroblast islands, 80, 82
erythroblast series, 82
erythroblasts, 80, 82
erythrocyte(s), 2, 3, 86–7
    aging, destruction, 87, 281
    antigens/blood groups, 93
    breakdown, bile pigment formation, 363
    cell count, 87
    decreased in leukemia, 92
    development, 79, 80, 82
    embryonic and fetal, 82, 83

erythrocyte(s) *continued*
lacking nucleus, 3, 68, 69, 86
number, 82, 85, 86
oxygen/carbon dioxide
transport, 87
properties, 86
shape, 86, 87
erythropoiesis, 79, 80, 82, 92
erythropoietin (EPO), 80, 82, 389, 410
esophagogastric junction, 332
esophagus, 329–30
abnormal conditions, 353
atresia, 353
Barrett's (metaplasia), 353
lamina propria, 329
mucous glands, 329, 330, 332
mucous membrane (mucosa), 329, 330
muscularis externa, 329
muscularis mucosae, 329
stratified squamous epithelium, 324, 329
submucosa, 329
espin, 456
estradiol, 247, 424
estrogen
bone growth in puberty, 247
bone-protective effect, 238, 248, 256
deficiency, 248
bone loss/fractures, 238, 256
lactiferous duct growth, 437
menstrual cycle, 413, 430, 431
receptors, 248
secretion by ovarian follicle, 410, 425
euchromatin, 14
eukaryotic cells, 1, 11
eumelanin, 211
eustachian tube, 472
exocervix, 433
exocrine cells, 97
pancreatic *see* pancreas, acinar (exocrine) cells
exocrine glands *see* glands
exocrine secretion, 114
exocytosis, 10, 26, 98, 172, 367
exons, 16
expiration, 297, 298, 302–3
external elastic lamina, arteries, 193, 194, 195, 200
extracellular, definition, 3
extracellular components, cells *vs*, 67
extracellular fluid, 118, 180, 202
volume, 121, 189
extracellular material, 4, 69
extracellular matrix (ECM), 71, 117, 121–6, 130
amorphous gel-like appearance, 121, 126
arteries, 194
bone, 223, 225
cartilage, 133
components, 117, 121, 125–6, 128, 131
fibers, 121–5, 128
see also collagen, fibers;
elastic fibers
macromolecules/proteins, 121, 125–6
extraglomerular mesangium, 379, 381, 386
extraocular muscle, 139, 149
eye, 476–90
anatomy, 476
disorders, 490
fetal and development, 476
newborn infants, 481, 490
see also specific regions of eye

eyeball, size, 479
eyelids, 476, 477
fused in fetus, 476

F
factor VIII, 201
Fallopian tubes *see* uterine tubes
(Fallopian tubes)
fascicles, 140
peripheral nerves, 176
skeletal muscle, 140–1
fat *see* lipid(s)
fat cells *see* adipose cells
(adipocytes); adipose tissue
fatigue, muscle, 149, 159
fatty acids, storage, 129
feedback control/loops, 393, 394
female reproductive system, 413–39
abnormal conditions, 438–9
see also individual structures
femur, 224
fenestrated endothelial cells
see endothelial cells
fertility disorders, 466
fertilization, 413, 422
fetus, 61
bone, 223, 227, 238, 239, 247
hands, 243
intramembranous
ossification, 239–40
long bone, 242, 244
onset of ossification, 239
skull, 239, 240
vertebral column, 254
erythrocytes, 82, 83
eye, 476, 482
fibrocartilage, 135
limb buds, 238, 241
liver, 79
ovary, 413, 415
skeletal muscle fiber formation, 142
see also embryogenesis
fibrillin, 123, 125, 126
fibrin, 87, 88
fibrinogen, 88, 125
fibroblast growth factor (FGF), 79
fibroblasts, 118
attachment and actin filaments, 40
collagen synthesis, 118, 121
in connective tissue, 117, 127, 128
corpus albicans, 427
elastic fiber synthesis, 123, 125
lamina propria of gut, 325
precursor, 119
proteoglycan synthesis, 125–6
fibrocartilage, 133, 135
intervertebral discs, 135, 255
fibroelastic tissues, trachea, 290, 291
fibromas, 136
fibronectin, 125, 464
Fick's law, 192
"fight or flight" response, 404
filaggrin, 209, 210
filopodia, 40, 41
filtration slit, 380, 381
fixatives, peripheral nerves, 174
flagella, 43–4
spermatid, 449, 450
fluid
absorption, 45, 353
volume, 323
transport, small intestine, 323, 344–5, 353
volume lost daily, 214
**fluorescence deconvolution
microscopy**, 54
**fluorescence in situ hybridization
(FISH)**, 14
fluoresterol uptake, enterocytes, 345

fluoride, 322
folic acid, 363
follicle(s)
hair *see* hair follicle
lymphoid *see* lymphoid follicles
ovarian *see* ovarian follicles
thyroid gland, 398, 399
follicle cells *see* granulosa cells
follicle-stimulating hormone (FSH), 395, 417
actions/functions/secretion, 425
folliculogenesis, initiation, 419, 420
menstrual cycle, 424
receptors, 419
Sertoli cell binding/proliferation, 455, 458
spermatogenesis, 441, 455, 458
follicular cells
anterior pituitary, 396
ovarian *see* granulosa cells
follicular dendritic cells (FDCs), 270, 276, 278, 279
follicular fluid, 420, 421, 422
folliculogenesis, 416
see also ovarian follicles,
development/growth
**folliculostellate cells, anterior
pituitary**, 396
fontanelle, anterior, 240
food allergens, 285
foot processes, podocytes, 380, 381
foreskin (prepuce), 466
formins, 40
fourth ventricle, 183
fovea, 476, 484, 486
foveola, 486, 488
fracture(s), 228, 230, 255
callus, 255
repair, and callus, 255
fracture gap callus, 255
FSH *see* follicle-stimulating hormone
(FSH)
fungus-derived drugs, 285
fusiform cells, cerebral cortex, 182

G
G cells, 335, 409
G-CSF, 80
gall bladder, 355, 364–5
disorders, and cancer, 371
gallstones, 371
gamma globulins *see* antibodies
(immunoglobulins)
ganglia (ganglion), 74–5, 163, 170, 171, 176–7
autonomic, 176, 177
dorsal root (sensory) *see* dorsal
root ganglia
enteric, 177, 325, 329
myenteric *see* Auerbach's
(myenteric) plexus
parasympathetic, 176, 177
satellite cells, 170
size variations, 177
sympathetic, 176
ganglion cells, 70
retinal, 484, 485, 486, 488
gap junctions (nexus), 45, 48, 104
cardiac muscle, 153
epithelial cells, 97, 104
hepatocytes, 360
osteocytes, 235, 236
Purkinje fibers, 191
smooth muscle, 154
ultrastructure, 48
gas exchange, 287, 297, 298, 300, 302
gastric acid, secretion, 334
gastric cancer, 353
gastric glands, 102, 112, 324, 330, 331, 332

gastric glands *continued*
cell types, 332, 333, 334
corpus of stomach, structure, 332, 333, 335
pyloric mucosa, 336
regions, 333
gastric juice, 331
gastric mucosa *see* stomach
gastric pits, 112, 330, 331, 332
gland arising from, and cell
types, 332, 333
pyloric mucosa, 336
gastric ulcer, 115, 353
gastrin secretion, 335
hypersecretion, 353
gastritis, 115, 353
gastrocnemius muscle, 149
gastroesophageal reflux, 353
gastrointestinal tract, 323–54
absorption/secretion, 323, 324, 344–5
adventitia, 323
basic architecture, 324–7
disorders, 353–4
extramural (external) nerves, 327
functions, 323
immune function, 337, 348
intramural nervous system
see enteric nervous system
(ENS)
motility/peristalsis, 325, 329, 330, 350
mucous membrane (mucosa)
see mucosa
muscle components, 323, 325–6, 326–7
muscularis externa
see muscularis externa
muscularis mucosae
see muscularis mucosae
neuroendocrine cells, 409
organization, 323, 324–9
serosa, 323, 326, 327
submucosa *see* submucosa
see also esophagus; large
intestine; small intestine;
stomach
gastrulation, 62, 64, 66
gene desert, 16
gene therapy, 93, 115, 285
genes, clustering, 16
genetic recombination, 57–8
spermatocytes, 448, 449
genioglossus, 305
genome, sequencing, 16, 17
**geographic tongue (erythema
migrans)**, 321
germ cell nuclear antigen (GCNA), 418
germ cell tumors
female, 438
male, 454, 467
germ cells, 54, 417
aplasia, 467
female, oocyte *see* oocyte
male, 443, 445
absence, 455, 467
clones, 447
coordination of
development, 451–3
Sertoli cells supporting, 443, 454, 455, 458
see also spermatids;
spermatocytes;
spermatogenesis;
spermatogonia
meiosis *see* meiosis
origin/formation, 64
primordial, 64, 413
germ layers, 64, 70
derivatives from, 65–7

germ layers continued
    examples listed, 66
    embryonic, 61, 62
    primary tissue origin, 61–7
    see also ectoderm; endoderm; mesoderm
germinal centers, 278, 279
    B cell affinity maturation, 266, 278
    B cell mantle, 278, 282
    lymph nodes, 277, 278
    mucosal lymphoid follicles, 283
    Peyer's patches, 348
    spleen, 282
    tonsils, 318, 319
germinal niches, 182
germinative cells, sebaceous cells, 215
ghrelin, 335
gigantism, 411
gingivae (gums), 312
gingival crevice, 312
gingival epithelium, 313
glands, 110–14
    branching, 71
    cardiac mucus-type, esophagus, 331, 332
    classification, 111, 112–13
        by mechanism, 114
        by morphology, 112
        by secretions, 113
        by secretory cells/structures, 113
    compound, 113
        acinar (alveolar), 111, 113
        tubular, 111, 113
        tubuloacinar, 111, 113
    derived from epithelia, 100
    development, 110
    endocrine, 71, 110, 114
    epithelial, 71
    exocrine, 71, 110, 112, 114
    multicellular, 111, 112
    sebaceous, 112
    secretory cells, 110
    simple branched acinar, 111, 112
    simple branched tubular, 111, 112
    simple coiled tubular, 111, 112
    simple tubular, 111, 112
    tongue, 138
    tubular, 113
    unicellular, 106, 110, 111, 112
    upper respiratory tract, 287
glands of Bowman, 471
glandular fever (infectious mononucleosis), 322
glandular metaplasia, 115
glandular tissue, 71
glans penis, 466
glassy membrane, 217, 218
glaucoma, 490
glia limitans, 180
glial cells, 2, 74
    neuroglia see neuroglia
    pituicytes, 398
    retinal, 486
glial fibrillary acidic protein (GFAP), 42, 167, 168, 486
glial processes, 180
"gliotransmitters", 167
globulins, 87
glomerular basement membrane (GBM), 381
glomerular capillaries, 198, 377, 378, 379
    basal laminae, 379
    fenestrated endothelium, 380, 381
    podocytes attached, 379, 380, 381

glomerular disorders, 392
glomerular filtration, 377, 381, 387
glomerular filtration rate (GFR), 385, 387
    reduced, renal failure, 390, 392
    regulation, 389
glomeruli (in cerebellar cortex), 185
glomerulonephritis, 392
glomerulotubular balance, 387
glomerulus, 374, 375, 379
    afferent/efferent arterioles, 379, 387
    basement membrane, 381
    blood flow, 387
    diseases, 392
    epithelial cells, 377
    filter, ultrastructure, 380, 381
    lacis cells, 379, 381, 386
    mesangium, 381
    organization, 377, 378
    origin, 378
    vascular network, 379
glucagon, 363, 370, 405, 407
    actions/functions, 367, 405, 407
    cells producing (α cells), 370, 405, 406, 407
glucocorticoids
    deficiency, 411
    synthesis, 403, 404
gluconeogenesis, 403
glucose, 407
    absorption/storage, 363
    ATP generation, 28
    blood, regulation, 407
    transport, 345
    in ultrafiltrate, 389
glucose transport protein, 345
glucuronide, 363
glycocalyx, 201
glycogen, 363
    granule clusters (rosettes), 32
    metabolism, 21, 407
    Purkinje myocytes, 191
    storage, 21, 32
    hepatocytes, 358, 360, 363
glycolipids, in plasma membrane, 11
glycoprotein hormones, 393
glycoproteins, 121, 351
    adhesive, 126
    in plasma membrane, 11
    zona pellucida, 419, 421
glycosaminoglycans, 126, 131, 223, 351, 491
glycosylation of proteins, 22
GM-CSF, 80
goblet cells, 71, 106, 110
    colon, 350, 351
    eyelid, 477
    rectum, 352
    small intestine, 338
        jejunum, 342, 343, 346
        ultrastructure, 346
    tracheal epithelium, 107, 108, 290, 291
    as unicellular glands, 106, 110, 112
    see also mucous cells
goblet-shaped cells, 2
goiter, 411
Golgi apparatus, 22–7
    autonomy and cell division, 27
    as central sorting station, 22, 23, 24, 25
    cis (forming face), 22, 23
    as dynamic organelle, 22
    in endocytosis, 26
    functions and location, 22
    movement of vesicles through, models, 24
    protein targeting, 21
    secretion/absorption roles, 25–7
    specific cells

Golgi apparatus continued
    epididymis, 463
    liver cells, 5, 7
    pancreatic cells, 6, 7, 24, 96
    plasma cells, 265
    spermatids, 449
    trans (maturing face), 22
    transport mechanisms, 24–5
    ultrastructure and structure, 22
Gomori's aldehyde fuchsin stain, 491
gonadotrophs, 395, 396, 397
gonadotropin-releasing hormone (GnRH), 425, 441, 458
gonadotropins
    ovarian follicle growth, 419, 420, 421, 422, 423, 425
    reduced secretion, 411
    see also follicle-stimulating hormone (FSH); luteinizing hormone (LH)
Goormaghtigh, cells of (lacis cells), 379, 381, 386
"goose bumps", 218
Gordon and Sweet's silver method, 491
gout, 256
Graafian follicles see ovarian follicles
graft-versus-host disease, 285
granular layer/cells
    cerebellar cortex, 183, 184
    epidermis, 209, 210
granulation tissue, 136, 160
granulocytes, 82, 86
    development, 82–3
    see also basophil(s); eosinophil(s); neutrophil(s)
granulocytopoiesis, 82–3
granulosa cells, 410, 413
    after oocyte release, 426
    apoptosis, 421
    corpus luteum, 426, 427
    primary follicles, 419
    secondary follicles, 419, 420
granulosa luteal cells, 410, 426, 427
granzymes, 267
Graves' disease, 411
gray matter, 178, 179
    cerebellum, 178, 182, 183, 184
    cerebral cortex, 178, 179
    spinal cord, 186, 187
gristle see cartilage
ground substance see cytoplasm, cell; extracellular matrix (ECM)
growth factors, hemopoiesis regulation, 80
growth hormone (GH), 395
    excess/deficiency, 411
growth plate see epiphyseal growth plate
growth spurts, 247
gut see gastrointestinal tract
gut-associated lymphoid tissue (GALT), 337, 348
gynecomastia, 439
gyri, gray matter, 178

H
H bands, 146
hair, color, 216, 217
hair cells, 472
    cochlea, 45, 473, 474, 475
    damage, 489
    vestibular apparatus, 472, 473
hair follicle, 102, 216–18
    bulb, 216
    cortex, 216, 217
    external/internal root sheath, 216, 217, 218
    matrix and medulla, 216, 217

hair follicle continued
    melanocytes, 217
    sebaceous glands associated, 214
hair root, 216
hair shaft, 216, 217
halitosis, 321
hand, fetal, growth, 243
haploid cells, 54, 56, 448, 449
hard palate, 320
Hashimoto's thyroiditis, 411
Hassall's corpuscles, 273
"hatching", 62
Haversian canals, 225, 226, 228, 229, 232, 235, 240, 250
Haversian system see osteon (Haversian system)
hay fever, 304
H&E staining, 174, 491
hearing, 472, 474, 475, 489
    threshold, 475
heart, 190–2
    action potential, 191
    blood pumped in lifetime, 190
    characteristic features, 190
    conducting system, 191
    as demand pump, 190
    disorders, 204–5
    fibrous "skeleton", 192
    valves, 190, 192, 205
    walls, 190–1
    see also cardiac muscle
heart failure, 160
heart muscle see cardiac muscle
heartburn, 353
heat loss, 201, 213
heat production, 129
heavy chains, immunoglobulin, 264
Helicobacter pylori, 353
helicotrema, 474
hematoxylin and eosin (H&E) staining, 174, 491
heme, 87, 363
hemidesmosomes, 47, 104, 212
hemodynamics, 192
hemoglobin (Hb), 82, 86
    adult, embryonic, and fetal types, 82
    anemia, 92
hemoglobinopathies, 92
hemolytic diseases of the newborn, 93
hemophilia, 88
hemopoiesis, 79, 80, 81
hemopoietic growth factors, 80
hemopoietic stem cells (HSC), 78, 80, 81, 271
    pluripotent, 77, 79, 80, 81, 262
    self-renewal, 271
    short-term, 80
    transplants, 93
hemostasis, 88
hemostatic plug, 85, 88
Henle, loop see loop of Henle
heparan sulfate, 127
heparin, release by basophils, 90
hepatic arterioles, 363
hepatic artery, 356, 359
hepatic biliary system, 356
hepatic encephalopathy, 371
hepatic sinusoids see liver, vascular sinusoids
hepatic stellate cells (Ito cells), 124, 359, 361, 371
hepatitis, 371
hepatocyte(s), 6, 356, 358–62
    absorption/secretion, 361
    clathrin-coated vesicles, 30
    functions, 363
    glycogen storage, 358, 360
    microvilli, 361
    mitochondria number, 27

hepatocyte(s) *continued*
    nuclei, 5, 7, 69, 358, 360
    organelles, 360
    polarity, 97
    stable (conditionally renewable),
        100
    surface specializations, 360
    ultrastructure, 5, 7, 30, 360
    volume and membrane surface
        area, 8, 9
herpes simplex virus infection, oral,
    321
Herring bodies, 398
heterochromatin, 14, 15, 16, 144,
    265
heterotopia, 65
hiatus hernia, 353
high endothelial venules (HEV),
    277, 279
hippocampus, 168, 182
Hirschsprung's disease, 353
histamine, 90
histology
    "best kept secrets", 69–70
    objectives, summary, 69–70
    pattern recognition, 70
histones, 14
HLA antigen, 268
    see also major
        histocompatibility complex
        (MHC)
holocrine secretion, 114, 214, 215
homeostasis, cellular, 32
homunculus, 181
horizontal cells/neurons, retina,
    484, 485
hormonal contraceptives, 439
hormonal cycle (menstrual), 424
hormone replacement therapy
    (HRT), 439
hormones, 111, 393
    ectopic production, 411
    mechanism of action, 394
    receptors, 394, 398
    renal secretion, 389, 410
    smooth muscle contraction
        control, 158
    steroid *see* steroid hormones
    synergistic action, 394
    synthesis and secretion, 393,
        394
    tissues secreting, 410
    transport and clearance, 393
    types, 393
Howship resorption cavity, 236, 237
Howship's lacuna, 236, 237, 250
human chorionic gonadotropin
    (hCG), 63, 410, 428
human placental lactogen (hPL), 410
hyaline cartilage, 126, 133–4
    articular, 133–4, 223, 252
    bronchus, 294, 295
    chondrocytes and matrix, 133
    epiphyseal ends, 242, 243
    nasal passages, 288
    proteoglycans, 133, 134
    trachea, 290, 291
    vertebral column, 254, 255
    zones, 134
hyalocytes, 485
hyaluronan, 126, 485
Hydra, 95
hydrochloric acid, secretion, 334
hydrocortisone, 404
hydroxyapatite, 135, 223, 234, 238
    bone, 136
    teeth, 312
    tidemark of enthesis, 135
hydroxyapatite crystals, 34, 135
5-hydroxytryptamine (serotonin),
    328, 347, 393
hyperglycemia, 412

hyperopia (far-sightedness), 490
hyperparathyroidism, 401, 411
hyperplasia, 114
hypersensitivity, immediate, 90, 285
hypertension, 160, 205
hyperthyroidism, 411
hypertrophy
    airway smooth muscle, 303
    epithelium, 114
    skeletal muscle, 143
hypoblast, 61
hypodermis, 207, 216
hypogonadism, 467
hypoparathyroidism, 411
hypophysis *see* pituitary gland
hypoplasia, 114
hypothalamic–hypophyseotropic
    area, 394
hypothalamic–pituitary axis, 394
    disorders, 411
    female reproductive function
        control, 413
hypothalamus, 178, 394–7
    disorders, 411
    nuclei, 394, 408
hypothyroidism, 411

I

I bands, 138, 144, 146, 147
    cardiac muscle, 150, 151, 152
I cells, 409
ileum, 348–9
imbrication lines of von Ebner, 313
immotile cilia syndrome
    (Kartagener's syndrome), 44,
    303
immune complexes, phagocytosis,
    381
immune-enhancing agents, 285
immune response, 257
    primary, 266
    secondary, 258, 265, 266
immune system, 257–85
    adaptive, 257, 258, 263–70
        dendritic cells and, 269–70
        features, 258
        innate system interaction,
            258
        specificity, 259, 263
    defense systems, 257–8
    effector phases/cells, 258
    evolution, 259
    gastrointestinal, 337, 348
    innate, 257, 258, 259–63
        adaptive system and, 258
        barrier protection, 260
        complement, 260
        extracellular killing, 261,
            263
        features, 258, 259
        intracellular killing, 260–1
        neutrophils role, 89
    lymphocytes *see* lymphocyte(s)
    medical importance, 284–5
    military analogy/attributes, 259
    overview, 270
immunity
    cell-mediated, 258
    humoral, 258, 265, 268
immunization, 285
immunoglobulin (Ig) *see* antibodies
    (immunoglobulins)
immunoglobulin A (IgA), 284, 295,
    307, 325
    tears, 477
immunoglobulin G (IgG), 264
immunoglobulin M (IgM), 264
immunological memory, 258, 270
immunological tolerance, 259, 263,
    274
immunomodulation, 285
immunopharmacology, 285

immunosurveillance, 269
inclusions, cell, 3, 31, 32–4
Indian hedgehog (Ihh), 247
indolamines, 410
infants
    bone marrow, 77
    see also neonates
infectious mononucleosis (glandular
    fever), 322
infertility, 44, 466
inflammatory reactions
    acute, 90, 260
    chronic allergic, 261
influenza virus, 285, 322
infundibular stalk, 178
inhibin, 422, 424, 425
innate immune response *see* immune
    system, innate
inner cell mass (ICM), 61, 62, 63
inner enamel epithelium (IEE), 315,
    316
inspiration, 297, 298
insulin, 363, 370, 405
    actions/functions, 367, 405, 407
    as hypoglycemic hormone, 407
    release (exocytosis), 406
    synthesis by β cells, 370, 404,
        405, 406
integrin receptors, 40
integrins, 126, 127
intercalated discs, cardiac muscle,
    150, 151, 153
intercellular bridge, spermatocytes,
    447, 448, 454
intercellular junctions *see* cell
    junctions
intercellular space, 10
interchromosomal domains, 14
interleukins, 80
intermediate filaments, 35, 36, 41–2
    categories, 42
    desmin, 147
    in desmosomes, 41, 42, 47
    function, 41–2
    self-assembly and, 41
    stratum germinatum, 209
    structure, 36
internal anal sphincter, 327, 352
internal elastic lamina (IEL), 124
    arteries, 124, 193, 194, 195,
        204
    arterioles, 195
    veins, 199, 200
interneurons, 166, 182
interphase, 49, 50
    meiosis, 56
interphase cells, 13–14, 39, 49
intersinusoidal spaces, bone
    marrow, 78
interstitial cells of Cajal (ICC), 328
interstitial fluid, 118, 202
    in lymph capillaries, 202, 203
    volume, 121
interterritorial matrix (IM), 134,
    252
intervertebral disks, 135, 253, 254,
    255
    herniation, 255
intestinal crypts, 102, 112
    loose connective tissue, 128
    see also crypts of Lieberkühn
intestinal epithelial cells
    see epithelium, intestinal
intestinal glands, 112
    jejunum, 340–3
    see also crypts of Lieberkühn
intestine *see* large intestine; small
    intestine
intima, synovial membrane, 253
intrafollicular cavities, 414
intramembranous ossification,
    238–9, 239–40

intraocular pressure, raised, 481,
    490
intrapleural pressure, 302–3
intraretinal space, 476
introns, 16
iodine, 398, 399
    deficiency, 398, 411
ion transport, 98, 99
iridiocorneal angle, 481
iris, 476, 478, 480, 481
    color, 479, 481, 490
    melanocytes, 480, 481, 490
    myoepithelial cells, 480
    root, vascularized stroma, 480
    stroma, 480, 481
iron, 87, 363
iron-deficiency anemia, 92
islets of Langerhans, 365, 370,
    404–7
    cell types, 370, 405
        alpha cells, 370, 405, 406,
            407
        beta cells *see* beta cells,
            pancreatic
    ultrastructure, 370
isogenous groups, chondrocyte
    clusters, 133
Ito cells, 124, 359, 361, 371

J

jaundice, 220, 363, 371
jejunum, 340–7
    crypt–villus axis, cells, 344–7
    intestinal glands (crypts of
        Lieberkühn), 340–3
    mucosa, 338
    plicae circulares, 338
    villi, 340–3
joint(s), 132
    disorders/arthritis, 256
joint capsule, 250, 253
joint space, 252, 253
junctional complex, 103, 107, 344,
    369
junctions *see* cell junctions
juxtaglomerular apparatus, 386, 387
    macula densa, 385, 386
juxtaglomerular cells, 386

K

K cells, 409
Kallmann's syndrome, 423
Kartagener's syndrome, 44, 303
karyokinesis (nuclear division), 49
karyorrhexis, 59
karyotype, 14
keloids, 221
keratan sulfate, 126, 134
keratin, 42, 109
    hair, 217
    nails, 218
    stratum corneum, 207, 210
    stratum granulosum, 209
    stratum spinosum, 209
keratin proteins, 42
keratinocytes, 208, 209
    desmosomes, 47
    migration and transit time, 210
    proliferation, psoriasis, 220
    stratum spinosum, 209
keratitis, 490
keratohyalin granules, 208, 209
kidney, 373–86
    basement membrane in, 127
    blood supply/flow, 373–4, 386,
        387
    collecting ducts, 374, 375, 376,
        383, 384, 385–6
    functions, 384, 388
    transverse/longitudinal
        sections, 384
    cortex, 373, 375, 376

kidney *continued*
corticomedullary junction, 373, 383
corticomedullary region, 383
medullary rays, 375, 376, 383
development, 374, 375, 376
disorders, 390, 392
as endocrine organ, 389
epithelial cells, basement membrane, 99
failure, 390, 392
functions, 373, 387–9
hormones secreted, 389, 410
interstitium, 387, 388
medulla *see* renal medulla
organization, 373–86
reabsorption processes, 389
sodium, 384, 385, 387, 389
water, 382, 384, 385, 387, 388, 389
see also entries beginning renal; glomerulus; nephron
kinesin, 38
kinetochore, 50
kinetochore microtubules, 39
Klinefelter's syndrome, 467
knee joint, fibrocartilage, 135
Krause end-bulbs, 220
Kulchitsky cells (neuroepithelial bodies), 297, 409
Kupffer cells, 359, 361–2
functions, 362

L

lacis cells (cells of Goormaghtigh), 379, 381, 386
lacrimal gland, 476, 477
lactation, 114, 413, 436, 438
myoepithelial cell role, 158
lacteals, 338
lactic acid, in muscles, 159
lactiferous ducts, 436, 437
lactiferous sinuses, 436, 437
lactotrophs, 395, 396, 397
lacuna (lacunae), 134
bone, 234, 235
Howship's, 236, 237
lamellae
bone *see* bone
elastic *see* elastic lamellae
lamellar granules, stratum granulosum, 209, 210
lamellipodia, 40
lamina densa, 127
lamina lucida, 127
lamina propria, 128
bladder, 390, 391
epiglottis, 320
gastrointestinal tract, 284, 325
esophagus, 329
large intestine, 350
small intestine, 337, 343
stomach, 333, 336
villi, 284, 343
olfactory epithelium, 471
seminiferous tubules, 443
tongue, 305
trachea, 291
ultrastructure, 284
lamina rara, 127
laminins, 99, 125, 127, 141, 195, 378
Langerhans cells, 211, 269
large intestine, 349–52
abnormal conditions, 353–4
appendix, 283, 352, 354
carcinoma, 354
crypts of Lieberkühn, 349, 350, 351
see also colon
laryngeal vestibule, 289

larynx, 289, 303
lateral geniculate nucleus, 181
lateral ventricle, 178, 182
leiomyomas, 160
uterine, 439
lens, 476, 481–3
capsule, 481, 482, 485
fetal, 482
shape, 482
age-related changes, 482
lens fibers, 2, 481, 482–3
cytoplasm and epithelium, 481–2, 483
mature, nucleus lacking, 69, 481, 483
leptin, 237, 335
leptotene, 57
leukemias, 92–3
leukocyte(s), 85, 86
agranular, 86
see also lymphocyte(s); monocyte(s)
in connective tissue, 119
granular *see* basophil(s); eosinophil(s); neutrophil(s)
margination (adherence to endothelium), 199, 201, 202
migration, 199, 202
leukoplakia, oral, 321
Leydig cells, 410, 441, 443, 446, 458
crystalloid inclusions, 34, 458, 459
fetal, 458
number and development, 458
testosterone secretion, 410, 441, 458, 459
ultrastructure, 458, 459
volume and surface area, 8, 9
whorled smooth ER, 21
LH *see* luteinizing hormone (LH)
Lieberkühn, crypts *see* crypts of Lieberkühn
ligaments, 132
collagen content, 123
elastic fibers, 123
tendons *vs*, 132
ligamentum nuchae, 123, 124, 125
light, detection by retina, 486, 487, 488
light chains, immunoglobulin, 264, 265
limb buds, 238, 241
lineage, definition, 67
lineage restriction, definition, 67
lingual glands, 305, 306, 307
lingual papillae *see* tongue, papillae
lingual tonsil, 307, 319
lipid(s)
cytoplasmic inclusion, 33, 403
metabolism, liver, 363
peroxidation, 34
storage, 33, 119
adipose cells, 33, 119, 129
Ito cells, 359
synthesis by smooth ER, 21
lipid bilayer, plasma membrane, 10, 11
lipochrome (lipofuscin), 33
lipocytes (hepatic stellate cells; Ito cells), 124, 359, 361, 371
lipofuscin (lipochrome), 33–4
lipofuscin pigment inclusions, 31, 33–4, 459
lipomas, 136
lipoproteins, 129
Littré, urethral glands of, 466
liver, 355–63
abnormal conditions, 371
acinar model, 356, 358, 359
adenoma, 371

liver *continued*
bile canaliculi, 356, 357, 360, 362, 363
bile flow in, 357, 358, 359
blood flow, 358, 359, 363
cancer, 371
cells *see* hepatocyte(s)
central vein, 356, 357
cirrhosis, 371
fatty (steatosis), 371
fetal, 79
functions, 79, 355, 363
histologic organization, 355–6
lobule concept, 355, 356, 357
lobules, structure/organization, 357
microvascular functional units, 358, 359
portal lobule model, 356, 358
portal triads/tracts, 356, 357
primary lobule concept, 358
radial cords, 355–6
reticular fibers, 124
storage disease, 371
structure, models, 356–8
vascular sinusoids, 124, 356, 358–62
endothelium, 361, 362
liver cells *see* hepatocyte(s)
loop of Henle, 382, 383, 384
countercurrent system, 388–9
thick ascending limb, 375, 383, 384
thin ascending limb, 375, 384
thin descending limb, 375, 382, 384
lower esophageal sphincter, 330
lower respiratory tract
see respiratory tract, lower
lung, 287
acini, 297–8
architecture, 294
blood supply, 295, 297, 300
developmental abnormalities, 303
histology, key markers, 294
infections, 303–4
inflammation, 303–4
macroscopic structure, 292, 293
neuroendocrine cells, 290, 409
neuroepithelial bodies, 297
oblique fissure, 292
parenchyma, 294, 297
tumors, 304
volume, 294
see also alveoli (alveolus); bronchi; bronchioles
lung buds, 102
lung root, 292, 293
lunula, 218
Luschka, ducts of, 364
luteal cells, 21, 410
see also granulosa luteal cells
luteal–placental shift, 428
luteinizing hormone (LH), 395, 417
actions/functions, 425
folliculogenesis, 419, 420
menstrual cycle, 424
receptors, 419
secretion, 425
spermatogenesis, 441, 458
testosterone secretion, 458, 459, 460
luteolysis, 427, 428, 432
lymph, 189, 202, 203
circulation, 276, 277
flow rate/circulation time, 203
formation in spaces of Disse, 361
lymph nodes, 72, 203, 276–9
architecture, 276, 277
B cells in, 276, 277, 278, 279

lymph nodes *continued*
cortex and medulla, 276, 277
dendritic cells, 269
enlargement, 276
functions, 276–7
germinal centers, 277, 278
lymphoid follicles *see* lymphoid follicles
medullary cords, 277
organization, 277
pericapsular connective tissues, 276
reactive hyperplasia, 277
reticular fibers, 124, 129
T cells in, 279
trabeculae, 277
lymph vascular system, 189, 202–3
cardiovascular system comparison, 189
characteristic features, 190
see also lymph nodes; lymphoid tissues/organs
lymphangitis, 205
lymphatic capillaries, 196
characteristic features, 190
lungs, 300
structure and function, 202
lymphatic sinusoid, 203
lymphatic vessels, 202, 203
characteristic features, 190
disorders/obstruction, 205
small intestine, 338
lymphoblasts, 84
lymphocyte(s), 86, 92, 257, 258
activation, 263, 270
antigen binding, 263, 266
clonal selection, 262, 263
development, 262
as effectors of adaptive immunity, 263
in esophagus, 329
functions, 92, 263
intraepithelial, 267, 284, 337, 338
colon, 350
functions, 338
jejunum, 342, 343, 346
life span, 92
lingual tonsils, 307
in lymph, 203
mucosal, 284
origin, 263
in Peyer's patches, 348
properties, 86
receptors, 263
small-/large-diameter, 92
in stomach, 332
structure, 262
in tonsils, 319
trafficking, 276, 277
ultrastructure, 262
see also B lymphocytes; T lymphocytes
lymphocytopoiesis, 84
lymphoid cell lineage, 80, 262, 271
lymphoid follicles, 129, 279
appendix, 283, 352
colon, 350
mucosal (MALT), 283, 284
Peyer's patches, 283, 348
primary, 276, 279, 280
secondary, 276, 278, 279, 280
small intestinal mucosa, 337, 339, 353
spleen, 280, 282
tongue, 307
tonsils, 283, 307, 322
upper respiratory tract, 289
lymphoid stem cells, 80
lymphoid tissues/organs, 271–84
follicles *see* lymphoid follicles
gut-associated (GALT), 337, 348

lymphoid tissues/organs *continued*
  mucosa-associated (MALT),
    265, 271, 283–4
  primary, 271
    see also bone marrow;
      thymus
  secondary, 271, 276–84
    see also lymph nodes;
      spleen
  stroma, 276
  in upper respiratory tract, 289
lymphoma, gastric, 353
lysosomal bodies, hepatocytes, 360
lysosomes, 5, 7, 23, 28–30
  autophagic, 31–2
  bone matrix degradation, 236,
    237
  enzymes, 29
  formation, 22
  heterophagic, 31
  immature *see* endosomes
    in macrophage, 31
  mature, types, 31
  in monocytes, 91
  retinal pigment epithelium, 488
lysozyme, 260, 346, 477

M
M (microfold) cells, 102, 283,
  348–9, 409
M-CSF, 237
M line, 144, 146, 147
macrophage, 91, 260
  activation, 261
  in alveoli, 300, 302
  antigen presentation, 260, 261
  bone marrow, 77
  development, 83
  functions, 119
  in connective tissue, 119, 120
  in lamina propria, 284
  in liver *see* Kupffer cells
  location and types, 260
  in red pulp (spleen), 281
  in testis, 458
  ultrastructure, 31, 260
macropinocytosis, 29
macula adherens *see* desmosomes
macula densa, 375, 378, 385, 386
  functions, 385, 386
major basic protein, 90
major histocompatibility complex
  (MHC), 267–8
  binding sites, 268
  class I, 268
    cytotoxic T cells and, 268
    on thymic epithelial cells,
      273
  class II, 268
    helper T cells and, 268–9
  functions, 268–9
  polymorphism, 268, 269
  transplant rejection, 268, 284
male reproductive system, 441–67
MALT (mucosa-associated
  lymphoid tissue), 265, 271,
  283–4
mammary gland, 102, 436–8
  see also breast
mammogenesis, 436
manchette, 450
Marfan's syndrome, 136
Martinotti cells, 182
Masson's trichrome stain, 491
mast cells, 80, 119, 128, 261
  dense granules, 119
  development, 80, 81, 83
  functions, 263
  mediators secreted, 263
  ultrastructure, 261
mastitis, 439
mastoid air cells, 472

matrix *see* extracellular matrix
  (ECM)
matrix metalloproteinases, 236
May–Grunwald–Giemsa stain, 491
mechanoelectric transduction, 475
mechanoreceptors, 218, 473–4
mechanosensory cells, osteocytes
  as, 236
Meckel's cartilage, 316
Meckel's diverticulum, 65
median eminence, 394, 395
mediastinum, testis, 441, 442, 460
medulla oblongata, 178
medullary cords, 277, 279
medullary rays, 375, 376, 383
megakaryoblast, 84
megakaryocytes, 2, 69, 78, 84, 85,
  271
  fragmentation, 84
  ultrastructure, 85
megakaryocytopoiesis (platelet
  production), 84–5
Meibomian glands, 477
meiosis, 54–8, 413
  arrested (oocyte), 57, 415, 418,
    423
  mitosis comparison, 56
  oocyte maturation, 423
  prophase stages, 56, 57
  spermatocytes, 445, 448, 449
Meissner's corpuscles, 219
Meissner's plexus, 177, 325, 329
melanin, 34, 211, 212
  functions, and types, 211
  hair, 217
  in retinal pigment epithelium,
    488
  synthesis, control, 211
melanocyte-stimulating hormone
  (MSH), 411
melanocytes, 211
  hair, 217
  iris, 480, 481, 490
  ratio to basal epithelial cells,
    211
  skin, 210
melanoma, malignant, 220
melanopsin ganglion, 485
melanosomes, 211, 217
melatonin, 408
membrane, plasma *see* plasma
  membrane
membrane discs, photoreceptive
  rods, 487, 488
membrane proteins, 10, 11
membrane recycling, 22, 23, 26, 28
"membrane ruffling", 29, 237
membranous (M) cells, 102, 283,
  348–9, 409
menarche, 423
Ménière's disease, 489
meninges, 180
meniscus, 251
menopause, 439
menstrual cycle, 413, 424
  breast changes, 436
  control, 427, 428
  endometrial changes, 430–1
  follicular phase, 413, 424, 428,
    430
  hormonal changes and details,
    424, 428
  luteal phase, 424, 426, 430
  ovarian cycle, 424
  proliferative phase, 430
  secretory phase, 430–1
  uterine cycle, 424
menstruation, 431, 432, 433
  volume of blood lost, 432
Merkel cells, 212, 409
merocrine (eccrine) secretion, 114,
  214

mesangial cells, 379, 381
  extraglomerular (lacis cells),
    379, 381, 386
mesangium, 381
  extraglomerular, 379, 381, 386
mesenchymal cells, 102, 118, 119
  adult connective tissue, 120
  of bone, 233, 239, 241
  of bone marrow, 233
  cell lines derived from, 118, 119
  chondroblast formation, 241
  fetal connective tissue, 120
  myoblasts derived from, 141
  origin/development (mesoderm),
    118, 120
  peritubular tissue, seminiferous
    tubules, 443
  as stem cells, 119
  ultrastructure, 120
  villi of jejunum, 342
mesenchyme, 102
  epithelial cell interactions, 102,
    120
  in tooth formation, 314, 315
mesentery, 72, 123, 130, 327
mesoderm, 64, 95, 118
  mesenchymal cell development,
    118, 120
  tissues derived from, 64, 65, 66
mesothelioma, 304
mesothelium, 104, 191, 327
metamyelocytes, 82, 83
metaphase, 50, 52
metaphase cells, ultrastructure, 51
metaphysis, 224, 242, 243, 246
metaplasia, 65, 115, 353
metarteriole, 196, 201
MG retinal ganglion cells, 486
MHC *see* major histocompatibility
  complex (MHC)
microbodies (peroxisomes), 5, 32
microfibrils, 123, 125
microfilaments, 3, 35, 36, 40, 41
microfold (M) cells, 102, 283,
  348–9, 409
microglia, 168
micropetrosis, 236
microtubule(s), 3, 35, 36, 37–9
  9 + 2 arrangement, 44, 99, 292,
    450
  abnormal aggregation, 37
  assembly and polymerization,
    37
  astral, 39, 52, 53
  axon/axonal transport, 166
  in centrioles, 39
  chromosomal, 53
  in cilia, 43, 292
  dynamic instability, 37
  functions, 37, 38
  growth (rescue), 37
  kinetochore, 39, 52, 53
  location, 38
  motor proteins, 38–9, 53
  networks, 37
  in platelets, 85
  polar, 39, 52, 53
  role in mitosis, 37, 39, 50, 52,
    53
  self-assembly, 37
  Sertoli cells, 456
  shrinkage (catastrophe), 37
  spermatids, 449, 450
  spindle, 39
microtubule-associated proteins
  (MAPs), 38, 166
  as motor proteins, 38–9, 42
  "walking", 38–9
microtubule-organizing center
  (MTOC), 38, 39, 267
microtubule-stabilizing protein, 419
microvasculature, 196

microvilli, 4, 42, 43, 98, 106
  actin microfilaments, 35
  brush border of *see* brush
    border (of microvilli)
  hepatocytes, 360
  immotile (stereocilia), 45
  intermediate filaments and, 42,
    43
  olfactory epithelium, 471
  proximal convoluted tubule,
    382
  simple columnar epithelium
    with, 106
  small intestine, 337
    jejunum, 343, 344, 346
    ultrastructure, 344
  taste buds, 469
  ultrastructure, 98
midbrain, 178
milk, breast, 158, 436, 438
mineralocorticoids
  deficiency, 411
  synthesis, 402, 403
  see also aldosterone (salt-
    retaining hormone)
mitochondria, 7, 27–8
  axon, 166
  cardiac muscle, 150, 151
  dimensions and compartments,
    27
  DNA, 27
  flagellum of spermatid, 450
  numbers, 27
  parietal cells, 334
  skeletal muscle, 139, 143, 145
  ultrastructure, 27, 28
  zona fasciculata (adrenal gland),
    403
mitosis
  in absence of centrosome, 39
  anaphase, 50–1, 52
  arrest, 100, 341
  cell cycle and, 49
  cytokinesis, 49
  epithelial cells, 100
  karyokinesis, 49
  meiosis comparison, 56
  metaphase, 50, 52, 341
  microtubule role, 37, 39, 50, 52,
    53
  myoblasts, 141
  prometaphase, 50, 52
  prophase, 50, 52
  spermatogonia, 445, 446, 447
  spindle
    dynamics, 52
    formation/structure, 39, 50,
      51, 53–4
  stages, 50–2
  telophase, 50, 51, 52, 54
mitotic figures, 68, 120, 217, 341
modiolus, cochlea, 473, 474
molecular motors, 37, 38–9, 166
Moll, glands of, 477
monoblasts, 83
monoclonal antibodies, 285
monocyte(s), 86, 91, 260
  development, 83
  properties, 86
  ultrastructure, 91
monocytopoiesis, 83
mononuclear phagocyte system
    see macrophage; monocyte(s)
morphological associations, 70
morula, 62
mossy fibers, 185
motion sickness, 489
motor and sensory peripheral nerve,
  175
motor cortex, 180
motor end-plates, 146, 148, 173,
  174

motor neuron(s), 163, 164, 166, 187
  alpha/gamma types, 148
  cell body, 74
  muscle contraction and, 148,
    173–4
  neuromuscular junctions, 146,
    148, 173–4
motor neuron disease, 187
motor proteins
  microtubule-associated proteins,
    38–9, 42
  in mitosis, 39, 53
motor units, 148, 174
mouth see oral cavity
mRNA, 13, 18
mucins, 333
  granules in colonic epithelium,
    351
  staining, 491
  synthesis, goblet cells, 346
mucoid-rich cells, duodenum, 339
mucoperiosteum, nasal cavity, 287
mucoproteins see glycoproteins
mucosa, 110
  gall bladder, 364
  gastrointestinal tract, 128, 323,
    324–6
    cell types and functions, 324
    colon, 349, 350, 351
    esophagus, 329, 330
    lamina propria, 325
    muscularis mucosae, 325–6
    rectal, and anal, 352
    small intestine see small
      intestine
    smooth muscle, 156, 325–6
    stomach, 330–2, 333, 334,
      335
    surface epithelium, 324
    tip for remembering, 352
    see also lamina propria
  olfactory, 470–1
  oral, abnormalities, 321
  respiratory tract, 287, 289, 294,
    295
  tongue, 306–7
  uterine tubes (Fallopian tubes),
    428, 429
  vagina, 434
mucosa-associated lymphoid tissue
  (MALT), 265, 271, 283–4
mucous cells, 112
  salivary glands, 308, 309, 310
  serous cell differences, 308–9
  stomach, 331, 332, 334
    corpus of, 332, 333
    neck cells, 332, 333, 334
    surface cells, 332, 333, 334
  see also goblet cells; mucus-
    secreting cells
mucous connective tissue, 130
mucous glands
  esophagus, 329, 330, 332
  gall bladder, 364
  tongue, 305, 307
mucous membrane see mucosa
mucous neck cells, 332, 333, 334
mucus, 309, 332
  cervical secretion, 433
  colonic secretion, 351
  intestinal secretion, 106, 346
  respiratory tract secretion, 287,
    303
  stomach, secretion from, 332,
    333, 336
mucus-secreting cells, 106, 112, 113
  salivary glands, 308, 309, 310
  stomach, 330, 331, 332, 336
  see also goblet cells; mucous
    cells
Müller cells, retina, 484, 485, 488
multicellularity, 61–7, 95

multiple sclerosis, 187
multipotent, definition, 67
multipotent cells, 65
mumps, 321, 467
muscle, 73, 137–60
  abnormalities, 159–60
  action potential, 146, 148, 174
  cardiac see cardiac muscle
  collagen, 123
  contraction, 137
    cardiac, 152–3
    see also skeletal muscle;
      smooth muscle
  coordination, cerebellum role,
    183
  delayed onset soreness, 159
  fatigue, 149, 159
  functions/actions, 137
  growth and development, 141,
    158–9
  loose connective tissue
    supporting, 128
  non-striated see smooth muscle
  skeletal see skeletal muscle
  smooth see smooth muscle
  spasm/rigidity, 159
  strength, 123
  striated, 73, 137, 150
    see also skeletal muscle
  tone, basal ganglia role, 182
  types and embryonic origins, 75
  voluntary see skeletal muscle
  weakness, 159
muscle cells (fibers), 2, 73
  contraction, and length, 137
  skeletal muscle, 68, 137, 141–2
muscle tissue, 73
muscular dystrophy, 147, 159
muscularis externa, 323, 326–7
  colon, 326, 349
  esophagus, 329
  myenteric plexus targeting, 329
  small intestine, 338
  stomach, 326, 330, 331
muscularis mucosae, 325–6
  colon, 349
  esophagus, 329
  small intestine, 338, 339
  stomach, 331, 332, 336
myasthenia gravis, 159
myelin, 174, 186
myelin sheaths, 68, 169, 170, 172
  loss in multiple sclerosis, 187
  spinal cord, 186
  staining, 174, 175
myelinated nerves, 68, 74, 139
  axons, 174, 175
  cerebral cortex, 180
  conduction velocity, 172, 175,
    176
  functions, 175
  peripheral nerves, 174, 175
  Schwann cells role, 169–70
  staining, 174, 175
  see also axon(s)
myeloblasts, 82
myelocytes, 82
myeloid cell lineage, 80, 81, 262
myeloid stem cells, 80
myenteric ganglia, 163, 328
  see also Auerbach's (myenteric)
    plexus
myenteric plexus see Auerbach's
  (myenteric) plexus
myoblasts, 118, 141, 142, 158
myocardial infarction, 159–60, 205
myocardial ischemia, 205
myocardial tissue necrosis, 205
myocardium, 152, 190
  see also cardiac muscle
myocytes, cardiac, 73, 137, 150–2,
  158, 191

myoepithelial cells, 158, 214
  apocrine glands, 214
  eccrine gland, 213
  iris, 480
  parotid gland, 308
myofibrils
  cardiac muscle, 150
  skeletal muscle see skeletal
    muscle
myofibroblasts, 158, 160, 342, 443
myofilaments
  cardiac muscle, 152
  Purkinje fibers, 191
  skeletal muscle, 140
  smooth muscle, 154
myogenic hypothesis, 196
myoglobin, 139
myoid cells, 99, 158
  epididymis, 462
  peritubular (seminiferous
    tubules), 443
  rete testis, 460, 461
myometrium, 429
myoneural junction
  see neuromuscular junction
myopathy, 159
myopia (near-sightedness), 490
myosalpinx, 428
myosin, 38, 149
myosin filaments, 147
  actin sliding along, 40, 137,
    147, 158
  cardiac muscle, 150, 152
  skeletal muscle, 140, 144, 146,
    147
  smooth muscle, 154
myotube, 141, 143

N
Nabothian follicle, 433
NADH, skeletal muscle metabolism,
  149
nail bed, 218
nail groove, 218
nail plate, 218
nails, 218
nasal cavity, 287, 288
  "respiratory" mucosa, 287, 288,
    289
  edema, 489
  roof, pseudostratified columnar
    cells, 287, 470
nasal passages, 287–90
nasopharynx, 287, 289
natural killer (NK) cells, 80, 261
natural killer T cell (pit cells), in
  liver, 362
necrosis, 58
neonates
  bone marrow, 77
  iris color, 481, 490
  jaundice, 220
  ovary, 413, 415
  respiratory distress syndrome,
    303
  testis, 446
neoplasia, 115
  see also cancer
nephrin, 42
nephron, 374–7
  functions/actions, 373, 374
  juxtamedullary, 377, 383
  long-looped and short-looped,
    377, 383
  number and length, 374, 376,
    377
nerve(s)
  conduction, 163
    mechanism, 171–2
    saltatory, 170, 172
    speeds, 172, 175, 176
    see also nerve impulses

nerve(s) continued
  loose connective tissue
    supporting, 128
  myelinated see myelinated
    nerves
  peripheral see peripheral nerves
  staining, 491
  types and embryonic origins, 75
  unmyelinated, 74, 175, 176
    conduction velocity, 172
    diameter, 175
    Schwann cells surrounding,
      170, 171, 176
    ultrastructure, 176
nerve cell bodies, 2, 74, 164, 166,
  177, 181
  dorsal root ganglia, 171, 177
  ganglia of Auerbach's plexus,
    328
  gastrointestinal tract, 323, 328
nerve cells see neurons (nerve cells)
nerve fibers, 73–4
  myelinated see myelinated
    nerves
  unmyelinated see nerve(s),
    unmyelinated
  see also axon(s); dendrites
nerve impulses, 161, 171–2
  action potential, 163, 171–2
    saltatory conduction, 170,
      172
  blocked/reduced, 187
  regulated by fibrous astrocyte,
    167
  resting potential, 171
  transmission, 172
  unmyelinated nerves, 175, 176
  see also nerve(s), conduction
nerve tissue, 73–5
nervous system, 161–87
  anatomy, 161, 162
  central see central nervous
    system (CNS)
  peripheral see peripheral
    nervous system (PNS)
nestin, 42
neural crest, 65, 66, 170
neural precursor cells, 182
neural tube, 167
neurilemma see myelin sheaths
neuroectodermal cells, 65
neuroendocrine cells, 290, 409
neuroendocrine system, dispersed,
  409
neuroepithelial bodies (Kulchitsky
  cells), 297, 409
neuroepithelial cells, 167
neurofibrils, tangled, 187
neurofilament proteins, 42
neuroglia (glial cells), 74, 161,
  166–71
  autonomic ganglia, 177
  cell number, 167
  cell types, 167–9
  cerebral cortex, 179, 180
  in CNS, 167–9
  dorsal root ganglia, 177
  enteric ganglia, 171, 177
  glial processes, 180
  nucleus, 168
  origin, 167
  in PNS, 167, 169, 171
  see also Schwann cells
  see also specific cell types
neurohypophysis see pituitary gland,
  posterior
neuromuscular junction, 146, 148,
  173–4
  muscle contraction, stimulus,
    148
neurons (nerve cells), 2, 73–4, 161,
  163–6

neurons (nerve cells) *continued*
  afferent and efferent types, 161
  Auerbach's plexus
    see Auerbach's (myenteric)
      plexus
  axons *see* axon(s)
  bipolar, 163, 164
  cell body (soma), 163, 165
  clusters *see* ganglia
  dendrites *see* dendrites
  function, 161
  integrative, 163, 164, 166
  intermediate filaments, 42
  motor *see* motor neuron(s)
  multipolar, 163
  nucleus, 163
  number, 161
  pseudounipolar (unipolar), 163,
    164, 176, 177, 186
  sensory, 163, 164, 166, 171
  structure, 161, 163
  types, 163
neuropathy, 159
neuropeptides, 409
neuropil, 163, 165
  cerebellar cortex, 184, 185
  cerebral cortex, 180
  spinal cord, 186
neurotransmitters, 167, 172, 173
  see also acetylcholine
neurotrophic factors, 167
neurovascular canal, bone, 228
neutrophil(s), 82, 89, 260, 261
  activated, 89
  adhesion/margination, 89
  development, 82–3
  functions, 89, 261, 263
  granules, 89
  life span, 89, 260
  migration, 40
  properties, 86
  ultrastructure, 89
neutrophil extracellular traps
  (NETs), 89, 263
neutrophilic series, 82, 83
nexus *see* gap junctions (nexus)
night blindness, 490
nipple, 437
Nissl bodies, 164, 165, 186
Nissl substance, 164
nitric oxide, 196, 201, 328
nocodazole, 37
node of Ranvier, 170, 172
non-specific urethritis (NSU), 467
norepinephrine, 129
  arterial constriction, 196, 201
  secretion, 404
  smooth muscle innervation, 158
normoblasts, 82
Notch pathway, 102
notochord, 254, 255
Noxa, 59
nuclear bag fibers, 148
nuclear chain fibers, 148
nuclear envelope (membrane), 12
  formation, during telophase, 51
  in metaphase, 51
  rough ER continuity with, 17
  spermatids, 449, 450
  torn, cell division, 13
nuclear lamina, 12
nuclear lamins, 42
nuclear pores, 12–13
nucleolar-organizing regions (NOR),
  13
nucleolus, 2, 13, 144
nucleonema, 13
nucleosomal fiber, 14, 16
nucleosomes, 14, 15
  3D structure, 16
  DNA in (models), 15, 16
  packaging/arrangement, 14, 16

nucleus (cell), 1, 2, 3, 7, 11–17, 67
  adipocytes, 68
  in apoptosis, 58, 59
  bilobular, basophils, 90
  cells lacking, 3, 68, 69, 86
  double, in hepatocytes, 69
  elliptical, 3
  envelope, 12
  exocrine pancreatic cell, 7
  liver cells, 5, 7, 69, 358, 360
  lobulated, 3
  mitotic figures lacking, 68
  multilobulated, 69, 82, 84, 85
  muscle cells, 132, 137, 138,
    139, 141, 145
    cardiac muscle, 150
  in necrotic cell, 58
  neurons, 163
  not visible in cells, 68
  pyknotic, 58, 59
  pyriform, 3
  shapes, in cell types, 2, 68, 69
  spermatids, 449, 450
  squamous-type cells, 68
  structure, 3
  translation in, 13
  see also individual cell types
nucleus pulposus, 255

O

obstructive airway disease, 296
occluding junctions *see* tight
  junctions (zonula occludens)
Oddi, sphincter of, 365
odontoblasts, 316–17, 318
  inward migration, curve, 313
  pre-dentin secretion, 312, 313,
    317
  tooth development, 314, 316
odors, and types, 471
olfaction, 471, 489
olfactory bulb, 471
olfactory ensheathing cells, 171
olfactory epithelium, 288
olfactory mucosa, 470–1
olfactory nerve, 470
olfactory receptors, 471
olfactory sensory cells, 471
oligodendrocytes, 168
  axon myelination (CNS), 168,
    170, 171
  injury, demyelination, 168
oligozoospermia, 466
oncocytes, 322
oocyte, 2, 64, 413
  antral follicles, 421
  diplotene/arrested, 415, 418
  fertilization, 413
  in Graafian follicle, 422, 423
  implantation, 428
  life history, 417
  mature follicle, 422
  meiosis, and 54, 57, 423
  origin, 413
  primary follicle, 417, 418, 419
  prophase, 415
  secondary follicle, 419, 420
  secondary oocyte, 423
  zygote formation, 61, 62
oocyte–cumulus mass, 422, 426
oogenesis, 413, 416
opioid peptides, synthesis, 404
opsin, 487, 488
optic chiasm, 395
optic disc (blind spot), 476, 488,
  489
optic nerve, 178, 476, 477, 489
ora serrata, 485
oral cavity, 109, 305–22
  abnormal conditions, 321–2
  lymphoid tissues *see* tonsil(s)
  soft palate, 320–1

oral cavity) *continued*
  see also salivary glands; teeth;
    tongue
oral epithelium
  mucosal lymphoid follicles, 283
  thickening, tooth development,
    314, 315
oral mucosa, 2
  abnormalities, 321
orchitis, 467
organ of Corti, 472, 473, 475
  hair cells, 473, 474, 475
organelles, cell, 3, 11–28
  see also specific organelles
organs, 61
  formation, 65, 75, 79
orodental tissues, 305–22
oropharynx, 289
ossicles, ear, 472
ossification, 239
  endochondral *see* endochondral
    ossification
  epiphyseal growth plate zone,
    246
  intramembranous, 238–9,
    239–40
  onset in embryo/fetus, 239
  primary center, 241, 242, 244
  secondary center, 243, 244
  time frame, 244
osteoarthritis/osteoarthrosis, 223,
  256
osteoblasts, 118, 231, 233–4
  bone remodeling, 250
  cancellous bone growth, 249
  endochondral ossification, 241
  fetal skull, 239, 240
  formation, 241
  intramembranous ossification,
    239–40
  matrix vesicle secretion, 234
  osteoclast communication,
    237–8
  periosteal, fracture repair, 255
  ultrastructure, 234
osteocalcin, 125
osteochondral progenitors, 239
osteoclastogenesis, 237
osteoclasts, 231, 236–8
  bone remodeling, 250
  bone resorption, 236, 237
  fetal skull/bones, 239, 240
  fracture repair, 255
  membrane ruffling, 237
  osteoblast communication,
    237–8
  recruitment, 236
  ultrastructure, 237
osteocytes, 2, 67, 72, 136, 234–6
  compact bone, 226, 227
  function, 235, 236
  gap junctions, 235, 236
  lacunae, 234, 235
  non-proliferative nature, 242
  processes, 227, 234, 235
  ultrastructure, 235
osteoid, 233, 234, 244
  development, 239
  mineralization, 234, 250
osteoid matrix, 233
osteomalacia, 256
osteon (Haversian system), 225,
  226, 232
  blind endings, 228, 229
  branching patterns, 228, 229
  cancellous bone lacking, 230,
    231
  collagen bundles, 228
  dimensions, 228
  formation, 227, 237, 240
    closing cone, 250
  generations, 251

osteon (Haversian system) *continued*
  Haversian canals, 225, 226,
    228, 229, 235
  number, 228
  overlapping, 228
  primary (first-generation), 249
  remnants, 228, 230
  resorption and renewal, 228,
    250
  structure, 227
osteophytes, 256
osteoporosis, 230, 256
osteoprogenitor cells, 232
otolithic organs, 472
otoliths, 472
ova *see* oocyte
oval window, 473, 474
ovarian cycle, 413, 424
ovarian follicles, 412, 414
  antral (tertiary), 414, 416, 417,
    420–3
    "dominant", 422, 425
    early, 420
    growth, 420, 422
  atresia, 420, 421, 422, 423, 426
    growth *vs*, 422, 425
  development/growth, 413, 415,
    416–25
    antral follicles, 420
    atresia *vs*, 422, 425
    failure, 438
    hormonal regulation, 420,
      423, 425
    life history, 417
    primary follicles, 419
    tonic (basal), 423
  Graafian (preovulatory), 416,
    417, 420, 422
    oocyte meiosis, 423
  hormone production, 423, 424
  maturation, 422, 423, 425
  non-growing (reserve), 414,
    415, 416
  numbers, 415, 416, 417
  pre-antral, 416, 417, 418,
    419–20
    primary, 70, 416, 417, 419,
      422
    primordial *see* ovarian
      follicles, primordial
    secondary, 416, 417, 419–
      20
  prepuberty, 422, 423
  primordial, 413, 414, 416, 417,
    418, 419
    intermediary, 419
    transition to primary
      follicle, 418, 419
    types, 419
  secondary, 420
  "selected", 425
  stratified cuboidal epithelium,
    109
  types, 416, 417
ovary, 413–28
  adult, 413, 414
  disorders, and cancer, 438
  fetal and neonatal, 413, 415
  follicles *see* ovarian follicles
  germ cell life history, 417
  hormones secreted, 410, 425
  menstrual cycle control, 428
  prepuberty, 422, 423, 425
  stroma, 413, 414, 415
oviducts *see* uterine tubes (Fallopian
  tubes)
ovulation, 413, 414, 417, 422, 423
oxidases, peroxisomal, 32
oxygen, diffusion, 87, 300
oxyhemoglobin, 87
oxyntic cells *see* parietal (oxyntic)
  cells

oxyphil cells, 400, 401
oxytocin, 398, 437
  disorders, 411
  lactation, 438

P

p53 protein/gene, 59, 220
pachytene, 57
Pacinian corpuscle, 171, 219
Paget's disease, 256
palate, hard/soft, 320
pancreas, 365–70
  acinar (exocrine) cells, 6, 7, 8,
    113, 365
    freeze-fracture EM, 369
    functions, 366, 367, 368
    secretions and, 366, 367,
      368
    structure and organelles, 7,
      24, 26, 366, 367,
      368
    ultrastructure, 7, 368
    volume/membrane surface
      area, 8, 9
    zymogen granules, 366,
      367, 368, 369
  acini (exocrine secretory units),
    71, 113, 365, 366, 370
    ducts, 366
    functions, 366
    secretory proteins
      pathway, 369
  centroacinar cells, 366, 367
  disorders, 371
  endocrine, 370, 404–7
    blood supply, 407
    disorder (diabetes mellitus),
      412
  endocrine cells, 6, 365
    see also islets of Langerhans
  endocrine–exocrine portal
    system, 367
  glucose levels and liver
    relationship, 407
  tumors, 371
pancreatic bud, development, 370
pancreatic ducts, 366, 367
pancreatic epithelial glandular
  cells, 96
pancreatic hormones, 370
  see also glucagon; insulin
pancreatic juice, 366–7
pancreatic polypeptide (PP), 370,
  407
  cells secreting, 370, 405, 407
pancreatic zymogens, 367
pancreatitis, 371
Paneth cells, 102, 324, 346, 348
pannus, 256
papillae, tongue see tongue
papillary dermis, 212
papillary muscle, heart, 150, 190
para-aortic splanchnopleure (PAS),
  79
paracellular transport, tight
  junctions and, 46
paracrine regulation, 393, 453
parafollicular (clear, C) cells,
  399–400
paraganglia, 410
paraluteal cells, 426, 427
paraneuron, 409
parasympathetic ganglia, 176, 177
parasympathetic innervation
  blood vessels, 201
  bronchioles, 296
  ciliary body, 481
  gastrointestinal tract, 327
  smooth muscle, 158
parasympathetic nervous system,
  161
parasympathetic paraganglia, 410

parathyroid gland, 400–1
  chief cells, 400, 401
  disorders, 411
  oxyphil cells, 400, 401
parathyroid hormone (PTH), 237,
  400, 401
parathyroid hormone related protein
  (PTHrP), 247
paraventricular nuclei, 394
paravertebral ganglia, 176
parenchyma, 118
  in exocrine glands, 71
  lung, 294, 297
  testis, 443
parietal (oxyntic) cells, 112, 331,
  333, 334, 335
  ultrastructure, 334
Parkinson's disease, 187
parotid gland, 308
  infections, 321
  striated duct, 310
PAS reaction, skeletal muscle, 149
PAS–AGM region, 79
patellar ligament, 251
pathogen-associated molecular
  patterns (PAMPs), 260
pathology, 70
pattern recognition, 70
penis, 465–6
peptide hormones, 393, 394
peptides, synthesis and folding, 18,
  19, 20
perforin, 267
periarteriolar lymphoid sheaths
  (PALS), 280, 281, 282, 283
pericapsular connective tissues,
  lymph nodes, 276
pericentriolar material (PCM), 39
perichondrium, 133, 241
pericytes, 158
  arterioles, 195
  capillaries, 197, 198
  postcapillary venules, 199
perikaryon, 163, 164
perilymph, 472, 474
perimysium, 140
perineurium, 169, 174, 175, 176
perinuclear space, 12
periodic acid–Schiff hematoxylin
  stain, 491
periodontal disease, 322
periodontal ligament, 311, 312, 313
  development, 313, 318
periodontitis, 312, 322
periodontium, 312
periosteal arteries/veins, 232
periosteal cells, 233
periosteum, 231, 232, 233, 242
peripheral nerves, 74, 162, 174–6
  conduction velocities, 175
  mixed motor and sensory, 175,
    176
  myelinated, 174, 175
  staining, 161, 174, 175
  unmyelinated, 175, 176
peripheral nervous system (PNS),
  161
  axon myelination, 169–70, 171
  glial cells, 167, 169
  see also Schwann cells
peristalsis, 329
  gastrointestinal tract, 325, 329,
    330, 350
  renal pelvis, 386
  urinary tract, 390
peritoneal fluid, 67
peritubular cells, 443
peritubular tissue, seminiferous
  tubules, 443
perlecan, 127
pernicious anemia, 92
peroxisomes, 5, 32

pertussis (whooping cough), 304
Peyer's patches, 283, 348
phagocytic cells, 119, 260–1
  microglia, 168
  mononuclear see macrophage;
    monocyte(s)
  neutrophils see neutrophil(s)
phagocytosis, 29, 98
  of apoptotic cells, 59
  lipid inclusions and, 33
  by monocytes/macrophage, 91
  by neutrophils, 89
phagolysosomes, 89
phagosomes, 31
phallacidin, 40
phalloidin, 40
pharyngitis, 322
pheomelanin, 211
phlebitis, 205
phosphatases, 234
phosphate
  homeostasis, 235, 236
  reabsorption, 389
phosphatidylserine, 59
photoperiod, hormone secretion
  control, 394
photopigments, 487
photoreceptor cells, retina, 483, 484
  cell bodies, layer, 484, 485
  distribution, 488
  function/mechanism of action,
    486, 487–9
  ratio to nerve fibers in optic
    nerve, 489
  see also cones (retina); rods
    (photoreceptive)
pia mater, 180
pigment epithelium, retinal, 484,
  485, 488
pigments, cytoplasmic inclusions,
  33–4
pineal gland, 408
pinealocytes, 408
pinocytosis, 29, 30, 98
pit cells, liver, 362
pituicytes, 398
pituitary gland, 394–7
  adenoma, 411
  anterior, 395, 396, 397
    cell types, 395, 396, 397
    cell ultrastructure, 397
    disorders, 411
    hormones, 395, 396
    "lateral wings", 395
    "mucoid wedge", 395
    staining, 396, 397
  development, 397
  intermediate lobe, 397
  posterior, 397, 398
    disorders, 411
    hormones, 398
    pituicytes, 398
pituitary stalk, 395
placenta, 434–5
placental lactogen (hPL), 410
plasma, 9, 77, 85, 117
  filtered by kidney, 374, 387
plasma cells, 258, 262
  in connective tissue, 119
  formation, 265, 278
  functions, 119
  in lamina propria, 284, 325
  stomach, 332
  ultrastructure, 17, 265
plasma membrane, 1, 4, 10, 67
  actin filaments beneath, 40
  apical, microvilli projecting
    from, 42, 43
  basal lamina contact, 127
  cell junctions, 45
  erythrocytes, 86
  functions, 10, 11

plasma membrane *continued*
  internalization, endocytosis, 29
  liver cells, 5
  movement of materials to, 22,
    24, 25
  receptors on, 30
  skeletal muscle fibers, 143
  structure, 10, 11
  surface area, 26
  ultrastructure, 10
  villi, in jejunum, 344
  zonula occludens (tight
    junctions), 46
plasma proteins, 85, 363
plasmablasts, 265
plasticity, definition, 67
platelet(s), 3, 69, 86, 88
  activation, 88
  adherence, 88
  circulation, 85
  granules, 85, 88
  nucleus lacking, 3, 69, 86
  production/development, 84–5
  properties, 86
  ultrastructure, 85
platelet-derived growth factor
  (PDGF), 85
platelet plug, 85, 88
pleomorphic salivary adenoma, 321
pleura, 302–3
  parietal, 302
  visceral, 294, 302
"pleural sac", 303
"pleural space", 302
pleurisy, 304
plexus of Henle, 325, 329
plica circularis, 337, 338
pluripotent, definition, 67
pneumonia, 304
podocytes, 379
  foot processes, 380, 381
podosomes, 236
Poiseuille's law, 192
polar bodies, 423
polychromatic normoblasts, 82
polycystic ovaries (Stein–Leventhal
  syndrome), 438, 439
polymorphonuclear leukocytes
  see granulocytes; neutrophil(s)
polymorphonuclear neutrophils
  see neutrophil(s)
polypeptides, synthesis, 18
polyribosomes, 18
pons, 178, 183
pores of Kohn, 299
portal hypertension, 205, 371
portal triads (portal tracts), 356,
  357, 359, 362
portal vein, 200, 359
portal venules, 363
post-translational targeting of
  proteins, 19, 20
postcapillary venules, 196, 198–9,
  204
  dimensions, 192
postcentral gyrus, 181
posterior chamber, of eye, 480
postsynaptic membranes, 172
postsynaptic neurons, 164
potassium ions
  efflux, from apoptotic cells, 59
  nerve conduction, 171
  reabsorption, renal, 389
pre-dentin, 312, 316, 317
pre-embryonic period, 61
prebone, 223
precapillary sphincter, 196
pregnancy, 413
  breast tissue, 437
  corpus luteum "rescue", 428
  ectopic, 439
  multiple, 439

pregnancy *continued*
  smooth muscle growth, 159
  vein disorders, 205
pregnenolone, 28, 459
pregranulosa cell, 413, 415, 418
preosseous tissue, 223
preprohormone, 393
preproinsulin, 406
prepuce (foreskin), 466
presbyopia, 490
pressure perception, 219
presynaptic neurons, 164
prevertebral ganglia, 176
prickle cells, 209
primary tissue types *see* tissues
primates, spermatogenesis, 452, 453
primitive endoderm, 61
primitive streak, 64
primordial germ cells (PGCs), 64
principal cells, epididymis, 107, 462, 463
principal piece, late-elongating spermatid, 450
pro-opiomelanocortin, 397, 411
procollagen, 118, 122
profilaggrin, 208
progesterone, 429
  luteal cell secretion of, 427
  menstrual cycle, 424, 427, 430–1
  synthesis, 410
progestins, 413, 429
progestogens, 429
programmed cell death *see* apoptosis (programmed cell death)
prohormone, 393
proinsulin, 406
prokaryotic cells, 1, 11
prolactin (PRL), 395, 437
  disorders, 411
  lactation, 438
proliferating cell nuclear antigen (PCNA), 100, 341, 415, 420, 447
promastocytes, 81
prometaphase, 50, 52
promonocytes, 83
promyelocytes, 82, 83
pronormoblast (proerythroblast), 80, 82
prophase, 50, 52
  meiosis, 56, 57
proplatelet clumps, 84
proprioception, 181
prostacyclin, 201
prostate gland, 464–5
  benign prostate hyperplasia, 114, 465, 467
  concretions, 465
  disorders, 467
  secretion, 465
  tubulo-alveolar glands, 464, 465
  tumors, 465, 467
  zones, 464, 467
prostate-specific antigen (PSA), 465, 467
prostatectomy, transurethral, 467
protamines, 449
protein(s)
  co-translational targeting, 19, 20–1
  in cytoplasm, 9
  extracellular matrix, 125–6
  fates, variations in, 20–1
  folding, 20
  glycosylation, 22
  incorrectly folded, degradation, 21
  membrane, 10, 11
  in nucleolus, 13
  post-translational targeting, 19, 20

protein(s) *continued*
  secretion, 18, 462
  sorting in cytoplasm, 19–21
  synthesis, 18–21
    close to nucleus, 12
    on free ribosomes, 18
    pancreatic acinar cells, 368
    rough ER, 12, 18–21
    sorting of proteins after, 19–21
  three-dimensional structure, 19
  transient storage/aggregation, 18, 21
protein hormones, 393, 394
proteoglycans, 121, 125–6
  aggregate, 126
  extraction from tissue sections, 126
  hyaline cartilage, 133, 134
  mucous connective tissue, 130
  synthesis by fibroblasts, 125–6
  turnover time, 126
prothrombotic compounds, 201–2
protofilaments, 41
proximal tubules *see* renal tubules, proximal
pseudopodia, megakaryocyte, 85
pseudostratified epithelium *see* epithelium
psoriasis, 220
puberty, bone growth during, 247
pulmonary artery, 300
pulmonary capillaries, 299, 300
pulmonary circulation, 189, 299, 300
pulmonary embolism, 205, 303
pulmonary vasculature, 294, 297, 300
pulmonary veins, 200, 300
Puma, 59
pupil, opening/closing, 480
Purkinje cells, 164, 165, 184
  cerebellum, 164, 184, 185
  dendritic spines/dendrites, 172, 184, 185
  synapses, 172, 185
Purkinje fibers, 153, 191
Purkinje layer, cerebellum, 184, 185
pus, 221
pyelonephritis, 392
pyknotic bodies, 58, 59
pyloric glands, 335, 336
pyloric sphincter, 330
pyramidal cells, 181, 182
pyramidal neurons, cerebral cortex, 163, 164

Q

quadriceps tendon, 251

R

RANKL, 237
RANKL/RANK pathway, 237
Rathke's cleft cysts, 397
Rathke's pouch, 395
receptors, 30
  hormones, 394, 398
reciprocal recombination, 57
rectoanal region, 352
rectum, 352
red blood cells *see* erythrocyte(s)
red pulp *see* spleen
Reinke, crystals of, 458, 459
Reissner's membrane (basilar membrane), 474, 475
renal calyces, 374, 385
renal columns, 373, 374
renal corpuscle, 374, 375, 377–81
  Bowman's capsule, 377, 378
  Bowman's space, 377, 378, 379, 387
  development, 375, 376

renal corpuscle *continued*
  distribution, 376
  filtration slit, 380, 381
  organization, 377, 378
  podocytes, 379, 380, 381
  polarity, 377
  slit diaphragm, 380, 381
  urinary pole, 377, 379
  vascular pole, 377, 378
  see also glomerulus
renal cortex, 373, 375, 376
renal failure, 390, 392
renal lobe, 373
renal medulla, 373, 375
  capillaries *see* vasa recta (medullary capillaries)
  inner/outer zones, 375
  interstitium, 387, 388, 389
  medullary rays, 375, 376, 383
renal papilla, 374, 375, 385
renal pelvis, 374, 385–6
renal pyramid, 373, 375
  apex, 385
renal sinus, 374
renal tubules, 376
  basement membrane around, 99
  collecting ducts *see under* Kidney
  connecting, 375, 385–6
  distal, 385
    length, 385
    thick ascending limb of Henle's loop, 375, 383, 384
  distal convoluted, 375, 376, 379, 384, 385
  functions, 382
  proximal, 382, 383
    functions, 382, 387
    length, 382
    microvilli, 382
    plasma membrane infolding, 382
    polarity of epithelial cells, 97
    ultrastructure, 382
  proximal convoluted, 375, 377, 382
    functions, 382, 387
  simple cuboidal epithelium, 105
  see also loop of Henle
renal vessels, 379, 387
  afferent/efferent arterioles, 379, 387
  corticomedullary region, 383
  see also glomerular capillaries; vasa recta (medullary capillaries)
renin, 378, 386, 389, 403, 410
renin–angiotensin system (RAS), 386, 387, 389, 403
reproductive system
  female, 413–39
  male, 441–67
residual bodies, 31, 33
  spermatids, 451, 452, 454
respiratory bronchioles, 294, 296, 297, 298
respiratory distress syndrome, 303
respiratory passages, 287–90
respiratory system, 287–304
  conducting zone, 287
  respiratory zone, 287
respiratory tract, 287–304
  disorders, 303–4
  divisions, 287
  epithelium *see* epithelium, respiratory-type
  infections, 303–4
  lower, 287, 292–8

respiratory tract *continued*
  bronchial secretions, 295, 296
  see also alveoli (alveolus); bronchi; bronchioles
  lung *see* lung
  upper, 287–90
    secretions/mucus, 287, 291
  see also individual anatomical regions
respiratory zone, 287
resting potential, nerves, 171
rete testis, 441, 442, 460, 461
reticular cells
  fibroblastic, 276
  fibroblastic, in lymphoid organs, 276
reticular fibers, 72, 125, 129
  bone marrow, 136
  liver, 124
  lymph nodes, 124, 129
  lymphoid organs, 276
  space of Disse, 361
  synthesis by Ito cells, 124
  thymus, 272
reticular lamina, 127
reticular layer, dermis, 212
reticular tissue, 129
reticulocytes, 82
retina, 477, 478, 483–9
  bipolar neurons, 164
  blood vessels, 486, 489
  central, 485–6
  color, of 485
  ganglion cell layer, 484, 485, 486
  glial cells, 486
  inner "limiting membrane", 484
  layers, 484
  light sensitivity, 488
  neural circuits, 485
  neuroepithelial layer, 485
  nuclear layers, 484, 485
  outer "limiting membrane", 484
  peripheral, 486
  photoreceptive layer, 484, 485
  plexiform (synaptic)layers, 484, 485, 486
retinal (visual pigment), 487, 488
retinal ganglion cells, 484, 485, 486
retinal Muller glia, 185
retinal pigment epithelium, 484, 485, 488
retinal vessels, 484, 489
retinopathy, diabetic, 490
retrograde transport, 22, 24, 25
Rhesus system, 93
rheumatic fever, 160, 205
rheumatoid arthritis, 136, 256
rhinitis, 304
  allergic, 285
rhodopsin, 485, 487
RhoGAM (anti-Rh gamma globulin), 93
ribosomes, 9, 37
  formation, 18
  outer nuclear membrane, 12
  protein synthesis, 18, 19
  rough ER, 17, 18
  subunits (40S and 60S), 18
  synthesis in nucleolus, 13
ribs, development and growth, 241
rickets, 256
rigor mortis, 159
ring of Waldeyer, 318, 319
RNA, 9, 82
  mRNA, 13, 18
  rRNA, 13, 18
  tRNA, 18
RNase, epididymis staining and, 461
rods (photoreceptive), 484, 485, 488
  defects, 490

rods (photoreceptive) *continued*
  function/mechanism of action, 487–9
  light sensitivity, 488
  rhodopsin, 485, 487
  ultrastructure, 487
Rokitansky–Aschoff sinuses, 364
Romanowsky stains, 87, 491
root canal (tooth), 311
rough ER *see* endoplasmic reticulum, rough
round window, 473, 474
rRNA, 13, 18
Ruffini corpuscles, 220

S
S cells, 409
saccules, 472
sacral nerves, 327
saliva, 322
  functions, 307, 322
  hypotonic, 310
  secretion, 307, 308, 310
  transport, 310
  volume, 308
salivary glands, 307–10
  disorders, 321–2
  ducts, 109, 309, 310
  functions, 307
  lobulated, 308
  major/minor, 308
  parotid *see* parotid gland
  secretory units, 308
  serous/mucus-secreting, 308
  sublingual, 308, 309
  submandibular, 113, 308, 309
  tumors, 321–2
salivary tissues, 305–22
Salmonella typhi infection, 353
salpingitis, 438–9
saltatory conduction, 170, 172
sarcolemma, 139, 143, 144, 145
  depolarization, 174
  depressions, motor nerve endings, 173
sarcomeres
  cardiac muscle, 150, 152–3
  skeletal muscle, 138, 140, 143, 146, 147
    assembly, myotubes, 143
    A bands, 138, 144, 146, 147
    contraction, 147
    H bands, 146
    I bands, 138, 144, 146, 147
    M lines, 144, 146, 147
    sliding filament model, 137, 147
    ultrastructure, 146, 147
    Z lines, 143, 144, 146, 147
  smooth muscle, 156
sarcoplasm, 143
  cardiac muscle, 150
  skeletal muscle, 143, 144
  smooth muscle, 154
  ultrastructure, 146
sarcoplasmic reticulum (SR), 143, 145, 146
  cardiac muscle, 152
  smooth muscle, 158
satellite cells
  ganglia, 170, 176, 177
  skeletal muscle, 143, 158
sawtooth-type glands, endometria, 431
scab formation, 221
scala media, 473
scala tympani, 473, 474, 475
scala vestibuli, 474, 475
scalp skin, 216, 218
scar tissue, and formation, 136, 221

Schmidt-Landterman clefts, 170
Schwann cells, 167, 169–71, 175
  cytoplasm, 68, 74, 170, 171
  Meissner's corpuscles and, 219
  membrane (myelin sheath), 169, 170
    ultrastructure, 169
  nucleus, 169, 170, 171, 174, 176
  origin (neural crest), 170
  surrounding unmyelinated nerves, 170, 171, 176
sciatic nerve, 162
sclera, 478, 479
scurvy (vitamin C deficiency), 136, 322
sebaceous cells, 215
sebaceous ducts, 215
sebaceous glands, 112, 214, 215
  ducts, 215
  ear, 472
  eyelid, 477
  hair follicle association, 214, 215
  overactivity, 220
  sites, 214, 215
  skin areas without, 215
sebum, 214, 215, 472
secretin, 367
secretion
  apocrine, 114, 214
  constitutive *vs* regulated, 25–6, 29
  eccrine (merocrine), 114, 214
  endocrine, 114, 393–4
  epithelial cell specializations, 98, 99
  exocrine, 114
  Golgi apparatus role, 25–7
  holocrine, 114, 214, 215
  mechanisms, 25–6
secretory cells, glands, 110
secretory granules, 22, 24, 477
secretory pathway, 21, 22, 23
  in pancreatic acini, 369
secretory vesicles *see* vesicles
self and non-self, 259, 266–7, 276
self-tolerance, 259
semenogelin, 464
semicircular canals, 472, 473
semilunar pockets, valves of veins, 200
seminal ducts, 461–6
  disorders, 467
seminal fluid, 441, 464
seminal vesicles, 441, 442, 464
  pseudostratified columnar epithelium, 107, 464
  tubulosaccular glands, 464
seminiferous cords, 458
seminiferous epithelium, 109, 442, 443, 445
  adult, 446
  basal/adluminal compartments, 455, 456
  cycle, spermatogenic, 452–3, 460
  spermatogonial mitosis in, 447
  ultrastructure, 444
seminiferous tubules, 441–5
  basal/adluminal compartments, 455, 456
  basal lamina, 443, 444, 446
  carcinoma in situ, 454, 467
  convolutions, 441, 442, 443
  diameter and length, 443
  germ cell development stages, 451–3
  intertubular tissue, 458
  lamina propria, 443
  multi-staged, 452, 453
  number, 443

seminiferous tubules *continued*
  peritubular tissue surrounding, 443
  termination, rete testis, 460
  see also spermatogenesis
seminoma, 467
senile plaques, 187
senses
  olfaction, 471, 489
  see also hearing; taste; vision
sensorineural deafness, 489
sensory cortex, 180
sensory ganglia *see* dorsal root ganglia
sensory innervation, tongue, 305
sensory (afferent) nerves, 161
sensory neurons, 161, 163, 164, 166, 171
sensory perception, free nerve endings, skin, 218
seromucous glands
  bronchi, 295
  nasal passages, 289
  trachea, 290
seromucous secretory acini, 308
serosa, gastrointestinal tract, 323, 326, 327
serotonin (5-hydroxytryptamine), 328, 347, 393
serous cells, 308–9
  salivary glands, 308, 310
  secretions, 308, 309
serous demilunes, 309
serous glands
  olfactory mucosa (of Bowman), 471
  tongue, 305, 306, 307
  of von Ebner, 306, 307
serous membrane, 110
Sertoli cell(s), 443, 446, 454–8
  androgen receptors, 455, 460
  crystal/lipid inclusions, 34, 457
  cytoplasm, 444, 445, 454, 457
    spermatids embedded in crypts, 450
  cytoskeleton, 456
  development and numbers, 458
  FSH receptors, 458, 460
  functions, 443, 454, 455, 458
  germ cell associations, 443, 454, 455, 458
  hormone synthesis/secretion, 443, 458
  junctional complexes, 103, 454, 455, 456, 457
  membrane, 456
  nuclei, 444, 457
  polarity, 97, 455
  spermatogenesis coordination role, 460
  tight junctions, 456
  ultrastructure, 457
  volume occupied by, 454
Sertoli-cell-only (SCO) syndrome, 467
Sertoli cells junctional complexes (ectoplasmic specializations), 450, 456, 457
serum, 85
serum-secreting cells, salivary glands, 308
sex chromosomes, 57
sex steroids, 441
  synthesis, 410
  see also androgen(s); estrogen
Sharpey's collagen fibers, 231, 232, 312, 313
short stature, 411
sickle-cell anemia, 92
sickle cell crisis, 92
signaling pathways
  bone growth, 246–7

signaling pathways *continued*
  epithelial stem cell control, 102
  Wnt, 239, 340–2
sinoatrial node, 153, 191
sinusitis, 304
sinusoidal capillaries, 197, 198
sinusoids
  liver *see* liver, vascular sinusoids
  lymphatic, 203
situs inversus, 44
skeletal muscle, 73, 137–49
  abnormalities, 159–60
  action potential, 146, 148, 174
  attachment to bone, 140
  A bands, 138, 144, 146, 147
  calcium release, 146
  cell length, 137
  cells *see* skeletal muscle, fibers (cells)
  characteristics, 137
  connective tissue continuity, 143
  contraction, 147
    control/mechanism, 147, 174
    speed, 149
    stimulus, 148–9
  development/embryogenesis, 141, 158
  endomysium, 138, 139, 140, 143
  extrafusal fibers, 148
  fascicles, 140–1
    ultrastructure, 143, 144, 145
  fatigue, 149, 159
  fibers (cells), 2, 68, 73, 137, 138, 141–2
    actin/myosin, 140, 144, 146, 147
    characteristics, 137
    cytology, 139
    cytoplasm (sarcoplasm), 68, 143
    fast glycolytic, 139
    growth, 141–2
    hypertrophy, 143
    length, 137, 141
    mitochondria, 139, 143, 145
    multinucleated, development, 141–2
    nuclei, 68, 138, 141, 142, 143, 145, 158
    nuclei, peripheral position, 132, 137, 138, 139, 142
    plasma membrane, 143
    polygonal shape, 139
    striations, 138, 141, 142
    structure, 141–2
    type I (red slow-twitch), 142, 149
    type IIA (intermediate fast-twitch), 149
    type IIB (white fast-twitch), 142, 145, 149
    types, and typing, 149
    ultrastructure, 143, 144, 145, 146
  fine control, 174
  growth and development, 141, 158
  H bands, 146
  I bands, 138, 144, 146, 147
  innervation, 148, 164
  intrafusal modified fibers, 148
  length, sensing, 148–9
  lingual, 305
  M lines, 144, 146, 147
  mitochondria, 139
  myofibrils, 140, 143–50, 145, 146

skeletal muscle continued
  number, 143
  thick filaments (myosin), 147
  thin filaments (actin), 147
  myofilaments, 140
  organization, 140
  regeneration after injury, 158
  rigor mortis, 159
  sarcomeres see sarcomeres
  satellite cells, 143, 158
  sensory receptors, 148
  spindles, 148–9
  tendon compared, 132
  tongue, 138, 305
  ultrastructure, 143
  Z lines, 143, 144, 146, 147
skeletal tissues, 223–56
  disorders, 255–6
  see also bone; synovial joints
skin, 109, 207–21
  architecture, 207
  cancer, 220
  cells, nuclei degenerating, 2, 209, 210
  color, 210, 211, 212
  dermis see dermis
  disorders, 220–1
  elasticity, 123
  reduced/loss, 125
  epidermis see epidermis
  functions, 207, 213
  inflammation, 220
  innervation, 218–20
  encapsulated nerve endings, 219–20
  free nerve endings, 218–19
  keratinized stratified squamous epithelium, 109, 208
  layers, 207
  neuroendocrine cells, 409
  pigmentation, 210, 211, 212
  abnormalities, 220
  scalp, 216, 218
  stem cells, 209
  thick/thin, 208, 210
  yellowing, 220
skull
  fetal development, 239, 240
  postnatal development, 240
sliding filament model, 137, 147, 158
slit diaphragm, 380, 381
small intestine, 336–49
  abnormal conditions, 353
  anatomical segments, 336
  epithelial cell turnover, 329
  epithelium, 10, 324, 337, 338
  fluid absorption/secretion, 323, 344–5
  ileum, 348–9
  immune system, 337, 348
  lymphoma and carcinoma, 353
  mucosa, 337–8
  duodenum, 339
  flattening, celiac disease, 353
  ileum, 348
  immune functions, 337
  jejunum, 340–3, 344–7
  microfolds, ridges and villi, 337, 338
  surface area, 337
  surface morphology, 337
  muscularis externa, 338
  muscularis mucosae, 338
  neuroendocrine cells, 409
  smooth muscle, 338, 353
  submucosa, 338
  villi see villi, intestinal
  see also duodenum; jejunum
smell, sense of, 471, 489

smooth muscle, 137, 153–8
  actin myofilaments, 154
  airway, 294, 295, 296
  hypertrophy in asthma, 303
  around ganglia of Auerbach's plexus, 177
  arrector pili, 216, 218
  arteries/aorta, 155, 193, 194
  autorhythmicity, 158
  bladder, 390, 391
  bronchioles, 296
  bronchus, 294, 295
  caveoli, 157, 158
  cell length, 137
  cells, 73, 153–4
  characteristics, 137
  cytoplasm, 154, 156
  elastic fiber synthesis, 124
  nuclei, 132, 156
  ciliary body, 481
  contraction, 154, 156, 157, 158
  appearance, 155
  calcium ion fluxes, 155, 158
  control, 155
  slowness, 154
  dense bodies/plaques, 156, 157
  development and growth, 159
  disorders, 160
  focal contact between cells, 157
  function, 154
  gall bladder, 364
  gap junctions, 154
  gut, 156, 325, 342
  innervation, 158, 164
  leiomyoma, 160
  longitudinal section, 156
  microfilament, 158
  modified, 158
  muscularis mucosae of gut, 325, 342
  myometrium, 429
  myosin filaments, 154
  relaxed, 154
  sarcoplasm, 154, 156
  seminal vesicles, 464
  sheets/bundles/layers of cells, 154
  sites, 154
  small intestine see muscularis externa; muscularis mucosae
  stomach, 330, 331
  tendon compared, 132
  transverse/oblique section, 155
  ultrastructure, 154, 156, 158
  uterine tubes, 428
  vas deferens, 463
  vascular, 157
sodium (ions)
  in nerve conduction, 171
  reabsorption, renal, 384, 385, 387, 389
  reabsorption from saliva, 310
  renal transport, 382, 384, 388
sodium channels, 171
sodium chloride
  renal transport, 384, 386, 388
  secretion, sweat, 213
sodium urate crystal deposition, 256
sodium–potassium pumps, 171, 382
soft palate, 320–1
soft-tissue tumors, benign, 136
solar keratosis, 220
sole of foot, 210
soleus muscle, 149
somatic hypermutation, 266, 278, 279
somatosensory cortex, 181
somatostatin, 370, 407
  cells secreting, 335
somatotrophs, 395, 396, 397
sound, detection, 472, 474, 475, 489

space of Disse, 124, 359, 361
sperm see spermatozoa
sperm acrosome reaction, 421
spermatids, 448, 449, 455
  acrosomal cap, 449
  acrosome-phase, 450
  cap-phase, 449
  cycle of seminiferous epithelium, 452
  cytoplasmic bridges, 454
  differentiation into spermatozoa, 445, 446
  early maturation-phase, 450
  elongated, 444, 445, 446, 449, 450
  excess cytoplasm (residual bodies), 444, 451, 452, 454
  flagellum development, 449, 450
  late cap-phase, 449
  late elongating, 450
  mature, 451
  microtubules, 449, 450
  nucleus and nuclear membrane, 449, 450
  round, 444, 445, 446, 449
  ultrastructure, 450
spermatocytes, 445, 448, 455
  cycle of seminiferous epithelium, 452
  intercellular bridge, 447, 448, 454
  leptotene, 457
  meiotic maturation, 445, 448, 449
  pachytene, 448, 449, 457
  primary, 444, 446, 447
  chromatin content, 449
  formation, 445, 448
  ultrastructure, 448
  secondary, 446
  formation, 445, 448
  synaptonemal complexes, 448, 449
  ultrastructure, 449
  zygotene (primary), 448
spermatogenesis, 441, 445, 446–54
  animals, 452, 453
  arrangement of stages, 451–3
  arrest, 467
  coordination, 451–3
  Sertoli cell role, 460
  cycle and stages, 452–3, 460
  differentiation phase, 445, 446
  disorders, 466
  duration/time required, 446, 452, 460
  hormonal regulation, 458–60
  FSH and LH roles, 458, 460
  testosterone, 458, 460
  meiotic maturation phase, 54, 57, 445, 446
  mitotic divisions, 445, 446
  Sertoli cell function, 458
  stem cells, 445, 447
  synchrony, 451–3
  see also spermatids; spermatocytes; spermatogonia
spermatogenic cells, 443
spermatogenic cycle, 452–3
spermatogonia, 445, 446, 448–50
  cycle of seminiferous epithelium, 452
  cytoplasmic bridges between, 444, 447, 448
  distribution and sites, 447
  mitosis, 445, 446, 447
  synchronization, 447
  as reserve cells, 445
  stem cells, 445, 447, 448
  type A dark, 445, 446, 447, 448

spermatogonia continued
  type A pale, 445, 446, 447, 448
  type B, 445, 446, 447, 448
  ultrastructure, 447
spermatozoa, 64, 441, 445, 448, 460
  maturation in epididymis, 462
  meiosis, 54, 57, 445, 446
  number, 441, 443, 466
  passage in uterine tube, 428
  phagocytosis in vas deferens, 463
  transport in epididymis, 462
  transport in rete testis, 460, 461
  transport to epididymis, 441, 442
  zygote formation, 61, 62
spermiation, 449, 456
spermiogenesis, 445, 446, 448
sphenoid bone, 395
sphincter
  internal anal, 327, 352
  lower esophageal, 330
  precapillary, 196
  pyloric, 330
sphincter muscle, ciliary processes, 480, 481
sphincter of Oddi, 365
spinal cord, 162, 186, 187
  anterior (ventral) roots, 186, 187
  central canal, 168, 169
  gray matter/white matter, 186, 187
  motor neurons, 148
spinal ganglia see dorsal root ganglia
spinal motor neurons, 186
spinal nerves, 161, 162, 187
spindle, mitotic see mitosis
spinous (prickle) cells, 209
spiral ganglion, 473, 475
spleen, 279–83
  B lymphocytes, 282, 283
  capsule, 279
  development, 79
  functions, 279, 281
  germinal centers, 282
  lymphoid follicles, 280, 282
  marginal zone, 282, 283
  organization, 280
  periarteriolar lymphoid sheaths, 280, 281, 282, 283
  red pulp, 279, 280, 281
  structure/architecture, 279, 280
  T lymphocytes, 282
  trabecula, 279, 280
  white pulp, 279, 280, 281–3
splenic cords, 281
splenic vasculature, 280
spongiosa, primary, 240, 242
spot desmosomes see desmosomes
squamous cell carcinoma
  oral, 321
  skin, 220
squamous cells, 104, 108
squamous epithelium see epithelium
squamous metaplasia, 115
squamous-type cells, 68
stab cells, 82, 83
stains and staining, 491
Starling hypothesis, 192
stathmokinetic technique, 341
steatosis (fatty liver), 371
Stein–Leventhal syndrome (polycystic ovaries), 438, 439
stellate cells, 68
  astrocytes see astrocytes
  cerebellar cortex, 184
  cerebral cortex, 182
  hepatic (Ito cells), 124, 359, 361, 371
stellate reticulum, tooth, 316, 318

stem cells, 49, 67, 79
  adult (AS), 67
  in bone marrow, 77
  CD34 antigen, 80
  cerebral cortex, 182
  characteristics, 80
  colonic epithelium, 350
  corneal epithelial, 115
  crypts of Lieberkühn, 340–2
  in culture, 80
  definition, 67
  embryonic (ES), 61, 64
  epithelial, 100, 102
  hair follicle, 216
  hemopoietic see hemopoietic
    stem cells (HSC)
  limbal, 115
  lymphoid, 80
  mesenchymal cells, 119
  myeloid, 80
  organs with, 67
  skin, 209
  small intestinal mucosa, 337,
    346
    crypts of Lieberkühn, 340–2
  for spermatogenesis, 445, 447,
    448
  stomach (corpus), 332, 333, 335
  transplants, 93, 115
  type II alveolar cells as, 300
stereocilia, 45, 98–9, 107
  epithelium of epididymis, 461,
    462, 463
  of hair cells of ear, 472
    cochlea, 474, 475
    vestibular, 472, 473
  sites, 45, 99
  ultrastructure, 98
steroid hormones, 363, 393
  synthesis/secretion, 21, 28, 393,
    403
    by adrenal glands, 402
    by ovary, 410, 425
    by testis, 410, 441, 458
steroidogenesis, 21, 28
steroidogenic acute regulatory
    protein (StAR), 28
stomach, 330–6
  abnormal conditions, 115, 353
  anatomical regions, 330
  cancer, 353
  cardia, 330, 332
    surface epithelium, 332
  corpus (body), mucosa, 332,
    333, 334, 335
  functions, 330, 331
  ganglia, 329
  gastric glands see gastric glands
  gastric pits see gastric pits
  lymphoma, 353
  mucosa, 330–2, 331, 333, 334,
    335
    cell types, 331, 332, 333,
      334
    gastric juice secretion, 331
    hyperplasia, 353
    regional variations, 330–2
    rugae, 330, 331
    see also chief cells; parietal
      (oxyntic) cells
  mucous neck cells, 332, 334
  mucus-secreting cells, 330, 331,
    332
  muscular externa, 331
  muscularis externa, 326
  muscularis mucosae, 331, 332,
    336
  neuroendocrine cells, 409
  pyloric region, mucosa, 336
  secretory epithelium, 324, 331
  smooth muscle, 330, 331
  submucosa, 331

stomach continued
  surface mucous cells, 332, 333,
    334
  ulcer, 115, 353
stomatitis, aphthous, 321
stratum basalis, 429, 430
stratum corneum, 208, 210
stratum functionalis, 429, 430
stratum germinativum, 208–9
stratum granulosum, 208, 209, 210
stratum lucidum, 210
stratum spinosum, 208, 209, 211
Streptococcus mutans, 322
stress, ACTH/cortisol secretion
    and, 403
stress fibers, 40, 281, 353
"stretch" cells (tanycytes), 169
stretch receptors, muscle, 148
stria vascularis, 109
stroma, 118
  cornea, 478, 479
  endometrium, 429, 431, 432
  iris, 480, 481
  lymphoid tissues/organs, 276
  ovary, 413, 414, 415
subarachnoid space, 186
subclavian artery, 193
subendocardial layer, 190, 192
subendothelial layer, blood vessels,
    201
subepicardial region, 191
sublingual glands, 308, 309
submandibular glands, 113, 308,
    309
submucosa, gastrointestinal tract,
    131, 323, 326
  colon, 349
  esophagus, 329
  ganglia, 177, 325, 329
  small intestine, 338
  stomach, 331
substantia nigra, 187
suckling stimulus, 438
sulci, gray matter, 178
sulcus terminalis, 306
sunburn, 221
suntanning, 211, 220
superior colliculus, 178
superior hypophyseal artery, 395
supporting tissue see connective
    (supportive) tissue
suprachiasmatic nucleus, 408
supraoptic nuclei, 394
suprarenal glands see adrenal gland
surfactant, 296, 298, 300, 302
  deficiency in premature
    neonates, 303
  secretion by type II alveolar
    cells, 299, 300, 302
swallowing, 320
sweat, 213, 214
sweat ducts, 131, 213
sweat glands, 112, 207, 213–14
  apo-eccrine glands, 214
  apocrine, 214
  ducts, 131, 213
  eccrine glands, 213–14
  see also apocrine glands; eccrine
    glands
sweating, control, 213
sympathetic ganglia, 176
sympathetic innervation
  arterial system, 196
  blood vessels, 201
  ciliary body, 481
  gall bladder, 364
  gastrointestinal tract, 327
  smooth muscle, 158
  veins, 199, 200
sympathetic nervous system, 161
sympathetic paraganglia, 410
symphyses, 253

symport carrier proteins, 345
synapses, 74, 172–4
  axodendritic, 172, 179
  axosomatic, 172
  chemical, 172
  dendritic spines and, 172
  dendrodendritic, 179
  dendrosomatic, 179
  density in cerebral cortex, 182
  peripheral, neuromuscular
    junction, 173–4
synapsis, in meiosis, 57, 448, 449
synaptic cleft, 172, 173
synaptonemal complexes,
    spermatocytes, 448, 449
syncitium, 63, 141
syncytiotrophoblast, 63, 435
synovial fluid, 253
synovial joints, 250–3, 251
  see also articular cartilage
synovial membrane, 130, 250, 253,
    256
synovium, 251
syntrophin proteins, 159
systemic circulation, 189
systole, 193

T
T lymphocytes, 80, 92, 258, 266
  activation, 267–8, 270, 279
  antigen processing and
    presentation, 266, 267–8
  antigen specificity, 266
  B cell interactions, 265
  CD markers, 266–7
  cytokines produced, 267
  cytotoxic (CD8+), 267
    activation, 279
    class I MHC and, 268
    transplant rejection, 284
  development, 84, 263
  diversity, 266–7
  double-negative, 274, 275
  γδ T cell receptors, 284
  helper (CD4+), 267
    B cell activation, 265
    class II MHC and, 268–9
    Th1 and Th2 types, 267
  intraepithelial see lymphocyte(s),
    intraepithelial
  in lymph nodes, 279
  maturation in thymus, 271, 272,
    273
  MHC restriction and, 268–9
  migration/circulation, 263, 276,
    277
    timeline, in thymus, 274,
      275
  in palatine tonsils, 319
  proliferation in Peyer's patches,
    348
  receptors (TCRs), 263, 266, 267
  regulatory (Tr), 267
  selection processes, 272, 273–6
    negative, 273, 274
    positive, 273, 274
  self-reactive, negative selection,
    273, 274
  single-positive (SP) (CD4 or
    CD8), 274, 275
  in spleen, 282
T-tubules, 146
T3 (tri-iodothyronine), 398, 399,
    400
T4 (thyroxine; tetra-iodothyronine),
    398, 399, 400
tanycytes, 169
tarsal plate, 477
tartar, 322
taste, 469, 489
  categories/types/mechanism, 470
  reduction in sensation, 489

taste buds, 306, 307, 469–70, 489
  apical pores, 469, 470
  function, 470
  structure and number, 469
taste receptor cells (TRC), 469, 470
taxol, 37
tear film, 477
tectorial membrane, 475
teeth, 310–18
  adult, 311
  within alveolus, 312
  crown, 311
  decalcification for studying,
    311
  decay (caries), 312, 322
  deciduous, 310, 314
  dentin see dentin
  dentinal tubules, 311, 312, 313,
    317
  dento-enamel junction, 316–17,
    318
  development, 312, 314–18
    amelogenesis (enamel), 312,
      314, 317–18
    bell stage, 314, 316
    bud stage, 314, 315
    cap stage (tooth germ), 314,
      315
    dentinogenesis, 312, 313,
      314, 316–17
    oral epithelium thickening,
      314, 315
  enamel see enamel
  enamel–dentine junction,
    316–17, 318
  loss, 312
  number, 310
  permanent, 310
  pulp, 311, 312, 316
  pulp cavity, 313
  root, 311, 313
  root canal, 311, 312
  sensory receptors, 312
  structure, 311–12
teloglia, 171
telomerase, 17
telomeres, 16, 17
telophase, 51, 52, 54
temperature, hormone secretion
    control, 394
tendon(s)
  collagen content, 123
  collagen fibrils, 121
  dense regular connective tissue,
    132
  enthesis, 135
  ligaments vs, 132
  light and dark bands, 132
  muscle attachment to bone via,
    140
  skeletal/smooth muscle vs, 132
  strength, 123, 132
tendon sheath tumors, 136
teniae coli, 341
teratocarcinoma, 67
teratoma, 438
terminal ganglia, 176
terminal hepatic venule, 357, 358
terminal web, 42, 43, 344
territorial matrix (TM), 134, 252
tertiary villi, 435
testicular cells see Leydig cells
testis, 441–60
  abnormalities, 466–7
  adult, 446
  cancer, 454
  carcinoma in situ, 454, 467
  descent into scrotum, 467
  ducts, 461–6
    see also efferent ducts,
      testis; epididymis
  endocrine cells, 410

testis *continued*
  exocrine/endocrine components, 443
  germ cell tumors, 454
  growth/development, 441, 446
  hormonal regulation, 441, 458–60
  immature prepubertal, 446
  intertubular tissue, 458
  Leydig cells *see* Leydig cells
  lobules, 441
  maldescent, 467
  mediastinum, 441, 442, 460
  neonatal, 446
  organization/structure, 442
  parenchyma, 443
  peritubular tissue, 443
  rete testis, 441, 442, 460, 461
  seminiferous epithelium
    see seminiferous epithelium
  seminiferous tubules
    see seminiferous tubules
  Sertoli cells *see* Sertoli cell(s)
  sex steroids secreted, 410
  spermatozoa formation
    see spermatogenesis
  tubules *see* seminiferous tubules
  tumors, 467
  tunica albuginea, 442
  tunica albuginea (capsule), 441
  tunica vasculosa, 441, 442
  volume, 441
testosterone, 441
  functions, 441, 455, 458
  secretion by Leydig cells, 410, 441, 458, 459
  synthesis, 459
tetanus (lockjaw), 159
tetraiodothyronine (T$_4$), 398, 399, 400
thalamic nuclei, 180, 181, 182
thalamus, 178
thalassemias, 92
theca albuginea, 422
theca cells, 419, 420, 421
  luteinization, 426, 427
theca externa, 419
theca interna, 419, 425
theca luteal cells, 426, 427
therapeutic cloning, definition, 67
thermogenesis, non-shivering, 129
thermoreceptors, 219
thermoregulation, 213
third ventricle, 394, 395
thoracolumbar nerves, gastrointestinal tract, 327
threonine, 346
thrombin, 88
thrombocytes *see* platelet(s)
thrombosis, 205
thrombus, 205
thymidine, radiolabeled, 341
thymocytes, 272, 273
  double-negative, 274, 275
  single-positive (SP) (CD4 or CD8), 274, 275
  timeline for migration, 274, 275
thymus, 84, 271–6
  birth to adulthood, 271
  cortex and medulla, 272, 273
  epithelial cells, 272, 273, 275
  functions, 272
  lobes and lobules, 272, 273
  reticular fibers, 272
  supporting tissue, 272
  T cell maturation, 271, 272, 273–6
    overview, 275
  T cell selection, 272, 273–6
thyroglobulin, 398, 399
thyroid cartilage, 289
thyroid colloid, 398, 399

thyroid gland, 398–400
  autoantibodies, 411
  disorders, 114, 411
  follicles, 398, 399
thyroid hormones
  receptors, 394, 398
  synthesis, 393
thyroid-stimulating hormone (TSH), 395, 398
  deficiency, 411
thyrotoxicosis, 411
thyrotrophin-releasing hormone (TRH), 398
thyrotrophs, 395, 396
thyroxine (tetra-iodothyronine; T4), 398, 399, 400
tidemark, of enthesis, 135, 252, 253
tight junctions (zonula occludens), 45, 46, 97, 103
  capillaries, 196, 198, 201
  endothelial cells, 201
  enterocytes, 345
  functions, 103
  Sertoli cells, 103, 455–6
  ultrastructure, 46, 103
tissues
  aberrant, 65
  dimensions, 1
  integration into body plan, 75–6
  labile, 49
  origin, 61–76
  permanent/non-renewable, 49
  primary types, 61, 64, 69–76
    classification and origin, 75
    embryonic germ layer, 65
    importance of knowing, 70
    similarities/differences, 70–1
    see also connective tissue; epithelium
  regeneration, 48
  stable, 49
titin, 147, 151
Toll-like receptors (TLRs), 258, 260
toluidine blue staining, 491
Tomes process, 317, 318
tongue
  abnormalities, 321
  geographic (erythema migrans), 321
  glands, 138, 307
    mucous, 305, 307
    serous (of von Ebner), 305, 306, 307
  histology, 305–7
  lymphoid follicles, 307
  papillae
    filiform, 306, 395
    foliate, 306, 307
    fungiform, 305, 306, 395, 469
    vallate or circumvallate, 305, 307, 469
  sensory innervation, 305
  skeletal muscle, 138, 305
  stratified squamous epithelium, 305, 306
  taste buds *see* taste buds
tonofilaments, 42, 209
tonsil(s), 318–19
  abnormalities, 322
  lingual, 307, 319
  lymphoid follicles, 322
  palatine, 283, 319
  pharyngeal, 318, 322
  tubal, 318
tonsillar crypts, 283, 319
tonsillitis, 319, 322
tooth *see* teeth
tooth bud, 314, 315
tooth socket (alveolus), 312
totipotent, definition, 67
toxoids, 285

trabeculae
  bone *see* bone
  liver cells, 358
  lymph nodes, 277
  spleen, 279, 280
trabeculae carnae, 150
trabecular arteries, 280
trabecular veins, 280
trachea, 290, 291–3
  cilia, ultrastructure, 291, 292
  function, 291
  hyaline cartilage rings, 126, 290, 291
  "respiratory" epithelium, 107, 290, 291, 293
  secretions, 291
  submucous glands, 291
  wall, 290
tracheo-esophageal fistula, 353
transcapillary diffusion, 197
transcellular transport, 46, 202, 345
transcytosis, 24, 98
transendothelial transport, 197
transfer RNA (tRNA), 18
transforming growth factor β superfamily, 79
transitional epithelium
  see epithelium, transitional
translation, nuclear, 13
transmembrane protein, 11
transmission electron microscopy, 4
transplantation
  bone marrow, 93, 285
  immune system and, 284–5
  rejection, 268, 284
"transplantation antigens", 268
transverse tubular (TT) system, 143, 146
  dyads, cardiac muscle, 152
  triads, skeletal muscle, 146
treadmilling, 40
triglycerides, 129
triiodothyronine (T$_3$), 398, 399, 400
trilaminar appearance, plasma membrane, 10
triskelion, 30
trophoblast cells, 435
tropocollagen, 118, 121, 122
tropomyosin, 140
troponins, 140
tryptophan, melatonin synthesis, 408
tuberculosis, pulmonary, 304
tubular glands, 111, 113
  large intestine, 324
tubules, renal *see* renal tubules
tubulin
  α- and β-types, 37
  dimers, assembly/polymerization, 37
tubulo-alveolar glands, prostate, 464, 465
tubuloacinar glands, 111, 113
  esophagus, 353
  lacrimal gland, 477
  salivary glands, 308
tubuloalveolar glandular unit, breast, 437
tubulosaccular glands, seminal vesicles, 464
tubulus rectus, 460
tumors *see* cancer
tunica adventitia
  arteries, 193, 194
  veins, 200
tunica albuginea
  penis, 466
  testis, 441, 442
tunica intima
  arteries, 193, 194, 201
  veins, 200

tunica media, 155
  aorta, 193
  arteries/arterioles, 193, 194, 195, 204
  veins, 199, 200
tunica propria, seminiferous tubules, 443
tunica vasculosa, 441, 442
Turner's syndrome, 438
twins, 439
  non-identical, 57
TWIST, 96
tympanic membrane, 472
typhoid fever, 353
tyrosine, hormones derived from, 393

U
ulcerative colitis, 353
ultrafiltrate, 377, 381, 387
  composition, 379, 389
ultraviolet light, skin pigmentation, 211, 220
umbilical cord, 130
unipotent, definition, 67
upper respiratory tract
  see respiratory tract, upper
urea, 384, 388, 389
ureter, 373, 374, 390
ureteric bud, 374, 376
urethra, 390
  female, 390, 391
  penile, 390, 391, 466
  prostatic, 465
urethral glands of Littré, 466
urethritis, non-specific, 467
urinary system, 373–93
  disorders, 390, 392
    see also kidney; urinary tract
urinary tract, 390
  infections, 392
  transitional epithelium, 110, 390, 391
urine
  concentration, 384, 387
  copious, in diabetes insipidus, 411
  production, 373, 374, 385, 387
  storage, in bladder, 390
  transport, 390
  volume per day, 373
uriniferous tubule, 374
urothelium *see* epithelium, transitional
uterine cervix *see* cervix
uterine cycle, 424
uterine tubes (Fallopian tubes), 413, 428–9
  ampulla, 413, 428
  ciliated cells, 428, 429
  disorders, 438–9
  isthmus, 428
  mucosa, 428, 429
uterus, 413, 429–33
  disorders, and tumors, 439
  endometrium *see* endometrium
  myometrium, 429
utricle, 472
uvea/uveal tract, 476, 478, 479–81

V
vaccines, 285
vacuoles
  basal, endometrium, 431
  condensing, 7
    pancreatic acinar cells, 367, 369
vagina, 434
vaginal mucosa, 434
vagus nerve, 176, 327, 367

valves
    heart, 190, 192
        damage, 205
    veins see veins, valves
valves of Kerckring (plicae
    circulares), 337, 338
van Gieson's stain, 491
varicose veins, 205
vas deferens, 441, 442, 462
    disorders/infections, 467
vasa recta (medullary capillaries),
    373–4, 376, 383
    arterial/venous capillaries, 386
    blood flow, 387
    countercurrent exchanger, 389
vasa vasorum, 201
    arteries, 194, 201
    veins, 200, 201
vascular canals, vertebral body
    development, 254
vascular endothelial growth factor
    (VEGF), 201
vascular sinusoids, 280
    bone marrow, 77, 78, 79, 271
    liver see liver, vascular sinusoids
    spleen, 280
vascular smooth muscle, 157, 196
    arterioles, 195
vascular system see blood vessels
vasculogenesis, 202
vasectomy, 463
vasoconstriction, 201, 387
vasoconstrictor nerves, 201
vasodilatation, regulation, 201
vasodilator nerves, 201
vasopressin see antidiuretic hormone
    (ADH; vasopressin)
Vaterian system, 365
veins, 198–201
    anastomoses with arteries, 201
    artery comparison, 204
    characteristic features, 190
    collapsed, 199
    dimensions, 192, 200
    disorders, 205
    distension, 200
    functions, 198
    large, 200, 204
    medium-sized, 199, 200
    small, 200
    structure variations, 199–200
    sympathetic innervation, 199,
        200
    valves, 200–1
        dysfunction, 205
    varicose, 205
    vasa vasorum, 200, 201

vena cava, 192, 200
venous plexuses
    nasal passages, 288
    penis, 466
venous sinus, nasal passages, 289
ventral root, 186
ventricles (brain)
    CSF circulation, 186
    ependymal cells lining, 168,
        169, 186
    fourth, 183
    third, 394, 395
ventricles (heart), 152, 190
venules, 199, 200
    anastomoses, 201
    characteristic features, 190
    collecting, 196
    dimensions, 192
    muscular, 196, 204
    ultrastructure, 199
vertebrae, development and
    growth, 241, 254
vertebral bodies, 254
vertebral column, 253–5
    development, 254
    ligamentum nuchae, 123, 124,
        125
vertebral ligaments, 123, 124, 125
vertigo, 489
very low-density lipoprotein
    (VLDL), 363
vesicles
    associated with Golgi
        apparatus, 22, 23
    clathrin-coated, 24, 27, 29, 30
    coated, 24
    condensing, 26
    destinations, 24
    endocytic, 28–32
    movement through Golgi, 24
    neuromuscular junction, 146
    neurotransmitter release, 172
    secretory, 22, 24, 26
        see also zymogen granules
    transport, 22, 23
    uncoated, 25
vesicular transport model, 24
vestibular apparatus, 472
    damage, 489
vestibular membrane, 474, 475
vestibular nerve, 472
vibration, sensing, 219, 473–4
villi, chorionic, 435
villi, intestinal, 128, 324, 337, 338,
    346
    blood vessels, 342
    cell types, 344–7

villi, intestinal continued
    core, 342, 343
    duodenum, 339
    jejunum, 340–3
    structure, 340, 343
    surface epithelium, 338, 340,
        343, 344
villous chorion, 434–5
vimentin, 42
vinblastine, 37
vincristine, 37
vision, 476, 490
    color, 487, 488
        red/green blindness, 490
    distant vs near, 481, 483
    light detection, 486
    mechanism, 181, 484–5
visual disorders, 490
visual field, 486
visual pigments, 485
vitamin A, 487, 488
    deficiency, 490
vitamin B$_{12}$
    absorption defect, 92
    storage, hepatocytes, 363
vitamin C, deficiency (scurvy), 136,
    322
vitamin D
    bone resorption, 237
    deficiency, 220, 256
    synthesis, 389, 401, 410
vitreous body, 476, 484–5
vocal cords (folds), 289
Volkmann's canals, 226, 228, 232
von Ebner
    imbrication lines, 313
    serous glands of, 306, 307
von Willebrand factor, 125, 201

W
W type, retinal ganglion cells, 486
Waldeyer's ring, 318, 319
warm spots, 219
Warthin's tumor, 322
water
    diurnal variations in intake, 373
    in extracellular matrix, 121
    reabsorption (renal), 382, 384,
        385, 387, 388, 389
    retention, 411
    total body volume, 121
water-clear cells, parathyroid gland,
    400, 401
    hyperplasia, 401
wax, ear, 472
white adipose tissue, 33, 128, 129
white blood cells see leukocyte(s)

white matter, 178
    cerebellum, 182, 183, 184
    cerebral cortex, 180
    spinal cord, 186, 187
whooping cough (pertussis), 304
Wiebel-Palade bodies, 201
Wnt/β-catenin pathway, 102
Wnt signaling, 239, 340–2
wound healing, 136, 160, 221
wounds, skin, 221
Wright's stain, 491

X
X chromosome, 448
    inactivation, 16
X type, retinal ganglion cells, 486

Y
Y chromosome, 448
Y type, retinal ganglion cells, 486
yolk sac, 79

Z
Z lines, 143, 144, 146, 147
    cardiac muscle, 151, 152
Zeis, glands of, 477
zero gravity, 489
Zollinger–Ellison syndrome, 353
zona fasciculata, 402, 403, 404
    ultrastructure, 403
zona glomerulosa, 402
zona pellucida, 62, 419, 421
zona reticularis, 402, 403, 404
    adrenal medulla boundary, 405
zonula adherens see adherens
    junction (zonula adherens)
zonula occludens (ZO) see tight
    junctions (zonula occludens)
zonular fibers, 479, 480, 481
zygomatic major muscle, ligament,
    123
zygote, 61, 62, 64
    passage, in uterine tubes, 428–9
zygotene, 57
zymogen granules, 7, 24, 26, 96,
    113
    chief cells, 335
    formation, 26
    immature, 24, 26
    mature, 26
    pancreatic acinar cells, 366,
        367, 368, 369
    ultrastructure, 26
zymogenic cells see chief cells
zymogens, 367